MW00779150

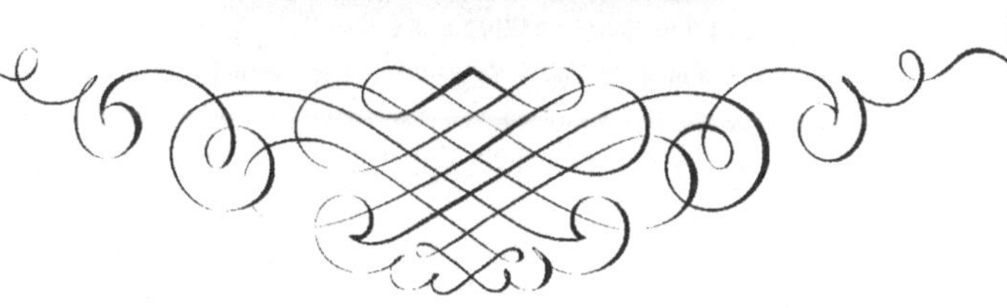

ISBN 978-1-333-81748-0
PIBN 10604678

VITALITY, FASTING

AND

NUTRITION

A PHYSIOLOGICAL STUDY OF THE CURATIVE POWER OF FASTING, TOGETHER WITH A NEW THEORY OF THE RELATION OF FOOD TO HUMAN VITALITY

BY

HERE WARD CARRINGTON

Member of the Council of the American Institute for Scientific Research; Member of the Society for Psychical Research, London; Author of "The Physical Phenomena of Spiritualism," etc.

WITH AN INTRODUCTION BY

A. RABAGLIATI, M.A., M.D., F.R.C.S.

Hon. Gynæcologist, and Late Senior Hon. Surgeon, Bradford Royal Infirmary; Consulting Surgeon to Bingley Hospital, to Bradford Children's Hospital, and to the Bradford Home for Cancer and Incurables, etc., etc.

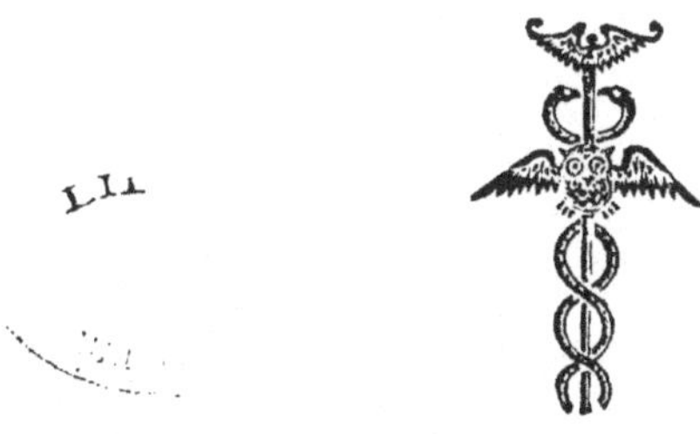

NEW YORK
REBMAN COMPANY
1123 BROADWAY

Printed in America

Dedicated to

THE MEMORY OF

EDWARD HOOKER DEWEY, M.D.,

RUSSELL T. TRALL, M.D.,

AND

SYLVESTER GRAHAM, M.D.,

Three Great Medical Philosophers

WHOSE PHILOSOPHICAL INSIGHT, ILLUMINATION,

AND UNTIRING ENERGY

HAVE SERVED TO LAY THE FOUNDATIONS

OF A TRUE

"SCIENCE OF MEDICINE"

PREFACE

IN PRESENTING the following work to the public—no less than to the medical and scientific man—I feel that a few words of explanation are necessary—if not of apology. The subject discussed is so entirely different from anything that has yet appeared in any language, and the subject-matter is frequently treated in so unusual a manner, that it will perhaps be necessary for me to indicate, briefly, what I propose to discuss in the following book, and why. It is not necessary to do this at any length, however, as the Contents page will doubtless prove more or less self-explanatory; and the theories will be found stated and defended in the text itself. I shall not attempt, in this place, to defend either myself or my theories, but must rest upon the text of my book allowing it to speak for itself, and will only ask that the book be read carefully and critically before any verdict is passed, either upon the theories advanced, or the sanity of the author! I admit that my position is at first sight revolutionary, to the extent, even, of being absurd; that, in attempting to overthrow the doctrine that we derive our strength and energy from the food we eat, I am attacking one of the fundamental postulates of science—and even, at first sight, attempting to overthrow the Law of Conservation itself. I have one, and only one, reply to all such critics: Read the facts and arguments advanced in the book, and when this has been done, I shall be only too glad to hear any criticism or fair-spirited attack that may be leveled, either at the book or at myself, as its author.

For the greater portion of this book I am tempted to claim originality. In the opening chapters, the theory of disease propounded is merely a re-wording of the theory that has been held for half a century by all expert hygienic physicians—it is merely a re-statement of the case; and, in the chapters on "Drug-Medication," and on "Stimulants," I have depended almost entirely upon the brilliant theoretical writings of the late Dr. R. T. Trall. The ideas concerning the germ-theory have also been advanced, in outline, by hygienic physicians; and the chapter on the physiology and philosophy of fasting I have borrowed largely from the writings of Dr. E. H. Dewey. In the chapter on "Vitality," also, I have received many valuable suggestions from the theoretical writings of Dr. Robert Walter—he and Doctor Dewey being the only two writers, so far as I have been enabled to discover, who did not believe that the bodily vitality was derived from the daily food, but for very opposite reasons. Doctor Dewey was forced to this conclusion owing to the facts presented by his fasting cases; as the result of clinical evidence; but he never followed up the suggestion in any detail, nor indicated the revolutionary effects such a theory would have on science, if true. Doctor Walter traced these out, to some extent; but his writings seem to me to be somewhat confused on this point, and the conclusions that flow from the theory are not drawn by this author either. Doctor Walter seems to be in considerable confusion regarding his theory of vitality, and its derivation from food. At times he seems to think that it is so derived; at other times not. Thus, on p. 161 of his "Vital Science," the following sentence occurs:

"That term 'physical vigor,' which most people will agree is a proper one, as coming from food, is itself a good answer to the doctrine that food gives vital power. Food yields to a living organism physical force for the performance of physical work, but only when that force is controlled by Vital Force." This seems to be somewhat confused, and also erroneous. Only by taking the broad stand that no energy whatever is derived from the food, can we see clearly the true relations of food and energy, as outlined in Book III., Chap. 1., to which I refer the reader for an exposition of the theory.

The only extended study of fasting cases I have ever come across is that contained in Dr. Joel Shew's "Family Physician," (pp. 783–97), published many years ago, in which the physiological effects of fasting are discussed at some length. The statements are somewhat crude in many ways, however, and the results vitiated by the fact that, in the cases studied, water, as well as solid food, was forbidden the patients; and consequently abnormal results were obtained—and studied. In the current books on fasting, only a brief reference is made, here and there, to these difficult problems; and no detailed study of the question has ever been attempted. It is to be hoped that the present work, if it does nothing else, will at least stimulate interest and enforce research in this highly important and interesting field of inquiry.

It may be thought by some that, in putting forward fasting as a virtual panacea, *e.g.*, as I do, (pp. 574-8), I am "extreme," and consequently to be distrusted in my conclusions. I shall not attempt to dispute these arguments here—merely asking my reader to peruse the chapters or passages themselves before arriving at any conclusion. They may be extreme, but if true, what does that matter? Like Doctor Trall, I, too, have "found truth to be both ultra and radical. It is *never* 'between two extremes,' but *always* one extreme or the other." Public opinion is worth nothing whatever in a scientific problem, which must always be determined by the facts in the case, and not by the opinions of any one—scientist or layman. And that is certainly not less true in such a case as this, in which next to nothing is known of the subject, even by the specialists!

Most certainly, fasting will never become a *popular* method of cure, for the reason that it involves too much self-denial! It is all very well to live "well" for a number of years, and then to think and feel we can avoid the results by taking a pill or a powder. That, unfortunately, is impossible. Nature does not work in that way, but always by gradual processes. As Doctor Keith so well remarked, ("Plea for a Simpler Life," p. 123), "A starving doctor would not, I fear, have as yet a very long career as a fashionable and popular physician in London." That is but too true!

In all the reported cases, I have refrained from mentioning names, except in some few instances—in which the permission had been obtained from the patient, or when the name had already appeared in print. I have all these names in my possession, however; and documentary evidence, in many cases, to prove that the statements made in this book are in every way correct, and that I have stated the strict truth in every case mentioned and discussed. Many of the patients I knew personally, and could doubtless soon reach, by mail, should the occasion for my doing so ever arise.

Before concluding, let me impress my reader with the importance of bearing in mind, throughout, the following facts. *First:* That the fasts undertaken, and studied in this book, were undertaken by *diseased* patients, and not by persons in health; and that I should not advise, but should, on the contrary, heartily deprecate any attempts at promiscuous fasting, by persons unfamiliar either with physiology or the philosophy of the treatment; or who are not diseased and in need of such a fast for the cure of certain ailments. I believe in properly conducted, therapeutic, fasting; but here, as in every other field, "a little knowledge is a dangerous thing." *Secondly*: The distinction between fasting and starving should be kept carefully in mind, throughout, and the two never confused. Fasting is altogether beneficial; starving precisely the reverse. I have, on page 564, stated what I conceive to be the radical distinction between these two processes, and I should advise my reader to peruse that passage before beginning the book, if he has not already a clearly formed idea of this distinction and difference between the two physiological processes. It is of the utmost importance that the distinction pointed out should be kept carefully in mind, throughout.

To my publishers I wish to express my thanks for their kind help, courtesy and assistance during the publication of this book. To my more than friend, Maurice V. Samuels, I owe a debt of gratitude I can never repay, for past help and encouragement, through years that seemed to betoken nothing more bright than failure and ridicule, and without whose friendly aid this book might never have been published. To Doctor Rabagliati I also owe a debt of profound thanks—which should be acknowledged here, as well as privately—not only for the full, kindly, and appreciative "Introduction" he has written, but also for the help and counsel he has given me, throughout the preparation of this work. I must record here, however, the fact that I find myself unable to agree with Dr. Rabagliati in his conclusions, after having read his Introduction carefully, and while in full sympathy with his aims. Every reader must, of course, select the theory that appeals to him the most. Finally, I wish to acknowledge that all that is of any value or worth in the book is due to the constant presence, acute criticism and sympathetic devotion of my wife.

H. C.

CONTENTS

PAGE
Preface vii
Introduction. By A. Rabagliati, M.D., F.R.C.S., etc. xiii

BOOK I

THE NATURE OF DISEASE

CHAPTER
I. Disease a Curing Process . . . .
II. Unity and Oneness of Disease . . . . . .
III. On Drug Medication . . . . . .
IV. Stimulants—Their True Action . . . .
V. The Germ Theory . . . .
VI. Nature's Law of Cure . . .

BOOK II

THE PHYSIOLOGY AND PHILOSOPHY OF FASTING

I Quality—The Question of Diet . . . . .
II Fasting as a Means of Cure—Historic Outline
III. The Quantity of Food Necessary to Sustain Life
IV The No-Breakfast Plan . . . .
V Theory and Physiology of Fasting . . . .
VI. Cases Cured by this Method . . . . .

BOOK III

VITALITY, SLEEP, DEATH, BODILY HEAT

I. Vitality:
§ 1. Present Theory of the Causation of Vital Energy by Food 225
§ 2. Weaknesses in and Objections to that Theory . 231

CHAPTER PAGE

§ 3. Author's Theory of its Causation 248
§ 4. Objections to the Theory and Replies Thereto 256
§ 5. Facts Supporting this Theory 267
§ 6. Fatigue: Its True Nature 278
§ 7. Additional Arguments Supporting the Author's Theory 282
§ 8. The Origin of Life: Criticism of Recent Attempts at Creation 284
§ 9. Practical Results and Theoretical Considerations 295
§ 10. Philosophical Conclusions 299

II. Sleep:
§ 1. Current Theories of Sleep—Their Unsatisfactory Nature 304
§ 2. Author's Theory of Sleep 307
§ 3. Objections to the Theory and Replies Thereto 310

III. Death:
§ 1. Theories of Death 324
§ 2. Author's Theory of Death, and Facts Supporting this Theory 326

IV. Bodily Heat:
§ 1. Current Theories of the Causation of Bodily Heat by Food 332
§ 2. Author's Theory of its Causation and Maintenance 333
§ 3. Facts Supporting this Theory 337

BOOK IV

HYGIENIC AUXILIARIES AVAILABLE DURING A FAST

I. Air and Breathing 351
II. Bathing 360
III. Clothing 370
IV. Exercise 378
V. Water-Drinking 388
VI. The Enema 406
VII. Mental Influences 424

BOOK V

STUDIES OF PATIENTS DURING THEIR FASTS

CHAPTER		PAGE
I.	The Tongue and the Breath	
II.	The Temperature	
III.	The Pulse	
IV.	The Loss and the Gain in Weight	
V.	Physiological Effects—I	
VI.	Physiological Effects—II	
VII.	Crises: And What to do When they Occur	
VIII.	How and When to Break the Fast	
	Reflections—Conclusions	572
	Appendices A, B, C, D, E, F, G, H, I, J, K, L, M, N	581
	Index	625

LIST OF ILLUSTRATIONS

OPPOSITE PAGE

Mr. George W. Tuthill, Figs. 1, 2, 3, 4, taken on the forty-first day of his fast 192

Mr. J. Austin Shaw, Fig. 5, taken on the fortieth day of his forty-five day fast 206

INTRODUCTION

PART I

A NEW THEORY OF ENERGY

Mr. Hereward Carrington, having asked me to write an Introduction to his interesting and scholarly book on "Vitality, Fasting and Nutrition," I have much pleasure in complying with his request. In doing so, it is necessary to say that although I agree with much that is in the book, and particularly with a main contention in it that neither the heat of the body, nor its energy, or power of work, come from the food, still it does not follow that my views are in harmony with those of the author in all particulars. That is, of course, not to be expected in any case, no two minds ever, I suppose, whether living now or at former times, being found to agree with each other in every particular. Mr. Hereward Carrington needs no help from me or any other man in defending his views. Any one who reads his book will see that. Further, it would be unbecoming in me, when writing a friendly Introduction to another man's book, to dwell on the points of disagreement between us. I write because we agree in a main contention, or perhaps in the main contention of the book, not because we disagree on other points. But I cannot refrain from mentioning one point on which our views seem to differ, although I do not propose to be guilty of the bad taste of criticizing his view, or of defending my own at present. Still, it seems necessary to draw attention to the fact that he strenuously (and also very ably no doubt) contends that *life* or *vital* force "is *absolutely alone, separate, distinct, per se,*" from all other forces. I do not take this view. To me, life is one form of the infinite and eternal energy by which all things do consist, and I think that, like other forms or phases of energy each of which procreates the form under which its manifestation or embodiment appears, life, whether under the forms of plant life, or animal life, procreates the form suitable for its manifestation. Each reader must settle in his own mind which of these views or what other view most commends itself to him in this question. Very much, as it appears to me, hangs on it. It is indeed vital, and therefore I was bound to mention, though unable to discuss it; and the reader will see if he cares to, the importance to be attached to the idea that Energy in all the varied phases of its ascending manifestation, procreates the mechanism fit for the embodiment of that manifestation. He will also see that I regard heat and light no longer as causes of energy, nor even as forms of energy, so much as they seem to be qualities of energy, and that this is in keeping with the ultimate conclusion that a study of organic life leads to the inference, not of a common ancestor, but to that of a common Author.

The author of this book is a vitalist of a sort. He has evidently read much in physiology and in that attempt at practical physiology known under the name of practice of medicine. His mind is not only critical, but it is also constructive, and on every page he may fairly be described as original. He accepts the main principles of physiology as generally expounded, though even as to some of these—witness for example his views on sleep—he has much to say that is out of the common purview; and various readers must determine, each for himself, how far they agree or differ from him. I have been asked to write this Introduction chiefly, or almost wholly, because I agree with Mr. Hereward Carrington in the belief that neither the heat of the body nor its energy for work come from the food at all. An attempt to realize this point of view leads to the perception of an interesting situation. Two men, neither of them experimental physiologists, allege that the ordinary physiological doctrines, reached by the labors of countless physiological workers after innumerable laboratory experiments, are wrong on an important or even a vital point. The balance of authority, being so tremendously on one side, the large majority of men will probably consider that the opinion of two or three men on the other side is unworthy of serious consideration, and will banish it from their minds without further ado. Although, however, this may be a natural course to take, it is not a wise one. Neither is it a scientific or philosophical[1] one, since the value of an opinion depends not so much on the number or even the importance of those who hold it, as on the evidence on which it rests. Now it so happens that the effect which I fear the statement of Mr. Hereward Carrington's view will have on the large majority of readers is exactly the one which it had at first on my own mind. When he first suggested to me that neither the work of the body nor its heat came from the food at all; I must confess that I

[1] The meaning of the word "scientific" is difficult to distinguish from that of "philosophical." Science is, properly speaking, the accumulation of facts, perception of their existence to us, knowledge of them by us. Philosophy is the explanation which we give of the perceived facts. A fact of sequence, as that day succeeds night; and night day, is scientific. Whenever we come to account for the succession, we enter the domain of philosophy; and yet the astronomical explanations given to account for the succession are generally classed among scientific phenomena. In point of fact, it is quite impossible to distinguish between science and philosophy, because no sooner do we perceive facts, than we begin to try to account for them. Religion arises when we push or try to push our philosophy to its ultimate conclusions.

But on the whole, although all these three domains of thinking are inextricably mingled and commingled with one another, we may consider science as dealing with facts and with their How and their occurrence, their sequence, their connections; while philosophy deals with the reasons for these or the Why of them. Religion on the other hand attempts to give the inquiry into How and Why a final unity. But it is almost impossible to separate these three domains from one another. Science should be philosophical; philosophy should be scientific; while religion should be scientific and philosophical, but transcending both. It is a poor sort of mind whose science, philosophy, and religion are not harmonious with one another.

the consideration of the idea away from me as unworthy of a moment's consideration or entertainment. The ordinary doctrine so universally held by a very large number, or even by the whole number without exception, of the physiological experimentalists, and further, as it seemed at first sight, entrenched impregnably experimental facts, and also behind the accepted scientific philosophical doctrines regarding the conservation of energy and matter, must, it was felt, be true. The very least which could be said for it was that it seemed to be inextricably bound up with those conclusions associated with the name of Lavoisier in the end of the eighteenth century, regarding the indestructibility of matter and force and carried to accepted certainty since by a crowd of experimental workers. How was it possible that on a vital point that great cloud of workers and witnesses could be mistaken? If, after more than a century's work, carried out with a zeal and industry never excelled in the whole history of human working and thinking —if after all this time and after the making of an almost infinite number of experiments, the general opinion on a fundamental principle were to be called in question—where, it might be asked, was or is certainty to be found? We may well ask. And yet, very recently, Gustav Le Bon has stated that, contrary to the views of Lavoisier and of the whole world of science since his time, matter at least is not indestructible or eternal, and that in certain circumstances, he has proved experimentally it dissociates and vanishes without return. This being so, the foundation of science is shaken; the law of the conservation of energy as at present understood and stated, is called in question. I am very unwilling to do it, or to set forth my own views on a subject which has racked the ingenuity of the greatest minds of all time, but I do not see how I can refrain, if I may hope to induce even a single mind to inquire into this question for itself, from stating shortly my conclusions as to the law of the conservation of energy. It is possible to agree that Energy, the power, is infinite and eternal, and omnipotent; and that it is neither increased nor diminished (it cannot, of course be either if it is infinite), and yet to agree with M. Le Bon that matter may vanish without return. This is indeed the conclusion to which I am compelled. Matter may be, and it seems to me to be, the effect of energy which may call matter into being for the purpose of expressing or declaring its own presence and power; and therefore, when the immediate purpose has been fulfilled, matter may again vanish into the nothingness from which it came. Energy or force, as it is sometimes called, seems to be neither more nor less than the power of the Infinite, and, like the source from which it emanates, it is infinite, eternal, changeful, and omnipotent, being limited, in the latter respect, only by the character of its Source or Origin, Who of course acts according to His own nature. The moral qualities of energy, though they may have to be referred to, are at present rather outside of our purview. Matter, on the other hand, seems to me to be phenomenal or apparent only. Le Bon himself says that matter is a variety of energy— which is exactly my view; or, if I might venture so to express it;

I think Energy calls matter into being, in order to manifest its own presence. Matter seems to me to be called into being in order to act as the embodiment or incarnation, or clothes of Energy; and it is continually in course of vanishing as it came. Matter seems to me to be a phenomenon procreated by the Noumenon Energy, in order that Energy may be able to manifest its presence to sentient creatures and to human beings. Energy wraps itself up in matter as a man puts on his clothes. If it were not for its embodiment in matter, so dense and dull are our apprehensions, that it seems to me we should probably fail to apprehend its existence at all. Energy, then, springing from an infinite and eternal source is infinite and eternal. (This is, of course, also Herbert Spencer's conclusion, and that of scientific philosophers generally.) Energy is one, but one with many forms and phases. It appears to be constantly struggling so to say, to express itself, knowingly or blindly, or ignorantly. (But the Power behind it is not unknowing, or blind, or ignorant; but on the other hand, knows and sees, and is purposive.) In order to express itself, Energy calls into being, or procreates, the vast variety of material things with which we are more or less familiar. The capabilities of the manifestations of energy are limitless; and higher and higher forms or manifestations of it are continually obtruding themselves on the observer. These manifestations of Energy appear to ascend as a hierarchy, and they seem to embody themselves in a corresponding hierarchy of forms which are procreated by Energy, or the various forms of manifestations of Energy, in order that Energy may declare itself and that our dull wits may appreciate its existence and presence. Energy appears always to exist in two forms: the kinetic, or active, or dynamic; and the potential or dynatic. And I wish to add here, as it will have to be considered or referred to from time to time, that all active or kinetic Energy, or dynamic Energy is warm, (and I think also luminous). It does not seem to me that heat and light are forms of Energy in the same sense as substance is, but they seem to be qualities of Energy. Whether they are also qualities of dynatic or potential Energy is another question. But inasmuch as kinetic or potential, or dynamic, or dynatic energy appear to be different degrees of the same power, I think warmth and luminosity are qualities of both. On this view, absolute zero of temperature or absolute and complete absence of heat and light would mean nothingness, for it would mean the withdrawal of the power whose manifestation they are; and this seems to me a justifiable and indeed compulsory conclusion, or opinion from the evidence of the facts. Although it is not necessary to insist on this view, I should not myself, I think, speak of thermodynamics, nor yet of photo-dynamics, although I should of hylodynamics, and hydro-dynamics, and chemico-dynamics, and the other forms of the universal Energy immediately to be named. Thermo-dynamics, or photo-dynamics, would, it seems to me, mean rather the statement of the facts and laws of *qualities* of Energy, than the facts and laws of the various forms of Energy itself. In saying that all kinetic or active Energy seems to be warm and luminous, I mean that when kinetic Energy is in action, heat seems always to be liberated, and light to appear. True, the light is often invisible—a statement which at once illustrates the impossibility of separating science and philosophy, and which we must not stay to discuss. Heat and luminosity appear to be qualities of kinetic Energy wherever it appears (and probably of potential Energy also).

The lowest form of Energy, or Energy acting in its simplest form may be named Hylo-dynamic (ὕλη substance) or the power of substance, *i.e.*, a power manifested by Energy through substance or matter, all sorts of matter, as clay, metals, even water and gasses (although it will be convenient to name separately the special forms of energy manifesting itself through these last). Energy seems to be itself imponderable, ubiquitous, omnipresent, omnipotent, but warm and luminous, and the procreator of substance and of the seen, of the audible or heard, the tasted, the smelled, the sensed or perceived, and generally of the qualified. Under all its forms Energy is never arbitrary, but works always according to laws, which may be discovered on inquiry, and when discovered, are capable of statement more or less precise, according as our knowledge extends.

Next in order after hylo-dynamic, appear what we may perhaps term hydro-dynamic, and aëro-dynamic with what we may call æthereo-dynamic.

2. Hydro-dynamic would be definable as the form of Energy which manifests itself through water and other fluids. The laws of this form of Energy are statable under the heading of "Hydrostatics," and "Hydro-dynamics."

3. Next in order seems to appear that form or phase of Energy which manifests itself through the various forms of airs and gases, to which may perhaps be joined the Energy manifesting itself through the presence of the æther, or ether, believed by most scientific inquirers to be universally distributed throughout the universe and to form the substratum or intermediary, by means of which Energy is conveyed. This we may name aëro-dynamic and æthereodynamic. The laws of the former would be Statable under the headings of "Aëro-statics" and "Aëro-dynamics." Æthereo-dynamic or ethereo-dynamic, I only name at present as it must be discussed later, and indeed should hardly be classed here.

4. The next form of Energy-manifestation may perhaps be considered to be crystallo-dynamic. Here there is required some complexity of power to be expressed, this complexity of power taking the form of separating crystals from the menstruum in which they lie dissolved. As when examining hylo-dynamics, we were impressed by the immense number of powers manifested through substance; the earths, the metals, the clays, etc., so here we are again impressed by the reappearance of an almost infinite variety of forms of crystallo-dynamic, in the variety of crystals—circular, obtuse-angled, rhomboid, prismatic, and of all kinds of shapes and forms found in nature. The modern evolutionary mind, being greatly impressed by this almost infinite variety of forms, is easily induced to assume that they are determined by various changes in environment—but

of course it is equally open to us to assume that the active crystalling power seeking its most suitable expression adapts the particular form or forms of crystallization assumed to the environment. Plainly, before crystallization is effected, the power to crystallize must have existed. The phenomena of polarization, right or left, seem to point to some preëxisting power which adapts the crystalline form to its own nature and character. The further question whether the almost infinite variety of crystalline forms are all modifications of one primitive original form arises here to our minds. Or are the numerous forms expressions each of closely allied crystallizing powers? Are they the proof at once and the effect of the earlier existence of a common ancestor? Or are they the manifestations of similar phases or forms of crystallo-dynamic? That is, do they rather point to a similar source? This question appears thus early; but the importance of it greatly increases when the higher manifestations of Energy come to be considered. My view, I must say, on the evidence is that they are immediately the effects of similar phases or forms of crystallo-dynamic, and that remotely they are the effects of a common Author. Energy is one, and its source one. Of course a similar question arises as to the various forms taken by hylo-dynamic. Are these, the earths, the alkalies, the clays, the metals, different forms of one primitive substance, or are they the effects of similar phases of hylo-dynamic? Are they the descendants of a common ancestor or are they the effects immediately of similar forms of hylo-dynamic, and remotely of a common Author? Between these alternatives, my mind is so made as that I have no hesitation whatever in making my choice. I am compelled to infer a common Author.

5. Next in order, probably, appears chemico-dynamic, in whose domain we come into relation with the attraction of opposites, as acids and alkalies (or earths) to run together and form new compound bodies, or as they may be considered, the embodiments of new phases of energy. Heat is noticeably liberated when chemico-dynamic functions, as for example when O_2 joins with C to form CO_2.

6. Next in order of Energy-manifestation seems to come electro-dynamic, where the positive and negative forms (apparently corresponding with acid and alkali in chemistry?) arrest our attention, as we observe that positive repels positive and attracts negative. In the manifestations of electro-dynamic also, heat is constantly being liberated, and we are greatly impressed by the observation that a copper wire along which an electric current is passing is warmer than one along which no current is passing. Of course there may be various verbal explanations of this, but one explanation may be that the wire is warmed by the current. This form of Energy, although it seems to be manifestable through all forms of substance, certainly travels much more readily through metals than through other media; and this fact must be particularly kept in mind when we wish to apply this power to human purposes. Before I pass on to the two next forms of manifestation of Energy in the ascending scale, the various forms of plant life and animal life, I think I ought

to mention a striking fact which may, indeed, already have obtruded itself on the reader's attention. Although these various phases or forms of Energy do seem to form an ascending series, each form being on the whole higher than the form immediately preceding it in the scale; still it invariably seems to appear that the higher manifestations of a lower form of Energy are higher in the scale than the lower forms of the higher. Electro-dynamic seems to be a higher form of Energy than chemico-dynamic, and its most active forms higher in the scale than the forms of chemico-dynamic—still there are lower and weaker manifestations of electro-dynamic, those for example perceivable through wool, or wood, or stone, which are much less active than many phases of chemico-dynamic, such for example, as may be seen in explosives. Explosions of gunpowder, nitro-glycerine, dynamite, etc., usually considered chemical in character, are generally on a much smaller scale than the electric explosions of a thunder storm; but a great chemical explosion might be a manifestation of a greater amount of Energy, if of a lower degree, than a small and limited thunder storm. The same reflection arose, although I did not mention it then, when we were considering hylo-dynamic or the power of substance. Hylo-dynamic, may on the whole be considered a lower manifestation of Energy than crystallo-dynamic, but the manifestations of the apparently unconsumable Energy expressed through radium may shew more energetic activity than the Energy manifesting itself through some crystals. This kind of reflection and observation becomes more important when we observe that although animals are on the whole unquestionably higher in the scale than plants, and therefore the phenomena of bio-dynamic higher than those of phyto-dynamic; still the higher plants are much higher in the scale than the lower forms of animal life. A beautiful flower for example with its division of parts; its corolla, its sepals, its stem and root, its stamens and pistil, and the fruit in which these culminate, are much higher than the homo-geneous un-differentiation and simplicity of the humble protozoön, although the manifestations of Energy shown in the mobile and responsive animal-series to which the protozoön belongs, is capable of reaching, and does in fact reach a very much higher manifestation and expression than any shown in plant or tree. In this respect, we make similar observations in other departments of nature. One form of power and Energy, and the material embodiment which it assumes, seems to merge into another by gradations so insensible that we cannot tell where one ends, or where the other begins. The connective tissues of the body—to take an example from a different sphere of Energy—are different from the synovial membranes, lining joints, or body-cavities; and these again differ from nerves; but on examining the connective tissues, and following them to their ultimate ramifications, we find connective tissue, periosteum, ligament, tendon, bursa and synovial lining of joint so inextricably blended and merging into one another; and also epimysium, peri-mysium, and peri-neurium so inextricably mingled and perfused that we find difficulty in describing the pre-

[illegible] and [illegible] of [illegible]

This kind of consideration is part of one even more general, from which it appears that nature is made up of a very large series of [illegible] whose [illegible] is that [illegible] is not mutually exclusive of its [illegible] but on the other hand merges into its [illegible] by gradations so insensible that we cannot say where one ends and where the [illegible] begins. Of such principle, examples are hot and cold, dry and moist, light and darkness, [illegible] and [illegible], [illegible] and [illegible], [illegible] and [illegible]. Between the varying and [illegible] degrees of which it is impossible to find a dividing line. [illegible] the whole of human experience, the practical [illegible] of life being always, or almost always, found in the answer to the question where the line is to be drawn. [illegible] on the other hand are mutually exclusive of one another. [illegible] of some [illegible] that A is exclusive of not A, [illegible] is the cause of energy, as modern science [illegible] assumes, or energy is the cause of substance. [illegible] without [illegible] the inconsistency between them. Sometimes we find [illegible] as determining our religious views, and [illegible] as determining our secular [illegible] is very [illegible].

[illegible] example of a pair of contradictories in material existence [illegible] is motion and rest, and no doubt this would [illegible] contradictory if there were in nature any [illegible] as non-motion or rest. [illegible] Nature is in a state of [illegible] and [illegible] and movement, [illegible] or [illegible] or imperceptible, [illegible] or non-motion [illegible] be, or can be. [illegible] a comparison of more motion and less motion, more [illegible] and less [illegible], more light and less light, more [illegible] and less [illegible], more [illegible] and less [illegible], more light and less light, more [illegible] and less [illegible] and so on. Energy is one with a variety of forms so vast and numerous that the human intellect altogether fails to comprehend them, or in comprehending for a moment, it passes on to the examination of some other domain, it too speedily forgets its former information and finds itself compelled to start afresh on its never-ending inquiry.

The next form of energy in its ascending hierarchy of manifestation is the energy of plant life, what may be called [illegible] energy. Here we enter on the consideration of the domain of biology as that term may be viewed as covering the domain of all life [illegible] plant life and animal life both. But it must not for a moment be forgotten that to confine life to these domains, and to exclude it from the domain of substance, crystallography, etc. is a purely arbitrary division. All Nature is alive; it [illegible] and [illegible] and moves and is moved by the working of a many-phased energy: the stones are only less alive than the chemical or electric atoms, while the latter are in turn less alive than the various forms of plant life, and of animal life. Still it is convenient, and in fact is even necessary to have terms to connote various differences that appear as manifestations of Energy, as we view ascending exhibitions of power. So we connote under the term phyto-dynamic and phyto-dynamic all the phenomena of plant life. Here we come into new revelations, as for example the sex-element whose existence enables the plant to be reproductive of its kind. This is perhaps not un-analogous to the reproduction of crystalline forms or of chemical phenomena, or electric phenomena in their respective spheres; but the differences are marked enough to demand special names. Very interesting questions arise under the heading of phyto-dynamic; as for instance the relations of the plant to air, to water, and to earth. I am not sufficiently acquainted with the phenomena of plant life to be able to say much about this; but if it be true, as I understand, that although a plant grows in the ground, it does not necessarily grow *from* it, but takes much of its nutrition from the air, this is a fact of extreme significance for us in our effort to understand the true inwardness of animal nutrition,—animal nutrition and its meaning, being of course, the objective toward which these preliminary considerations are intended to lead on.

In plant life, then, I think we have the forms which the phase of Energy called phyto-dynamic generates for its own manifestation. Phyto-dynamic appears to generate all plants in order to manifest its special powers; and in root, stem, leaves, the various parts of the flower, and the reproductive organs, we find the embodiment of differing powers. Another question which obtrudes itself on us now with greater force than before is as to whether all plants are modifications of one original form or whether they may not rather be generations of similar forms of phyto-dynamic, which as it emanates from the One Source of all Energy, must in the nature of things work similarly and so generate forms similar and similarly behaving. Adaptation and environment count for much, no doubt, but the power or capacity of the plant to modify itself as the environment alters and in accordance with changes in the environment, must, it seems to me, have preexisted in the plant, or no change or adaptation could have occurred at all. Hybridization raises also very many and most deeply interesting questions with which it is impossible here to deal, even if I knew sufficient of the facts to justify me in attempting to do so. But as in the case of animals, no naturalist, I believe, has suggested that all plants have been modifications of one original form. Several forms, at least, are required to account for the vast variety of plant life: and if this be so, to me it appears more likely that the various forms of plant life are generations of similar forms of phyto-dynamic than that they sprang from a common aboriginal form. Instead of inferring a common ancestor after the Darwinian-Haeckelian suggestion, I infer first the action of similar phases of the power of phyto-dynamic, and secondly a common Author.

8. I have so often now stated the mental attitude, I am compelled to assume in discussing the general question of the relation of Energy to things and forms, that probably I need say little as to the view forced on me regarding the action of bio-dynamic, and bio-dynatic (βίος=life). Bio-dynamic is, therefore, the power of animal life (just as phyto-dynamic stands for the power of plant life), phyto-dynamic and bio-dynamic appear to me to be lower and higher manifestations of the one universal, eternal and changeful Energy by which all things do consist. Bio-dynamic appears to procreate the various animal forms through which it reveals its presence and existence. If it is not likely that all forms of phyto-dynamic came from a common ancestor; but if on the other hand it appears more likely that they were procreated by similar phases of Energy, so that a common Author is a far more justifiable inference than a common ancestor, still more does this conclusion seem to force itself on us in the case of animals. Four or six primitive forms of animal life were demanded by Darwin in order to account for the existence of the vast variety in animal life which he knew. He did not see how else he could account for the protozoa, the cœlenterata, the radiata, the annulata, and the vertebrates. He could not conceive them all as having sprung from one original form or common ancestor. It is doubtful whether even the vertebrata can be so accounted for. But if four or six original species are required, why may not a much larger number be posited? And evidently between this much larger number and the idea of a separate procreation for each of the very numerous now existing species, only a difference of degree and not of kind is involved. My mind finds it easier to account for existing species and existing animals (as well as for extinct ones) on the view that they have been procreations of similar forms of bio-dynamic than on the view that they have sprung from a common ancestor. Hybridization here also is very instructive. First of all, very widely separate species cannot be crossed at all; and second, artificial hybrids either tend to die out because they are unproductive; or they tend to revert to some more primitive form. But dogs do not pass into apes, or even into cats, although within the genus dog, there is an almost infinite variety of gradations from the Newfoundland to the toy-terrier; and within the genus cat there is in turn again an almost infinite variety of gradations from the tabby to the Persian. And dogs and cats are made alike with paws and claws, and vertebræ, and tails, and skulls, and brains, not because they sprang from a common ancestor, but because they were procreated immediately by like forms or phases of bio-dynamic which worked alike in all cases because it emanated from a common source. The more natural inference to my mind is undoubtedly a common Author than a common ancestor. This also explains and easily explains the similarity of the construction of apes and men. In the one case pitheco-bio-dynamic procreated apes; in the other anthropino-bio-dynamic procreated men, and their forms therefore bear on them the marks not of a common ancestor, but immediately of a similar procreating power, and remotely of common authorship. The

Darwinio-Huxleyan hypothesis is evidently no more tenable that men are an ascent through apes, than the suggestion or theory of some tropical peoples that apes are degenerated men. The one is quite as likely as the other. But the view that different forms of bio-dynamic procreated both, accounts for their similarity and offers far less violence to our reasoning faculty in its suggestion of a common Author than does the impossible view of a common ancestor. It also enlightens us as to the meaning or significance of the search for intermediate forms, if such forms exist. If they do, what do they prove? Is it not evident that intermediate forms may as readily be accounted for on the view that they are procreations of similar phases or forms of Energy, as on the view that they are the descendants of common ancestors or of a common ancestor? To me this is plain, and as it is so simple I adopt the inference.

G. Le Bon speaks of the variability of chemical species, and says that they are as variable as animal species. This may readily be admitted. They are as variable, as much so, and no more, and perhaps no less. But the sense in which M. Le Bon uses the phrase is not quite the same as that in which it is used by me. The difference will be manifest to any reader who may have cared to have followed me so far, and I need not therefore say any more about it.

The comparatively simple ideas which we term phyto-dynamic and bio-dynamic become most complex when we inquire into their characteristics. To keep to the latter, which concerns us most nearly, bio-dynamic contains in it a vast variety of the forms and powers of life. These we require to separate in our minds for purposes of study, yet we feel that they are inextricably blended and mixed up with one another. Mere naming of them seems to imply that they are distinct, while, in fact, they merge into one another by insensible degrees. There is, for example, (A) Tropho-dynamic (τρέφειν= to nourish) or the power of assimilation or nutrition by means of which an animal restores the waste of its body from food, assimilating in a remarkable way its food into its body-stuff. This power, as every physiologist knows, is itself exceedingly complex, to understand it completely requiring the devotion of a whole lifetime and more. Even to name the various organs involved in the powers is a labor and demands time and space we are unable to give now and here. Then (B) bio-dynamic carries with it the power of perception or feeling—what we may call æsthetico-dynamic (αἴσθησις, αἰσθητικὸς= perception, and perceptional or æsthetic). How complex this is, no student of psychology needs to be told, since it compels the introduction of various differentiations of nervous matter through which æsthetico-dynamic may be carried on. Closely allied to æsthetico-dynamic is the power of movement or kinetico-bio-dynamic, which I merely name.

Then (C) bio-dynamic implies or rises to the power of noetico-dynamic (νοητικὸς=knowing) or of knowledge. (D) Then, boulo-dynamic (βουλὴ=will) implies will-power. Further (E) bio-dynamic, or at least its human embodiment, anthropino-bio-dynamic, implies the existence of a religious sphere, what we may call psychodynamic (ψύχη=spirit or soul) by which spiritual things are apprehended. Unfortunately the term psycho-bio-dynamic has already been appropriated to a series of phenomena not connected with spiritual or at least not with religious ideas; and we require another term to indicate this sphere of consciousness. If the Greeks had possessed such an idea as the religious one (but they do not seem to have had the idea at all!) it seems as if it might have been expressed by the name εὐσεβεία, and hence we might perhaps name the religious part of man as eusebio-bio-dynamic. And finally when anthropino-bio-dynamic has risen to a faint perception of its place in the universe, and aspires to the lofty position of consciously aiding in the scheme or plan of things seen to be carried on and to be developing in one unbroken and majestic and orderly sweep of progression from generation to generation, and from century to century, and from one eternity to another, we perceive the existence within us of another faculty or power for which we require a name. Might I suggest Synoidal anthropino-bio-dynamic (σὺν=together, and οἶδα=I have known) for the name of the faculty which aspires to be a co-worker, drawn, attracted, and inspired by the unspeakable majesty and orderly harmony of the scheme of things of which it feels itself an integral and willing part. This also, like all the other parts of bio-dynamic and particularly of human bio-dynamic is seen to comprehend an infinite variety of forms which can only be hinted at, as they cannot be uttered or described. When I add that each of these powers (all of them of course—let me repeat this—modifications of the one universal and infinite Energy) procreate, each of them, the organs suitable for their expression, it will be perceived dimly how very varied and complicated these are. Nerve and nerve-cell, ganglion and connections, fiber and cell, in diversity of collocation and arrangement; impossible of unravelment by the finest instruments of the anatomist and physiologist, taxing his powers of investigation from generation to generation, these are some of the facts of the inquiry which stimulate while they oppress and humiliate the intellect and the soul of man, which nevertheless feels itself a dimly glowing point and faintly flashing spark emanating from the source of that infinite and eternal and omnipotent Energy by which all things do consist.

9. I fear I must say something regarding the æther or ether which is supposed by most physicists to fill all space and to act as the medium for the conveyance of Energy. I have classed æthereo-dynamic with aëro-dynamic, but evidently some further discussion is necessary, for there is no science of ethereo-statics and ethereo-dynamics as there is of hydro-statics, and aëro-statics and aëro-dynamics. According to M. Le Bon the ether seems to be the link between the ponderable and the imponderable. According to M. Sagaret, whom M. Le Bon quotes approvingly, the positing of the ether responds to our yearning for unity. "It sets up a unity than which it would be impossible to imagine anything more complete, and it focuses our knowledge on the following principle; one substance alone exists which moves and produces all things by its

movements. This is not a new conception, it is true, for the philosopher, but it has remained hitherto a purely metaphysical speculation."

Does the scientist then mean to imply that "purely metaphysical speculations" are any less metaphysical in the mouth of the scientist thinking to prove their truth through experiments, than in the mouth of the philosopher thinking to prove them by reasoning? The scientist is on very dangerous ground if he does think this. He would realize this better if he would reflect more about it and about the results of his experiments, for it is not his experiments that are important so much as the conclusions, always metaphysical, which he draws from them. It is not so much facts and experiments which sway and modify us, as the interpretation of the same—and the interpretation always is and must be metaphysical. Surely those old thinkers who named metaphysics because they were τὰ μετὰ τὰ φυσικά, *i.e.*, after the physical, were not so far wrong. But I pass on:

"The scholar has till now stopped at the atom without perceiving any link between it and the ether. The duality of the ponderable and the imponderable seemed irreducible. Now the theory of the dematerialization of matter comes to establish a link between the two.

"But it realizes scientific unity in yet another way by making general the law of evolution. This law, hitherto confined to the organic world, now extends to the whole universe. The atom, like the living being, is born, develops and dies, and Dr. G. Le Bon shews us that the chemical species evolves like the organic species." So much for M. Sagaret and M. Le Bon. Alas! that one should be compelled to point out that "evolution" is being used in two incompatible senses here. To say that the atom or anything else "is born, develops, and dies" is not original to Darwin and Huxley. It has always been known. It could not fail to be known because the simplest observation has always been competent to show it. Birth, development, and death are suggestive of the true evolution which exists in nature, *viz.*, the evolution of higher and higher manifestations of power—power procreating the increasingly complex forms in which its ascending manifestations shall be exemplified or embodied. But this evolution Darwin and Huxley hardly saw, so little have they said about it. The evolution on the other hand which they did see and commended to us to see also, may almost be said to be a myth, for they implied, if they did not say it, that dogs pass into cats, horses into zebras, elephants into hippopotami, apples into pears, and apes into men; and set us on a futile search after intermediate forms which probably do not exist, and which would prove nothing if they did—nothing that is, which cannot be as well proved without them. For a true interpretation of such facts (if there were or are any such) would more reasonably suggest common authorship than common ancestry.

But now let us examine M. Sagaret and M. Le Bon more closely. "One substance," we are told, "alone exists which moves and produces all things by its movements." Is this so? This is called the realization of "scientific unity" although it ought to be called philosophic unity; and it is reached, if at all, by those very metaphysical speculations to which we have referred, and on which the scientist foolishly sets such small store. But let this pass. Suppose we said that "one principle or power alone exists" (not one substance) "which moves and produces all things by its movements." Would not this be a better solution and one nearer to apprehensiveness than M. Sagaret's, approvingly quoted by M. Le Bon? Suppose we said—this is what I submit, ought to be said: "Energy is the one existence which procreates substance or matter in order to manifest itself." And when Energy, having stored itself up in prodigious or colossal quantity in the atom to form what M. Le Bon calls intra-atomic energy, or better, let us call it end-atomic energy—when Energy leaves the atom in which it had stored itself up, the atom vanishes to the original nothingness from which it came. According to M. Le Bon, matter comes from the ether, and it goes back by dissociation and by vanishing into the ether from which it came. But what is this ether? M. Le Bon tells us, or at least suggests to us, that it is a solid, without density or weight. Some scientists, indeed, suggest to us that the ether has density and no weight, while others say it has weight and no density. These are the men, be it observed, who speak somewhat disparagingly of purely metaphysical considerations. They deduce their conclusions from "experiments." But are not the definitions purely metaphysical? and are they any less so because deduced from experiments? It is a highly interesting state of mind which uses metaphysical expressions and justifies them because they are alleged to have been come to by experiments, and not from philosophical considerations. "A solid without density or weight." What is such a body? Is it nothing? I suggest that it is—nothing. But according to the thesis, it is the origin, and it is again the grave of the atom. The atom then came from—nothing, and it goes back to—nothing! But is not this the very proposition which, when it has been stated by philosophic or religious men, has been sneered at by the scientists? It is the very proposition. But then it was made from metaphysical speculation! But now that it is stated from physical speculation—(is that it?) or from experiments—it is allowable; nay we must yield our consent to it! All I can say is, that never have I been asked to believe anything more transcending reason by any philosopher. The scientific men and the physicists, and the experimentalists seem, certainly, to have got themselves into a quagmire regarding this solid without density or weight, and I wish them well out of it. But I think it is not unreasonable, all the same, to suggest that a conclusion come to by philosophy from metaphysical considerations, and now reached by physicists from experiments, the conclusion namely that things have been made out of—nothing, is not improbably correct. It is certainly very remarkable that it should have been reached by two modes or methods of inquiry so very different from one another. As to the cause of the infinite and eternal Energy which procreates all things out of—nothing, and which, when its procreating power is removed, allows them to go back to—nothing: as to the cause of this infinite and eternal Energy, I at present can say nothing, for it is not necessary to my present purpose to do so. There is, however, one other point to which I wish to refer, before leaving consideration of the ether, the solid without density or weight, which is alleged to be at once the mother and the grave of the atom. It is imagined to be the vehicle along which Energy is conveyed. In reference to this, I have to say that I do not feel the philosophic difficulty confessed to by so many minds of admitting that Energy may act without the intervention of an intermediary. I do not know why attraction, for example, may not pass from sun to earth without any intervaring ether on which it may be carried or conveyed; or why the majestic order of the heavens, more distant than our sun, may not be maintained similarly by power acting through absolutely empty space. I do not say it does so act; for I do not know—but why may it not do so theoretically? My mind feels no difficulty here. Of course I feel the force of the reasoning that if light is an undulation, there must be some medium in which it undulates. Undulations can hardly undulate on nothing, and yet as we have seen the ether is nothing. But light and warmth appear to me, not energies, but qualities of Energy. That seems to me to make a difference.

But granting the intermediary's existence; how is it defined? Very differently, as we have seen, by the different physicists who have spoken in such diverse and contrary senses, about it; some of them even calling it a solid or a fluid indiscriminately.

But further, if we grant for argument's sake that an intermediary is necessary to intervene between power or Energy, and the substance on which it acts—if such an intermediary is necessary, why may not Energy procreate it in order that it may act through it? I confess I see no reason why it should not, and much reason on the other hand why it should. Energy seems to me to procreate substance in order to manifest the powers of hylo-dynamic; water in order to manifest the powers of hydro-dynamic, chemical elements in order to manifest the powers of chemico-dynamic, etc., etc.; and if so, why may not Energy procreate the ether in order that it may pass without let or hindrance in space—if, that is, (which for my part I do not feel) such an intermediary is a necessity? For why, it may be asked, may not power leap out to substance, its own procreation, without the intervention of any intermediary at all? Similarly it appears to me, power may leap into communication with power in the same way, one phase or form of Energy with another, without any intermediary. When we consider the higher forms of intelligent powers, those that have embodied themselves in animals and men, the various forms of bio-dynamic, this possibility becomes increasingly likely. Various facts indeed, as action at a distance, what is called telepathy and so on, render this suggestion by no means unlikely. But to discuss this question here would carry me much beyond my limits, although it would also open up considerations which will not, I think, be much longer excluded from the field of science, which is at present viewed in far too limited ways. True, the various forms of bio-dynamic, and particularly the human embodiment of it—what may be called the different forms of anthropino-bio-dynamic (ἄνθρωπος=human being; and ἀνθρωπινὸς or ἀνθρωπικὸς=human) do not now as a rule act in this way. They maintain the embodied form in their action on substance and on other powers. But this universal or all but universal experience implies no logical necessity why it should always be so, or why a soul must necessarily be always trammelled by the existence of a body.

I am indeed encouraged to think that M. Le Bon himself might perhaps agree with me in this suggestion from passages like the following at the bottom of page 12 of the "Evolution of Matter." "It would no doubt be possible," he says, "for a higher intelligence to conceive Energy without substance, for there is nothing to prove that it necessarily requires a support; but such a conception cannot be attained by us." Why cannot it? M. Le Bon refers to it. In doing so, he surely attains to it. If not how could he refer to it? If he followed his own line of thought a little further, he might come to think (as I do) that he might substitute for his conception of end-atomic-energy that of Energy which is atom-procreating. That is, instead of thinking of Energy as emanating from matter he might think (as I venture to do) of Energy taking to itself or procreating a material body in order to declare or reveal itself. Instead of classing himself, as M. Le Bon unconsciously does, as a materialistic monist; in making Energy emanate from matter (intra-atomic or end-atomic-energy) why might he not consciously class himself as an idealistic monist and make matter depend on Energy? "Intra-atomic-energy" or end-atomic-energy would then become atom-generating power or hylo-generating-dynamic, *i.e.*, matter procreated by Energy or dynamism procreating substance, in order that it may declare itself. Evidently the experimental facts on which his expression is based would not be altered by the new term; only the interpretation would be altered, but it would be spiritualized and, to my mind, much improved, because brought much more closely into relation with the fitness of known things. I suppose there always will be human minds which will approach the discussion and the attempted solution of questions like these from two opposite and contradictory aspects. This being so, I wish to put in a plea that every man be fully persuaded in his own mind, and modestly, yet emphatically to state that for the position of the immaterial or idealistic monist, everything can be urged and every fact accepted which the materialistic monist can urge for his own conclusion, and in addition there seems to arise an afflatus of warmth and color and light,—a something interspersed with the whole nature, that is in harmony with the glories of rising and setting suns, and that warms and elevates and spiritualizes the whole being of man.

PART II

METABOLISM AND NUTRITION

Having thus cleared the ground by stating my view that Energy in its various infinitely numerous phases and forms, procreates the substance or mechanism, or organism best suitable for any and each particular phase of its manifestation, I proceed to apply this principle to the action of the human body. I have little doubt that the same view would also explain the action of other animal bodies, and even of plants; but happily I am not compelled to consider the application to any except the human body. Now the general principle or proposition which I believe to be the true one in this matter, is that the direct metabolic changes in the human body are nutritional or trophic only, and that any phenomena of work or heat-liberation are indirect, and attributable to the action of Energy acting through or by means of the body. I am sorry to be obliged to use new terminology, but it is unavoidable if we have to express new ideas, and also if we are to escape wordy repetitions which will be apt to have the effect of confusing both the writer and the reader.

Translating then my proposition into the terminology already suggested in the first part of the Introduction, it is this. The metabolic changes which occur in the human body are examples of bio-tropho-dynamic only and not of bio-erg-dynamic, nor of bio-thermo-dynamic. It being understood that my remarks refer to the human body only, I omit the prefix anthropino—in order to keep the terminology as short and concise as possible. In other words I am quite certain that the author of the book is correct in his view that neither the mechanical work of the human body, nor its heat come from the food at all. In Book III the author has argued this view at great length; his first two books leading up to the study and arguments for this proposition; and the reader who wishes to understand on the one hand, or who may feel himself called upon to argue in favor of the general scientific view on the other, must seriously address himself to what the author says in his work, and particularly in Book III. Whoever sets himself to do this will have his occupation cut out for him, because there seem to be very few publications on this subject which the author has not read. More than that, he has given to them all a discriminating consideration, as every reader will see for himself. This being so, it may be asked, what is there left for me to say? Or in what way are any remaks of mine likely to confirm a proposition which appears to me to be established in the book? This is a pertinent question; but the answer is that it seems to me that I can hope to put some of the scientific facts in the case in a new way, and in another light. Further, there has been published this year the English translation of a most elaborate three-volume work on this subject by Professor von Noorden of Vienna. The title of this work is "Metabolism and Practical Medicine," a most suggestive title by the way, and one indicating great advance in knowledge of the subject; since it seems to imply that if we can understand metabolism in the human body, we at once and thereby are able to formulate for ourselves a body of rules for the conduct and determination of medical practice. This is entirely, I may say, my view. It might have been put otherwise, *viz.*,—it might have been said that practical medicine ought to be applied physiology, and this proposition, if it is not original to me, is at least one which I have often formulated, and which I hold very strongly. Professor von Noorden and his coadjutors, Magnus-Levy, *etc.*, mean by the term metabolism all the changes which they conceive to take place in the body, of food into body-tissue, and of food into the Energy of work (what I call erg-dynamic) and heat (thermo-dynamic—but heat seems to me not to be a form of Energy, but a quality of all kinetic or active Energy). As I take for correct, Mr. Carrington's view that neither the work of the body (its erg-dynamic) nor its heat come from the food at all, in my use of the terms metabolism and metabolic, I think of nutritional changes only. Nevertheless whoever deals with the subject of the functions of food in the body must consider Professor von Noorden's book, and as Mr. Hereward Carrington has not done this, it is necessary to make some reference to it. It is, of course, impossible to do this completely in the space at my disposal, but the first thing to be said, is, it seems to me, this: Even the mental functions effected through the human body, the phenomena of noetico-dynamic, æsthetico-dynamic and boulo-dynamic, or perception and knowledge of perception, of feeling and of will are held by some writers to be functions of the brain, and the nervous system, whose changes are again held to be determined by the food, and to be forms of food-metabolism. But no proof regarding the occurrence of chemical changes when these functions are being exercised is brought forward or alleged. Mr. Carrington discusses this question at some length when dealing with the views of the late Professor Bain, although he does not discuss the chemical question. The failure on the part of Professor Bain and others to adduce the evidence for the existence of chemical changes coincident with the occurrence of these functional manifestations seems to me to be a remarkable thing. I have little doubt myself that this is primarily due to the failure of physiologists and scientists to realize the signification of the behavior of the brain in reference to the blood-circulation. This, as is well known, moves not with the general circulation, but when the internal carotid artery enters the jugged opening in the skull, which conducts it to the brain proper, the circulation at once becomes synchronous with the respiration and not with the general circulation. That is, the brain circulation proper moves at the rate of, say: 12 to 20 times a minute, while the rate of the general circulation is from 60 to 90 times a minute. Even so, I have little doubt myself that if we had instruments fine enough to detect them, or if we were subtle enough to infer them, we should find fine changes occurring in the brain-mechanism coincidently and concomitantly with the occurrence of functional mental changes. This discovery, if we made it (and probably some day we shall make it) would not in the least prove that these changes were the *cause* of mental functioning, any more than it is now proved that chemical changes which always accompany nutritional functionings are the causes of those nutritional functionings. Neither constant concomitance nor constant succession are necessarily the same as cause and effect. Otherwise the constant concomitance of day with light, and the constant succession of night on day would prove that day was the cause of light on the one hand, and the cause of night on the other. We know in fact, that the rotation of the earth on its axis and its behavior to the sun, are the causes both of the constant concomitance of day with light and of the constant succession of night upon day. There is a casual nexus no doubt between these four phenomena, but the nexus is not the crude one which we were at first disposed to imagine. We shall have to consider this fallacy of inference again when we come, as we shall do immediately, to the constant concomitance of increased O_2 intake, and of increased CO_2 output, with the appearance of the phenomena of erg-dynamic and of tropho-dynamic in the body, or of the doing of work and the performance of digestion changes in it.

I must say one word more before I pass on to the further examination of the prevailing scientific view as to the relations of the food to the work and heat of the body. As Lavoisier in the end of the eighteenth century formulated the statement that neither Energy nor matter are increased nor diminshed, and as this statement has come to be universally accepted by scientific men,[1] obviously it is not competent for us to speak of the production or generation of Energy Now Professor von Noorden's book above referred to (as indeed do most other scientific writings) constantly refer to the "production" of Energy, and of Energy being "derived" from this or that sort of food, when all that can be meant is the *liberation* of Energy. As, according to received views in science, heat is a form of Energy, it must be incorrect for us to speak of heat being "produced;" yet the expression "heat-production," in place of "heat-liberation," is being constantly used also in "Metabolism and Practical Medicine." No doubt, it may be said that these are conventional expressions, but from time to time, it seems to me, they cover the fallacy that Energy may be "produced" or "generated,"—such an idea being totally opposed to the view of modern science, and of (probably) true science for all time to come. That matter on the other hand may be found

[1] Yet note the views of M. Le Bon already referred to in Part I. of this Introduction.

to vanish without return, into the nothingness from which it came, will probably before long be an opinion accepted by Science.

The following statements appear to be true:

1. Whenever food is taken into the body, there is an increase in the amount of O_2 inspired, and a corresponding increase in the amount of CO_2 expired.

2. Whenever mechanical work is performed by the body, there is an increased amount of O_2 intake and a correspondingly increased amount of CO_2 output. These are the facts. The inferences drawn from these facts are that just as in the fireplace of a steam engine, an increased amount of CO_2 output is coincident with (not the generation) but the liberation of a certain amount of heat, the same occurs in the human body. But this does not follow. It does not follow that because heat is liberated in a fireplace in proportion to the amount of O_2 intake and of CO_2 output, it will be the same in the body. In point of fact there is no proof that an increased CO_2 output in the body is accompanied by any increase of heat-liberation. If it were, the blood in the pulmonary artery, which carries the blood to the lungs for the separation of the CO_2, ought to be warmer than that of the rest of the body. But although for some time physiologists, being carried away by the force of the analogy between the steam engine and the human body, believed that the lungs were the seat of the fire in the body, and that therefore the blood in the lungs was warmer than anywhere else in the human body, they found after a time that they were mistaken, and that the blood in the lungs was not any warmer than was the blood of any other internal part of the body. The analogy between the steam engine and the human body then breaks down at this point. Pursuing the same analogy, physiologists still believe that because the fire of the steam engine both heats the water and generates the steam which works the machinery, so the food of the body corresponds to the fuel of the steam engine, and supplies the material both for maintaining the body-heat (thermo-dynamic) and also forms the source of the work done (erg-dynamic). The analogy breaks down entirely. The body is far liker to an electric tram-car than it is to a steam engine. In the electric car, the motors at the bottom of the car work the car, no doubt; but they could not make a revolution if the trolley were off the wire; nor even if the trolley were on the wire, could they be got to work, if no current were passing. The truer analogy (but even *this* analogy is not perfectly complete) is that, as Electric energy runs the motors which run the car, so vital-energy (bio-dynamic) runs the body, which does the work. Then nextly, as a copper wire along which an electric current is passing is warmer than a similar wire along which no current is passing, and as the wire is warmed by the passage of the electric current along it, so the body is warmed and kept warm by the passage through it of the life-current or bio-dynamic. It is no answer to say that we know the source of the electric current which came from the nearest generating (liberating?) station, while we do not

know the source of bio-dynamic or the life-current. This is beside the question, especially as, if we inquire further into the source of the electric current about which we thought we knew so much, we find that it was not generated but only liberated through the chemical changes in the coal consumed (chemico-dynamic) at the generating (liberating?) station. And remotely, the electric current was liberated in the sun whose heat was stored up in the coal through which the station was worked, while the source from which the sun got it, or even what the sun is, is entirely beyond our knowledge. It is very dangerous, and proves very fallacious as we thus see, to argue from an analogy between the action of chemico-dynamic in a cold fireplace before the coal is set into oxidation, to the action of chemico-dynamic acting in an apparatus which is already warm, like the human body. The analogy fails so completely that there is no proof at all that what takes place in the one will be like what occurs in the other. And a further failure of the analogy between the body, not only to the steam engine but even to the electric motor is that while the body is self-regulating, self-rectifying and self-repairing, neither the steam engine nor the electric tram manifests any of these powers.

It has been alleged that food burned in a laboratory liberates exactly the same amount of heat as the same food oxidized in the body. This is a very doubtful statement. The only way in which the proposition can be proved are by:

1. Burning the food and finding out how much CO_2 is given off by a given amount of it; and

2. By analyzing the chemical composition of a given amount of the food, and calculating how much CO_2 ought to be liberable by its combustion. But as we have seen, and however the results might be as to the CO_2 and heat liberated in the laboratory, or as to the possible production of CO_2 from the C, in the chemical composition of the food, these facts by no means determine the heat liberable, by oxidation of the same food in the body. The conditions of the experiments are so entirely different that we cannot reason from one to the other.

I will proceed, however, to the further examination of the two propositions already made, and for reasons which will appear as we proceed, will begin with the second one, *viz:* that, whenever mechanical work is performed by the body, or, as I prefer to say, through or by means of the body, there is an increased amount O_2 intake and coincidently and proportionately an increased amount of CO_2 output. The ordinary view asserts that this increase of metabolism (wholly nutritional or trophic as it plainly is, or at least, as it appears to me to be) is so certainly the cause of the work done, that it holds that all that it is necessary to do in order to prove this assumption, is to state the facts. Now I do not dispute the facts of increased O_2 intake in the circumstances, nor of the coincident increase of CO_2 output, but I deny the validity of the inference from them. It is usually said that the increased CO_2 output in such circumstances is caused by the breaking down of the glycogen stored up by the liver, and this may be admitted as correct; that is, I admit that glycogen does break down to furnish the carbon which in combining with the O_2 of the inspired air forms the CO_2 expired. But this seems to me to be a trophic change only and the consideration determining it is the following: Whenever Energy acts upon substance, it seems to me, substance wastes. Now, in the bodily machine (procreated, as it appears to me by bio-dynamic for the exercise of its powers) whenever erg-dynamic or the power of mechanical work, uses the body for the expression or the manifestation of its power, the body at once begins to waste; and as it is a self-repairing and self-rectifying machine, at once there are started trophic changes to make good the waste. Obviously the increased CO_2 output does not come immediately from the food ingested, because by the supposition as to the conditions of the experiment, no food was taken. This, however, matters little on the ordinary view, because, admittedly, the glycogen stored up by the liver, from which proceeded the C of the CO_2 output did come from the food. Still, for all that, and admitting also, as I do, that the CO_2 output is proportionate to the work done or the erg-dynamic at work, I do not admit that the CO_2 output is the *cause* of the work done, but contend, on the other hand, that it is the effect of the work done; or rather that it is the effect of the waste effected by the action of erg-dynamic on or through or by means of the organism, and of the trophic or the nutritional changes which are at once set up in the organism to replace the waste. To take an analogy, it seems to me it would be as pertinent to argue that because the strings of the violin or piano or harp waste in proportion to the quantity of the music evolved through or by means of them, therefore the strings are the causes of the music, while in fact it is the hand of the player, and even the spirit behind the hand which is the real and efficient cause of the music. So the form of the infinite and universal Energy which we may call erg-dynamic is the cause of the waste of the body through which it works; and this is at once made good by the increased trophic metabolism which occurs to replace the waste, this increased trophic metabolism shewing itself in increased O_2 intake and coincidently or correspondingly with increased CO_2 output. If the strings of a musical instrument were self-repairing, we might perhaps be induced to think that the material which fed the strings was the cause of the music, since in that case some measure of the waste would probably be discoverable in the *debris* emitted; and we might imagine that the *débris* was the measure of the music, while what it really was, was the measure of the waste of the strings, when they were made the instrument of the music. If a spade is used in digging, the spade wastes in proportion to every spadefull of earth it is made to lift. The more it digs, the more it wastes. If we could arrange that a stream of fine steel particles flowed into the spade to replace the waste caused by each act of digging, we might perhaps come to think that these fine steel particles were the cause of the digging, especially as the quantity of them required would always be exactly proportional to th amount of work done. Nevertheless this would be a very incon sequent assumption. So it would be also, if we were to infer, be cause the motors at the bottom of the electric tram-car waste a they are used by electric-energy as the means of doing work, an if we could arrange that this waste should be made good by som self-acting mechanism—as well might we imagine that the stee particles flowing in were the cause of the work done, as that th food is the cause of the work done by the human body. Yet thi is the assumption invariably made by modern scientists, and s universally and invariably that any one arguing as I am doing now has the utmost difficulty in getting a hearing at all. Scientists eve go into raptures when writing on this subject. The "brilliant re sults" of experimentalists are referred to, as when it was shown tha within certain limits the food-stuffs each represent a relation to th amount of heat arising in the organism from them. The "brillian results" referred really to the proportion found to obtain betwee food-ingestion and the O_2 intake, food-ingestion and CO_2 output But the statement as made overlooks the facts already stated (1 that the organism is no warmer after food-stuffs have been ingestec than before, the healthy human organism having a temperature o 98.4° F., both before and after eating; and (2) the fact that th blood in the pulmonary artery or lungs is no warmer than the blooc elsewhere in the body is also overlooked. That "heat cannot main tain life" is a proposition made by M. Magnus-Levy himself, a coadjutor of Professor von Noorden, and this statement, might, think, have opened the eyes of some to the inconsistency of th general view on this subject. Another expression which may no unfairly be termed going into raptures is when the "furnishing o decisive results" is spoken of. These references are to the future no doubt, but already we have "the brilliant results" of experi menters described; and the "decisive results" already obtainec are so little decisive that some authorities actually state proteid-food requirements at three times the amount said to be necessar) by other authorities. That something must be wrong is quite evi dent when disproportion so serious exists; and what is wrong, have no doubt, is the unproved assumption that the Energy of th body comes from the food. According to Magnus-Levy "som sources of error are present." So they are indeed. Never, it ap pears to me, was an assumption made, so little warranted by th evidence. And yet notwithstanding the disparity of results, M Magnus-Levy speaks of these results being "a standard," bein "decisive" and "sufficing for the the claims of hygiene." Whicl is the standard? The one part or the three parts? Is it not reall extraordinary to see the same writer using such inconsistent expres sions? On page 188, Vol. I, M. Magnus-Levy, talking of the wate given off by the lungs and skin, goes on to say: "This is less impor tant for the estimation of the Energy exchange, than for the determi nation of a water balance." In the same way it might have beer said, and I think ought to have been said, that the O_2 intake and CO_2 output in the body are less important for the estimation of the Energy-exchange than for the determination of a nutritional or trophic balance.

I come now to deal with the first proposition formerly made, whenever food is taken into the body, there is an increase in the amount of O_2 inspired, and a corresponding increase in the amount of CO_2 expired. It is often assumed that the increased CO_2 output comes from the food, that is, that the C of the CO_2 expired does so. It may do so, of course. But it may come from the body. If the latter, then remotely the C must have come from the food, because the body is made, or makes itself, through trophic-energy, out of the food. My own view is that the C comes from the body, at least as a rule in the first place, and that the function of food is to be made into blood and to be assimilated into the body by this means. Whenever food is taken into the body, work is thrown on the organism to effect the assimilation of food. And just as we saw before, that whenever erg-dynamic acts on the body, the body-substance begins to waste, which waste has to be restored by increased trophic metabolism, so when tropho-dynamic acts through the body, when the labor of assimilating ingested food is thrown onto it, the action of tropho-dynamic causes waste of the body-substance, and this waste at once calls on the nutritional power of the body to make it good. This is very noticeable and very intelligible when ordinary foods are ingested, which take a long time, often many hours (from 7 to 11 or 12) to digest. The feeling of stimulation from taking food is felt often long before any of the food taken can possibly have been assimilated. It is well known even that human beings may and do occasionally experience a feeling of stimulation which enabled them to start fresh work in walking, after filling the stomach with stones, or even earth. Tightening the belt even, without putting anything into the stomach, is frequently the cause of comfortable stimulation which can be converted into doing work. And any time that any of these processes are put into operation, no doubt increase of O_2 intake and increase of CO_2 output concomitantly and coincidently occur. So that it does not follow that the increased O_2 intake and of CO_2 output which admittedly accompany the ingestion of food are caused by that food, as we see by considering all these conditions and circumstances. This was the reason why I considered the action of erg-dynamic through the body, before I considered that of tropho-dynamic. Since admittedly erg-dynamic does not supply the material through which its processes are carried out, but acts by stimulating trophic activity to repair the waste which the substance of the body sustains, in being made the medium of conveying energy, —so, it seems to me, the action of tropho-dynamic acts similarly. But I fear if I had begun by discussing the action of tropho-dynamic in wasting the bodily substance, which waste has to be made good by increased nutrition, it might not have been possible to get the point considered. Now, after considering the action of erg-dynamic in wasting the bodily substance, and after reflecting that Energy always wastes substance when it acts through it, it may be more possible to get the question duly considered. A question, or rather several questions, arise here. Suppose a person is in a state of collapse from shock or any other cause, and that such person has some sugar and hot water administered to him, with or without the addition of a few drops of brandy, in order to effect relief. At once, no doubt, increased O_2 intake and increased CO_2 output occur. I suppose it would be universally held that this was so because the sugar or hydro-carbon was directly burned in the organism? The action is so immediate and the stimulating effects so noticeable that this seems the most likely explanation. Well, it may be so; but in view of the considerations advanced, it seems to me doubtful whether it is, and whether the true explanation may not be that the heat supplied may not have stimulated the body to use its own flagging powers, and call upon tropho-dynamic to make new exertions. Even mental stimuli may have this effect, as when a teacher in charge of tired and hungry and flagging children, when neither food nor rest could be given them, safely stimulated them to the fresh exertion necessary to complete their journey by getting them to cut branches of trees to be used as hobby horses. Another interesting point arises when we consider that M. Magnus-Levy calculates that alcohol is a food to the extent of 7 calories for each gramme. For protein his statement is 4.1 calories and the same for starch, while that of fat is 9.3. A calorie is the quantity of Energy, as measured in heat, which will suffice to raise 1 c.c. of water through 1° C. in temperature, and M. Magnus-Levy's extraordinary statement is that, when used in the body, 1 gramme of alcohol will suffice to liberate 7 calories, while 1 gramme of protein or starch will liberate each 4.1 calories. As, according to modern scientific views, heat is energy, we are here face to face with a very interesting but at the same time very extraordinary view of the nutritional or trophic processes that occur in the body. As to the combustion or the oxidation of sugar in the organism, a recent traveler in Norway has recommended the use of hot water and sugar for walking and climbing with very little food indeed, in addition (a sandwich or two). The question again arises whether the sugar is directly oxidized or whether the hot water and sugar supplied may not stimulate the trophic energy of the body to convert carbonaceous stuff already stored up in the form of say glycogen to a larger intake of O_2 and a larger output of CO_2. It seems to me that this is the more likely explanation, although so subtly is the bodily machine made, and so wonderfully does it work, that it may be able both to oxidize sugar directly and to use its presence as a means of stimulating the nutritional powers of the body to oxidize stored-up glycogen to increased metabolism.

As to the thousands of experiments referred to in the four hundred scientific journals quoted in Professor von Noorden's book, they all assume that O_2 intake and CO_2 output are the equivalent of heat-production in the organism, and also that they are the cause of animal heat. Whether they are even the cause of heat-liberation is very doubtful, but the cause of heat-production, they certainly are not. We may make the experimentalists a present of an amount of accuracy which they do not allege they have yet attained, and we may assume that they have succeeded in showing that the waste of the organism is exactly proportioned to the O_2 intake and the CO_2 output. So much accuracy is not possible, for whenever Energy acts on substance, substance wastes, and not all of it can be restored. But supposing within the limits of human error, such a position had been experimentally attained, what then? It would be still open to us to maintain that the increase of O_2 intake, and the correspondingly increased CO_2 output were the effects of Energy acting through the organism. When either erg-dynamic or tropho-dynamic act through the organism, the organism wastes and at once the self-repairing, self-rectifying machine starts an increased nutritional metabolism to restore the waste caused. This view explains, and it seems to me that it is the only one which does explain, the enormous differences in the amounts of food which are recommended by different authorities as proper to be taken by man. As the body works more, or as it is made the medium through which Energy performs its work, the body wastes more, and as the waste has to be made good, a little more food is needed by the working than by the resting body. But a much smaller addition is required than has been supposed. How else are we to explain the very different amounts of food said to be necessary by different physiological authorities?

In the matter of proteid food, one-half or one-third of what is usually recommended was found sufficient to maintain athletes in sound condition, and this for months together—as we see from Chittenden's experiments. And there is much reason to believe that the carbonaceous food also is taken greatly in excess of requirements. So that the inference, to my mind, after viewing the question from all points, is that very much too much food, both nitrogenous and carbonaceous, is ingested into the body and is recommended to be ingested into the body, than is really required. The intellectual reason for this conflict of authority is, I believe with Mr. Carrington, the universally held scientific belief that the work of the body and its heat come from the food, while in fact they are manifestations of the powers of life. But there is another reason for the persistence of this unsound view of the functions of the body, a moral reason to which I will draw attention in closing this Introduction. On page 304, Vol. I, of his book, Professor von Noorden or M. Magnus-Levy thus expresses himself, talking of Chittenden's experiments. After showing that, on a restricted diet, the thirteen men of the second group, who engaged in gymnastic exercises for one and a half hours daily, showed more than an increase of 100 *per cent.* in their dynamometric records; and that even the athletes who had been previously in training showed an increase of 50 *per cent.* in muscular power, and that there was no sign of any deterioration in the composition of the blood, nor in the reaction for hearing, etc., he goes on to say: "Just as in Chittenden's book, so also in the writings of Ludovico Cornaro and Hufeland, the advantages that accrue from moderation in diet are emphasized. The doctrine of the sufficiency of small amounts of protein in the dietary has been expanded by Chittenden to a doctrine of the advantages to be gained by lowering the protein intake." And then he adds: "However, such a doctrine will not attract too many admirers, or at least will not bring them in as adherents, for the majority of men, even with the tempting prospect of a prolongation of life, or at least rejuvenation, prefer to enjoy the comforts of this life." If ever a doctrine was entirely given up, this seems to me to be a good instance. If "the comforts of this life" really depended on a large food intake, men might justify themselves in continuing their present habits. But when the comforts of this life are greatly interfered with, when much pain and untold miseries are the consequence, and a variety of diseases ensue which not only destroy the comforts of this life, but greatly shorten its duration, is it not high time to reconsider and to attempt to rectify the perverted reasoning which has led humanity into such a false position? If Mr. Hereward Carrington's book will not induce us to make this attempt at reconsideration, it seems to me nothing will.

A. Rabagliati.

BOOK I

THE NATURE OF DISEASE

VITALITY, FASTING AND NUTRITION

BOOK I

CHAPTER I

DISEASE A CURING PROCESS

Before it is possible for us to proceed to a consideration of "fasting as a cure for disease," it will be necessary for us to consider the primary question: What is disease? If, in our perplexity and quest for knowledge, we turn to the medical profession for our answer to this question, we find that they very frankly confess that, in the vast majority of cases, practically nothing is known of the nature—the real essence of—disease. We shall learn that its nature is still unfathomable and mysterious, and that next to nothing is known either of disease (its essence), its true causation or effective cure. My reader may, perhaps, doubt that statement, or even believe it to be incorrect. In reply, I would ask him to consult any medical authority upon this point—the higher the authority, the better—and to ascertain if he, or the medical profession as a whole, considers that disease has ever been satisfactorily explained; inasmuch as its very essence is no longer a mystery. See whether or not you will find explained and rendered clear to you the whys and the wherefores of the genesis and the progress of disease, and the multiform and complicated symptoms that invariably arise; why some are "susceptible" to disease, and others not; why one disease is frequently followed by another of a totally different character; what is "predisposition"; what constitutes "idiosyncrasy;" whether you will find explained to you the *rationale* of the action of drugs and of stimulants upon the organism. If the authority whom you have consulted (and the higher the authority, the more surely will my statements be borne out) is conscientious in the expression of his opinion, there can be no possible doubt as to the answer you will receive to every one of these questions; he will frankly admit his ignorance on *all* these points.[1]

Hear, *e.g.*, the word of Austin Flint, M.D., LL.D., one time Professor of the Principles and Practice of Medical and Clinical Medicine in the Bellevue Hospital Medical College of New York, etc., when he says:

"The definition of disease is confessedly difficult. It is easier to define it by negation, to say what it is *not*, than to give a positive definition; that is, a definition based either on the nature or essence of the thing defined, or on its distinctive attributes. Disease is an absence or deficiency of health, but this is only to transfer the difficulty, for the question at once arises, how is health to be defined? And to define health is not less difficult than to define disease."[2]

Dr. Samuel Wilks, F.R.C.S., lecturer on medicine at Guy's Hospital, told his class plainly that the method which he had to teach them was unscientific. His words are:

"All our best treatment is empirical. . . . I should have preferred to have offered you some principles based on true scientific grounds, and on which you could act in particular cases. . . . At the present day this cannot be done, nor is it wise to speak of 'principles' when framed from conclusions whose premises are altogether false. To say that I have no principles is a humiliating confession. For my own part, I believe that we know next to nothing of the action of medicines and other therapeutic agencies. There was a time when I scarcely dared

[1] Much is heard nowadays about exact diagnosis, etc. But of what benefit is the diagnosis, after all, unless the physician can cure the disease he finds? Says Dr. T. L. Brunton, F.R.S. ("Modern Developments of Harvey's Work in the Treatment of Diseases of the Heart and Circulation," p. 463), "diagnosis alone is not the aim of the physician, whose object must be to prevent, to cure, or to control disease." Precisely! It does not matter *how* a man has become ill, after all; the practical and immediately necessary problem is that of curing him. Thus; if we should find a man cut and bleeding, lying by the wayside, we should not stop to inquire how he received his injuries, but would immediately devote ourselves to the practical side of the question, and concentrate our efforts in attempting to relieve the individual so disabled.

[2] "Treatise on the Principles and Practice of Medicine," p. 22.

confess these opinions to myself, and this is the first occasion in which I have been bold enough to assert them before my class."—*Lancet*, February, 1871.

Again, Professor Gross says:

"Of the essence of disease very little is known; indeed nothing at all."

Prof. George B. Wood, M.D., of the Jefferson Medical College, Philadelphia, Pa., says (in his "Wood's Practice of Medicine.")

"Efforts have been made to reach the elements of disease, but not very successfully, because we have not yet learned the essential nature of the healthy actions and cannot understand their derangement."

Quotations such as the above might be multiplied indefinitely (See *Appendix A*), but they serve to show the actual position of the medical world, when frankly admitted. Young doctors, who have just come from college, and who are primed to the brim with vast stores of (quite useless and largely erroneous) theoretical knowledge, are, to be sure, confident that they know all about the nature of disease and its proper "treatment," under every conceivable condition, for have they not a drug for the cure of every disease? But, with the older physicians, such is by no means the case. Says Prof. Alexander H. Stevens, M.D., of the New York College of Physicians and Surgeons:

"The older physicians grow, the more skeptical they become of the virtues of medicine, and the more they are disposed to trust to the powers of Nature."

Says another author:

" the most distinguished doctors, who are also scientific men, have found it to be invariably the case, that the more they saw of disease, the less they believed in the efficacy of the drugs they had been using for years, and the more they believed in the natural forces of the body, and the more inclined were they to be content with playing a waiting game, instead of forcing their Great Partner's hand."[1]

[1] "Mad Doctors," by One of Them, p. 12. See also Flick: "Consumption," p. 65.

And if medical science of to-day does not know what is the nature of disease, how can it be successfully treated? How can we expect to treat and cure diseases the nature of which are entirely unknown to us? Would this not lead us to think that much—indeed, we might say the vast majority of—medical treatment to-day is purely empirical, and really a vast series of experiments upon the patient, while suffering from various diseases? Indeed, it would appear so.

But I must go yet further in my criticism of the medical profession—or rather of their methods of treatment—for with them, as men, I have no quarrel whatever. I shall endeavor to show that what little the medical profession is supposed to know of the nature of disease is totally wrong; that their theories of the origin and nature of disease are erroneous *ab initio,* and that every new discovery made, which they have considered an unmixed blessing and a sign of progress, has, in reality, only led them further and further from the truth, and away from an understanding of the real cause and cure of disease. These remarks will, no doubt, appear most extraordinary, if not absurd, to those of my medical readers who are unacquainted with modern hygienic (nature-cure) literature, but I ask, merely, that, for the present, they keep their judgment in suspense, and follow my argument carefully through this and the following chapters. This done, I have no fear of the ultimate result.

To begin with, then, I must state that there are, broadly speaking, two and only two schools of healing in the world; the hygienic, on the one hand, and every other school, sect or system, on the other. No matter what the physician may be —allopath, homeopath, osteopath, eclectic, faith-curist, mind-curist, Christian Scientist, or what not, he is not a hygienist, in that he does not know the real cause and cure of disease. The theory, or the philosophy of disease which the hygienist defends is totally opposed to all other medical systems, being directly opposite to them in theory.

And now, that I may not keep my readers longer in suspense, I shall state, in as clear and precise a manner as possible, the fundamental differences between these two schools, as to the nature of disease—how caused, how cured. With this object in view, I cannot do better than to quote, in full, the very excellent résumé of these differences as stated by Emmet Densmore, M.D., in his work entitled "How Nature Cures." In that brilliant (though apparently little known) work, he remarked (p. 9):

"An examination of the methods of operation of orthodox old school medicine shows that these physicians, although able, learned, earnest, and scientific, have been utterly misled as to the nature of disease. They have considered disease as an organized enemy and positive force, which has taken up a position within the body and is carrying on a warfare with the vital powers, and the legion of heroic remedies (so-called) which the orthodox physicians have prescribed and are prescribing for suffering invalids are the shot and shell hurled at the invisible enemy, in the hope of dislodging and expelling it."

The hygienist, on the other hand, regards disease as a "curative action on the part of the ruling (vital) force." (p. 7.)

"All disease and all manifestations of disease are friendly efforts and curative actions made by the organism in its efforts to restore the conditions of health.

"The law of cure may be defined as an unfailing tendency on the part of the organism toward health, and since disease, as above defined, is but the expression and result of a disturbance of the conditions natural to life, the only useful office of the physician is to restore those conditions, and there will be seen to follow, as a result of the law of cure, the disappearance of disease and the establishment of health." (p. 8.)

"There are two methods of treating dyspeptics; one aims to cure the disease; the other endeavors to cure the patient. All drug medical systems profess to cure the disease, and they can do it, whatever becomes of the patient. The hygienic medical system is based on the fundamental premise that *disease should not be cured*, but that its *causes* should be removed, to the end that the patient may recover health. All drug systems teach that disease is an entity or substance; a something at war with vitality which should be suppressed, opposed, counteracted, subdued, expelled, killed, or cured; hence it is opposed with all of the missiles of the drug shop. The hygienic system teaches that disease is a *remedial effort*, a struggle of the vital powers to purify the system and recover the normal state.[1] This effort should be aided, directed and regulated, if need be, but never suppressed. And this can always be better accomplished without medicines than with them."[2]

Again, Doctor Densmore, in showing that the true healing power lies within the organism, in opposition to the idea that it lies outside the body, in some bottle or substance, says ("How Nature Cures." pp. 5-6):

"These everyday occurrences (healing bones, etc.) are as familiar to the laymen as to the physician, but the strange part of it is the fact that almost no one—laymen or physician—seems to understand that these and like processes of nature are *all the healing force there is.* It does not matter what the trouble may be—a sliver in the flesh, or a lodgment within the organism of the poison germs of typhoid fever—no medicine is required or will benefit; all that is needed is that the conditions demanded by nature be supplied, and the same mysterious force which we call 'life,' which builds a bone-ring support whenever and wherever it is needed, and at once places a most admirable protection in the shape of a scab wherever there is an abrasion of the skin, will prove itself as well able successfully to handle an attack of typhoid fever as a broken bone, or an abrased skin."

"There are, aside from accidents—mechanical injuries—but two sources of disease in the world, *viz.*, poisons or impurities taken into the system from without, and effete or waste matters retained. In either case the result is *obstruction.* These extra neous particles are the *causes* of disease, and, aside from mental impressions and bodily injuries, the *only* causes.

"What is this mysterious thing, disease? Simply the effort to remove obstructing material from the organic domain, and to repair damages. Disease is a process of purification. It is remedial action. It is a vital struggle to overcome obstructions and to keep the channels of the circulation free. Should this struggle, this self-defensive action, this remedial effort, this purifying process, this attempt at reparation, this war for the integrity of the living domain, this contest against the enemies of the organic constitution, be repressed by bleeding, or suppressed with drugs,

[1] We thus see the force of Mr. Macfadden's remark that it requires more energy to be ill than to be well. ("Strong Eyes." p. 62).

[2] "Digestion and Dyspepsia," by R. T. Trall, M.D., p. 114.

intensified with stimulants and tonics, subdued with narcotics and antiphlogistics, confused with blisters and caustics, aggravated with alteratives, complicated and misdirected, changed, subverted and perverted with drugs and poisons generally?"[1]

Again, Doctor Trall says:[2]

"Some authors tell us that medicines cure disease, and other authors tell us that the *vis medicatrix naturæ* cures. They are both wrong. What is the *vis medicatrix naturæ?* It is vital struggle in self-defense; it is the process of purification; it is *the disease itself!* So far from the disease and the *vis medicatrix naturæ* being antagonistic entities, or forces at war with each other, they are one and the same. And if this be the true solution of this problem, it is clear enough that the whole plan of subduing or 'curing' disease with drugs is but a process of subduing and killing the vitality. We see, now, the *rationale* and the truth of the remark of Professor Clark: 'Every dose diminishes the vitality of the patient.'"

Says Miss Florence Nightingale:[3]

"Shall we begin by taking it as general principle that all disease, at some period or other of its course, is more or less a *reparative process,* not necessarily accompanied with suffering; an effort of nature to remedy a process of poisoning or decay, which has taken place weeks, months, sometimes years beforehand, unnoticed, the termination of the disease being then, while the antecedent process is going on, determined?" "The same laws of health or of nursing, for they are in reality the same, obtain among the well as among the sick. The breaking of them produces only a less violent consequence among the former than among the latter—and this sometimes, not always." (pp. 9–10.)

I cannot too strongly impress my reader with the importance of grasping and making part of his mental viewpoint this fundamentally important distinction. It is upon its thorough understanding, and an appreciation of its implications that the hygienic system of medication is based. A full acceptance of this theory means such a complete and wholesale revision of our

[1] Trall: "True Healing Art," pp. 43–4.
[2] "True Healing Art," p. 66.
[3] "Notes on Nursing," p. 7.

views of the nature of disease, and of its cure, that it is small wonder that the student of hygiene—upon first encountering the theory, thus boldly stated, should hesitate to take the step —even if he thoroughly understood the principle. Yet the step must be taken if we are to make any progress whatever in our knowledge of the essence of disease, and its successful cure. The student must "think into" this great truth, by reading and reflection. A gradual change of opinion and mental attitude must always come about in this way. A lifelong habit of viewing any subject from a certain mental standpoint cannot be changed instantly—very often not at all! Prejudice is here exhibited in an astonishing degree, in most persons. The trait of open-mindedness—the willingness to receive new truths, new impressions, is as rare a possession as a truly great musical or poetic or artistic temperament. The conviction of the correctness of any theory must, of necessity, be gradual, in most cases; "Certainty," says Prof. Charles Richet,[1] "does not follow on demonstration; it follows on habit." And I must impress upon my readers that it is only by continual study, reflection and experiment that the truth, in this matter, will finally be appreciated. Aside from advising my readers to peruse the works herein quoted for themselves, therefore (the best course), I can only ask them to divest his or her mind of all prejudice, in this matter, and to read and weigh what arguments are brought forward here with an open and candid frame of mind. If this much is granted, I have no fear of the ultimate result.

And now let us turn back, in our argument, to the point emphasized some time ago, *viz.*, that all disease, as we know it, is a curative action on the part of the organism; a reconstructive process; and that, what we know as "disease" is really the outward symptoms of this cleansing process, going on within the organism. It is the process of cure itself—we but observing the outward signs of such curative action. As Mr. Macfadden remarked:[2]

"It is disease that saves life. It is disease that actually cures the body. By means of disease poisons are eliminated, which might have caused death, had they been allowed to remain."

[1] "*Proceedings* of the Society for Psychical Research," Vol. XIV., p. 157.
[2] "Natural Cure of Diseases," p. 10.

This may be most readily seen in cases of epidemics, *e.g.*, when the mortality is frequently *lower* than in the preceding years, when no epidemic was present—showing that the disease actually *saved* many lives! See, *e.g.*, Doctor Wallace's "Cholera," p. 2; also his "Necessity for Smallpox," etc.

Now consider what this implies. The "orthodox" medical treatment consists in doctoring or smoothing these symptoms, which are mistaken for the real disease, and, in fact, in *attempting to cure a curing process!* Further, by checking or subduing or retarding these symptoms (by drugs, etc.), they actually retard and hinder the process of cure, to just the extent to which they are "successful" in supposedly "curing" the disease; *i.e.*, the more successful their palliative treatment is, the more they have, in reality, hindered the true process of cure! Physician and patient have alike mistaken the true disease, and assumed the outward symptoms of its cure to be the disease itself. The real disease is the *cause* of these symptoms—not the symptoms themselves; it is that which lies behind the phenomena observed —the phenomena being really the outward and visible signs of the general cleaning-up process proceeding within the organism. As Doctor Trall so well expressed it:[1]

"All morbid actions are evidences of the remedial efforts of nature to overcome morbid conditions or expel morbid materials. All that any truly philosophical system of medication can do, or should attempt to do, is to place the organism under the best possible circumstances for the favorable operation of those efforts. We may thwart, embarrass, interrupt, or suppress them, as is usually the case, with allopathic practice, or we may direct, modify, intensify, and accelerate them, as is the legitimate province of hydropathic practice. But we must confess to the paradoxical proposition, that the symptoms of disease are the evidences of the restorative effort; the effort, however, may be unequal to the end in view, and hence the powers of nature are to be assisted in removing obstacles, diverting irritation, etc."

And now, what is it that lies behind these symptoms? What is the real cause of disease? To this, I answer—It is the poisonous and effete matter which has collected within the organism—

[1] "Hydropathic Encyclopedia," Vol. II., p. 64.

the accumulation of which we have been repeatedly warned of, by headache, lassitude, (physical and mental) pain, unhealthy accumulation of fatty-tissue, etc.; and the elimination—the getting rid of, this poisonous matter constitutes the series or "set" of symptoms mistaken for disease, and treated as the disease itself.[1] To suppress these symptoms—which is the whole aim, goal, and ambition of the medical fraternity—is to stop this elimination, to check the system's remedial efforts, and to "lock up" as Doctor Trall expressed it, "the disease within the organism." Or, as Dr. K. S. Guthrie said:[2] "People die of disease not because the disease is fatal, but because the system is not permitted to throw it off. . . ." The entire medical world having utterly mistaken the true nature of disease—have thus directed their energies and skill to the *suppression of symptoms—rather than to the removal of cause,* while the hygienic system of cure is based solely upon the removal of the cause—the effete matter collected within the organism—regarding the symptoms as altogether insignificant, and, in fact, they temporarily aggravate or increase the symptoms, purposely in some cases (making the disease "worse" according to accepted theories), in order to affect thereby, a more rapid and true cure.

It will be noticed that, upon this theory, it would be quite impossible for any really healthy person to be "attacked" by disease, since disease, as such, is not an entity, but the symptoms we see are the result of long processes of *accumulation,* going on for—we do not know how long within the system. Disease and death are never *sudden,* though they may appear to be so. The long-continued line of causes have passed unnoticed. Says Doctor Brouardel:[3]

"I have shown that, in spite of an excellent outward appearance, sudden death is the termination of very different diseases, which develop secretly, quite unknown to the patient and those around him; such as certain affections of the kidneys, arterio-sclerosis, diabetes, etc."

[1] Reinhold: "Prevention and Cure of Tuberculosis," p. 8.
[2] "Regeneration Applied," p. 209.
[3] "Death and Sudden Death," p. x.

And again, (p. 122)

" . . . We will define sudden death as the termination of an acute or chronic disease, which has in most cases developed in a latent manner."[1]

This idea was the cornerstone of Doctor Dewey's philosophy of disease—to be outlined in detail presently—and he said:[2]

" . . . disease is never an attack, but always a *summing-up*. . . . Disease is a curative condition of bodily sins that, borne to the limit of endurance, must needs to be settled or death will come." (p. 224.)

To all this it may be replied:

"How, then, are we to know that a real cure has ever been effected? If a drug is administered, to 'cure' rheumatism, and the rheumatism shortly disappears, it is claimed that this is because the symptoms have been suppressed; whereas, if, *e.g.*, exercises, baths and diet are recommended and tried, and the symptoms disappear, it is claimed that this is because the cause of the disease has really been eradicated! How do we know that, in such cases, the symptoms have not been suppressed also; how do we know that a 'real' cure has been effected by these means any more than in the other case?"

To this I reply, that we must depend upon our reason for the answer. Drugs are given with the avowed object of removing the symptoms (though this may be denied, it is a fact) and depends upon the mistaken idea that the symptoms of the disease are the disease itself; whereas the exercises, baths, etc., are *per se*, beneficial, physiological, and are devoted altogether to the removal of the *cause*. They do not directly attack the symptoms—the pain, etc.—that is disregarded, and the treatment devoted to removing the cause. If now, under this treatment, which does not at all aim at removing symptoms, they do, nevertheless, subside and finally disappear altogether, it is obvious that it is because the removal of the cause has, at the same time, and incidentally, removed the symptoms. There has been no attempt at repression, and consequently their dis-

[1] See also Doctors Tebb and Vollum," Premature Burial," p. 160.
[2] "New Era for Women," pp. 29–30.

appearance could not have been due to that cause. A true cure has been effected, and the above method of reasoning will always indicate whether such cure has been accomplished or not; it depends upon whether the symptoms have, or no, been made the object of treatment.

This fundamental distinction, then, must lie at the root of all our further considerations, *viz.*, the recognition of the fact that, in treating a visible disease (what is known as the disease), the physician is, in reality, treating only the effects of the underlying, hidden cause, and that only in the removal of the cause, is any true cure effected. That we must always bear in mind —the fact that all disease is *itself* a curing process or method of elimination, and, as such, cannot possibly be cured! Thus, a cold is merely a process of expelling, through the nose, impurities that should have been gathered up and eliminated through other, more natural, channels (See *Appendix B*). A boil is but the same process in operation in a little different way;[1] a cough is merely the effort of nature to expel solid material from a locality where it has no right to be;[2] a pain is only a symptom, and not a disease at all—merely an indication of such (pp. 25-9); a fever is simply a natural process of rapid combustion—the "burning up" of this material—unduly retained within the organism; a night sweat is merely another attempt on the part of nature to eliminate this material through the skin, and so on, throughout the list. Every so-called disease can thus be shown to be a friendly, curative effort on the part of the bodily organism, and this idea (although I cannot stop to prove or elaborate it here) must be grasped and accepted before we proceed—as it is a point of cardinal importance. For those who require further, detailed proof, I can but refer to the references given, where they will find such proof in abundance. Beautiful examples of this theory can be found in Lionel Beale's

[1] This view is now regarded by many as the obsolete idea of a century ago, which modern science has outgrown. It is not that; the principle is still as sound as ever, but the truth is that this elimination may take place without involving such radical means of cure.

[2] "Cough often serves a very useful purpose in removing excessive secretions or irritative substances from the windpipe or bronchial tubes, and people have been known to die, practically drowned in their own secretions, because for some reason they could not remove them by coughing." "How Can I Cure My Catarrh?" by J. R. Tillinghast, Jr., M.D., p. 36.

"Life and Vital Action in Health and Disease," pp. 83–4; "Liver Complaint," p. 40; Reinhold's "Pulmonary Consumption," p. 8.

I shall close this chapter by a quotation from a recent address by Sir Frederick Treves, Sergeant-Surgeon to the King of England, at the Edinburgh Philosophical Association, and reported in the London *Times, Weekly Edition,* November 3, 1905, in part, as follows:

"Sir Frederick Treves' subject was disease. The foundation of any system of medicine, he said, was a right appreciation of disease. He ventured to think that the conception of disease which was the basis of medicine *a la mode* was not in accord with facts. If the patient were sick the sickness must be stayed, if he coughed the cough must cease, if he failed to take food he must be made to eat. But disease was one of the good gifts, for its motive was benevolent and protective. He could not express that more precisely than by saying that if it were not for "disease," the human race would soon be extinct. The lecturer demonstrated his proposition by instances. His first was that of a wound and supervening inflammation, which was a process of cure to be imitated, rather than hindered. Peritonitis, which had always been spoken of as the operating surgeon's deadliest enemy, was in reality his best friend. The general mortality of the common disease known as appendicitis was low. This fortunate circumstance was due to peritonitis, for without that much-abused ally every example of the disorder would be fatal. Another instance given was that of the common cold, which was, no doubt, a so-called bacterial disease. According to popular medicine, the phenomena constituting the disease were purposeless, profitless, and wantonly distressful, so that the victim demanded from the physician a means for stamping the trouble out. These symptoms however, were in the main the manifestations of a process of cure, and were so far benevolent that without them a common cold might be a fatal malady. The catarrh, the persistent sneezing, were practical means of dislodging the bacteria from the nasal passages, while the cough removed them from the windpipe. The lecturer described the symptoms of malaria and bubonic plague, both of bacterial origin, and also discussed the question of immunity, and said that the success of the serum treatment of diphtheria was now beyond all question. The whole of the manifestations of tuberculosis were likewise expressions of an unflagging effort on the part of the body to oppose the progress of an invading bacterium."

CHAPTER II

UNITY AND ONENESS OF DISEASE

"BUT," I hear my reader exclaim, "every disease a curing process. Why, that is equivalent to saying that there is but *one* disease in the world—while everyone knows that there are scores, nay, hundreds of such diseases![1] The second of these statements is self-evident; the first is obviously absurd from the fact that these innumerable diseases must spring from as numerous sources, and be due to a variety of causes."

This reasoning is entirely erroneous. It is based upon the false premise that the symptoms we observe are the actual diseases themselves—instead of merely the curing processes. What we really observe are *the various modes of cleansing the system* which Nature adopts, in her efforts to rid the organism of the corrupt matter it contains. This basic material itself—the real cause of the disease—might thus be the same in all cases, but, owing to the differing methods of its elimination, might be, and in fact *is*, mistaken for so many different and distinct diseases. But is it not obvious that they are, at basis, due to the same cause—having essentially the same general characteristics? As Doctor Dewey expressed it:

> "New diseases? What is there essentially new that can be treated with remedies, in the coated tongues, foul mouths, high temperature and pulse, pain, discomfort, and acute aversion to food, that is to be found in the rooms of the sick? Are there really specifics for these conditions?"[2]

[1] Eleven hundred, according to one authority! A. T. Schofield, M.D., "Nerves in Order," p. 21.

[2] "No-Breakfast Plan," p. 14.

All disease may thus have one common cause, which is equally the cause of all disease, and this I shall endeavor to both illustrate and prove as we proceed.[1]

Let us see if we can trace all diseases to one primary cause—the cause of all disease, equally—somewhat more clearly. Louis Kuhne, a German, has written a lengthy treatise entitled "The New Science of Healing; or the Doctrine of the Unity and Oneness of All Disease"—a remarkable work that has been translated into no less than twenty-five different languages—in which he has worked out, in great detail, this idea that all diseases are but the various modes, or methods of elimination of the morbid material—his doctrine being that "There is only one cause of disease, and there is only one disease, which shows itself under different forms." (pp. 32–33.) He traced their origin and growth to one basic cause.[2] With the utmost ingenuity he succeeded in showing wherein all disease is essentially *one;* arising from the presence of effete, morbid matter within the organism, and pointing out, in detail, how much morbid accumulations give rise to the phenomena we term "disease." He even succeeded in tracing a close connection between the kind, amount and location of the "encumbrance"—as he called such material—and the disease which might follow such an accumulation in any certain locality; and, as the result of a vast series of experiments and observations, he deduced his theory of "The Science of Facial Diagnosis"—a system in which it is only necessary to observe the character and the location of the encumbrance in order to determine, with great accuracy, the character of the disease to which the patient is most liable—this forming, also, a method by which we can *foresee* the disease from which a patient is likely to suffer—quite impossible by any other means what

[1] Parenthetically, I may observe that, though there is nothing to prevent the supposition that the basic, corrupt material is the same in all cases, I consider it quite improbable that it is the same. In fact, it is possible that the differing chemical compositions of the effete matter, may, in some way, determine the avenue by which it is most easily eliminated—Nature choosing the path of least resistance for its elimination in each case; but for a further discussion of this question, I would refer my readers to the chapter on the Action of Drugs.

[2] In this, however, he was anticipated by Dr. Samuel Dickson, who, in 1838, published a treatise on "The Unity of Disease," and he defended this idea throughout his "Fallacies of the Faculty."

ever. A brief résumé of this scheme will be found outlined in *Appendix C.*

I conceive, then, that all disease is essentially *one;* that an identical cause is operative in every case, which is equally the cause of all disease. And it may prove interesting to many of my readers to know that there is a distinct tendency among modern medical writers to adopt this view. Thus; Doctor Rabagliati writes:[1]

"Disease is *one;* it is one fundamentally, with many different phases or manifestations. The essence or property of a disease is that it is present; its accident is the place in the body where it appears."

Says Dr. Joseph Wallace:[2]

"All diseases in men are simply the results of decomposition in one form or another."

Again Dr. C. E. Page stated that:

"The naming and classifying of 'diseases' is calculated to mystify and mislead; sickness is the proper term for describing them all; self-abuse, in the broadest sense of the word, is the cause of them; and obedience to law, the only means of prevention or cure."[3]

Again, Dr. G. H. Patchen writes·

"The established custom of giving different names to similar abnormal conditions, simply because they manifest themselves in different parts of the system, is unfortunate from the fact that it is liable to cause the suffering part or organ to be treated as if it were an isolated entity, having no intimate connection through the nervous and circulatory channels with all the other parts of the body."[4]

Says Dr. A. F. Reinhold:[5]

"There is but one disease; *i.e.,* deposits of foreign matter.

[1] "Aphorisms, Definitions, Reflections, and Paradoxes; Medical, Surgical and Dietetic," p. 174.

[2] "Fermentation: The Primary Cause of Disease in Men and Animals," p. 8.

[3] "Natural Cure of Consumption," etc., p. 131.

[4] "How Should We Breathe? A Physiological Study," pp. 32–3.

[5] "Nature *vs.* Drugs," p. 54.

The special ailments are produced in the particular place where the matter happens to be deposited."

How much this conception differs from that of the orthodox medical man is illustrated by the following extract from Dr. Floyd B. Crandall's "How to Keep Well," p. 27, where he says: "Diseases do not result from a single cause, and they cannot be cured by any single method of treatment." As I shall presently try to show, they are ultimately traceable to one cause or source, and can all be treated in precisely a similar manner.

For consider. Every single part of the organism is and must be connected with every other part, since it is an organic whole. Every part is affected by the same means—the blood-supply—for better or worse, each passing moment. The whole organism is, through the blood, made essentially *one;* and no one part of the body can possibly be affected without all other parts being also involved—even in cases where this is apparently not the case. No one part of the body can be diseased, and the remainder be healthy; that is a most certain error. It is either connected through and by means of the blood stream, or the nervous mechanism, or both, and this should be so apparent as to need no proof whatever. It is only the weight of medical "authority" which prevents everyone from accepting that statement as axiomatic. Says Dr. Sylvester Graham:[1]

"The function of no one organ can be impaired, without involving the whole system in the consequences. Such is the dependence of each organ upon the whole system, and of the whole system upon each organ; and such are the fixed and important laws of constitution and relation appertaining to the economy of the human body "

Or, as Dr. Durham Dunlop expressed it:[2]

"The primary effect of a morbific impression on the individual constitution, is to call forth an excess of vital normal action, to resist and remove it; and the disturbance thus created constitutes general disease. Should this state continue, through the inability of nature to throw off the morbific taint and readjust

[1] "Science of Human Life," p. 272.
[2] "Philosophy of the Bath," p. 236.

the balance, then the tendency is, for the general disturbance to eventuate in local disease. 'All local diseases,' observes Dr. Edward Johnson, 'with the exception of accidental injuries, some virulent poisons, and malformations, are only the symptoms; that is, the morbid results of general disease.'"

Were the body *spherical* in shape, it might, perhaps, be more readily perceived and granted that an affection of any one part of the body would necessarily involve all the remainder of that body (provided that it was connected throughout by a freely circulating medium—such as the blood) and that no part could be diseased without involving and diseasing all the rest of the organism. In the orange or apple, this rule does not apply, for the reason that, in these cases, there is no such freely circulating medium; hence any one part may be diseased, without involving all the other parts, but in the human body, such is not the case. But, since the blood does in reality, form this intimate connection; and supply, in turn, every tissue and cell throughout the body —connecting and unifying the whole—it is most certain that no part of the body can be diseased without infecting the blood which bathes that portion, and that the blood, thus infected, must of necessity, in turn, infect or disease every other portion of the body it feeds and bathes. It would be inconceivable for this *not* to be so—since the tissues depend for their nutriment and their consequent character altogether upon the character of the blood which bathes them. It will thus be seen that no one part of the body can be diseased without the entire body becoming diseased—and consequently, *there is no such thing as a "local" disease.* Says Dio Lewis, M.D.:[1]

" A local disease is an impossibility. Every disease must be systemic before it can assume any local expression. Or, in other words, every local pathological manifestation is an expression of systemic pathological conditions."

Doctor Rabagliati asserts that:

" . . . most local diseases are the local expressions of general states; and that, for their successful treatment, therefore, it is not and cannot be enough to confine our attention and

[1] "Weak Lungs," p. 15

efforts to the organ or part affected, but that, if any real or permanent benefit is to be achieved, we must treat the organism as a whole."[1]

Dr. Samuel Dickson, as far back as 1861, wrote:

"Properly speaking there never was a purely local disease."[2]

And Dr. T. J. Pettigrew, F.R.S., stated that:

"Every individual part is essentially connected with the whole —governed by the same laws, operated upon by the same influences and circumstances; nothing in the human body—either in health or disease—can, strictly speaking, be called local."[3]

All talk of "local diseases" then, is nonsense pure and simple, and implies either ignorance or short-sightedness on the part of any man who uses the term as to what constitutes the real nature or essence of disease. The whole organism is always involved, and necessarily so; and all local treatments—ignoring constitutional treatment—are merely so many attempts at suppressing the symptoms in that one locality (generally by driving them inwards or to another locality) and quite ignoring the fact that such symptoms are, invariably, merely the localized manifestations of the condition of the entire body. Local treatments are worse than useless—they are positively injurious, and must always be so; the only logical method is to strike at the root—the *cause* of the evil—the blood—by constitutional treatment—and so benefit this as to render it normal; and, when once this is effected, healthy tissue in every part of the body must necessarily result, since every part of it is dependent upon, and is enabled to exist solely through its blood supply. The diseased portion must, therefore, be thereby rendered normal, as is every part of the body; these tissues—as all others—being dependent upon the composition of the blood supplying them, for their healthy or diseased condition. The logic of this method, as compared with the prevailing treatment, should surely appeal to all thinking persons, and practically prove the contention made without further elaboration.

[1] "Air, Food and Exercises," p. 128.

[2] "Fallacies of the Faculty," p. 17.

[3] "Superstitions Connected with the History and Practice of Medicine and Surgery," p. 45.

CHAPTER III

ON DRUG MEDICATION

A LONG and an interesting chapter might be written on this subject of drug medication, but the limited space at my disposal for that purpose effectively prevents my doing so in the manner I should like. Yet perhaps this is not so much to be regretted since the ground has been so well and completely covered already by a great number of eminent and able writers on the subject that it will be hardly necessary for me to give more than a very brief résumé and outline of the theories already advanced and held by hygienists, or of their arguments against drug-medication. So ingrained is this popular and direful superstition, however—so ingrained is this belief in the curative powers of "medicine"—that it will be necessary for me—at the risk of some tediousness—to trace in brief outline the origin and growth of this extraordinarily grotesque idea, and to show that this whole notion of deriving benefit or of becoming "cured" through the taking of "medicine" in any form, or under any circumstances, is one of the most disastrous, as it is one of the most ludicrous fallacies; one of the most harmful beliefs extant, and one which the coming generations of freethinking medical men will have to most vigorously combat.

In the first place, then, I would point out that the whole theory of drug medication is based, primarily, upon the false conception of the nature and essence of disease; and that when once our ideas in this direction have undergone a change, the whole magnificent edifice, reared by patient labor, comes tumbling about our ears. For, when once we realize the true nature of disease—that it is itself a curing process—and, as such, cannot possibly be cured!—to what has this theory of drugging, in order to "cure" the patient come? And this one single objection—the right understanding of the nature of disease—is, in itself, enough to condemn utterly and forever all drug-medication, without any additional or supplementary argument whatsoever.

For what are drugs supposed to do? Obviously, to "cure" the disease: with that object they are administered, and for that reason they are taken. But this whole theory is based upon the idea that a disease is a thing that can be attacked, or driven out, or suppressed or subdued, or in some way affected by the drug; but when once we realize that the disease is in reality not an entity at all; that it is not, in fact, what we must fight or combat, but that it is *itself* the process of purification—of "getting well" —when this grand truth is once thoroughly realized and appreciated, its true significance grasped—then drug medication will take its rightful place in the history of science—and be classed with the other vulgar superstitions, than which it is no less pathetically amusing.

Yet the whole science of "medicine" is based upon the notion that drugs possess this very power—which prompted their administration. From the very earliest times this idea has prevailed, and the drugging system of to-day is based upon exactly the same false notions as it has always been based upon. Drugs are "the shot and shell," as Doctor Densmore so well described it,[1] "hurled at the invisible enemy in the hope of dislodging and expelling it."

It would be an interesting study to consider the historical side of this question and to show that the present methods of regarding disease, and the means pursued in order to effect its cure—are, in reality, nothing more than the modernized counterpart of the more ancient notion of looking upon all diseased conditions as the result of the presence, within the body, of a devil or demon of some sort, which the conjurations and incantations and administering of "remedies" to the patient were supposed to expel or drive out—in just the same manner, and for precisely the same reason, as the drugs of the schools are administered to-day—in order to expel, or to drive out, the disease which has taken up a foothold or a lodgment within the system;[2] and though the medical man may not like to admit this, the idea is no more

[1] "How Nature Cures," p. 9.
[2] "Perfect Health," by H. B. Weinburgh, p. 83.

ridiculous, and can, in fact, be shown to be the direct outgrowth of the earlier idea—descending from it, by a directly traceable and irrefutable chain of evidence. It is but a modernized version of the older theory, from which it is derived, in reality, by a distinct process of evolution.[1]

But now this whole notion has received its death blow from the modern, hygienic theory of disease; the idea has been turned completely inside out, and we must regard drug medication as an obvious absurdity, and most necessarily untrue, for this reason, if for no other, as I have stated above.

But, quite apart from such considerations, drug medication can be shown to be absolutely without logical foundation or support, for other reasons entirely. First, drugs are admittedly *poisons;* either they are poisonous *per se* (snake virus, *e.g.*), or they become poisons simply because of their presence within the organism. It must always be distinctly remembered, in this connection, that any substance, present within the organism, which is not a food, is, strictly speaking, a poison;[2] *i.e.*, it is either appropriable material for tissue-building (a food), or it is not; and if not, then it is a foreign substance—a poison—and as such can only damage and cannot possibly ever benefit the organism. And just here I must break off to make one or two remarks which are of cardinal importance to a true and rational understanding of our problem.

"In the living world there are," as Professor LeConte pointed out,[3] "four planes of material existence which may be represented as raised one above another — animal, vegetable, mineral, and elements. Now, it is a remarkable fact that there is a special force whose function it is to raise matter from each place to the plane above and to execute movements on the

[1] "Superstition in Medicine," by Dr. Hugo Magnus, pp. 32–3; "Medical Essays," by Oliver Wendell Holmes, p. 187.

[2] "In a strict sense, everything which is not a food is a poison. Drugs and medicines of all kinds, whether derived from the animal, mineral, or vegetable kingdom, are poisons, and nothing else. Every chemical substance in the universe is a poison to the living organism. . . . The rule to determine whether a substance has a normal or abnormal relation to the living organism—whether it is a food or a poison—is simply this: If it is *usable* in the normal processes—if it is convertible into tissue—it is food; if not, it is abnormal and poisonous." "Water Cure for the Million," by R. T. Trall, M.D, p. 41.

[3] "Conservation of Energy," pp. 173–4.

latter. Plants cannot feed upon elements, but only on chemical compounds; animals cannot feed upon minerals, but only on vegetables. . . ."

This is emphatically insisted upon by Dr. Burney Yeo—a most "orthodox" lecturer, for he says:[1]

"It is a characteristic of the members of the vegetable kingdom that they are able to feed on inorganic substances. Animal organisms are unable to do so; they are dependent upon vegetable organisms to provide them with food that they can appropriate."

Science has now definitely accepted this as a fact, and allowed it to become axiomatic; and the statement that inorganic substances of any kind cannot directly nourish the animal organism—but only organized matter—must be thoroughly recognized, and allowed to become part of our mental selves and shape our view-point. Now, such being the case, what is its practical applicability? What position does this statement occupy in my argument?

Simply this: since inorganic, mineral substances cannot possibly be utilized by the vital economy; since they cannot become appropriated by it, and form a part of its organic structure, its presence there must, of necessity, act as a foreign substance—a *poison*—and, as such, call for elimination—just as any other poison would do.[2] And, in fact, this is precisely the case. The hygienic physician is much more concerned, invariably, in eliminating the drug poison from his patient's system (put there by the regular physician in his attempt to cure the disease!) than he is in removing the disease itself. The medication is far worse than the original malady! This is, as a matter of fact, actually the case. For, whereas the diseased condition is, in itself, a simple *condition*—an attempt at cure—the latter is a deep-seated, positive and dangerous entity—a poison or substance—calling for active and positive hygienic treatment, in order to remove it and effect a cure.

The fundamental truth is that any substance which is not a food is a poison—necessarily. Either the material ingested is

[1] "Food in Health and Disease," by Burney Yeo, M.D., F.R.C.P., p. 3.
[2] "Medical Essays," by Oliver Wendell Holmes, p. 254.

capable of being appropriated and utilized by the system, as food, or it is not; and if not, then it is a foreign substance—a poison—to the organism. There is no halfway ground between the two; the line of demarcation is distinct, clear-cut, absolute; and since drugs belong to the latter category, they must of necessity be a foreign—and consequently injurious—substance. That such material should be *voluntarily* introduced into the system, in the hopes, too, of benefiting the patient, seems almost too ludicrous for words.

Besides, Nature does not cure in that way. Her efforts at cure are not *chemical* changes, but *vital* ones; so that the last support of the champions of drug medication is effectually knocked away. The reparative action of the organism, the *vis medicatrix naturæ*, that which heals, is not a *chemical action* but a *vital tendency.*[1] It is an effort of the life-principle to right a wrong. Apart from all other considerations, therefore, this objection should hold good. The method of cure adopted by Nature is one and constant—it is a vital process—as distinct from a chemical one. As Doctor Dewey pointed out:[2]

"We may rightfully believe that the generation of new structures to take the place of the dying and the dead ones, is due to cell-multiplication, involving the same creative forces which operate in the body of the growing, developing, unborn child; and more, that these life energies have no more need of the action of drugs than does the growing, unborn body, the growing infant, child, youth. This suggestion ought to impress you all the more when you are reminded that the blistering and the bleeding of a hundred years ago was as strongly orthodox as the only less barbarous milk, whiskey, and the still-crucifying drugs of to-day—treatments ever changing, but Nature ever going on in her life-and-death evolutions in the same changeless ways."

[1] Unfortunately, the modern germ theory has caused the medical world to turn further and further from the truth, in this direction—the tendency being more and more to disregard entirely the vital element, and to consider the body solely from a chemical point of view. Thus, Snyder ("New Conceptions in Science," p. 286) says: "the problem of immunity is, at bottom, a chemical problem." Though this may be rather a crude statement of the case, it at least illustrates the tendency of modern medical thought on these questions, and how far removed they are from accepting any such thing as a vital principle.

[2] "Chronic Alcoholism," pp. 42-3.

One other, and very grave, objection I must urge against the practice of drug medication, in this place. This is that drugs as commonly administered, tend to *suppress symptoms* rather than to *remove causes.* If any set of symptoms arises, a drug is administered, and the symptoms subside—and the drug is administered with the precise and definite object in view of causing such cessation of symptoms. It is, in fact, commonly supposed to be the real "cure." But a real cure is based upon altogether different principles. It should be remembered that symptoms are *such* only, and are not the real disease—the cause—which must itself be removed, if any true cure is to follow. Suppression of symptoms, such as that afforded by drugs, is by no means a true cure, since the cause is not removed; the symptoms are not the disease, but the evidences of such, and should not be removed or suppressed. Doing so can only encourage the faith of the patient in spurious "cures" and divert his mind from all true methods of regaining his health.[1]

A good instance of the lack of appreciation by the medical profession of the true theory of disease and of what constitutes the real cure, as opposed to mere suppression of symptoms, is illustrated in their theory and treatment of *pain.* In their view, pain is a morbid sensation, due to a variety of causes influencing the nerves to such an extent that pain becomes manifest—a sensation of pain is present, in other words, which must be disposed of. This they proceed to do by administering opiates, narcotics, anæsthetics, etc. When the pain is subdued, the disease is (supposedly) cured, and the patient goes on his way rejoicing![2]

But is this a true cure? Is it not rather a suppression of symptoms than a removal of causes? Pain must be a symptom of

[1] Dr. Oliver Wendell Holmes saw the true point established by the introduction of the homœopathic practice, when he wrote ("Medical Essays," p. xiv): "While keeping up the miserable delusion that diseases are all to be cured by drugging, Homœopathy has been unintentionally showing that they would very generally get well without any drugging at all." A striking coincidence in thought is the following passage from the writings of Dr. Isaac Jennings, in which, speaking of homœopathy, he said: "a harmless chimera, serving the purpose of exposing a deep-rooted and dangerous delusion, and establishing the fact that diseases of all sorts can be cured better, cheaper and quicker without any drugs whatever."

[2] See "Massage," by Geo. E. Taylor, M.D., pp. 83–4.

something—of some internal and abnormal condition. "Nature is never absurd;" nothing ever happens without just cause for its happening; if pain exists there must be a cause for the pain, whether we find it or not. It is true that very little is known of pain and its significance, how little becomes manifest when we peruse such work as, *e.g.*, Dr. E. C. Hills' "Pain and Its Indications." In this we notice that any discussion of real or possible causes of pain are almost entirely avoided—yet another eminent authority has stated that "every pain has its direct and pregnant signification, if we will but carefully search for it."[1]

Pain is merely a *symptom.* Can suppressing the symptom remove the cause (since there must be a cause for the pain, otherwise there would be none)? It is the hygienist's duty to seek out and remove this cause; and, this accomplished, pain will cease, simply because the cause of the pain is no longer present. Let us consider the question from that standpoint.

"Pain," says Doctor Trall,[2] "denotes the presence of some morbific agent, or some abnormal condition. . . . The practice of 'curing' pain by means of opiates, narcotics, bleeding, etc., is founded on an erroneous theory of the nature of disease. Opium is more extensively employed in medicine than any other drug because it is the most convenient agent to allay pain. But it does this by silencing the outcries of Nature. The vital instincts of Nature proclaim that there is an enemy within the vital domain, and in the language of pain they call for help—for such materials and influences as they can use in expelling the morbific cause and in repairing the damages. The doctor poisons them with the drug, which is resisted with such intensity in another direction as to suppress the original effort—and this he calls a cure! The whole process is resolved into curing the disease by killing the patient. Hygienic agencies relieve pain by supplying the conditions which Nature requires to overcome or expel its *cause.*"

Such considerations as these doubtless prompted Doctor Reinhold to write:[3]

"The introduction and use of anæsthetics, upon which the drug

[1] "Lectures on Rest and Pain," by John Hilton, M.D., p. 499
[2] "Hygienic Hand Book," pp. 209–10.
[3] "Nature *vs.* Drugs," p. 254. "Consumption Curable," etc., p. 393.

advocates pride themselves so much, has been the greatest drawback to the progress of the true art of healing ''

Now, it is a well-recognized fact that *fasting* will relieve pain of almost every description. Says Doctor Shew:[1]

"Very seldom will toothache withstand twenty-four hours' entire abstinence from all food."

And again:[2]

"If a person has a toothache—no matter how bad—provided there is not swelling and ague in the face, it is cured with certainty within twenty-four hours by abstaining from all food and from all drinks, except water. At any rate, I have known no case where such treatment has failed of complete success."

Again, it has frequently been observed that neuralgia has been cured by fasting; while Doctor Oswald says:[3]

"Rheumatism, like gout, is a consequence of dietetic abuses. Counter-irritants, hot baths, etc., can effect a brief respite, but the only permanent specific is fasting."

Until we understand the *rationale* of pain, it is not easy to explain such cases, and an explanation only becomes possible, I think, when we accept some such theory as the following. Pain, I contend, is usually if not invariably due to the presence of foreign, encumbering matter in the system, and *the pressure of this foreign matter upon the nerve-tissue is the true cause of what we term pain.* In almost every instance we can call to mind would this explanation be complete and satisfactory. Whether the abnormal pressure comes from a hammer, a dentist's forceps, or other external causes; or whether the foreign matter presses against the nerve-tissue from within, the effect is precisely the same, *viz.*, pain; and the cause is the same—the pressure of foreign material upon the nerve—which material was not in its proper and rightful place.

It has frequently been suggested that cross nerve-currents, etc., would occasion pain. This may be a *vera causa* in a few cases, but in a few only—being limited, mostly, to cases of mental

[1] "Water Cure in Pregnancy and Childbirth," p. 63.
[2] "Family Physician," by Joel Shew, M.D., p. 796.
[3] "Household Remedies," p. 228.

influence. Pain from such causes would undoubtedly be more or less instantaneous (the effects wearing off almost immediately), and the pain would, in such cases, partake more of the nature of *shock*. For the steady, continuous, or dull pains, this explanation is obviously most unsatisfactory. These same objections might also apply to Doctor Patten's theory that "pain . . . is due to the sudden transformation of sensory into motor nerves."[1] Again, it may very possibly be true that, in its ultimate analysis, pain is nothing but a "psychological fact, a psychosis connected with definite bodily states and physical antecedents in the same sense as are other mental states which are subsumed under the category of the sensations;"[2] but what of the "definite bodily states" that give rise to this sensation? What are they?

In cases of headache, *e.g.*, the cause of which is certainly due in nearly every case to cerebral hyperæmia—the blood carrying with it the excess of encumbering material[3] the remedy is obviously to cleanse or free the blood from this matter, and a cure will follow—the same explanation and treatment sufficing for all such so-called diseases as neuralgia, rheumatism, etc.—themselves mere symptoms.

"When all the functions of the body are rightly performed," says Doctor Reinhold,[4] "we are not conscious of them; hence, any unpleasant sensation or pain is a sign of disorder. Just as the presence of a splinter in the finger, or a grain of sand in the eye, causes irritation and suffering, the presence of any matter not needed for growth or strength in any part of the body, will eventually cause fever and pain. . . . . Pain is nothing to be feared, but should be welcomed as a kindly signal—dangerous only when its warnings are neglected.[5] The suppression of pain

[1] "Over-Nutrition and Its Social Consequences," p. 38.

[2] "Sensation of Pain and the Theory of the Specific Sense Energies," by Anna J. McKeag, p. 9.

[3] "By far the larger share of headache . . has its origin in that foul state of the system, particularly the stomach and bowels, caused either by bad dietetic habits, or by an insufficient elimination of morbid matter through the bowels, skin, lungs, or kidneys. . . . The headaches of old age are generally caused by taking too much food—more than is required by the work done and more than can be digested." "Liver Complaint, Dyspepsia, Headache," by M. L. Holbrook, M.D., pp. 113, 131.

[4] "Nature *vs.* Drugs," pp. 220–4.

[5] "Bodily pain prompts us to many actions which are necessary for the maintenance of security of life, and warns us against things that are hurtful." ("The Mystery of Pain," by James Hinton, p. 17.)

by pain-killers is not only useless but highly injurious. The pain *ought* to continue so long as there is any disorder. Cure consists in removing the *cause* of the disorder."

It may be objected, of course, to all the above, that, although drugs do undoubtedly suppress symptoms in this manner, in many cases, yet they also assist in curing the disease, by removing the cause. I ask: how do they do this? Do they supply any of the necessary conditions of health—sanitary and hygienic—which would enable the body to recuperate the more quickly? Certainly not! They actually do the reverse. Drug medication adds impurities and poisons to the system—the causes of the diseased state. And how can adding impurities to the system help it to become well, when its sole trouble is that it is overburdened and surcharged with impurities already? As Doctor Trall said:[1]

"To give drugs is adding to the cause of disease; for drugs always produce disease. Indeed, they cure one disease, when they cure at all, by producing others. Can causes cure causes? Can poisons expel poisons? Can impurities deterge impurities? Can Nature throw off two or more burdens more easily than one? No! Poisoning a person because he is impure, is like casting out devils through Beelzebub, the prince of devils. It is neither scriptural nor philosophical."

There is one class of medicines which might, perhaps, be claimed as beneficial in that they *do* help to cleanse the system of corrupt material by stimulating the eliminating organs to extra work. I refer to such medicines as purgatives, emetics, diaphoretics, etc. I have shown (pp. 409–10) wherein are the great objections to all such medicines (taking purgatives as a typical example), and shall only state here that precisely the same results as any of them afford can be equalled, if not excelled, by the water cure methods—internal and external—together with other hygienic agencies—and without any of the disastrous after-effects which invariably follow the taking of the drug.

The whole system of drug medication, then, is fundamentally wrong—in that it is based upon an erroneous theory of disease—

[1] "True Healing Art," p. 44.

mistaking the effect for the cause; an erroneous theory of vitality, of the true method and nature of cure; and upon the mistaken idea that suppression of symptoms indicates a true benefit—a removal of cause—when in fact, it means nothing of the kind. All these objections are, I believe, perfectly valid and just. The lack of confidence in Nature's recuperative powers; the absurd idea that we must "do something"—we have no idea *what* it should be, but something—whenever a person is ill; and the ingrained impression that that something must be the administration of a drug[1] and preferably a nasty one; above all, the fundamentally erroneous and exceedingly harmful belief that what is good for a well man is not equally good for a sick one, and *vice versa*,[2] instead of perceiving that the same vitally beneficial, hygienic agencies are and must be equally good for both; these are the fundamental fallacies upon which the whole system of drug medication is based. This latter factor, perhaps, deserves special consideration. The medical man well knows that drugs, milk-and-whiskey diet, alcohol, and other abominations are not only unhealthful but actually poisonous to a healthy man; and yet he argues that because *the same man is engaged in getting well*, then such substances are, of necessity, and by some magical transformation, which he cannot even attempt to explain, at such times actually transformed into a substance capable of benefiting and even curing the system of its diseased condition! Says Doctor Ryan:[3]

"It may be stated generally that a medicine in a large dose is a poison, and a poison in a small dose, is a medicine."

[1] "Neither physicians nor patients have yet got rid of the idea of curative virtues residing somewhere in some *thing*." ("The Exact Science of Health," p. 256). The truth is, of course, that all the reparative effort resides in the organism and in no external thing whatever. As Miss Florence Nightingale remarked ("Notes on Nursing," p. 9): "Another and the commonest exclamation which will be constantly made is—Would you do nothing, then, in cholera, fever, etc.?—so deep-rooted and universal is the conviction that to give medicine is to be doing something, or rather everything; to give air, warmth, cleanliness, etc., is to do nothing. . . ." See also Doctor Oswald's "Physical Education," pp. 244–5.

[2] Dr. O. W. Holmes called this ("Medical Essays," p. 442) "the old rotten superstition that whatever is odious or noxious is likely to be good for disease." On p. x, he refers to "the old barbarous notion that sick people should be fed on poisons."

[3] "Homœopathic Infinitesimal Doses," by John Ryan, M.D., LL.D., etc., p. 29—quoted from "Guy's Hospital Reports," Third Series, p. 381.

Could any position be more inherently and palpably absurd and illogical? As Doctor Trall remarked:[1]

"No physician has ever yet given the world a reason that would bear the ordeal of one moment's scientific examination, why a sick person should be poisoned more than should a well person and I do not believe the world will endure until he finds such a person." "If a medical man with good intentions administers one of these drug poisons, or a hundred of them, and the patient dies, he dies because the medicine can't save him. But if a malefactor with murderous disposition gives the same medicine to a fellow-being, and the fellow-being dies, he dies because the poison killed him! Does the motive of the one who administers the drug alter its relation to vitality?" (p. 73).

But there is one and, for me, a final and crushing objection to drug medication which absolutely disproves the correctness of this system—even in the absence of any other arguments or proofs whatever. All other considerations aside, all other objections apart; this final objection is to my mind complete and irrefutable. The significance of this objection once realized, I do not see how drugs can ever be conscientiously administered again by anyone understanding the *rationale* of their true action—their real *modus operandi*.[2] Drugs are always supposed to effect their cures, of course, by acting upon the various tissues or organs of the body, directly or indirectly, and hence benefiting them, by means of their chemical action thereon. If not, their administration would be sheer nonsense. The whole theory, then, is based upon the fundamental idea that drugs do act upon certain tissues, organs or localities, and to their action is ascribed their beneficial effects. But now I take the broad stand, and defend the philosophic principle, that such supposed "action" is itself altogether a myth, and does not exist in reality at all. The real *modus operandi* of medicines is altogether differ-

[1] "True Healing Art," p. 22.

[2] Lawrence tells us that "although we cannot point out the *modus operandi* of a medicine, we are not, on that account, to withdraw our confidence in its power. 'It is enough,' he remarks, 'for us, in medical science, to know that certain effects take place!'" (Lect. on Surg., *Lond. Med. Gaz.*, Vol. V., p. 769). Needless to say, I disagree with this as much as it is possible for any two minds to disagree upon anything; the reason for my own belief will presently appear.

ent. The cart has again been placed before the horse. Let me once again quote Doctor Trall, since he is the discoverer of this fundamentally important and most revolutionary truth. I quote the following passage from his "Water Cure for the Million" (p. 4), and it is to my mind one of the most immensely important passages—not only in the philosophico-medical writings of Doctor Trall, but in the entire English language; for, with the truth it outlines truly grasped, and realized, drug medication would cease at once and forever. It would become a barbarity worthy of the middle ages. The passage is:

"It is further taught, in all the books and schools of the drug-systems, that medicines have specific relations to the various parts, organs or structures of the living system; that they possess an inherent power to 'elect' or 'select' the part or organ on which to make an impression; and that, in virtue of this 'special', 'elective' or 'selective' affinity, certain medicines *act* on the stomach, others on the bowels, others on the liver, others on the brain, others on the skin, others on the kidneys, etc. This absurd notion is the groundwork of the classification of the *materia medica* into emetics, cathartics, collagogues, narcotics, and nervines, diaphoretics, diuretics, etc. Now, the truth is exactly the contrary. So far from there being any such ability on the part of the dead, inert drug—any 'special affinity' between a poison and a living tissue—the relation between them is one of absolute and eternal antagonism. *The drugs do not act at all.* All the action is on the part of the living organism. And it ejects, rejects, casts out, expels, as best it can, by vomiting, purging, sweating, diuresis, etc., these drug poisons; and the doctors have mistaken this warfare *against* their medicines for their action on the living system."[1]

[1] The only real action of drugs—their chemical action, in the case of some compounds—is altogether a different thing from their vital action—which latter is what we perceive and call "the drug acting." That is, we do not see, in a set of external symptoms, this chemical action, only its vital action, which is all that is known to us as its action. The chemical changes and combinations, etc., which the drug may undergo, in the system, in certain rare cases, is an altogether different thing from this, and upon an altogether different plane. The body, it must be remembered, is merely the medium or vehicle through which vital force manifests (pp. 250–2); and the changes in that body deal only with this material medium. Chemical changes may, and of course, do take place in it, in addition to vital changes, but it is never these chemical changes we perceive, always the vital changes, which ultimately rule and govern the body. Just as the horse and his jockey are, in a sense, essentially *one*—the muscular power coming from the horse, the directive

I cannot go into the proofs of this statement here. Doctor Trall argued his position logically throughout his writings, and should the mere statement of the theory not carry conviction to my readers, I must refer them to the works in question, and ask them to read the arguments for themselves. But the mere statement of the case should be enough to carry conviction, when once our eyes have been opened to the true significance of the facts—to the real *modus operandi* of medicines.[1]

And so, since drugs do not "act" at all, in any case, and since they cannot possibly benefit the system by supplying it with any of the hygienic requirements it needs in order to regain health; since it must, because inorganic, always remain a poison to the organism; and since Nature does not cure, in any case, by chemical action, but by vital growth—by cell replacement—what becomes of the whole theory of drug medication?—especially since drugs are administered to "cure" a "disease" which does not in reality exist at all!

effort from the man—so, I conceive, does chemical action take place in the same body as vital action—but they are in a different plane. Vital and chemical action may take place in the same body—yet their action is always separate, and in no wise inter-related.

[1] See especially "Hydropathic Encyclopedia," Vol. II., pp. 17-19—physiology distinctly proving the case *ad oculos*, in a sense, as follows: "If you divide the pneumo-gastric nerves of a living dog—nerves which, as their name imports, connect the brain with the lungs and stomach—arsenic will not produce its accustomed effect on either of these organs." ("Fallacies of the Faculty;" by Samuel Dickson, M.D., p. 135.) Inasmuch, further, as all drugs of the tonic variety seem to increase the energy of the body, and hence are *stimulants*, they should be tabooed as wasteful to the bodily energy, for the reason that all other stimulants are tabooed.

CHAPTER IV

STIMULANTS—THEIR TRUE ACTION

THE explanation of the action of drugs that has just been given is equally the true one for all alcoholic and other stimulants. The basic error is just in the fact that it has always been believed and taught that the alcoholic or other stimulant *acted upon the body*, whereas the true explanation is that the *body reacts against the alcohol*—or whatever other poison is introduced directly or indirectly into the circulation. I do not wish it thought that I am now introducing this question of the theoretical action of stimulants for the mere purpose of discussing the temperance question, for such is by no means the case. I speak of it here, and at some length, because a correct understanding of this question of the action of stimulants is in fact most important and necessary, and forms, as we shall see later, the crucial turning point of my whole theory of vitality, outlined on pp. 225–303.

We shall be better able to appreciate its significance when we reach that part of our argument. For the present, then, let it be accepted that this discussion of the question of stimulants, and the nature of their "action," is by no means unimportant or subsidiary, but is, on the contrary, a most important link in my chain of argument.

First, however, let me clear away some few misconceptions under which the general public is laboring with regard to the supposed action of alcohol and other stimulants.

1. *Alcohol never imparts strength to the system.*—Says Dr. Benj. Ward Richardson:[1]

"It is assumed by most persons that alcohol gives strength, and we hear feeble persons saying daily that they are being 'kept up' by stimulants. This means actually that they are being

[1] "Diseases of Modern Life," p. 234.

kept *down;* but the sensation they derive from the immediate action of the stimulant deceives them and leaves them to attribute passing good to what in the large majority of cases, is persistent evil. The evidence is all-perfect that alcohol gives no potential power to brain or muscle. During the first stage of its action it may enable a wearied or a feeble organism to do brisk work for a short time; it may make the mind briefly brilliant; it may excite muscle to quick action, but it does nothing substantially, and fills up nothing it has destroyed, as it leads to destruction. A fire makes a brilliant sight, but leaves a desolation. It is the same with alcohol."

Says Dr. James C. Jackson:[1]

"All the popular stimulants, refreshing drugs, and 'pick-me-ups' have two distinct and opposite actions—an immediate exaltation, which lasts for a certain period, varying with the drug and constitution of its victim, and a subsequent depression proportionate to the primary exaltation, but, as I believe, always exceeding it either in duration or intensity, or both, thus giving us as a net or mean result, loss of vitality."

2. *Alcohol does not aid digestion, but, on the contrary, hinders it.* —In this connection Dr. B. W. Richardson says:[2]

"It has been urged as a last kind of resource and excuse, that alcohol aids digestion, and so far is useful. I support, in reply, the statement of the late Doctor Cheyne, that nothing more effectually hinders digestion than alcohol. That 'many hours and even a whole night after a debauch in wine it is common enough to reject a part or a whole of a dinner undigested.' I hold that those who abstain from alcohol have the best digestion; and that more instances of indigestion, of flatulency, of acidity, and of depression of mind and body, are produced by alcohol than by any other simple cause."

3. *Alcohol does not warm the body, but, on the contrary, cools it.* —Says Doctor Richardson:[3]

"Test the animal body under the action of alcohol, and see your findings. Your findings shall prove that, under the most

[1] "Tea and Coffee," pp. 18–19.
[2] "Researches in Alcohol," by B. W. Richardson, M.D., F.R.S., etc., p. 20.
[3] "Moderate Drinking," pp. 269–70.

favorable conditions, the mean effect of the alcohol will be to reduce the animal temperature through the mass of the body. There will be a glow of warmth on the surface of the body. Truly. But that is cooling of the body. It is from an extra sheet of warm blood brought from the heart into weakened vessels of the surface, to give up its heat and leave the whole body chilled, with the products of combustion lessened, the nervous tone lowered, the muscular power reduced, the quickened heart jaded, the excited brain infirm, and the mind depressed and enfeebled."

Again, he says:[1]

"The ultimate action of alcohol is to reduce the temperature."

Inasmuch as the surface of the body is flushed with blood, the ultimate effects must be to cool the general mass of blood, since more of it comes in contact with the cooler air.

4. *The feeling of warmth is due to partial paralysis of the nerve centers—not to added heat.*—It is, in fact, due to partial anæsthesia. I cannot stop to consider this at length here. See Richardson's "Researches," pp. 16–17; Dewey: "No-Breakfast Plan," pp. 177–79.

5. *Alcohol is not and cannot be at any time a food.*—Says Doctor Richardson:[2]

"The popular prevailing idea that alcohol, as a food, is a necessity for man, has no basis whatever from a scientific point of view."

Says Dr. R. T. Trall:[3]

"Alcohol passes through the system unchanged. Unless it is in some way altered, decomposed, diminished, changed or transformed, it can impart nothing. It cannot be used. It can supply neither the element of combustion nor of tissue. . . . Alcohol is not digestible. It is taken into the system as alcohol; it is carried through the system as alcohol, and it is expelled from the system as alcohol. If a potato, an apple, a piece of bread, or beef, was expelled from the system as potato, apple, bread, or beef, no

[1] "The Medical Profession and Alcohol," p. 306.
[2] "Researches," p. 11.
[3] "True Temperance Platform," p. 60.

one would think it acted or served the part of food. Is it not passing strange that medical men will confess that alcohol passes unchanged through the system, and yet insist that in some marvellous and incomprehensible manner, it does something, or imparts something?"

The one fact that alcohol enters the body *as alcohol,* and leaves it *as alcohol,* without undergoing any chemical changes whatever is certain proof that alcohol cannot impart anything to the system—for it has no vital or spiritual essence to impart, aside from its purely chemical properties. Since it is in no way changed, however, how can it possibly give or impart anything to the system?

I know that of late it has been claimed that part of the alcohol *is* oxidized—a very small part, it is true, but just enough to account for the increased energy noticed—just as food, when thus oxidized, is supposed to supply it.[1] I cannot now go into this question; first, because I have not space to discuss it here —important as it is, but principally because Doctor Trall has so completely and convincingly demolished these arguments in his various writings, and especially in his two booklets "The True Temperance Platform" and "The Alcoholic Controversy," that I feel it is only necessary for me in this place to refer the reader to the above-mentioned books, asking him to investigate the question for himself, to completely refute this position, and disprove the idea that we do at any time, derive any strength or energy whatever from the stimulant, thus introduced into the system.

But now I must reply that it is rather amusing for me to find physicians contending so stoutly that alcohol does actually impart strength to the organism because it is, in part at least, oxidized in the body *in the same manner as food,* because, *even were this point established,* and proved beyond all reasonable doubt (which it is not), even then, it does not prove what it sets out to prove, for, as I shall endeavor to show later on, we do not (in spite of the generally accepted ideas), derive any strength from the oxidation of food, so that all attempts to prove that

[1] See, *e.g.*, "The Cycle of Life According to Modern Science," by C. W. Saleeby, M.D., p. 90.

alcohol, *e.g.*, furnishes strength to the organism, because it is oxidized in the same manner as food, must of necessity prove a failure, since the food itself does not furnish our strength or energy; so that the comparison is by no means helpful to my opponents, as it was thought to be.

But, apart from the fact that, even were such oxidation established, it would in no way prove the point made—since oxidation of food, does not in any way supply us with energy—I must insist that no respectable evidence has ever been forthcoming to show that such oxidation has actually taken place. Any alcohol that has not been eliminated as alcohol, is simply lodged in the tissues, and there it must remain until it is eliminated at a later date—perhaps days or weeks later.

6. *Alcohol does stimulate the appetite, and for that very reason I consider it bad!*—Doctor Gully summed up this whole question when he said:[1]

"Either the stomach has appetite, and does not require the stimulus of alcohol to make it digest, or it has not appetite, and should not have food put into it to digest. Where, then, is the necessity for daily wine-bibbing?"

Having now cleared the ground, so to speak, let us at once raise the question: *What is stimulation?* We know that it is an induced condition in which the organism can, temporarily, perform a greater amount of muscular, vital or mental work than would normally be performed in the same period of time, and this increase in its ability to work is undoubtedly traceable to the "stimulus" it has received. There is a greater capacity for work (implying a greater nervous force being expended in such action), and it is generally known that there is invariably a "reaction" or prostration, more or less profound and noticeable, following upon such stimulation. But beyond this, how much is known of the *rationale* of stimulation? Is it known how this extra force is imparted or given to the system? What is the real nature of such action? and why does the reaction invariably follow? In what manner is the (apparently) added force related

[1] "Water Cure in Chronic Diseases," p. 370. See also "Total Abstinence," by Canon Farrar, D.D., F.R.S.

to its source—the stimulus? In short, why do stimulants stimulate at all? A completely satisfactory answer has never been given to any of these questions, and it could not possibly have been given without an initial understanding of the action of drugs, outlined above, and of the true relations of living and dead matter.

But now, having once grasped the true significance of the facts, we are enabled to explain all these puzzling questions relating to the supposed action of alcohol, and its relation to the organism, and I cannot do better than to quote the words of R. T. Trall, the original great discoverer and ingenious defender of this theory.

". . . We see how it is that alcohol is an element of force. . . . It *occasions* force to be wasted, that is all . . . If a small draught is taken, only a little force is wasted (not supplied) in defending the system from it, and the individual is but slightly excited; that is, a little feverish. If much is taken, a greater amount of force is necessarily wasted (not supplied), and greater excitement is manifested in stimulation, fever, delirium, madness, etc."[1] "The system expends its force to get rid of the alcohol, but never derives any force, great or small, good, bad, or indifferent, *from* the alcohol." (p. 64). "Stimulation does not impart strength; it wastes it. Vital power does not go out of the brandy into the patient, but occasions vital power to be exhausted from the patient in expelling the brandy."[2]

Now, in the light of these facts—this true and philosophic explanation of the "action" of alcohol—we can easily see how absurd it is to talk of alcohol "agreeing" with one person and

[1] "Alcoholic Controversy," p. 63.

[2] "True Temperance Platform," p. 35. Elsewhere ("Alcoholic Controversy," p. 68), Dr. Trall says: "When alcohol or other poison is taken into the system, we have, instead of the digestive juices, an outpouring of a watery and viscid fluid (serum and mucus) from the whole mucus membrane, contemplating the expulsion of the enemy from the system." The "alcoholic thirst" is doubtless explained by this fact. Since the secretions are poured out in abnormal quantities whenever alcohol is drunk, for the purpose of resisting the alcoholic poison, a call for liquid is made by the system, in order to replace the amount expended in this manner, and this craving is gratified (?) by more alcohol, which, in turn, necessitates the outpouring of more of the secretions, and so on *ad infinitum*. The ultimate effects of such a course can be imagined, and it will be seen, moreover, that the only substance capable of replacing the liquid of the secretions—and so quenching the thirst—is cool, pure water.

not with another. Or that the alcohol is "necessary" in some cases of extreme prostration, weakness, etc. Is it not enough to make any sane man not only impatient but disgusted to hear such rubbish talked (and even taught!) by persons who should know better? For, why does alcohol differ in its "action" in the two cases supposed? *Merely because the particular or peculiar mode of reaction—the degree of resistance—by the two nervous systems, is different,* and not at all because the real "action" is, in its essence, at all different in the two cases; the difference is purely one of degree, not of kind, and the result is necessarily harmful in both cases—only not equally so. It is "equally" a poison in both cases, the difference noted being solely in the degree of vigor with which the system is able to expel such poison; the difference is due to the differing degree of vitality present and available for such purely wasteful purposes. And so we can clearly see that the weaker the system—the greater the degree of prostration—the less force should be or could be expended uselessly; and consequently we should be *more* careful not to administer (in fact, to actually prevent the administration of) any stimulant whatever at this time! The weaker the patient, the greater the danger of administering alcohol! And that this is not seen, merely proves how unphilosophical and perverted are the prevailing ideas on these subjects, and how completely ignorant is *everyone* on these questions, who has not thoroughly mastered and appreciated the true philosophy of Doctor Trall's teachings.

Now what is the net result of our argument thus far? Summing it all up, and bearing in mind the philosophic principles underlying the argument, we reach this conclusion—a conclusion the importance of which is so great as to completely overshadow every other consideration bearing on this problem; a conclusion whose true significance and vast and far-reaching importance cannot be appreciated at first sight, but which will become more and more obvious, no less than significant, as we proceed. And as it is, in fact, the very *crux* of my future argument, I cannot too strongly emphasize the necessity of permitting it to sink into the very core of the mind, and of allowing it to become a part of the mental make-up. It is this:

Under all circumstances, vitality or energy of any character whatever is invariably manifested or noticed by us, as energy, in its expenditure, never in its accumulation.

I do not think it is necessary to support this plain statement with a great showing of proof, because it is so obviously self-evident that it should require no proof whatever. A body may contain any amount of potential energy, but it is never perceived by us until it is being expended, and the only way we can possibly know that it has that energy is for that body to expend it. A miser may possess untold wealth, yet, so long as it is never spent, and remains purely potential, so to speak, it is never known that he has the money to spend, and the only way in which he can convince the world at large that he has this wealth is, again, to spend it. And so in every department of nature. Suppose a storage battery is being charged with electricity. We do not, in this case, perceive the passive, accumulating energy, as energy; it may be there, but it is unperceived by us; what we *do* perceive is the active expenditure of energy in the machine charging the battery. And so it is the vital or life realm. During sleep, while the vital activities are becoming potentially stronger, and we are accumulating energy, we perceive it least—we are apparently the weakest, and during the periods of tense excitement or exertion, when the energy is being rapidly and forcibly expended in nerve and muscular power, we are apparently at our strongest, but we are really weaker at that moment than before.[1] It is because it is so being expended, that we do notice it; always in its expenditure, never in its accumulation. And

[1] I do not wish to be misunderstood in this connection. Of course the body which is exerting a certain amount of strength or energy at a given moment, is stronger, in one sense of the word, than when it is not doing so; *i.e.*, more energy is being brought into activity and expended. But, because of this expenditure, we are and must ultimately be the weaker. What I mean by the above remark, therefore, is this. If we call the present moment of time X; and the moment at which the body gives out from exhaustion Y; then the space or period from X to Y will be a certain length, and this length will depend upon the amount of reserve force the body contains. It is obvious, therefore, that anything that tends to shorten that period—the time or distance from X to Y—must render the body, ultimately, weaker to that extent. What is meant, then, is that all exercise renders the body weaker, in the sense that it expends a certain amount of reserve force; and hence, tends to shorten this X to Y period or distance; and not that the body was actually weaker at that moment—which is the meaning in which most persons would interpret the sentence, and is obviously absurd.

mark this! The greater the extent of this expenditure, the less actual or potential energy is there left; the greater the expense, the outlay, the less capital always remains.

I might call attention, perhaps, to the analogy that exists in all such cases, to the bank account, and the manner in which the money is drawn therefrom. A man has a certain amount of money; he can only convince others of that fact (that he is "rich") by spending it, and people think that, the more he spends, the "richer" he is. As a matter of fact, of course, the poorer he is, (in capital), since all expenditure is so much outgo, pure and simple, and the smaller is the amount of his credit at the bank. The more he spends, then, the poorer he is, in reality, but *apparently*, the more he spends, the richer he is—because wealth is not measured by its potential value, so to speak, but by its actual expenditure. The greater the outlay, the less the reserve, and *vice versa*; appearances are altogether deceptive—indicating, indeed, precisely the reverse of the actual fact. And so it is with the "bank of human energy." The only way in which we can convince others that we have energy to expend is to expend it —to lose it, and during the process of expenditure, we are apparently stronger, and have more energy than formerly. In reality, the reverse of this is the case; we are *weaker*, and weaker in exact proportion to the extent of the outlay of force. Says Doctor Walter:[1]

"It can be proved beyond reasonable controversy that the appearance of strength—the feeling of strength—is always coincident with, and the result of, its expenditure, while the conservation of energy in a patient, as in every other natural object, is coincident with its disappearance."

The law of action and reaction is one of the most misunderstood laws in the Universe. The weaker the person is, generally speaking, the more he feels he must do for himself; in order to gain strength; *what*, he does not know exactly, only he must do something—actively! But this activity most obviously means energy expended, and consequent loss by reaction. We cannot *force* recovery; that truth cannot be too emphatically insisted upon.

[1] "The Exact Science of Health," p. 67.

The very fact that he is weak indicates most plainly, in reality, that he must do *nothing*, and the importance of his doing nothing is exactly proportionate to the extent of his weakness. The delusion that "something must be done," in cases of sickness, is the cause of hundreds and thousands of premature deaths. The fear of being obliged to wait passively; the lack of faith in the healing powers of Nature, is one of the greatest causes of medical mal-practice of to-day. We must bear in mind, always, that no action can possibly occur without an equal and opposite reaction; that the pendulum of human energy cannot, by any possibility, swing in one direction indefinitely; but must, at some time, turn and swing in the other. Rest must always follow effort, and effort rest; and this law of rhythm applies, of course, to the human body, so far as its energy is concerned. This being so, is is not most obvious that the digestive organs need their periods of rest—just as all our other organs call for rest? And is it not obvious, also, that the only way in which such a rest can be furnished is by *fasting?* The common sense aspect of this argument should, I think, appeal to everyone of my readers.

Bearing all the above facts in mind, the question might, perhaps, be raised: Can there be any such thing as real, uninjurious stimulation? At first sight, it would appear that there can be but one answer to this question—the negative. And indeed, as stimulation is generally understood, I believe this to be the case. But there is a species of stimulation which does not, perhaps, fall under this classification. It is not the artificial and injurious calling-forth of force; it is not a diversion of it into another—useless or injurious—channel; for, as we have seen, all this is a waste of energy, and can lead to no good end. No, it is a species of *vital reinforcement*, so to say; *i.e.*, an inrush of energy, due to a natural or artificially induced condition of the nervous system—allowing a peculiar and characteristically beneficial influx of energy—never experienced save in these moments of physical exaltation, or extreme receptiveness—of the nature of which we are still in the blankest ignorance. This form of "stimulation," then, I believe we occasionally encounter, and it is decidedly beneficial, and not injurious to the organism. It denotes life-force added to the system, not force abstracted from it; and though, even here, it would be noticed only in its expenditure, the source of the energy would be different in the two cases; the one being the energy already stored in the body; the other, energy derived from external sources—a form of *vis a tergo.* But this would not be noted, as energy, at the time of the inrush, in all probability. The question is too deep and complicated for discussion here, of course; I merely offer this as a suggestion, which may, perhaps, be profitably worked out in detail on some other occasion.

CHAPTER V

THE GERM THEORY

On p. 15 I made the definite statement that all diseases are, in reality, but the varying modes, faces, or expressions of the one underlying cause—equally the cause of all disease— it being the effete material unduly retained within the system, and I then promised to consider, at a later period, the objection to this theory which "germs" apparently offer—since there are, undoubtedly, many scores of varieties of germs, each variety of which is, it is claimed, capable of producing, and in fact, does actually produce, the specific disease for which its presence is responsible. Here, at least, we have an undoubted variety and plurality of cause. Again, on p. 5 I asserted that all disease is merely a negative condition, never a positive entity, and the fact that germs are, beyond doubt, entities, and as they do, it is claimed, cause diseases of various characters, my philosophy of disease seems at least open to question upon this point. Apparently, then, diseases are (sometimes, at least) both entities, and due to various causes—instead of being conditions, and due to one primary cause, as it is claimed. If the teachings of modern medical science are not altogether and totally wrong, on this point; if their premises are not false, this certainly is established beyond all reasonable doubt.

As the reader may have already suspected, I shall take the broad stand that the premises *are* wrong; that the teachings of medical science are erroneous *ab initio*, in this question of the causation of disease by micro-organisms, and that, consequently, my philosophy of disease—its causation and nature—is not in any way overthrown or disproved, for the very reason that the diseases in question are not, in reality, caused by the micro-organisms which are found to be present in every "germ disease" at all, but are due to precisely the same cause as all other diseases whatever; *viz.*, the effete material in the system, that should have been eliminated.

Now, how am I to make good my position? In each of the various germ diseases there is undoubtedly present a particular germ, and that these germs are actually present I do not for one moment deny. That would be merely a denial of an obvious fact. But the point I wish to make is this: that their presence within the system, on such occasions, is not the *cause* of the disease, but merely one of its accompaniments; they are not that which causes the diseased state; they merely happen to be present during such a state; in short, they are not *causal*, but *coincidental*.

It need hardly be pointed out that if germs were the causes of diseases, they must *always* be present in the organism, *before* the disease they occasion appears; yet such is by no means the case! Dr. R. L. Watkins examined the evidence for this fact, and found that there was no positive proof that the germ (of tuberculosis) ever existed before the disease, and further points out that, although "it is claimed that these bacilli are carried to the tissues by the blood, . . . it is acknowledged that they have never been found in the blood."[1] Dr. Liònel S. Beale also contended that there was no evidence whatever for the belief that the bacilli invariably existed first, while there was strong evidence to the contrary.

It is a well-known fact that any germs must have, before they can successfully propagate and thrive, a suitable soil or "medium" in which this can take place; and unless such suitable soil or medium is present, germs can never live, nor can they propagate. It would be an utter impossibility. My readers must bear this well-ascertained fact in mind, throughout the following argument.

Now, what constitutes this soil or medium, favorable to their growth and perpetuation? Most certainly it is the presence, in that locality, of their suitable food; for germs—no more than any other living thing (be it sponge, roach, bird, camel, or man!)—most assuredly will not and cannot voluntarily establish themselves in a locality in which there is no suitable food. Such would be against all reason, and is, in truth, opposed to the actual

[1] "Diagnosis by Means of the Blood," p. 77.

facts. They would not enter into such a region; and if they, by any chance, did do so, they would be quite incapable of supporting and sustaining their own lives—much less propagating their species, and continuing to exist under such conditions. Obviously, the thing is impossible. And so we very clearly perceive that, so long as their proper and suitable food is lacking, germs are totally unable to establish themselves—to live and propagate their kind—in such a locality.

Now, the great point is this. *So long as the body is sound and healthy, this food material is entirely lacking;* there is none of it in the system upon which germs can possibly feed—no medium or soil in which they can, by any chance, flourish; and consequently, their growth and presence within the organism is rendered possible only by ill health; and so long as good health, a normal standard, is maintained, no germs on earth—no, nor in air or water!—can possibly harm the body, for the very reason that, even did they gain access to it, they would instantly be killed, or die from sheer lack of food.[1] We are, beyond doubt, breathing, eating, drinking germs—germs of consumption, of diphtheria, of typhoid, of cholera—all the time; and at the rate, it is said, of some 14,000 per hour![2] We cannot possibly keep them out of any system; the most healthy body doubtless contains the germs of the above-mentioned diseases—if not this minute, then probably, the next, or the next—for we eat, drink, and breathe them constantly. Why, then, do we not all have typhoid, and consumption, and cholera, and diphtheria? Simply because there is no suitable soil in our bodies in which they can flourish; no food material upon which they can sustain themselves; and that is the sole and the only reason why we do not all have these diseases, and all others supposedly caused by germs. The great principle, the grand truth, is that, so long as the body is kept sound and vigorous, germ diseases of any sort, no less than any others, become impossible; the body is rendered totally immune. Professor Rosenbach summed up the whole question when he wrote:[3]

[1] See Beale: "Life and Vital Action," p. 49; Holbrook: "Consumption," p. 31.

[2] "Eating and Drinking," by A. H. Hoy, M.D., p. 36.

[3] "Physician *vs.* Bacteriologist," by O. Rosenbach, M.D., pp. 260–1.

"The danger does not lie in the fact that an enemy is close at hand, for then we all were to perish; but usually in that we, under conditions of existence unfavorable to us, furnish a medium for our enemies, hence accord to them the conditions of existence which nature either withholds from us, or renders more difficult to us. The micro-organisms cannot harm us so long as our organism functionates normally; they are harmless if the defensive measures of our body are in good conditions. We cannot be infected because the infective agent cannot find a soil, as fire becomes extinguished if the fuel does not ignite. Hence the danger does not lie in the fact that we are surrounded by enemies, but in that an organism cannot offer any or adequate resistance to prevent their colonization, so that they, as it were, live at the expense of the affected body."

So perverted is the view of many men on this subject, however, that they seem to voluntarily turn away from the truth, after having seen it. Thus, it is stated,[1] that "the diseases of infancy the fatal diseases of childhood relate, not so much to states of the system then in the fullest vigor of vital reaction as to the accidental liability of exposure to morbific agencies current among populations, such as the contagions of the catching diseases, as, for example, scarlet fever, smallpox, measles, typhus, etc." I cannot conceive anything more opposed to all true reason, no less than the actual facts in the case, than is this statement.

For consider: upon what sort or character of food do these germs live and thrive? Is it upon healthy tissue? Most certainly it is not and cannot be; for if it were, we should all be the victims of one or more germ diseases, and there would be no possible help for us. Health would then be no guarantee of immunity, and hygiene would sink into a meaningless chaos. No! Germs cannot thrive in a healthy soil; a certain predisposition must be present in order to render their growth possible. So much is generally admitted. Besides the presence of the germ, the predisposition must also be present, in order to render possible any form of germ disease whatever.

Now, what is this predisposition? The medical profession has,

[1] "Premature Death," p. 13. *App.* 'Health Primers."

to this question, no answer. It does not know in what it consists, and consequently does not know how it originates, nor how it is to be removed. But surely the answer is simple enough. *Impure material,* in the body, *must* be the food of such germs, since we have just seen that healthy tissue is not and cannot be their food. And it is only the presence of this effete, retained, gross material which renders their growth possible—since it is their food, and without their suitable food, life, for them, would be impossible. The real danger, then, is in harboring within the system, this impure material, upon which such germs feed, and on which they can increase and multiply; and this is, as a matter of fact, the "predisposition" of the medical fraternity; and the degree of the predisposition corresponds to the amount of this material unduly retained. Were this not present, the germs would not be present either—their presence would be impossible. And from this reasoning we arrive at the ultimate view-point that, *the true disease is the predisposition,*[1] and that the germs are merely attracted by such a condition—their presence being rendered possible by the predisposition—the retained effete material. As Doctor Rosenbach put it:

"What we call predisposition to infection is nothing but the capacity for furnishing a suitable soil; absence of this tendency points to an unfavorable condition of the nutritive soil."[2]

And from this we are led to the following important definition of germ diseases as—*not a disease, caused by the presence of a specific germ, but, as that condition of the organism which renders possible the growth, within it, of that particular germ;* and the difference between such ideas is, it will be seen, truly immense. Thus; cholera is not caused by the bacillus to which it is generally attributed, but is, in reality, that condition of the body—and especially of the intestines—which renders possible its life and growth within the body. The "soil" is ready, prepared; the real cause of cholera is present, within the body, before the entrance of the germ renders its presence noticeable by setting up the characteristic disturbances associated with cholera, and taken as its symptoms. The presence of the germ here, as elsewhere,

[1] *Vide* "Nature *vs.* Drugs," by A. F. Reinhold, M.D., p. 251.
[2] "Physician *vs.* Bacteriologist," pp. 70–1.

is merely coincidental, not causal. Such is the conclusion, also, of Professor Rosenbach.

It must always be remembered that microbes are *scavengers*, attacking only impurities in the system.[1] It is therefore manifestly ridiculous to try to free the body of these minute beings, and at the same time to make no effort to cleanse it of their real cause. Such a procedure would betray the greatest short-sightedness, because we now know that any attempt to kill the germ in the living body must have disastrous consequences to the living tissue itself. "Remedies that in a certain concentration are sure to exterminate some varieties of microbes would of necessity, even in comparatively small quantities, destroy the component parts of animal tissue." And indeed, as Doctor Floyd M. Crandall pointed out:[2]

"Increased knowledge regarding bacteria and their action in producing disease renders it more and more probable that but little is to be expected in the actual prevention and cure of the infectious diseases from any known chemical compound or antiseptic. They are either poisonous to the animal body, or are decomposed and rendered inert before they reach the germs at the seat of the disease."

We must also remember that if we do not deprive germs of their food, and render the soil unsuitable for their growth, we shall in no wise effect a real cure, for the reason that such germs as survive, or their progeny, or at any rate, such fresh germs as are introduced into the organism, will always continue to thrive and multiply—so long as the soil be not removed; and, instead of directing their efforts toward removing this soil—the cause—we have simply endeavored to discover new germs—which seem to be endless in their variety.[3] Hence we see the folly of trying to kill the germs with germicides, antitoxins, etc.—using the body as a battle-ground-royal for such deadly chemical experiments—poisoning it, and exhausting its vitality, and in no wise

[1] "That bacteria are general scavengers is now generally acknowledged. . . ." "Bacteria and Their Products," by German S. Woodhead, M.D., p. 15.

[2] "How to Keep Well," p. 41.

[3] "Photography of Bacteria," by E. M. Crookshank, M.D., F.R.M.S.

effecting a real cure eventually—inasmuch as the soil, or predisposition, the real *cause* of the disease, has not been removed.

Indeed, it may here be pointed out that the fact that micro-organisms have been found to exist, in various diseased conditions, merely accentuates and adds to the reasonableness of the fasting theory, since we can now see that we, by depriving them of their food, starve them (the supposed cause of the disease), and so rid the system of its enemies. As Doctor Walter expressed it:[1]

"The nourishment of the germs is not the patient's blood, but the organic materials in the blood which obstruct circulation and nutrition because they cannot be assimilated by the patient. Give the liver, bowels, kidneys, skin, opportunities to gather out of the system these impurities, and the germs soon starve."

When it is a contest between their lives and the life of the faster, they will always be the first to succumb, and this can readily be proved by direct experiment.

But I must go yet further in my denunciation of the existing practice. I believe that it is not only totally wrong, in its treatment of such "germ diseases," but that the truth has actually been completely inverted, and that every supposed advance in medical science along these lines of recent years, is actually a step in the wrong direction and away from the truth! They are journeying further and further from the true goal—the real explanation of the causes and cure of such diseases. And I think this will become clear as we proceed.

It will now be acknowledged, I hope, that germs invariably feed upon the effete material in the body; that is their natural food, and upon that only can they live at all. Beyond all question this is the fact. Now, as the prime object in the cure of all disease is the elimination of offensive material; and since germs do help in its elimination, by actually feeding upon it, it follows that all germs are our actual friends or *benefactors* in such diseases, helping and aiding us rid the system of the effete material that it contains, and that we do, as a matter of fact, get well largely on account of, and certainly not in spite of, their presence—as it has always been taken for granted. As Doctor Page put it:[2]

[1] "The Exact Science of Health," pp. 211-12. [2] "Natural Cure," p. 81.

"The idea of being eaten alive by myriads of little vermin from which there is supposedly no escape, is enough to strike terror to the mind of a patient; but let him know that his disease is of such a nature that (with the *aid* of the bacilli, perhaps) a radical change in his manner of living affords great assurance for the hope of its entire eradication, and he has at once an all-suffi cient motive for reform."

So now it will be seen why I regard all supposed modern ad vance in these lines as retrogression, and a step away from the truth. Again, we have a case of the putting of the cart before the horse. Germs are not our enemies, to be combated, and killed, and poisoned, but our friends and aiders, in the cure of such diseased conditions! They—by feeding upon such material —assist the body very greatly in recovering its health, and in completing this elimination of the true cause of the disease.[1] There need be no fear of the germ itself, since, when its food is gone, it will no longer find it possible to live; it will be starved out—just as would any other living thing, under the same circumstances.

It may be asked—if germs really help Nature, as is claimed, instead of retarding her efforts, how is it that disease ever kills —that the patient ever dies? Surely the patient should recover more surely still, were this the case—were the germs assisting Nature's efforts, instead of retarding them. All this is very true, and the patient *would* recover more quickly were it not for the fact that we are, at the same time, continually adding to the cause of the disease (by constant feeding, etc). and thus negativing the curative efforts of the micro-organisms. Nature's efforts may, in every case, be ultimately overcome, if we persist in abusing the organism for a sufficiently long period of time, and in a sufficiently injurious manner.

The real danger, then, is not in the introduction of such germs into the system (since we could not possibly prevent their entrance under any circumstances), but in having present. in the system, such material as these germs, when introduced, can feed upon. And this material (which is the predisposition) is the

[1] "Consumption Curable," by A. F. Reinhold, M.D., p. 6.

same effete material which is equally the cause of all other diseases, so that my philosophy of disease is in nowise disproved, but, on the contrary, confirmed by this modern germ theory of disease, when rightly understood.

Diphtheria, *e.g.*, is not a "local" disease at all, any more than any other disease whatever. The germs are present in the throat, almost exclusively, for the very good reason that it is only at that particular point or locality that their food is supplied to them in the greatest quantities—the impure material on which they feed being brought there from every part of the body and deposited at that spot. The impure material is scattered more or less throughout the body, however, and that explains the presence throughout the blood, of these micro-organisms—where they frequently are present.[1] Dr. James C. Jackson, indeed, had no hesitation in calling diphtheria a "blood disease."[2] Dr. R. T. Trall,[3] and Doctor Black[4] both took the same view.

Thus we see that there is an economy in this process; that it is, in fact, a salutary and a purifying process, just as are all other diseases. For, instead of scattering this impure material throughout the body—poisoning it, and leading to disastrous consequences; this material is all gathered up and carried to one spot; is deposited there, and to this localized region the germs are confined, and are busily engaged in feeding upon, and so ridding the system of this foul material. Again, we see that germs are our benefactors; and again we see that disease is salutary—a cleansing and purifying process—adapted to the best ultimate welfare of the organism. Says Professor Rosenbach:[5]

"Is the danger for a patient with the bacillus greater than for one who is without it? Certainly not; for the cases of so-called scarlatinal diphtheria, in which the characteristic bacillus is entirely absent or is covered by proliferations of other microbes, are especially dangerous. Besides, there are plenty of healthy individuals who have the bacillus and remain healthy. Neither is there reason to believe that such carriers of the bacillus endanger their environments more than those who have no bacillus . . ."

[1] "Diphtheria," by J. H. Kellogg, M. D., p. 12.
[2] "Diphtheria," p. 4.
[3] "Diphtheria; Its Nature, History, Causes and Prevention," p. 228.
[4] "The Throat and the Voice," p. 12.
[5] "Physician *vs.* Bacteriologist," pp. 295–6.

What we must fear and guard against, then, is, not the germs themselves, but that condition of the organism which renders their presence and growth possible.[1] And the means we should adopt, in order to effect this, are the same means that should be adopted in removing all other diseased or morbid conditions whatever—having a common cause, they must necessarily receive identical treatment.

There are only two objections to this theory of germ diseases which can reasonably be raised, or which demand serious consideration. The first of these is the fact that germs, when thus present in the tissues, secrete a certain poison, or "toxin" which is detrimental to the organism;[2] and, while they might, perhaps, assist in removing diseased conditions, by disposing of their cause (the effete material present) still, such poisons as they secrete would be most detrimental to the organism, and so their good services be far outweighed by their deleterious effects. Such is, I believe, the generally prevailing idea.

I do not by any means share this opinion. For, while I can readily believe that, *under existing medical treatment*, this toxin might accumulate, and produce disastrous results, I am positively convinced, from practical observation and demonstration, as well as by reason, that, were such patients treated as they should be (on the hygienic plan), no such effects would be at all noticeable—no such results possible. Treated on the hygienic plan, all such diseases as these (the group of so-called germ diseases) are speedily, effectively, and permanently cured; and without showing any of those "deadly" effects of this toxin, which are so much feared. And simply because the plan of treatment is a rational one—the body being purified and cleansed, and the depurating organs kept constantly active, in their attempts to eradicate such poisonous material as may be in the body—it has been altogether ignored by the medical world of to-day. Yet, if this plan be carefully followed, and a fast undertaken (the significance of which we shall see presently), a little more or less poisonous material thrown into the

[1] "Bacteria and Their Products," p. 230.

[2] "Recent Advances in Science, and Their Bearing in Medicine and Surgery," by Prof. R. Virchow, p. 577.

circulation can scarcely count for any serious harm—especially as, under this régime, the germs are frozen,[1] or starved out almost before they have begun to seriously affect the system, and its stock of poisons. It must be remembered, in this connection, that the body is constantly and spontaneously producing poisons of all kinds, all the time—these being thrown into the circulation. The body has, in fact, been called a "factory of poisons," and it is only because such poisons are being constantly eliminated that we do not poison ourselves and die at once. In order to make this clear, take the cases of death from suffocation, *e.g.*, consequent upon strangulation, let us say. In such cases, it is not the want of air that has killed the person, as is generally supposed, but it is due to the fact that, once the action of the lungs has ceased, the carbon-dioxide normally exhaled at each breath, at once begins to accumulate within the system—to such an extent that death results from this poisoning. In such cases, the blood of the person so strangulated is almost *black*—due to the lack of oxygen. This should show us most forcibly how soon we should die, were not our depurating organs constantly and vigorously at work, and what a tremendous mass of poison is being hourly—aye, every minute—thrown into the circulation and being eliminated. And we know that blockage of the pores of the skin will produce the same result; while Bouchard tells us that "if the secretion of urine ceases for about fifty hours, sufficient waste materials and poisons (made in the body) will accumulate to cause death."[2]

Now, if these facts be true, how can the minute amount of toxic matter secreted by the few germs seriously affect the health—so long as the depurating organs are kept well open and active—and no more poison be put into the system? Perish the idea! It is quite unthinkable, and has gained credence simply and solely because—under the existing treatment—in which the action of the skin and other depurating organs are completely neglected, and *fresh* poisons, in the shape of food and drugs constantly introduced—any addition to the existing stock of poison is bound to be followed by grave and serious

[1] "The development of microscopic parasites can be arrested by the influence of a low temperature." See Oswald: "Household Remedies," p. 215.

[2] Cutter: "Physiology," p. 96.

consequences. Let the attention be directed, however, to the ridding of the system of *all* poison, and to depriving the germs present of their food, and a cure will be rapidly and surely effected in every case.

The second and only remaining serious objection to this theory is that it is, at first sight, hard to reconcile with the facts of *infection*, and the supposed spread of infectious diseases by their respective germs. It is easy to see how, if the germ be the actual carrier of disease, its entrance into the body (containing the suitable medium for its growth and propagation) would impart to that body the disease carried with it—thus readily accounting for epidemics and kindred outbreaks of so-called infectious diseases; and this is, in fact, the theory all but universally held. But if I adhere to my former convictions—that disease is not an entity or thing at all, and consequently cannot be carried from one person to another; and further, that germs are not the true causes of the disease, in any case, but merely its accompaniments—I am at first sight forced into rather a hopeless position, in attempting to account for the undoubted *fact* of sudden epidemics, since—although there is doubtless much exaggeration always present in such cases—epidemics undoubtedly do exist. How, then, on my theory of the non-transmission of disease, are these epidemics to be accounted for?

This is truly a most perplexing and baffling problem. It was one that puzzled me for many weeks before I found what I now believe to be its correct solution. I was thoroughly convinced that my general philosophy of disease, as herein outlined, was fundamentally true, and that all contradictory facts were so in appearance only; and were not such in reality. When rightly understood, I was convinced that the facts would turn out to be no disproof of the theory at all, but merely difficulties *within* the problem. I am now convinced that such is, indeed, the case; and I accordingly offer my theory, which I believe, will be found to solve the difficulty and explain the facts.

Let me first fairly state the case as the scientist believes it to stand. In the case of an epidemic, we have a great number of cases of the same disease present in one locality—the disease having been spread or carried from one individual to another by the specific germ of that disease; they are, moreover, its true cause, as well as its medium of transmission, and are invariably present, of course, during such disease.[1]

Now, the fact that they are present does not at all prove that they are its cause, as we have seen (p. 46); it shows, merely, that the germs invariably *accompany* such disease; they are, in fact, coincidental, not causal. Still, their invariable presence has to be accounted for, undoubtedly, and that I propose to explain as follows.

Specific germs flourish in their own suitable medium, and there only; and when—or where—ever that soil or medium is present, they do, or at least might, flourish. Diseased, effete material in the organism is that material upon which they feed, and upon that only. So that, when—and where—ever such diseased material is found, germs will, or might be, present—not necessarily by infection from another person, but spontaneously. But since, in cases of epidemics, the number of such germs is increased enormously, and since the probability of their finding an entrance into a human organism is also increased, in proportion to their numbers, it follows that (since they undoubtedly can travel some distance through the air, and yet live) they will find an entrance into many *more* organisms than they would under normal conditions—simply because of their greater numbers; and, if there were present in such organisms as they invade, the soil or material suitable for their growth, then there would naturally be a greater number of cases of that particular disease than formerly—for the very reason that the entrance of the germs into the body *would determine the form of disease necessary, in order to rid the system of such effete material—since it must be gotten rid of, by some means—by some disease (cleansing process) or we should die.*

Now, I have only to suppose that there is present, in each one of the bodies of a very large proportion of the inhabitants of any locality, just such suitable food material (soil) as would render the growth of such germs (once introduced in considerable numbers) possible. That is, all such persons would be

[1] The fact that such is *not* invariably the case really disproves the doctrine at once and forever. However, we let that pass, for the present.

more or less diseased already, and their bodies more or less saturated with foul material. On p. 63 I advance this theory, and adduce some proofs of its correctness. Now, if this is so, it would only be necessary for the germ of the specific disease, in each case, to find its way into such an organism, in order for it to set up, therein, the characteristic symptoms associated with the disease; *i.e.*, the germ would determine the form the disease would take—in order to rid the system of such material. We must not forget the primary consideration—disease is always a beneficial reparative process, an expulsive effort, a curing process. And the germ merely assists in this effort, but, while doing so, helps to determine the method of elimination; the form the disease will take; meanwhile (and incidentally) causing the appearance of certain symptoms (and among them, its *presence*) which symptoms characterize the disease, in each case. That is, the disease is not actually communicated from one organism to another; but takes the same form in two or more organisms, for the reason that the same factor was introduced into each at the same time, and determined, in each case, the method of elimination necessary (the character of the observed disease) in order to effect a cure. Just as rain will wet two persons at the same time, or sea-sickness affect two persons at an identical moment—so does disease attack two persons at precisely the same period of time; it is not because the disease has been transmitted from one organism to the other, any more than, in the former cases, the wetness or the sea-sickness was transmitted; but because the external, acting stimulus is identical in each case. It is merely that the same external cause (the presence of germs, let us say) acting upon two individual organisms, which are in very much the same state, at the same moment, can affect both of them at once, and independently of each other, just as the other external causes—the rain, or the motion of the vessel—affected them; and there is no more evidence to show that the disease was "caught" in the one case than in the other.

Thus, in epidemics, the disease is never "caught," but is, in each instance, contracted anew; and is due, in each case, to the presence of the same external cause—the micro-organisms—

acting in conjunction with the same internal cause—the predisposition. But it must be remembered that, if this predisposition be lacking, the possibility of contracting such disease is always lacking also, and perfect immunity is present. In a word, then, my theory is this: granted a number of more or less diseased individuals, living together in any one locality, whose bodies are more or less encumbered with effete material, *for the elimination of which some form of disease is necessary*; the introduction, into such a system, of the specific germ which can live upon the particular form of effete material there present, *will determine the particular form or mode of disease* (the special method of elimination) *necessary in order to effect a cure.* Thus, it merely determines the character of disease necessary—some form of which would be necessitated, in order to regain health, and in no sense *causes* the disease.[1] And it should be more than ever apparent, also, that, unless the body is in such a condition as to render some form of disease necessary, in order to regain health, germs would be quite impotent to "cause" their own or any other form of disease—or even to determine the form the disease shall take—since no disease at all would be necessary, or even possible. The *causes* of disease being absent, their manifestations in any one form or in any other would be an utter impossibility.

[1] It is interesting to note that I had written the above passage before Doctor Rosenbach's "Physician *vs.* Bacteriologist" was published; since, on p. 52 of that book, the following sentence occurs: "An epidemic breaks out, not because at other times no germs were transmitted or had developed, but because at stated periods communities or nations, owing to influences unknown to us, are in a condition that is particularly adapted to cause an infection by a certain microbe." The close similarity of thought will be observed

CHAPTER VI

NATURE'S LAW OF CURE

THE real nature of disease should now be apparent. It is the encumbrance of the system with effete, mal-assimilated, foreign material—and the degree of "susceptibility" of any person exactly corresponds to the amount of this morbid matter within the organism—it is, in fact, the degree of actual disease present. As Kuhne put it:

"The one common cause of all disease is the presence of foreign substances in the body."[1]

This is the real and the only cause of disease. The disease itself is merely the process of ridding the system of these impurities; and any real cure, must, therefore, be based upon this philosophy, and have for its successful accomplishment, the sole object of assisting nature to rid the system of these impurities. This is, in fact, the hygienic theory of disease and of its cure in a nutshell.

The great, underlying truth, then, is that all disease is but a curative crisis—a method adopted by Nature to rid the system as rapidly and energetically as possible of the effete, encumbering material it contains. Our organism is more or less encumbered or saturated with this material perpetually—owing to our artificial methods of living—*i.e.*, we are chronically more or less diseased—and, as Doctor Page pointed out ("Natural Cure," p. 184):

" the various acute diseases, so-called, are in point of fact acute *remedies* for chronic *disease*."

It may be asked, perhaps: "why, then, does disease ever remain chronic?" My answer to this is that the prolonged

[1] "Facial Diagnosis," p. 11.

sickness and attempt on the part of Nature to cure, have so depleted and so de-energized the system and wasted the vital powers that a radical and sudden method of cure is no longer possible. As Dr. Robert Walter expressed it:[1]

"An acute disease is a vigorous effort of the vital organism to resist injuries, to repair damages, and to restore health; while a chronic disease is a prolonged and subdued ailment in which the power of cure has been so depleted that active manifestations are not possible."

It cannot be doubted that if it were possible to change or convert the slow attempt at cure—a chronic disease—into a more rapid and vital process of cure, it would, ultimately, be far better for the system, in that it would be a tremendous saving of the vital forces. And, since we know an acute disease is but one method of cure that is undertaken in order to rid the system of the effete material it contains—our first object, in all chronic diseases, should be *to convert the chronic into an acute disease.*

As Doctor Oswald has pointed out:[2]

"A chronic disease, properly speaking, is nothing but Nature's protest against a chronic provocation."

It indicates a chronic cause. The one is continuous because the other is continuous, and when one is discontinued, the other ceases. It is simply a question of cause and effect, and the "cure" of such diseases thus becomes one of the simplest and most obvious of processes. We know the cause of the diseases—it is the same as the cause of all acute diseases—effete material; and to effect a cure, the rule is merely: Cease adding to the cause; cease introducing into the system those materials which act as the cause of disease.

But this philosophy of disease would imply that the whole human race is more or less diseased—and that continually! This conclusion I do not shrink from; in fact, I must insist upon it as most certainly correct and true. We are all of us diseased—all the time. The various diseases from which humanity

[1] "The Exact Science of Health," p. 178.
[2] "Physical Education," p. 241.

suffers are but the various means Nature adopts in order to cure humanity of its conditions. If any person is not in the *best* health—in the finest physical condition—then he is diseased, a little, perhaps, yet diseased. The majority of persons imagine that they are "perfectly well" if they are not actually in bed, or wracked with pain, or in the throes of some acutely diseased condition; but everyone is, in reality, diseased, who is not in the best of health, *i.e.*, in actual training—the "pink of condition." All states below that necessarily indicate some degree of disease.

I have long contended that even very grave states and dis eased conditions might exist without giving the least hint of their presence by any external noticeable sign. The case of Doctor Beaumont illustrates and indeed demonstrates this view. He says:[1]

" . . . The lining membrane of the stomach might be so inflamed and broken out, and filled with eruptions and ulcerations, as not only to secrete pus, but to bleed, without the subject of so much disease being conscious of the least suffering, and without his health being in any way affected 'in any sensible degree.' Extensive active or chronic disease may exist in the membranous tissues of the stomach and bowels, more frequently than has generally been believed. In the case of the subject of these experiments, inflammation certainly does exist to a considerable extent, even in an *apparent* state of health."

Again, Dr. James M. Gulley stated that:

"The most serious ulceration of the stomach and bowels—nay, cancerous ulceration of those organs—may go on without the smallest amount of animal pain. How often have I seen medical men pronounce positively the absence of all inflammation of the digestive organs, because pressure on them with the hand elicited no *pain!* and this at the very time when apoplectic fullness of the head from extension of chronic irritation of stomach kept the patient tottering on the brink of the grave; yet was speedily relieved bv hot fomentations over the stomach, and spare diet."[2]

[1] "Tea and Coffee," by Wm. A. Alcott, M. D., pp. 52–3.
[2] "Water Cure in Chronic Diseases," p. 19.

A *perfectly* healthy man does not, in all probability, exist; perfect health is an ideal state—an imaginary condition. Says Dr. Joel Shew:[1]

"Perfect health, at the present day, among civilized nations, is probably nowhere to be found. It exists only as an ideal thing."

Almost ideal health is the nearest we can ever hope to come to that ideal condition, and every stage below that is disease. Who can doubt the truth of this remark when we see the yellow, wizened, colorless, blotched, bloated or emaciated faces everywhere about us, in the streets—instead of the clean, healthful, pink complexions that should encounter us on every hand? How many of the human family are in perfect health—possessing buoyancy of spirits, clear skins, and possessing the energy and activity characteristic of those in health? And, if such conditions are not present, then that individual is diseased. *The whole human race is sick!* Death and disease, misery and suffering, are on every hand, where there should be nothing but health and strength and comeliness. Says Doctor Smidovich:[2]

"I began to regard people surrounding me with a new and strange feeling, and I was more and more struck by the rarity in their midst of healthy individuals; nearly every one of them had some ailment. To me the world began to assume the aspect of one gigantic infirmary; normal man was sick man; the healthy person merely represented a happy freak, a sharp deviation from the normal; this fact was ever becoming more plain."

Again (pp. 198–9):

"The appalling number of bad teeth that we see in civilized communities speaks for this. (The prevalent ill-health). . . . Eighty per cent. of the population of highly cultured communities are affected by dental corrosion. Pray give this your full attention: the living organism is a state of rot and corruption in the living man! There is nothing exceptional about this—on the contrary such is the rule, with but insignificant deviations."

[1] "Family Physician," p. 9.
[2] "The Confessions of a Physician," p. 7.

Yet, as Dr. R. T. Trall pointed out:[1]

"If the teeth are properly treated, they would never decay. There is no more reason, except abuse, why the teeth should ulcerate or become loose, than there is for the fingers or toes, or the ears or nose, to rot and fall off. The teeth are the densest, firmest of all organic structures, and should be the very last, instead of the first, to decay."[2]

Surely, it is plain enough that there must be some great error in the habits of the people which brings all this to pass! And is not the reason, the cause, obvious enough? It is simply that man has so far digressed from his normal manner of living; has become so morbid throughout, owing to his departure from the natural, physiological modes of living—that disease and death are everywhere prevalent, instead of health and happiness. As Dr. Dio Lewis so well remarked, ("Our Digestion," p. 229):

" Short life and a merry one, indeed! That's a grim joke. Merry! Why, a temperate man, who eats just what he needs, and enjoys the harmonious play of all his powers and faculties of body and soul, has more happiness in one day than one of these 'short-and-merry-life' fellows has in a year. The temperate man's life is one continuous flow of solid enjoyment."

Now, let us return again to a consideration of disease—its nature and true cure—since we have found it to be so universal. What is it that cures, in cases of disease? *Nature* is the only curative agency. It is that alone that cures, and we cannot force her to cure either. All curative, expulsive effort must come from within, and depends altogether upon the amount of the patient's vitality. We can only assist nature, by removing the obstacles that prevent, or retard its active operation. This much is, I believe, granted by most up-to-date physicians at the present day. All good physicians probably acknowledge this; but they do not follow the chain of important deductions that may be drawn from that fact—revolutionizing, as they do, the whole of medical science. Thus, their acknowledging these

[1] "Digestion and Dyspepsia," p. 18.

[2] See also Dr. C. S. Weeks: "The Causes of the Decay of Teeth," p. 6. See also *Appendix D.*

facts, implies that they acknowledge the curative powers of Nature, and the importance of hygiene and the hygienic treatment; but they do not see or acknowledge that the other part of the treatment—and all treatment other than the hygienic, is *per se* injurious and harmful; that all that is and can be good about their own treatment is the hygienic advice that is given at the same time as the medicine! That they do not see. It might be said, indeed, that the medicine is decidedly harmful, and that the hygienic advice counteracts the ill effects of the medicines and other treatment—which is a great detriment and exceedingly harmful. However, for this point, I refer the reader to the chapter on "Drug Medication."

It may be objected to all that I have said that, though the *vis medicatrix naturæ* is very powerful, and doubtless of great assistance in "the cure of disease," it is not, unaided, powerful *enough* to accomplish everything. If it could, without assistance, perform these cures, and is the only thing that ever does cure, as it is claimed, why is it that physicians have never found this out—have, in fact, apparently found that it is not sufficiently powerful to overcome and conquer disease, and effect a cure?

My answer to this is simple. It has never been fairly and properly tried, by regular physicians—since many of the hygienic appliances and aids are unknown to them, for all practical purposes, and consequently, they do not know how best and most effectually to utilize and direct the energies of the body into the proper channels, and to obtain their full, concentrated and most powerful action in the curative effort. They have always allowed but a fraction of these forces to be utilized, and have kept a very great part of them diverted into other channels (the digestion and elimination of food, *e.g.*). But let this be once dispensed with, and the full force of the *vis medicatrix* directed into the curative effort, and we shall see a speedy and effective cure, in every instance, and this I shall presently attempt to prove in detail. We cannot, at the present time, set any limit upon the undiverted power of this force.

But while it is now, I think, becoming more and more universally recognized that all disease is a curing process, the puzzle to many minds is: Why do we die at all? If the disease is merely the expulsive effort, the process of getting well, why should we die while doing so, when we did not die before; and why is any sort of assistance or medication necessary at all? The answer to this question is simply this: Although Nature always attempts a cure, still, *this attempt is not always successful*—especially if the vital, expulsive effort is not assisted and properly directed.[1]

And it is to the *direction* of this vital, expulsive action that the physician should most closely attend; upon this problem he should bend all his energies; for it is only by a delicate adjustment of the vital energies, and of the circulation, that a successful cure can be effected, and this is the true and the only service the physician can render his patient. I do not by this intend to minify the physician's importance nor the value of his services; but it must always be remembered that all curative action must come from within and thence only; and the idea that the physician can in any way "cure" you is the grossest of superstitions. As Dr. James C. Jackson stated, in speaking of his patients:

> " . . . Through the whole range, from Allopathy clear down to Hydropathy, these patients of mine had been left under the impression that the curative power resided in the doctors, and not in the vital element which God had implanted in their organisms."[2]

The doctor cannot even assist you in getting well—save for whatever brightening influences he may bring with him. All he can possibly do, in reality, is to direct this blind, expulsive effort of the vital force; to balance such effort and to give each eliminating organ its proper share; and for that he requires much special skill and knowledge—not the knowledge generally given and acquired at medical colleges, but that acquired by a constant and close study of the laws of vital action—both in health and disease.

The only remaining difficulty is the question of "incurable

[1] See Dunham: "The Science of Vital Force," p. 156; Barlow: "Reserve Force in Relation to Disease," p. 304.

[2] "How to Get Well and How to Keep Well," p. 15.

diseases"—surely they are not processes of cure, too? And why are they not cured—or rather, why do they not terminate in the cure of the patient? Now, I do not believe that there is any such thing as an "incurable disease." This is not saying, be it observed, that every *case* must recover. As Kuhne remarked:[1]

"There is no disease, whatever name it may bear, which cannot be cured; though there are patients, whose physical strength is too far gone to complete the process of cure."

Now, when we come to consider the question: How can we best assist Nature?—we come to a "dividing of the ways," where the regular medical practitioner and the hygienist part company forever. It is owing to the prevalent false medical teaching that diseases are entities (that they can "pass through" or "attack" or "leave" a patient, etc.),[2] and that drugs may in some way antidote or drive out this mysterious thing—or, at most, assist Nature in expelling it—that prevents the regular physician from perceiving the true philosophy of disease and its cure. *The disease is the cure!* That must be realized once and finally. Disease is merely a *condition*—not a *thing*. As Doctor Trall so well pointed out·[3]

"How much longer will medical men expend brain and labor, and waste pen, ink and paper, in looking for a thing that is no thing at all, and in trying to find a seat for a disease which has no localized existence? As well might a physicist point his spy-glass to the moon to discover the whereabouts of the electrical

[1] "Am I Well or Sick?" p. 27.

[2] It may be objected that the idea that diseases are entities and not the effects of cure, is no longer held by the leading medical men to-day. I can only say that this is not the case—at least, if they know it, they have not grasped the true significance of the fact. Dr. William Osler, *e.g.*, stated that "the control of physical energies, the biological revolution and the good start which has been made in a warfare against disease, were the three great achievements of the nineteenth century. . . ." ("Science and Immortality," pp. 6–7.) Here the term "warfare against disease" clearly indicates the lack of appreciation of the fact that disease is *itself* the process of cure. Again, Professor Metchnikoff ("The Nature of Man," p. 211), speaks of the poison produced by the microbe of diphtheria, which, he asserts, is capable "not only of protecting those in good health from diphtheria, but of curing those who have been attacked by the disease." Haeckel, on the other hand ("Wonders of Life," p. 107), states that disease can no longer be considered an entity.

[3] "True Healing Art," p. 69.

force, as for our doctors to turn their mental microscopes to any given locality in the vital domain, to ascertain the local habitation of a fever."

Disease is an attempt to clean the system from the foul material with which it is overloaded—and from which it must be rid, if life is to be maintained. Were there no disease (curative crises) and were the effete matter (which is the cause of the disease—and which the disease, as we know it, merely expels from the system—this process of expulsion being the so-called disease) retained within it—death would invariably result—due to tissue-poisoning. The disease is thus the curative measure Nature employs in order to prevent death—which would otherwise follow with extreme rapidity and certainty. Having once fully grasped this conception, we are in a better position to answer the question just proposed: How can we best assist Nature, in her efforts to rid the system of the impurities it contains—the real cause of the disease? Certainly not by adding more impurities; that would be the height of folly! Yet this is what is almost universally done! No; to assist Nature, we must use natural, not unnatural methods; we must use physiological, hygienic agencies; not unnatural ones.

"Any person who can explain the philosophy of sneezing has the key which may be applied to the solution of all the problems before us. Does the dust or the snuff sneeze the nose, or does the nose sneeze the dust or the snuff? Which is acted on or expelled, and what acts? Is sneezing a healthy or a morbid process? No one will pretend that it is normal or physiological. No one ever sneezes unless there is something abnormal in or about the nasal organ. Then sneezing is a remedial effort, a purifying process, a disease, as much as is a diarrhœa, a cholera, or a fever.

"And this brings me to the rule for the successful treatment of all diseases. Disease being a process of purification, I do not wish to subdue it, but to regulate it. I would not repress the remedial action, but direct it. Patients are always safe, as the remedial action is nearly equally directed to the various depurating organs, or mainly to the skin. They are in danger just to the extent that the remedial action is determined from the skin and concentrated on some internal organ. Our rule, then, is to balance the remedial effort, so that each organ shall perform its due share of the necessary labor, and no part be disorganized and ruined by overwork. And to direct and control the remedial effort, we have only to balance the circulation; and to balance the circulation we have only to regulate the temperature, and for these purposes, we have no more need of drugs than a man has of a blister on his great toe to assist him to travel. He wants useful, not injurious, things. . . ." ("True Healing Art," pp. 64–5).

"We are told that Nature has provided a 'law of cure.' Here is another vexed question for us to settle, and I meet it by denying the fact. What is this law of cure? The Allopaths say it is *contraria contrariis curantur*—contraries cure opposites. The Homœopathists proclaim *similia similibus curantur*—like cures like. The Eclectics declare that the law exists of or consists in 'Sanative' medication, and the Physio-Medicals believe that the law is fulfilled in the employment of 'Physiological!' remedies.

"They are all wrong; there is no 'law of cure' in all the Universe. Nature has provided nothing of the sort; Nature has provided *penalties*, not remedies. Think you, would Nature or Providence provide penalties or punishment as the consequences of transgression, and then provide remedies to do away with the penalties? Would Nature ordain disease or suffering as the corrective discipline for disobedience to the laws of life, and then permit the doctor to drug and dose away the penalties? There is a condition of cure, and this is *obedience*." (pp. 70–1).

And, in this connection, I would point out that this unbalancing of the circulation is due to (1) mental influences, and (2) to physical causes. These latter are of two varieties: (a) External causes—cold, heat, pressure, etc.; and (b) internal causes—the collection of impure material in one locality—drawing the blood to that spot, in order to rid it of such a condition (inflammation, congestion), and consequently leaving the other parts bloodless and anæmic. And the cure for such a condition is thus also double; (1) *suggestion*—hypnotic or other—directed to the balancing of the circulation—through the mental influences; and (2) the adoption of such physical remedies as will tend to equalize the temperature and the circulation by purely mechanical and physical means. The former process *forces* the circulation to certain parts by vital action; the latter *draws* the blood to the same parts (and consequently away from the other parts) by physical action—both processes thus having their legitimate uses. The latter process, perhaps, saves, to some extent, the vital powers; otherwise the processes are identical. But whereas I believe that suggestion will be extensively practiced, in future years, for this purpose, I think it safer to rely, for the present, and until the effects of suggestion are more universally recognized—and until the human family has progressed sufficiently far—I should certainly think it advisable in most cases, to apply merely the physical means, for such balancing of the circulation. Until our larger powers are realized and understood, they cannot be employed, and the attempt to employ them, prematurely, is, I fancy, the cause of almost all the trouble with which we are met in the mental treatment of disease.

I might point out, here, that fasting, by relieving congestion upon the internal organs—by drawing the blood away from these organs, and allowing it to circulate more freely and readily throughout the periphery of the body—thereby assists in balancing the circulation, and restoring the normal condition. Feeding determines the vital power, and consequently the blood, largely to the internal organs, while fasting allows this vitality, and the blood correspondingly, to be distributed to the extremities and surface, thus equalizing the circulation and removing congestion.

And now, if all this be true, if what we know of disease is, in every case, merely the outward symptoms of an internal cleansing process; if it is an indication, merely, of a cleansing, rectifying, purifying process going on within the system; if the prime object of medication is, therefore, to let the symptoms alone, and to aim at the removal of their *cause;* if we can appreciate the fact that there does not exist a multitude of diseases, but only an innumerable number of modes, faces, or expressions of one primary disease—a variety of methods of eliminating the one underlying cause; that there is, in reality, a unity and oneness of all disease, due to a single cause, which is known to be the retention, within the system, of waste, effete, poisonous material; if we but realized that in the elimination of this material consists the true and only rational method of cure—applicable alike to all diseases; if this were once recognized as true, it will readily be seen how far from the truth is the average practitioner in his theory of disease. In all his text books, in all his previous training, he has been taught to search for disease, and treat it as a thing that should be searched for and destroyed. But there is no "thing" to be found; disease is not an entity, but a *condition*—the very symptoms he treats as the disease itself—quite ignoring and ignorant of their cause. And when he has suppressed or palliated the outward symptoms, a cure is deemed to have been effected! Only when a complete revision of the existing theories of disease (and, consequently, its treatment) shall have taken place, will medical science commence to be such in reality, and medical men to treat disease with the confidence of knowledge, as to its essence and true method of cure. Then and then only will it be placed upon a secure and permanent basis—and be deemed an exact science, worthy of a place beside chemistry and physics, botany and astronomy.

It may be objected, perhaps, that such statements as those made above are merely dogmatic statements of a theory or view-point—and that it lacks the support of facts substantiating and proving it. That I admit; my defense being that, in a work of this character, this branch of my subject (which is only reviewed at sufficient length to enable the theory to be grasped by the reader, as it is essential to the argument) must necessarily be stated in somewhat dogmatic form, in order to render it terse and clear; and if I attempted to prove, here, each statement made, I should fill the whole book with facts and arguments, establishing these theories alone, while this has been done over and over again by hygienic authorities—to whose works I must refer the reader for such proofs—should he seek them. But I wish it to be distinctly borne in mind that I am not, in this section of my book, attempting anything more than a *statement* of the case—without bringing forward the facts that would prove the correctness of these theories.

But, it may be urged, what proofs have you to show that your theory is correct, any more than the generally accepted theories are correct? To this I reply: I think it correct for two reasons. *First,* because the explanation is more logical; more common sense; more philosophical; more explanatory; and, for all open-minded persons, carries an intuitive sense of its own correctness. The mere fact that it includes and explains a large mass of facts hitherto unclassified, unexplained and inexplicable—should force its acceptance for these reasons alone. The Copernican system of astronomy replaced the Ptolemaic theory, in all thinking men's minds, for precisely the same reason and for none other; not that it had—or could have—any experimental facts in its support, at that time, but because it explained, in a simple manner, what otherwise required a very complicated and not altogether complete hypothesis to explain the observed facts. And precisely the same rule applies here, it seems to me. *Second,* because we have actual experimental evidence and facts to show that disease—treated upon this system, and according to these theories—actually is cured more rapidly, effectually and permanently and in a greater percentage of cases than under any other system whatever. Statistics returned from various hygienic institutes, health homes, etc., prove this so conclusively that it would be useless to argue the point further. A system which is sound in its philosophy, and certain in its practice should need no defense from any source—other than its own innate, and obvious correctness.

As a proof that the facts and arguments advanced in this book are correct, I shall adduce one or two statements from the writings of those men who have treated their patients on these lines, in hygienic hospitals, and have had an opportunity to note and compare the results. Dr. R. T. Trall,[1] *e.g.,* says:

"It is now more than fifteen years since I prescribed a particle of stimulus of any kind, and although I have treated hundreds of cases of all the febrile diseases incident to New York and its vicinity, including measles, scarlatina, erysipelas, small-pox, remittent typhus, typhoid, congestive and ship-fevers, pneumonia, influenza, diphtheria, child-bed fever, dysentery, etc., etc., I have

[1] "True Temperance Platform," p. 139.

not lost one. And this statement I have repeatedly published in this city, where the facts if otherwise than as I represent, can be easily ascertained."

Again:[1]

"We have not yet known a single instance of death under hydropathic treatment, although the experience of the physicians of our school has been most extensive. I have myself treated many hundreds of cases, in young and old, strong and feeble, without losing any."

Says Doctor Dunlop:[2]

"Of the 7,500 patients who visited Grafenburg (a Nature-cure resort) up to 1841, or twenty years, . . . there were only thirty-nine deaths."[3]

The only other appeal that the medical man can make is to "experience." When so much has been achieved in the past, it may be said, how can it be that so much of the present-day practice is false? But to this it may be replied that experience always shows only one side of the shield, and never the other

"Experience," says Doctor Trall:[4] "What is experience? It is merely the record of what has happened. It only tells what *has been* done, not what *should be*."

It does not prove to us what results might have been obtained if other, and better, methods had been pursued. That remains for the future to demonstrate; meanwhile, in view of the many and terrible blunders that have been made in the past, perhaps it would be as well for the medical man not to insist too much on what past experience has shown—lest the showing be other than they expect!

If, now, it be granted that the only way in which we can "cure" a disease is by assisting Nature; the question naturally arises: How can we best assist her? This is a simple question, simply put. We must now endeavor to find an answer to that question.

[1] "Diseases of the Throat and Lungs," p. 37.
[2] "Philosophy of the Bath," p. 267.
[3] See also James C. Jackson: "How to Nurse the Sick," p. 4.
[4] "True Healing Art," p. 71.

Of course the correct and full answer would be an immediate solution of our problem—of the much-vexed problem of the treatment of the sick. This book endeavors to answer the question in a decided and final manner; but for the reasons and arguments I must refer the reader to the text of the book itself. Meanwhile, let me draw attention to one or two fundamental principles which must ever be kept in mind, in considering these questions.

How can we best assist Nature? The most obvious answer to that question would be, by natural—not unnatural—means. It may be stated definitely that, so far as a healthy bodily organism is concerned, all that is natural is beneficial, and all that is unnatural and artificial is injurious. This position I believe to be impregnable—and if challenged, as it has been—puts the person so challenging it in the position of one asserting that life is not adapted to its environment, as modern evolution teaches, and so crosses the full tide of modern scientific thought, in that particular. Further, this can be shown to be true in every case, even where it apparently does not hold good. A fuller understanding of the nature of disease would very soon prove to us that even here this statement is true. In regaining health, man needs healthful, not injurious things. All those things which are in themselves healthful—those influences and factors which keep the body in health—are, *ceteris paribus*, those which will restore it to health, when diseased. This is a truth of fundamental importance. Yet, according to the prevailing ideas, it is anything but the truth! Hygienic physicians have been pointing out this common-sense aspect of the problem for nearly two thousand years, but it has not even yet gained general acceptance! So great is the force of example and precept!

Thus: the fundamental principle upon which the hygienic system of medication is based, is this: The laws of health, the laws of its preservation, and the laws which, when followed, enable the organism to maintain its health, are unalterable and unchangeable. All disease is the result of transgression of these laws, and the result of disobeying one or more of them—consciously or unconsciously. The only way in which health can be maintained, therefore, is to conform to these laws in every respect, and when health is lost, as the result of their transgression, the only way in which it can possibly be regained, is by ceasing to transgress, and by again conforming to these laws; and in this manner, only, is the return of health rendered possible. All other ways of gaining it are illusory, and, when viewed in a rational light, obviously impossible. It follows from this, moreover, as a natural consequent, that the laws of health govern the well and sick equally; that those practices which are good for the well are equally good for the sick. What is good for the well man is equally good for the sick man and *per contra*, what is injurious and hurtful to the well man, must, of necessity, be equally hurtful and injurious to the sick man.

These simple truths contain all that need really be known of the theory of disease; and upon them the whole hygienic system of disease, and its cure, is based. Yet, self-evident, and palpable, and common sense, as they appear, the whole of present-day medical science is founded upon exactly opposite and contrary principles! The assumption that the medical world goes upon is that—what is good for the well man, is *not* good for the sick! and that what is good for the sick man is certainly injurious and hurtful to the man in health! and upon this absurd and utterly false idea is reared the whole fabric, the whole "science" of drug medication. That drugs (admittedly poisons), are detrimental to the health of the normal man is too obvious to deny; yet the idea prevails that these injurious substances, these poisons, are, for some mysterious reason, actually beneficial to the man diseased! Of course this idea is based upon the false notion that diseases are *things*, and can be attacked, subdued, or driven out by the medicines administered. This is, of course, merely a relic of mediæval superstition, which pictured demons, devils, etc., as the causes of the various diseases, and the rites, ceremonies, etc., were the various means employed to expel these demons. But once realize that the disease is *itself* the process of purification, the process of "getting well," and the absurdity of the generally accepted theories on the subject become manifest. (*v.* pp. 21–22 "Drugs".) The only way in which we can possibly assist the organism in its process of self-purification, is by supplying the most healthful physiologic conditions possible. As Doctor Trall so justly remarked: "the body wants healthful, not injurious things," and injurious things, I may point out, are always equally injurious at all times, and under all circumstances, while the healthful influences are invariable and easily recognized. And since the hygienic system is based upon the simple laws of Nature, they must forever remain unchanged, unalterable, and equally efficacious—so long, at least, as the laws themselves remain unchanged.

The great laws of hygiene are never "out of date;" its principles are the same, and as true as when they were first propounded twenty-five hundred years ago. The simple advice given by every true hygienist has always been the same, since they understand the laws of nature, and work with, and not against them. Air, light, rest, exercise, bathing, proper diet—the understanding and right application of these factors constitute all that is required for a successful cure (now, as it did a thousand years ago), simply because these are the true, natural and only real curative agencies in the universe, set there by Nature, whose laws are unchangeable. Yet how has medical treatment varied in that time! Scores, hundreds of methods—of whole systems—have been devised; schools have arisen, flourished and sunk into oblivion; the medical practice of to-day differs hopelessly from the practice of only a generation ago,[1] and it is surely no vain supposition that the treatment of to-day will be looked upon as crude—even barbarous—in the years that are to come. And, throughout all this change, this clash of opinion, the hygienic school has stood unshaken; its principles have been the same, and its practice equally efficacious throughout. And to-day it is receiving the indorsement of more brilliant thinkers than ever before. It is becoming recognized—"respectable." Surely this fact in itself, should prove the correctness of the hygienic theory of disease; that this method is Nature's own; and that, by following it, we are led only to that which is correct and true.

And following, as a practical conclusion from the above, is the immensely important consideration, that the hygienic sys-

[1] It is acknowledged that practically nothing was known of the real laws of disease and its cure, even forty years ago! ("New Conceptions in Science," by Carl Snyder, p. 287.)

tem presents this great advantage. No matter what the disease may be, we can, in every case, commence treatment *instantly*, and without waiting to see what form the disease will ultimately take. No matter what the symptoms may be; no matter what disease will ultimately appear; the treatment adopted in each case will and must be practically identical, for the reason that we know that, whatever the disease, whatever the symptoms, they are, *in every case*, due to the one ultimate cause, and require practically identical treatment; and this treatment must be equally beneficial for all the so-called diseases. We should, in every case, be removing the cause of the disease noted by thus striking at its root. We should not have to wait for the symptoms to develop before knowing what to prescribe; "yes, wait and wait," as Kuhne said:[1] "until disease and the decomposition of the juices are so far advanced, as to render real aid, in most cases, impossible."

And what a relief that would be! No matter what the disease may ultimately prove to be, no matter what form it assumes—to feel that we have, in fasting, and kindred hygienic agencies, an absolute, safe and certain cure in every single instance! It would surely be impossible to overestimate the value of such a conclusion—of such knowledge. Yet such is what the hygienic plan of medication offers!

Now, if we grant the validity of the above argument and the conclusions drawn therefrom, the next question is: What are natural means? Granting that these measures are the only ones to be pursued, how are we to ascertain what rules these are?

In answer to this, I would reply: Turn to first principles; revert to Nature; look to the animals—wild, preferably—who live nearer to nature than does man, and see what animals do under such circumstances. In following them, we cannot go far wrong; and were we implicitly to follow the dictates of Nature, there would be but little sickness in the world, and that little easily and rapidly cured.

Now, what do animals do when they are diseased? If we observe them closely, we notice that they rest and sleep an unusual amount; that they drink a far greater quantity of

[1] "Am I Well or Sick?" p. 30.

water than they usually do; and that, in all cases of real sickness, *they totally abstain from all food.* This is invariably the case. There are apparent exceptions to this rule, but they are such only. Thus dogs, *e.g.*, eat grass, sometimes, when ill, and do not fast altogether. But to this I would reply (1) that dogs are domestic animals—hence more or less perverted—so far as their instinct is concerned; only in *wild* animals is this preserved in a perfect condition—and we should accordingly study wild animals if we are to base our conclusions no observations made on the animal world; as Dr. J. H. Rausse pointed out, in answer to the objection that dogs eat medicinal herbs, when ill:

"This fact has not been proved; grass, which dogs sometimes eat, is no medicine. Even if the fact had been proved, it would not be favorable but unfavorable to the medical method of healing. For our principal objection to the latter is that medicine is antipathetic to human instinct, which has even a horror of it. If animals seek medical herbs, they instinctively want them, he detests them."[1]

Again, dogs only eat grass when they are slightly sick—"out of sorts," as we say, and possibly need the salts and other ele ments the grass contains, in order to restore them to health. When *seriously* diseased, however, the dog will invariably fast, completely. A very good example of this is Dr. Felix Oswald's dog, a little dachshund, which fasted twenty-six days in order to cure himself from the effects of a fall, which had broken several of his ribs, and inflicted severe internal injuries. The dog recovered perfectly, nevertheless—though it is exceedingly doubtful if he would have done so had he been artificially fed, and otherwise treated according to the latest medical and scientific knowledge. Lives more valuable than that of this dog have been sacrificed by premature feeding, as we well remember.

Instinct, therefore, knows when there is no need for food—no power to digest it, and hence no craving is experienced for it. Hunger is abolished. We notice this, more especially, in cases of colds, and kindred affections, where the sense of smell

[1] "Health and the Various Methods of Cure," p. 96.

—and consequently of taste—is almost or quite abolished; but in all cases this lack of appetite is experienced, if we but knew it. (*v.* p. 551.) Here is the operation of instinct—the guidance of Nature—and this guidance may be safely followed so long as the appetite is not present. Hunger will dictate when food is needed (p. 555), and, until that signal is received, none should be eaten. Only benefit will result from such abstinence.

A total abstinence from all food, when diseased, is, therefore, one of our primary and most powerful instincts. The fact that this instinct is right, and that the theory of fasting is supported by facts and logic irrefutable, I shall endeavor to show in the succeeding book.

To summarize: It will be seen that if this theory of disease —its nature and cure—be correct (and I hereby challenge anyone to successfully disprove it); if there be a "unity and oneness" of all disease, all originating in one common cause, the different diseases, so-called, being but the varying faces, aspects, or modes of expression, of this primary disease; and if the *cause* of this primary disease be due (apart from mental influences and mechanical injuries), to an undue retention, within the system, of effete, excrementous material, and the disease itself merely the active process of expulsion of this material; if all this be true, we can readily perceive that there is but *one method of cure*—to remove the cause; to expel from the system this overload of superfluous impurities—the "bad stuff" of Seb. Kneipp, which is thus equally the cause of all disease. The old water curists recognized this truth, and all their efforts were directed into this one channel, the results being, as we know, that they constantly made the most marvelous cures—in cases, too, which had been given up by the "regular" physicians as incurable.

Now there are, normally, but two ways in which this impure material can enter the system—through the lungs, by breathing impure air; or through the stomach, in swallowing improper food and drink. In no other way are impurities (normally) ever introduced into the circulation—and so into the system.[1]

[1] I have purposely omitted mention of the possibility of introducing foreign substances by purposive, or voluntary inoculation, or through wounds, etc. I have also—in order to simplify and clarify the statement—omitted to men-

And there is only one method by which this material may be expelled—through the eliminating or depurating organs. By balancing and regulating the efforts of these organs, and by keeping them at work constantly—their functions stimulated to the highest degree—in this way and in this way only can we ever hope to cure disease—by removing the *causes* of the disease. A treatment devoted to any other end, for any other purpose, is purely wasted effort, and will in nowise assist in effecting a true cure—even if it does no actual harm.

And we can readily see, also, the means for the *prevention* of all disease. Cease taking impure material (solid, liquid, gaseous) into the system. Breathe pure air at all times—a rule simple enough to follow. Drink the purest of water—also simple enough. Eat only the purest of foods—ah! now we encounter the question of *diet;* the question, *i.e.*, of the quality of food eaten—as distinct from the question of its quantity. As the latter question is the one that is dealt with throughout the remainder of this book, I must break off, just here, to consider, briefly, this question of quality—returning to that of quantity in the succeeding chapters.

tion that poisons are frequently *generated* within the system through bad food combinations; also the question of heredity, as this is discussed on pp. 150–1.

BOOK II

THE PHYSIOLOGY AND PHILOSOPHY OF FASTING

BOOK II

CHAPTER I

QUALITY—THE QUESTION OF DIET

"And God said, Behold, I have given you every herb bearing seed, which is upon the face of all the earth, and every tree, in the which is the fruit of a tree yielding seed; to you it shall be for meat."—"Genesis," I. 29.

To many of my readers it will doubtless appear something of a paradox—if not highly amusing—for me to devote a whole chapter to the subject of diet, when I am, throughout this book advocating no diet at all! But it must be remembered that all fasts of however long duration must terminate some time or other; and from that time on, eating will be resumed regularly. Further, many persons who, either from business or social engagements, or through lack of complete faith in the system advocated, cannot or will not enter upon a complete and protracted fast, may yet be persuaded to take a series of short fasts, alternated by days of light eating. On all such occasions, food is, of course, required—as throughout the regular course of life it is required. Only in diseased conditions is food harmful, it must be remembered; constant deprivation or semi-starvation while in health I deprecate and disbelieve in as heartily as the most adverse critic could possibly wish. Such being the case, then, the question before us is this: Given a fairly healthy organism which is capable of assimilating and utilizing food to advantage, and granting that the food supplied is thoroughly masticated, and is not ingested in too great quantities, granting all this, what is the *best kind* of food to supply such an organism, in order to obtain the best results from it? In other words, what, *ceteris paribus*, is the best food to allow the convalescent and the healthy, since there must be *some* choice in the materials allowed—all foods most obviously not being equally wholesome?

Doctor Dewey, and, in a lesser degree, Mr. Fletcher, and others are of the opinion that this is of small matter, provided that the quantity is sufficiently reduced and mastication sufficiently practiced. To a certain extent this plea is, of course, feasible; but I think that even better results would follow the adoption of a more natural diet, eaten subject to the same rules. To put it squarely, my contention is this: Some foods must be more healthful and more normal than others; further, many foods are known to be injurious (not to mention the fact that they are not nutritious) in however small quantities they may be taken. Again, many foods may be considered more or less natural and beneficial at all times and under all circumstances (when eating is advisable at all), while other foods are unnatural and detrimental to the organism at all times and under all circumstances—the degree of harm depending upon the amount ingested; the more food eaten, the greater the harm.

Let me make my meaning a little clearer by means of examples. It would hardly be questioned, I suppose, that rattlesnake virus, *e.g.*, is harmful and detrimental in every case, under every conceivable condition. Conversely, it may safely be said that a slice of bread made from whole wheat flour is good food, wholesome and nutritious, in all conditions, under all circumstances (where eating is advisable at all).

Similarly, I conceive every article of diet must be more or less healthful or more or less injurious; and philosophy, reason and experience should determine for us to what extent which is which. This being so, only those foods which have been proved the most wholesome should be eaten if health and strength are to be retained, since the fact that the body can assimilate and utilize and, without any apparent ill effects, eliminate certain food stuffs not so healthful (or even grossly unhealthful) merely proves that the system can *withstand* the bad effects of these latter foods, and by no means proves that a higher degree of health, strength and vitality would not have been present if the more normal foods had been eaten—and in that case such energy as had been utilized in overcoming and expelling the unhealthful food material, could have been utilized to better advantage elsewhere in maintaining the structural integrity.

Further, I am convinced that what is good and healthful food for one person is necessarily good and healthful for another. *The same foods are alike detrimental or beneficial for all.* Only the erroneous beliefs and false teachings of the medical fraternity prevent us from perceiving the complete rationality of this statement. They have invariably and steadfastly maintained that what is good and wholesome food for one is not necessarily good and wholesome food for another; that the individual idiosyncracies differentiating the organism of one from the organism of another are complete and absolute enough to justify the assumption that food may be beneficial to one person—harmful to another. In short, they propound and defend what Doctor Page so cleverly called "the most foolish of all aphorisms"—*viz.*, "one man's meat, another's poison." As generally understood, this sentence is, I am convinced, one of the most erroneous, and harmfully erroneous, sentences in the English language. As generally accepted, it enunciates a false doctrine, supports a false philosophy, and is illogical and erroneous throughout. Its harmful effects can scarcely be overestimated. I shall now attempt to justify these somewhat sweeping charges, and to prove the correctness of my position.

It must be noticed, then, that, with the single exception of man, every class of animal feeds upon its own particular and especial kind of food. All dogs, for example, eat practically the same food, and about the same amount of it (when in health—they fast when ill!), at all times and under all circumstances. When a dog is fed upon milk, meat and biscuit in certain amounts when living in England, we do not think of modifying his diet to any appreciable degree should we take him with us to America or to the Tropics. The diet might, in the latter case, be somewhat *lessened*, but that would affect its *bulk* only, not materially affecting the *quality* of the food supplied. Again, we should be surprised to find dogs fed upon altogether different substances in any portion of the globe to which we might travel; if, *e.g.*, they were fed upon turnips, oysters, mince pie, hay, and sauerkraut!—yet I must earnestly insist that this unholy combination is no more bad and unnatural than some that supposedly "civilized" men and women take into their stomachs in the course of twenty-four hours! To be sure, there might be modifications or alterations in the diet, but the changes would not be of *kind*, merely of *degree*, and we should feel, doubtless, that these dogs, having their diet altered to an altogether different kind, live under such abnormal and altered conditions rather *in spite of* than *on account of* their newly acquired régime, and would be inclined to feel that the same dogs might be infinitely more healthy and live longer lives on their more normal diet. Similarly, with every other species of animal; each *genus* has its proper and natural food, allotted by nature, and any attempts to depart from this diet, and to live upon other and altogether unnatural food must of necessity weaken, devitalize, and eventually destroy the organism of the animal so attempting to live contrary to Nature's unchanging dietetic laws.

Now, if this be true of every other species of animal, it must be true of man also. Although there are great individual differences and idiosyncrasies that must be allowed for, still as Doctor Page pointed out:[1]

"All men are *rudimentally* alike; and the body of each human being is made after a certain pattern, which pattern is in accordance with the general principles which apply to all individuals."

They belong, that is, to the same *genus*, and consequently, their food must be, *within certain limits*, alike also. There is a natural food for man, as there is for any other animal, and any departure from this diet will, and must, sooner or later, show itself in some form of disease. The contrary would be inconceivable. Were it possible, it would mean that there is a law in Nature that can be broken with impunity and with no consequent evil effects. Man has never yet discovered such a law, and it never will be discovered—since it does not exist.

My main contention, then, is this. With man, as with every other animal, a standard or normal food exists in Nature, and (within certain limits) man must confine his diet to this food if

[1] "How to Feed the Baby," by C. E. Page, M.D., p. 56.

health is to be maintained. Any *absolute* divergence from this system of diet, such, for example, as the continued feeding upon food intended for another class of animals altogether, will inevitably result in disease and death. Says Doctor Wait·[1]

"Individuality appeared to have much less effect upon the digestion than might be expected."

It may be replied to all this that practical experience has shown us that the same foods will *not* agree with everyone; but that it is, on the contrary, one of the commonest of experiences to observe that one article of food can be eaten and enjoyed by one person, while it causes grievous indigestion or other troubles in another. Or, that food which nourishes one person and seems to agree with him perfectly, causes a rash, diarrhœa, or other symptoms in another. I freely admit all this, but I do not think that it alters or affects my position in the least. It does not in any way disprove the fundamental principle that the human race should feed altogether upon its normal food. What it *does* prove is that, *in their present physical condition* they are unable to profitably assimilate and digest those particular food stuffs. It does not by any means show that, if

not be easily and profitably digested—as they are in the majority of cases. What it proves, in other words, is that the system is, in such cases, in an abnormal or pathological condition—perhaps of a particular chemical composition—and that this abnormal organism, reacting perforce abnormally, produces abnormal results. Doctor Jackson, in fact, went to the very heart of the problem when he said:[2]

" if I had his ultimate good in view, I should seek to change the state of his stomach that he might eat what was in itself better for him, rather than have his morbid necessity say what he should be compelled to eat."

But granted a healthy and normal organism, and logic and experience both go to prove that, reacting normally, normal

[1] "Experiments on the Effect of Muscular Work upon the Digestibility of Food and the Metabolism of Nitrogen," by Charles E. Wait, Ph.D., F.C.S., p. 39.

[2] "The Whole and the Hulled Wheat," by James C. Jackson, M.D., p. 10.

conditions would follow; in which case the normal food of man is easily and perfectly digested without any untoward results, which could not be expected and actually does not happen in the case of unnatural food.[1]

Now, if it be granted that some foods are necessarily better for us than others—a statement which will hardly be challenged, I fancy—the next question to be decided is, *what is* the best food for man? From the foregoing reasoning, we are in a position to state definitely, in answer to this question; the most natural.

If, then, it be granted that the most natural foods would be, *ceteris paribus*, the best, the question then arises, in turn: What is the most natural food? and, in attempting to answer this, we at once enter one of the most bitterly contested battle grounds in the history of medicine. The question, whether or not man is naturally a vegetarian; whether or not meat is a normal, wholesome food; whether, in short, man is carnivorous, herbivorous, gramnivorous, frugivorous, or omnivorous by nature, is one of the most hotly disputed points in the history of medical science. But it is a point into which I cannot enter here, interesting as the discussion of this question might be. I will only say that, from every conceivable standpoint do the arguments for vegetarianism (or fruitarianism) become stronger and stronger the more they are examined and inquired into, and the more ephemeral and lacking in reason do those become which are advanced against the practice. That "too much meat" is now consumed is generally admitted; but that man can do without meat altogether, and be better, healthier and stronger from a total discontinuance of its use—this may strike my readers as, at first sight, overstating the case. Such however, is by no means the fact. Meat is not man's natural food, since he is not either a carnivorous or an omnivorous animal—whatever the physiologists may say. Every argument drawn from comparative anatomy, from physiology, from chemistry, from

[1] Our instinctive tastes have, however, become vitiated, as Doctor Wallace pointed out ("Dietetic Advice," etc., p. 1), disqualifying them as our guides—though it is probably true, as Mr. Macfadden stated ("Physical Training," p. 91), that we may "eat what we like best" *if the appetite be normal.* This should be carefully borne in mind.

experience, from observation, and, when rightly used, from common sense, as well as the arguments from the agricultural, the hygienic, the ethical and humanitarian standpoints—all agree in proving that man is not a meat-eating animal; and that, if he does indulge in this practice, it is to his own detriment; and, in fact, he keeps well in spite of, not on account of, such an unhealthful, unnatural and abnormal habit. Our discussion on p. 83–4, relative to the lower animals, applies also to man; with him also marked deterioration follows—must follow—this radical departure from his normal diet. He can never be *as* healthy under the prevailing "mixed" diet as he would be were he to follow the dictates of Nature, and to live upon his natural food—fruits and nuts, eaten in their uncooked, primitive form.[1] Every element the system needs can be shown, by chemical analysis, to be present in these foods, in their proper proportion, while, being *live* foods, instead of mere "dead ashes"—which is all the cooking process leaves—they will be found to supply a degree of vital life and energy which no cooked foods ever supplied, or could supply. It is man's natural diet, and should be the universal one.[2]

I know that there will be almost innumerable objections raised to this advice, on very many grounds. I cannot stop to consider these here, as I hope to do so at length in a further volume on vegetarian diet generally—in which I shall go into the quality of foods in the same manner as I have discussed the quantity in the present book. I must, however, in this place, answer one objection—the one most frequently raised to its adoption—since I am sure it will occur to the average reader

[1] See *Appendix E.*

[2] Says Doctor Holbrook ("Eating for Strength," p. 86): "Cooking destroys life. I do not say that these articles should never be cooked, but only that there is loss in cooking them, especially if we can eat them perfectly fresh and alive. . . . The life and soul of fruits are lost in cooking." Doctor Schlickeysen also says ("Fruit and Bread," p. 116): "Finally—and this is a point that physiologists have hitherto quite overlooked—the food must contain a certain *electrical vitality.* Although the real origin and nature of the vital force is not yet known, we believe that it is closely related to electricity; not less so, indeed, than to light and heat. . . . The same vitality is stored up in uncooked plants and fruits, but is greatly impaired by all our culinary processes." Mr. Christian argues for the use of uncooked foods throughout his book, "Uncooked Foods;" Doctor Susanna Dodds agrees with the main contentions put forward by these authors; while Mr. Otto Carqué, in his "Foundation of All Reform" (pp. 32–4), strongly urges the value of the raw-food diet, as opposed to cooked foods.

at once. It may be asserted—and this is a very common, and to many minds a very grave objection—that man, having lived so many ages upon the cooked, or supposedly unnatural diet, is now more adapted to that diet than to his original, uncooked foods—and that an attempted return to such a diet would be attended with grave, and disastrous consequences. As Doctor Goodfellow remarked:[1]

> "The conditions of life have so altered that the natural food of our ancestors would be unnatural now, living as we do under such different conditions."

But this objection is completely refuted by the facts in the case, which are that those who have attempted the reform and to return to original and natural conditions, so far as their diet is concerned, have done so easily and rapidly—with nothing but marked benefit to themselves—physically and mentally. As usual, appeal to the actual facts in the case disproves the *à priori* theories. Again, the contention is disproved, it seems to me, by the fact that *no anatomical change whatever* has taken place in man's digestive apparatus since the most primeval times. If the body had gradually "grown accustomed" to the cooked and unnatural foods, this, surely, could never be the case—Nature's adaptive capacity being far too great, in all cases, where such adaption is really necessary, or in any sense "natural." The system has not, as a matter of fact, become adapted to the new diet at all—nor is it any the less detrimental to the organism now than it ever was. To argue that an unhealthful thing can become healthful—simply because repeated generations have lived in that manner, and in spite of such detrimental effects, is to me, frank nonsense. We should rather suppose, *à priori*, that the effects of such a course would be to deteriorate the systems of the persons so living—which is exactly the case. Let me illustrate my meaning a little more clearly: Suppose that a family had always been brought up in an impure atmosphere—rarely or never breathing the pure atmosphere in "God's out of doors." Suppose the progeny of this family were also reared in the same conditions—and their children likewise, and

[1] "Dietetic Value of Bread," by John Goodfellow, F.R.M.S., p. 166.

so on, for a number of generations. At the end of that time, what should we expect to find? If any members of such a family existed at all, should we not expect to find in them a deteriorated, diseased collection of individuals? Most assuredly we should! And we should hardly be tempted to assert that continued subjection to this foul air had in any way rendered it more normal or more healthful than pure outdoor "natural" air. Would not any physician assert that nothing but good, and immediate good, could possibly result from the transition of such a person from the foul to the pure atmosphere? Would he be tempted to claim that any number of generations, living in such an atmosphere could render it better and more normal for the last generation than for the first?[1]

And why should this not apply also to food? What logical ground is there for asserting that the law applies in the one case and not in the other? No matter how many generations have lived on the abnormal, perverted diet, a return to the original, natural diet can only be accompanied by great and permanent benefit to the patient.

All that is required to prove the point here so dogmatically stated is the setting aside of preconceptions and prejudices; and a few weeks' fair *trial* of the fruitarian diet. Once given a fair trial in this manner, and there is no possible doubt as to the final verdict. Life will be found in a fullness hitherto undreamed of—a degree of vitality sustained, of which the experimenter was till then quite unaware; an added zest will be found in life—in short, he will "add life to his years and years to his life." By all means I should advise the patient, who is breaking his fast—and whose appetite may then be considered normal—to adopt this fruitarian diet, to give it a fair trial, at least. He will find that it is all that is here claimed for it, and doubtless more. Further, it will render him practically immune from all diseased conditions in the future!

[1] Extraordinary as this statement may appear, and so perverted are some men's minds on medical matters, that this view actually *has* been defended! Thus, Doctor Stockton-Hough, in his "Relative Influence of City and Country Life," p. 10, says: "The citizen of the town is fully acclimated to its atmosphere, but cannot spend a single night in the country without serious risk of life . . . "1

CHAPTER II

FASTING AS A MEANS OF CURE—HISTORIC OUTLINE

Having now studied briefly the effects of an unnatural diet upon the organism—the question of the quality of the food ingested—we must now turn to a consideration of the main theme of this book, the question of the amount of food ingested, and its effects upon the organism when excessive; the question of *quantity*. Here, my object will be to show that even the best of food, eaten in excess, is the cause of the clogging of the system, and of consequent disease—the more unhealthful and grosser foods being naturally quicker and more certain causes of fouler and worse diseases.

What is commonly known as a "fast" may, perhaps, be defined as a complete abstinence from all food or nourishment—liquid or solid—for a greater or lesser period of time; the process of abstaining from food, for whatever reason, constituting "a fast," and the duration of such abstinence constitutes its "length." Of course we all fast the greater portion of our time, since we are, in a sense, fasting whenever we are not feeding, and the very term "breakfast" is supposed to imply the breaking of the long (!) term of fasting—since the meal of the preceding evening. But we do not, of course, generally associate this idea with the word "fast;" we say that a man has fasted one day, or one week, or one month, or whatever the period may have been—or even that he has been "fasting since early morning" (whereas now it is the evening) but hardly that a man has been fasting for two hours! From all of which we may conclude that, generally speaking, a man is understood to begin his fast *with the omission of the first meal.* Thenceforward, he may be considered as fasting, until nourishment is again administered.

Now this practice of fasting is one of the most ancient customs of which we have any record. More than two thousand years ago the fasting cure was advocated by the school of the natural philosopher Asclepiades,[1] who also applied the water cure, etc. And we know that Plutarch said: "Instead of using medicines, rather fast a day." It was practiced as a rule in connection with religious ceremonies, and so came to be considered an inseparable part of almost all such observances, and a most important factor in any religious ceremony. Thus, we read in a queer old book, entitled "Of Good Workes, and First of Fasting" (published in the 16th century) that the Church of England speaks of fasting, and of its treatment by the Council of Calderon, as follows:

"The Fathers assembled there decreed in that Council that every person, as well in his private as public fast, should continue all day without meat and drink, till the evening prayer. And whosoever did eat and drink before the evening prayer was ended should be accounted and reputed not to consider the purity of his fast. The canon teacheth so evidently how fasting was used in the primitive Church, as by words that cannot be more plainly expressed."

Here then we see that fasting was considered to be a highly important part of the religious ceremony, and of spiritual salvation; and we find the same idea expressed throughout the Scriptures in passages too numerous to mention: see, *e.g.*, Neh. IX., 1; Esther, IV., 3; Judges, XX., 26; I Sam. VII., 6; II Sam., XII., 16; Dan., X., 2, 3; Jonah, III., 7; Isa. LVIII., 3–6; Matt., IV., 2; Matt., VI., 16–18; Matt., XVII., 21; Mark, IX., 29; Acts, X., 30; Acts, XIII., 3; Acts, XIV., 23; Acts, XXVII., 9; I Cor. VII., 5; etc.

In every other religion likewise do we observe this practice followed; the Mohammedans, the Buddhists, the Brahmins, and many — if not all — others have their periods of strict fasting. The saints of mediæval times set great store by this method; Catholics of our own day follow it more or less strictly; while individual cases of protracted fasts may be found in the

[1] "Household Remedies," by Felix L. Oswald, M.D., p. 215.

history of any nation whatever.[1] Again, we read in the "Peregrinatio Silviæ (the writer is describing how Lent was observed in Jerusalem, when she was there, *circa* 386 A.D.):

"They abstained entirely from all food during Lent, except only on Saturdays and Sundays. They took a meal about mid-day on Sunday, and after that, they took nothing until Saturday morning. This was their rule through Lent."

Christians need hardly be reminded that Christ himself fasted forty days.[2]

Many other cases might be cited, were it necessary; but, as we shall presently see, such a marshalling of historic evidence is not at all necessary, since we have cases of similar and even of considerably longer fasts recorded within the past few years; and, indeed, such fasts are now being constantly undertaken. Doctor Tanner aroused the whole scientific world some years ago by fasting forty and again forty-two days, on two separate occasions; and, though charges of "fraud" were, of course, circulated at the time, and believed in by many, even to the present day, anyone who cares to take the pains to thoroughly investigate the origin of such stories, and to read the current medical and other accounts—contemporary and otherwise—as I have done—will find that there is absolutely no foundation whatever for these stories, and that Doctor Tanner was never directly accused of fraud by anyone who was in possession of

[1] See Lowell: "Occult Japan," pp. 11–12, 116; Howitt: "History of the Supernatural;" Mrs. Crowe: "Night Side of Nature," p. 481.

[2] "Robert de Moleme, the founder of the Cistercian brotherhood, was overcome with grief on learning of the death of a female friend, and like General Boulanger, resolved to follow her to the Land of Shades. Being averse to direct suicide, he retired to the mountain-lodge of a relative, and abstained from food in the hope that one of his frequent fainting fits would fade into the sleep that knows no waking. But finding himself alive at the end of the *seventieth* day, he reconsidered his resolution and began to suspect a miraculous interposition of Providence. By resuming his meals, in half ounce installments, he contrived to recover from the condition of frightful emaciation, and in the supervision of an ever-increasing number of scattered monasteries, led an active life for the next fourteen years." ("Fasting, Hydropathy and Exercise," p. 59.) Said Luigi Cornaro ("The Art of Living Long," p. 147.): "I do not know whether some desperate degrees of abstinence would not have the same effect upon other men, as they had upon Atticus, who, weary of his life as well as his physicians, by long and cruel pains of a dropsical gout, and despairing of any cure, resolved by degrees to starve himself to death, and went so far, that the physicians found he had ended his disease instead of his life!"

the facts of the case. Great as was the prejudice in professional circles; bitter as was the feeling at the time; no direct charge of fraud—no atom of proof of such—was ever forthcoming, for the good and sufficient reason that no such proof existed. But we digress.

The point I wish to make is this: These cases (particularly that of Christ's fast—which will be accepted, I suppose, by most Christians), though they may be accepted as true—as isolated instances, or cases that have actually occurred—are, as a matter of fact, looked upon as curiosities, rather than as actual, vital facts, by the majority of persons. Christ's forty day fast is, for them, sufficiently explained by his supposedly Divine power. It was, in short, a "miracle," which would be impossible under any ordinary circumstances, and for any other man. Doctor Tanner's case and the few other "classical" or universally known cases are looked upon as, perhaps real, as having actually occurred, but as purely historical eccentricities; as isolated and extraordinary facts that have occurred from time to time, in the world's history, but are entirely unrelated to the general order of events—sporadic cases that have occurred, and may possibly, under very exceptional circumstances, occur again; but quite impossible under ordinary conditions—for the ordinary man. The cases have been looked upon as historical "freaks," in short; not as cases that may occur, and the exact duplicates of which are occurring (and that continually) to-day; in our very midst—and which the reader himself might, perhaps, undertake, as we shall presently see, with naught but distinct advantage. The general view is, probably, well summed up by the Reverend Puller, when, in discussing the previously mentioned cases of fasting during Lent in Jerusalem, he remarks that:

"Such fasting is certainly, for the mass of English people, impossible now. It seems to me that this great difference in the power of fasting, which is quite indisputable, must be taken into account, when we are considering how to apply the Apostolic rule to modern circumstances."[1]

[1] "Concerning the Fast Before Communion," p. 36.

Now the question I raise is this: Why is it impossible now? If men and women once lived for these extended periods without food or nutriment of any kind, why may they not do so to-day? (I am not discussing the *advantages* of such fasting, be it observed, merely its *possibility*.) Is there any evidence—physiological or other—to prove—any ground for supposing—that these individuals were especially favored of Heaven, or especially constructed anatomically or vitally, to enable them to undergo such an ordeal—better than any, average, person to-day? None whatever! As Doctor Page so cleverly remarked, *à propos* of this point:[1]

"It is commonly supposed that these are uncommon men: they are uncommon only in possessing a knowledge as to the power of the living organism to withstand abstinence from food, and in having the courage of their opinions."

These cases are not necessarily "historic" at all, and are not exclusively so. There is no "miraculous" element whatever surrounding them; and the average man of to-day—any reader of this book—could, without any doubt, live for a period of from thirty to ninety days, without partaking of any food whatever—a fact which I shall presently endeavor to prove both by physiological argument, and by the citation of actual, recent cases of a similar character. Says Doctor Holbrook:[2]

"Fasting is no cunning trick of priestcraft, but the most powerful and safest of all medicines."

I fully realize that this statement may sound strange—perhaps absurd—yet it is a great and certain truth, as we shall presently see.

Granting, then, for the sake of argument, that it is *possible* for man to thus live without food of any kind for this length of time, the question arises; what will be the results of such a protracted abstinence? Certain physiologic or pathogogic symptoms must necessarily follow any such abrupt and complete departure from the routine of our daily life. Will the results be beneficial or otherwise? What will be the condition of the

[1] "The Natural Cure," p. 74.
[2] "Eating for Strength," p. 96.

patient's body? of his mind? of the various organs and tissues throughout the body? A study of such symptoms should at least prove interesting, and it is just such a study that this book essays to make. Up to the present time, there has been practically no book published that deals with this question at any length; in no book has there been any attempt whatever to study and record the phenomena observable in fasting patients; to note the conditions of the pulse, the temperature, the tongue, its effects upon the various bodily organs—their functions and disturbances; upon the mind, and the senses; no detailed clinical study whatever of the bodily organism while undergoing a fast. I have searched through our libraries, and the records of medical literature, in vain; and (with the exception of Doctor Dewey's writings in America and Doctor Rabagliati's in England, and a few other scattered references, to be referred to later) I have found nothing on "fasting" from the physiologist's standpoint. I sincerely hope that my initial studies will stimulate inquiry along this highly interesting—though all but neglected—line of investigation and inquiry.

It must be understood, however, that my observations of the effects of fasting have been almost entirely limited to its effects upon the *diseased;* not upon those who voluntarily impose a fast upon themselves, when in a state of health. Were a really healthy person to commence going without food, and continue this course for a number of days, we can easily picture the result in our imaginations—a starved and shrunken body; hollow, staring eyes; parched and shrunken skin; perhaps a wandering mind; emaciation; weakness; and a ravenous, uncontrollable appetite—these are a few of the many symptoms we can imagine as following upon this outrage upon Nature. What the exact symptoms would be; how long life could be sustained under the circumstances; these are questions I am totally unable to answer—since I have never had the opportunity of observing the effects of starvation upon the healthy body. My experience has been limited to those who were ill—diseased; and this side of the question I have studied attentively and long; in the hope that I might, thereby, add something of permanent interest to the scientific literature of our day. I have closely watched many cases of sick persons who were fasting, and this book is largely the result of my observations; but I have never studied any cases of real *starvation*—since, as I shall show presently, *fasting is a totally different thing from starvation.* This is a paradox which I cannot hope to make clear at present, but merely ask my reader to bear this statement in mind, and remember that my observations have been confined to the effects of complete abstinence from all food in cases of extreme sickness; in chronic and acute disease.

I have just drawn the picture of the effects of starvation in the case of the well person: would the effects of fasting be the same in the case of the sick man? In other words, would the same symptoms appear as the result of complete abstinence from food, in such cases, as result when we withhold food from a well man? My answer to this is a decided No! The effects of fasting, in such cases, are very different. Now we should almost expect this *à priori,* since the effects of anything would doubtless be different in healthy and in diseased bodies; and, in practice, such proves to be the case. But my next statement will be considered far less obvious when I make the assertion that, so far from weakening the patient, and rendering him less liable to make a safe and speedy recovery, I am positively convinced that this simple practice of omitting the daily food (for a longer or shorter period, according to necessity and the requirements of the case) will invariably and necessarily result in an increased amount of bodily vigor; and a more rapid, easy and effectual recovery. In other words, I ascribe to it, as will be seen, an immense *curative* or *therapeutic* value.

That the mere omission of our daily food should be such an extensive and potent factor in the restoration of health to the sick, will, I am aware, meet with anything but a cordial reception from scientific men—both medical and lay. "How is it possible," they will ask, "that this should be the case? How can such a simple—such an absurdly simple—remedy be possessed of such tremendous worth? Besides, it is quite opposed to everything that we know at present of disease and its treatment? Do we not derive our strength and our energy from the food we eat? and is not this strength, this vitality, doubly necessary when the system has disease to fight; as well as its existence to maintain? Would food not be *more* necessary, therefore, at this time than at any other—since we must 'keep up the patient's strength' for the reason just given? The position is absurd, illogical, ridiculous! The arguments must obviously be wrong, no matter what may be said!"

This, I take it, will be the position of the average scientific reader, whose attention has been called to this book. I have endeavored to state their side of the case fairly, and feel assured it represents the average scientific man's opinion upon this subject. It is the task of this book to examine that opinion—these arguments—and to demonstrate wherein lies the fallacy. I shall endeavor to prove that these statements do not, by any manner of means, represent the actual facts, but mere current and generally accepted opinion—which, in turn, is based upon dogmatic affirmation and erroneous inferences drawn from the observable phenomena presented; that such a theory does not coincide with true philosophy, or with the actual facts, or with the teachings of Nature; but that it is founded upon an inverted and false conception of the nature and source of vitality, of the essence of disease, and of its consequent, successful treatment. All this I shall elaborate in the succeeding chapters; for the present, however, I shall content myself by strengthening my position from another, and negative standpoint. The question as to whether fasting is or is not efficacious in diseased states, cannot be decided *à priori*, but must be put to an actual test. In the present condition of medical science, no man, however great, is entitled to consideration unless he has actually tried—put into practice—and found to fail, a system that he condemns. It is impossible to state, *à priori*, what may be advantageous to the organism, and what may not. Experience has been too limited; practice far too uncertain to permit of any premature dogmatic assertions. Unless the system has been fairly tried and "found wanting," it cannot (or should not) be condemned. Prejudice—that "hydra-headed monster" that dwells in all of us—and to which the human race, I verily believe, owes nine-tenths of its suffering and misery; prejudice, and the bigotry that exists in many minds which have preconceived ideas and opinions—this, I hope, will be resolutely set aside by the reader while perusing the remainder of this volume. I am fully aware of the immeasurable difficulty most persons experience in doing this. It is but natural that it should be so; their whole nature revolts against accepting, as truth, something which upsets all their previous habits of thought, their very outlook upon life. Yet I must plead with my reader that he, at least temporarily, may do so; that he may lay aside all preconceived ideas, all prejudice, and read what I have to say with an open, and in an unbiased frame of mind. Since it is very largely due to chance that I have had the opportunity of studying the cases mentioned in this book, I feel that I can speak of its contents in this way without involving the charge of egotism, which might otherwise be made.

One word further, in this connection: It may be objected that this method of treatment (fasting) cannot be truly beneficial for the reason that, if it were, physicians would have adopted and used it long before now. To this I would answer: by no means, necessarily. Were not electricity and hydropathy and hypnotism and many other potent and generally accepted methods of cure at first rejected with contempt and scorn? Were not their champions ridiculed and persecuted, even to the extent of being deprived of their practice, and hounded from the locality in which they practiced? Is not all this history? And is not its like being repeated—in a lesser degree, perhaps, but still repeated—to-day? Physicians have often proved themselves to be a very prejudiced set of men and strongly averse to accepting any theory that threatens to upset the fundamental principles of their science. Their sincerity and devotion to science and the cause of Truth may sometimes be gravely doubted; but of this I shall not speak at present—though I can offer proof for my assertions, if need be, in every case.

But the principal reason for this prejudice is, doubtless, that physicians have been, till now, all but quite *ignorant* of this subject of fasting.[1] And it must necessarily be so. Apart

[1] This has frequently happened in the past, in other connections. Thus: "The Hyderabad Chloroform Commission, which in 1889 thoroughly investigated the causes of death under chloroform, has proved that *all such deaths*

from Doctor Dewey's books, which, owing to the fact that they were privately printed, no less than the character of their contents, are necessarily known to but a small minority of the profession—there has been nothing authoritative and scientific published which can, in any sense, be considered an exposition or a defense of the subject. It speaks volumes for the reasonableness and truth of the system that it has, in spite of this complete lack of scientific backing, in the literary forum, attained as great popularity as it has, and that so many physicians are now advocating this method of treatment, more or less openly.

Because any system of treatment is new, it does not necessarily prove that it is false—as the majority seem to think. Far from it! A new system invariably has the support of facts—for without these it would be impossible, nowadays, to champion any new cause. In this book, and in the others I shall mention, will be found many such facts—which I leave to the consideration of the reader, to explain as he may. The facts, I conceive, will hold good, whatever view may be taken of the theory I advance to account for them.

But is this idea of fasting new after all? To those unfamiliar with the literature of hygiene, it may seem that it must be so; but further knowledge would very soon dispel such an idea. Fasting in disease has been recommended by certain reputable and even noted physicians for nearly a hundred years back. Says Doctor Oswald:[1]

"A germ disease, as virulent as syphilis, and long considered too persistent for any but palliative methods of treatment (by mercury, etc.,) was radically cured by the fasting cures, prescribed in the Arabian hospitals of Egypt, at the time of the French occupation."

are preventible, if a different mode of administration is adopted. And its conclusions have been confirmed by the independent researches of four medical men—two English and two American physicians. Yet the old method of administration is still common in this country, no less than seventy-five deaths having occurred from this cause in 1896, while the Registrar General records seventy-eight deaths from anæsthetics (almost all from chloroform) in 1895. There is thus a terrible amount of mortality due, apparently, to the ignorance of medical men on a subject as to which they are supposed to have exclusive knowledge." ("The Wonderful Century," by Alfred Russel Wallace, F.R.S., etc., pp. 147–8.)

[1] "Fasting, Hydropathy and Exercise," p. 55.

Even so "orthodox" a practitioner as Dr. Robert Bartholow, in his "Materia Medica and Therapeutics," (pp. 31–2), admits the value of the method in such cases; Doctor Shew, *e.g.*, writing:[1] "The hunger-cure is nowhere more applicable."

In his "Family Physician" (p. 190), Doctor Shew stated his conviction that the hunger-cure was the most potent of all remedies. It is curious to note, in this connection, that Andrew Jackson Davis had a very clear idea of the true essence and nature of disease, and advocated the fasting cure on several occasions; see his "Harbinger of Health" (pp. 4, 311, 382). Doctor Dewey, for more than a quarter of a century, allowed practically no other treatment in his hundreds and thousands of cases—which he conducted both personally and by mail, in almost every part of the civilized world. Doctors Keith and Rabagliati, in England, have both written spirited and brilliant defenses of the method, while the growing testimony of hundreds of successful cases that have been cured by this method, and the increasing acceptance of the theory by the medical world to-day, all indicate that the fasting cure is anything but a new and untried method; but is, on the contrary, one that has been more or less recognized for years, has received the sanction of some of the most brilliant minds in and out of the medical profession, but that it is now just beginning to receive that wide and unhesitating support which it has deserved, and for which it has been striving for so long. I trust this book may, in some measure, assist in drawing the attention of the scientific world to the real and immense importance of this question, and induce some men, at least, to investigate, with a free and unbiased mind, the method of treatment here advocated—the importance of which, I am convinced, cannot be overestimated.

[1] See Macfadden's "Virile Powers of Superb Manhood," p. 231, where a number of statements to like effect are gathered together.

THE QUANTITY OF FOOD NECESSARY TO SUSTAIN LIFE

BEFORE attempting any detailed defense of the fasting treatment, or any statement of the physiology upon which such treatment depends, it will be necessary for us, first of all, to consider the primary question of the amount of food that is necessary, in order to nourish the organism, and to maintain it in health. It may be objected that my whole theory of fasting, and the whole of the preceding and following argument is based upon the idea that such an excess of food is constantly eaten as to render fasting necessary; and, it may be objected, the majority of persons do not eat any such excess as I have indicated, nor over-eat to the extent I have contended they do and must. "In fact," the patient may exclaim, "I have always been considered a very moderate eater by my friends; my food is not exceedingly rich or indigestible, but plain and wholesome; I eat but three average meals a day, and never feel distressed after any of them. How, then, can you substantiate the claim that all disease is the result of over-feeding, and that, in such cases as my own (which, after all, probably is a very average case), disease and death, and such foul conditions as you represent are present—simply as the result of my food habits? It cannot be the case; it is incredible! No doubt there are many persons who over-eat (have we not the authority of Doctor Hemmeter that "the average American in the better classes of life eats entirely too much?")[1] but, in such cases as my own, you will have to find a different explanation of my disease; it is not right nor fair, moreover, to claim that any such foul conditions are present or possible—as those you maintain *are* present before disease is possible; it may be so in *some* cases, it is certainly not so in my own!"

[1] "Strength and Diet," by the Hon. R. Russell, p. 380.

This, I take it, is the line of argument most persons would follow when first reading over the theory of the causation of disease outlined above; particularly its relation to excessive nutrition. It is human—if not logical—and indicates the very natural disinclination we all have for believing that our sicknesses are brought upon us by ourselves—our own transgressions of physiological law; by our excessive love for eating,[1] and are not attributable to germs, nor "miasma," nor heredity, nor to any outside and uncontrollable influences or conditions whatever. It is a natural position to assume, but alas! an altogether unjustifiable one, and one that melts away in the light of the actual facts, as we shall presently see.

For the position is simply this. The question is not—how much a person can eat and keep well, but *how little he can eat and retain his physiological integrity and mental powers.* The object is—not to see how much food can be consumed with safety, and without engendering disease, or prostrating the vital energies; but it is to sustain life on as little food as we possibly can; and this for the reason that that amount accurately represents the actual requirements of the body, and any quantity of food over and above that amount would be just so much food which the system did not need, but which was got rid of by the system—passed through it—at the expense of the vital energies. Every ounce of food passed through the body which is not actually needed by it is thus a great, a tremendous tax upon the vital power—a waste of our energies. How great a waste this is will presently appear. And, that I may not be thought to be alone in this position, I quote the following passages, which strongly bear out my contention. Says Dr. T. L. Nichols:[2]

"A man may be able to digest and dispose of three times as

[1] Says Dr. Dio Lewis ("Weak Lungs," p. 113): "Few spectacles are more painful than the struggle often seen among the poor to keep their table supplied with the 'best in the market.' Foregoing books, periodicals, a good house, good clothes, the healthful luxury of a summer trip, etc., they devote everything to supplying their table. They are ashamed to be seen eating plain, cheap food; not ashamed to live in a poor house, to wear insufficient clothing; to have no library, to have no pew in church, to have nothing, to be nothing, if only their table is well supplied! I declare it a low, vulgar ambition—pride on the lowest plane of life."

[2] "Diet Cure," p. 22.

much food as he really requires. One ounce more than he requires is a waste of force, a waste of life. We waste life in eating more food than we need, in digesting it, and then in getting rid of it. Here is a triple waste. We have other work to do in this world than eating unnecessary food, and spending our strength for naught."

Says Doctor Dewey:[1]

" Think of it! Actual soul power involved in ridding the stomach and bowels of the foul sewage of food in excess, food in a state of decomposition, to be forced through nearly two rods of bowels and largely at the expense of the soul itself!"

Says Doctor Graham:[2]

" . . . Every individual should, as a general rule, restrain himself to the smallest quantity which he finds from careful investigation and enlightened experience and observation will fully meet the alimentary wants of the vital economy of his system, knowing that whatsoever is more than this is evil. . ."

It may, perhaps, be thought that I am overestimating and exaggerating the amount of nervous or vital force which is thus used up for digestive purposes; and that the amount of energy actually expended would be nothing like that amount, or be of such great importance. I can only say that I do not agree with this view, and that, so far from overestimating it, I have, if anything, far under-rated the quantity of force thus daily utilized for purposes of digestion.

The extent of this digestive tax is indirectly admitted by physicians when they prescribe "easily digested foods" for their weak patients—thus tacitly admitting the enormous loss of nervous energy necessitated in all digestive processes. Unfortunately they do not grasp the deep significance of this fact. "Easily digested" foods are always considered those calling for rapid *stomach* digestion, without taking into consideration the ultimate effects of the food, when thus digested—which might be far less beneficial than those calling for a more prolonged digestive effort. As Dr. R. T. Trall pointed out:[3]

[1] "No-Breakfast Plan," p. 80. [2] "Science of Human Life," p. 581.
[3] "Hydropathic Cook Book," p. 121.

"It is a common error that such articles of food as are soonest dissolved in the stomach are most easily digested. It is well known that tainted meat, or that which has become putrescent by decomposition, will 'pass along' through the stomach and be resolved into a chymous mass sooner than will fresh meat, or even the best of bread. But it would hardly comport with common sense to call such half-rotted flesh most wholesome or most digestible on that account."

Again, it is emphatically insisted upon that the bowels must have a certain amount or "bulk" of food upon which to work, and if this "bulk" is not supplied, evil results will follow! Then again, with singular inconsistency, foods are prescribed that call for practically no digestive effort at all in the intestines—all being absorbed in the stomach! Would it not be better, I ask, to administer those foods that call for a more or less equal effort all along the digestive tract and only at times when such food is called for and may be readily assimilated?

Let us return, however, to the question of the amount of energy that is expended in the digestion and elimination of food material. I think it can be made clear that this amount is enormous by a very simple illustration. Suppose we place a leaden or iron ball—weighing, say, one pound—on the palm of the hand. Now let us imagine that we are, under compulsion, made to move that ball continuously for two hours, without in any way ceasing or slackening in our manipulations; that we must turn and twist and revolve and rotate that ball, and move it in all possible directions continuously for the allotted period. How do you think we should be enabled to perform such a task; and would not the muscles and nerves become fatigued long before the appointed time was "up"—aye, even after the expiration of a few minutes? And would we not appreciate the tremendous outlay of nervous force required thus to manipulate and handle this weight—even once a day? And yet this is exactly what we require of our poor stomachs whenever we ingest a pound of food! *That* has to be churned and rotated and manipulated by the muscles of the stomach, also, and the power which actuates them is, in that case also, nervous or vital. And we not only require this of our stomachs once a day, but constantly, and think we are actually injuring the stomach if we even give it any rest at all! Is it not obvious what a tremendous vital power is here being constantly utilized, and how this power could be utilized elsewhere—to perform bodily and mental work, or to cure diseased conditions—if it were but given the opportunity to do so? As Dr. F. M. Heath said:[1]

"Thousands there are—yes, millions—who eat more than they can digest, and whose Life Power is so worn down in the endless struggle with waste food, that existence is a hopeless, dragging misery."

Too true!

I know that it will be objected that, in the former of the above examples (in which the ball was revolved in the palm of the hand), the *voluntary* muscles are employed, and in the latter, it is the involuntary; and that anything like an equal outlay of nervous force is not required in the two cases. All that I know and recognize; my point was merely to illustrate, by analogy, that the one must necessitate a constant outlay of nervous force—just as does the other; and that the amount of this force is undoubtedly far greater than is generally supposed. How much greater, the phenomena of fasting illustrate most forcibly.

But to return to a consideration of the actual physiological needs of the body—so far as its nutrition is concerned. As before stated, our object is to ascertain, by direct experiment, just how little food is actually required by the body, in each individual case—that amount representing our real organic needs. Food over and above that amount would simply be passed through the body without in any way benefiting it—but, on the contrary, directly and permanently injuring it.

Let us consider this question from another point of view. One great proof, to my mind, that we were intended by Nature to receive a scanty supply, and not a superabundance of food, is the fact that the lymph vessels seem to be constructed almost solely for the purpose of collecting and bringing back, to be

[1] "Why Do Young People Die?" p. 16.

reabsorbed, all food material that had failed to be properly digested and assimilated, in its original passage through the system. They will not allow any waste to take place in the system if they can help it. Any nutrient materials, whose powers have not been completely exhausted, are re-collected by these vessels, and carried by them to join the thoracic duct, charged with the products of digestion. They may thus be utilized again without waste. This would all be readily enough intelligible were we adapted by Nature to subsist upon a very scanty food supply—since these vessels seem to be adapted for that very purpose; but it is not intelligible to us if we were adapted and suited by Nature to receive—not a constant and adequate supply, but such continued over-nutrition and excess of food as we habitually do receive and constantly indulge in. I venture to think this a very strong reason, indeed, against the constant over-nutrition we observe on every hand—showing how contrary to our nature such an excess must be.

It is true that many of the lower animals feed more or less continually, with no other results than continued, normal growth; but, because this is so, can it therefore be argued that man can do likewise, with anything but disastrous results? Obviously not. Indeed, it is very doubtful if man could possibly spend more than two hours daily in his feeding, for purely physiological reasons, let alone the fact that disease would undoubtedly follow any such attempt. For at least twenty-two hours a day, therefore, man is compelled to fast; while it has been demonstrated that this period may be extended to more than twenty-three hours and a half—and this, not with any detriment to the organism, but, on the contrary, with decided benefit.[1] This allows man, it will be seen, almost his entire waking day to devote to other, intellectual or spiritual, pursuits. It would thus seem that, in man, the animal functions are reduced to the minimum—affording the maximum opportunity for the cultivation of his higher self. And the more highly developed, the more æsthetic, the man is, as a rule, the less need he eat; while the grossly animal man invariably ingests and disposes of an astonishing—even disgusting—amount of

[1] "New Glutton or Epicure," p. 119.

food. From all these and similar considerations we may, I think, deduce the following law:

The higher in the scale of evolution we proceed, the less the time that is actually required for the nutrition of the body; and consequently the more time has he to devote to the cultivation of his other interests—his mental, moral and spiritual powers. And, as the greatest mark of distinction between man and the lower animals *is* his mental characteristics, we may briefly express ourselves in the formula:

The greater the mentality, the less the need for food; or, *as men tality increases, the need for food decreases.* I am unaware that this observation has ever been made before—or such implications as it involves recognized; yet this statement is, I am persuaded, demonstrably true.

We all know that the lower forms of life spend almost their entire time in the search for, and devouring of, food; they are "all stomach and no brain." But as we ascend the scale of evolution, we find less and less predominance given to the digestive organs, and more and more to the intellectual side of the animal. And finally, in man, we find the mental side so largely predominant, the purely animal side so far reduced, in relative bulk and importance that, in the ideal "economic and æsthetic nutrition (as well as for the highest bodily comfort and good health) we can, as we know, reduce the time required for feeding purposes to but a small fraction of the time; and it is surely not an absurd or even an extravagant supposition to think that, as we continue to develop along the lines of mental growth, this time may be still further reduced—almost to nothing in fact. And that this may actually have been accomplished, in some cases, may be contended, when we consider the cases of those Yogis of India who have been enabled to live for very considerable periods without food of any kind; while, owing to their otherwise most abstemious lives, it cannot be contended that *fasting* this lengthy period would be necessary or possible, without signs of starvation resulting. Yet such signs are seldom or never noticed. The physical side of such trance states should be as carefully studied in the future as the psychological side has been studied in the past. From the point of view of the student of fasting, such cases are of intense interest, no less than to the psychologist, or to the psychical researcher.

An interesting account of such trance conditions is to be found in Dr. T. J. Hudson's "Law of Psychic Phenomena," pp. 312–13; and in various works devoted to the subject. Swami Abhedananda tells us[1] that:

"All Hatha Yogis eat very little, but they can also go without food for days and even for months, and succeed in conquering sleep."

Doctor Oswald and Mr. Macfadden write:[2]

"Reptiles, with their small expenditure of vital energy, can easily survive dietetic deprivations; but bears and badgers, with an organization essentially analogous to that of the human species, and with a circulation of the blood active enough to maintain the temperature of their bodies more than a hundred degrees above that of the winter storms, dispense with food for periods varying from three to five months, and at the termination of their ordeal emerge from their dens in the full possession of their physical and mental energies."

It is practically acknowledged that human hibernation is "a condition utterly inexplicable to any principle taught in the schools."[3] And it is interesting to note that the time for such hibernation is the *winter*, when we might almost expect it to be the summer months, if the accepted theories were correct as to the causation of heat by food—which doctrine we shall presently examine. Kuhne called attention to the fact that many animals eat far less in the winter time than they do in the summer,[4] and Doctor Oswald remarked that:[5]

"Winter is not the worst time for a fast, it may even be the best, to judge from the phenomena of hibernation."

Still, I agree with Mr. Purinton when he advises all prospective fasters to "choose summer or spring for the conquest fast."[6]

[1] "How to Be a Yogi," pp. 45–6.
[2] "Fasting, Hydropathy and Exercise," pp. 60–1.
[3] Tebb and Vollum: "Premature Burial," p. 43.
[4] "New Science of Healing," p. 120.
[5] "Fasting, Hydropathy and Exercise," p. 65.
[6] "Philosophy of Fasting," p. 104.

The whole subject should be closely studied, and is well worthy of serious consideration from scientific men.

Let us return, however, to the main theme of this chapter—the discussion of the amount of food that is required by the body, in order to maintain and preserve it in a high state of health. The point I wish to emphasize is this. If this lesser amount of food is all that is necessary, in order to maintain the body in health, it follows that more than this amount must be injurious; must clog the system and waste the vital forces. *The proper amount and more than the proper amount cannot possibly have exactly the same effects upon the organism;* that would be a physical impossibility; and the effects must be injurious because the food supply is not the normal amount, and the normal amount is always the best. It *must,* therefore, be injurious; and probably injurious, *ceteris paribus,* just to the extent that the excess passes the normal limit. How and in what ways this is injurious we shall presently see.

Of course it is possible for us to be underfed, though the chances are, I believe, so slight that they need hardly be taken into consideration.

Undoubtedly it is *possible* for us to impoverish the blood, and to starve the tissues, by under and improper, feeding, and I am not contending for a moment that such is not the case. That numbers of the poor should have a greater amount of, and better, food I fully admit. Even in the majority of *these* cases, however, I am convinced that it is the quality rather than the quantity of food ingested which is below the proper standard. Doctor Rabagliati takes a very decided positive stand in this question. He says:[1]

"If he (the reader) should whisper to himself—what about poverty, then?—do the very poor also eat too much and too often? It seems to me that they do. The poor, it seems to me, eat poor food too often and too much, and the rich eat rich food too often and too much, and they are both ill."

He contends that the babies of the poor are invariably overfed (p. 239). Still, I conceive that under-feeding may, occasionally, be

[1] "Air, Food and Exercises," p. 237

a very great and pressing menace both to the individual and to the community; and that starvation is not, of course, impossible. My contention, throughout, is that the evils arising from the practice of under-feeding, in any case, are so immeasurably eclipsed by the extent of the opposite practice as to sink into utter oblivion, and to be hardly worthy of consideration. My distinction between fasting and starvation should make that clear. (p. 564.)

But, after all, the chances of under-feeding—for the average person—are very slight. Over-feeding is the great curse from which civilization suffers to-day. I consider it is far more important than drink; both because it affects a far greater *number* of persons—both young and old; men, women and children, afflicting them with its consequences—diverse and grievous diseases—but also because the craving for drink is a natural result of and consequent upon this continual over-feeding. The surplus of food in the stomach—particularly if it be of an irritating and stimulating quality—sets up a constant irritation of that organ, which is temporarily allayed by the greater stimulant, alcohol. It is a great truth that every stimulant calls for a higher and more powerful one. Thus the inter-relation of alcoholism and meat-eating is fast becoming recognized; and is well and tersely stated by Doctor Keith where he says:[1]

"I have long been convinced that there is a cause and connection between a free use of flesh foods and inclination for stimulants, especially in the young. Roast beef is, perhaps, the most sapid food that exists; desire gratified leads for a demand for something higher in the same line. This cannot be had from food, but it may from drink."

To eradicate this evil, then, once and for all, it would not be necessary to send out an army of reformers; moral suasion will not answer in cases of disease (and alcoholism undoubtedly is a disease), but merely to introduce a rational system of feeding the masses; supplying them with a limited supply of simple, wholesome, non-stimulating food. Alcoholism could no more

[1] "Fads of an Old Physician," p. 42.

persist on such a diet than could the winter's snow resist the influence of the warm, spring sun. The root, the *cause* of the evil would be removed, eradicated; the craving would no longer be present; and until this cause is discovered and removed, the crusade against alcoholism will be in vain.[1]

It will thus be seen that a fast is one of the easiest methods known for the cure of alcoholism, and for this reason: When such a patient enters upon a fast, the lack of food is the first and the temporarily over-ruling sensation, to which everything else is subordinated. All else is lost sight of, so long as food is permanently withdrawn; while every new and abnormal sensation or craving will be put down to the lack of food. In reality, it is due to the lack of the stimulus of the alcohol; but so accustomed are we to believe that our strength comes from food, that any weakness or depression following the commencement of the fast would be put down to that cause, and cheerfully acquiesced in—so long as a fast is undertaken at all. It is not appreciated that this depression is due almost solely to the withdrawal of the alcohol. When once this craving has subsided, however, and the fast has been terminated, and feeding resumed, it (the alcoholic craving) is no longer present—since its *cause*—the abnormal condition of the stomach and system generally—will have been removed. Thenceforward, the appetite will have disappeared—since the cause of the appetite is no longer present.

What has just been said regarding certain physical cravings and conditions, applies equally to the mental characteristics. The "cross, irritable dyspeptic" is a combination of words too deeply rooted in the English language ever to be entirely eradicated; and who does not know the cheerful optimist who never feels a pain nor an ache, and who "never realizes that he has a stomach?" To be sure there are exceptions to this, as to every rule, but it must be remembered that they *are* the exceptions —*not* the rule. In the vast majority of cases my argument holds good. Evil temper, vicious disposition (aye, and even

[1] See H. P. Fowler: "Vegetarianism, the Radical Cure for Intemperance;" Doctor Dewey: "Chronic Alcoholism;" Schlickeysen's "Fruit and Bread;" Dr. Anna Kingsford: "The Perfect Way in Diet;" James C. Jackson's "How to Cure Drunkards;" also his "Four Drunkards;" "The Drink Problem," etc.

worse vices), spring, it can readily be shown, from this single habit—a habit that affects everyone of us from the cradle to the grave, and whose far-reaching evil consequences we are just beginning to realize.

The question thus narrows itself down to this: what is, approximately, the amount of food needed, in each individual case, in order to keep the body's vital and physical powers in equilibrium? And to this question I must at once say that I have no definite answer. I have attempted on p. 471, to give a tentative answer to this question, but science has no means of determining it other than that of direct, personal experiment, and observation. And it is easy to see why this should be so. Until quite recently, no man has made the experiment, and scientifically recorded the results of an attempt, to see how far this reduction of food is possible; of how little food, *i.e.*, can be eaten daily for an indefinite period, without harmful results following therefrom; but the moment one such attempt was made, it was found that the actual bodily requirements were very greatly below or less than the standard set up, as being necessary, in the text-books of physiology (whose supposed "facts" were at once proved to be erroneous); and that this reduction was so great that only about *one-third* as much food was necessary, in order to properly sustain life—as has been universally taught by the physiologists, whose views are now held to be "incomplete, unsound and unscientific";[1] while the Voit standard of minimal nitrogen requirement for a healthy worker, has been proved to be grossly incorrect. And when we remember that the vast majority of people eat a very great deal *more* food than even the physiologists say is necessary, we at once perceive the enormous disproportion between the bulk of food actually required and that which is almost universally eaten.[2] Probably from four to six times as much food is eaten as the body actually requires, and this great amount of excess must be disposed of at the expense of the vital powers. I shall now adduce, briefly, the evidence upon which the above statement is founded, and shall bring forward, first, the classical case of Louis Cornaro.

[1] "Humaniculture," p. 8.

[2] "In a Nutshell," by Dio Lewis, M.D., p. 37.

Cornaro, a Venetian nobleman, was born in 1464, and lived about one hundred and two years—dying in 1566.[1]

In the first forty or so years of his life, Cornaro lived very much as did his companions of the nobility, with the consequence that, at that age, he broke down completely and almost died—being saved only through an adoption of those habits he outlines and defends in his little book, "The Temperate Life." To this I would refer the reader for a full statement of his own case and also for a most philosophic and masterly defense of the doctrine of reduction of diet for the cure and prevention of all disease. Cornaro reduced his daily allowance of food to 12 oz. —with 14 oz. of light Italian wine—and on this diet he subsisted for practically the remainder of his wonderfully active and brilliant life—to his death at the age of 102. (p. 55.) Only once or twice did Cornaro even slightly increase the amount of his daily food supply, and on both occasions did he become ill, and was forced to resume his former lower diet—on which he quickly recovered. I should like to quote largely from this most scholarly and philosophical author, but lack of space unfortunately forbids my doing so.

But it is not necessary, fortunately for this argument, to refer to this classical case for proof of my contention—since we have living to-day, a "modern Louis Cornaro," *viz.*, Mr. Horace Fletcher—whose case has aroused the interest of the whole scientific world, and whose experiments will surely tend to revolutionize medicine and physiology—if they have not, indeed, already done so.

I regret that I cannot offer more than a brief résumé of this case. Mr. Fletcher himself has treated the subject in an excellent manner in his two books—"Glutton or Epicure," and "The A. B.—Z. of Our Own Nutrition." Briefly, the case is this: Mr. Horace Fletcher was first led to experiment upon himself through illness. He conducted a series of experiments upon himself in nutrition and food supply, and turned his attention largely to thorough mastication, and the quality and quan-

[1] There is considerable uncertainty as to the year of Cornaro's birth, also that of his death, and the exact age of the venerable old man cannot be given. The majority of modern authorities seem to give from a hundred to a hundred and two years, however.

tity of food required in order to properly sustain the human organism in weight and health. By practicing *very thorough* mastication (regarding the effects of which he has much of interest and moment to tell us)[1] he was enabled to reduce the amount of food eaten very far below the bulk usually consumed, and considered necessary; and this, without lowering the tone of health, the strength and vitality—or, when once the superfluous fatty tissue had been removed, and normal conditions restored—no further loss of bodily weight. On the contrary, a vastly improved physical and mental condition became manifest—exalted mental powers, greater mentality and stamina, and the increased ability to undergo almost any amount of physical exertion without fatigue. The reason is obvious enough. All the bodily energy, which, heretofore, had been utilized in digesting and eliminating food material in excess, now became available for other—bodily and mental—purposes.[2] Since it thus appears that the less we eat, the more energy we have (within certain limits), it should be our logical conclusion, from this, that, were we to eat *nothing at all*, we should have very much more energy than usual—since none would be used for digestion, and we should be able to use it all for the daily activities. This should be our conclusion, arguing logically. And, indeed, such is the stand I shall presently take, and in Book III., Chapter I., I shall endeavor to prove that this is the actual state of affairs, and that we do, as a matter of fact, have more energy while fasting than at any other time. As the argument is there stated, however, I leave that branch of our question for the present.

Now, if this case stood alone, it might perhaps be questioned

[1] It is not sufficiently appreciated that mastication not only breaks up the food into small particles, but is a very important first step in the chemical transformation of food. ("Glutton or Epicure," p. 6.) And it is highly essential that these changes should take place in the mouth, where we have control of the food—and not involve the digestive energy of the body in this useless work—since, as Doctor Edinger pointed out ("Have Fishes Memory?" p. 389): "Human beings may take or refuse to take food, but as soon as a bite passes the arch of the palate and enters the domain of the swallowing apparatus, properly speaking, it is beyond their control." Mr. Fletcher often insisted upon this. How important it is, then, to see that this initial state of digestion is thoroughly performed!

[2] For accounts of this case, see Reports of Sir Michael Foster, F.R.S., Professor Chittenden, Dr. Wm. G. Anderson, etc.

as being universally applicable; but, I may state, this is not the case. For years it did so stand, but, fortunately for my argument, Professor Chittenden, of Yale, has furnished the "missing link" in his two books, "Physiological Economy in Nutrition" and "The Nutrition of Man." Here, we find detailed and abundant proof that the body can sustain its weight and increase its vitality on at least *one-third* the amount generally considered as necessary for the healthy man. ("Physiological Economy in Nutrition," p. 41.)

Not only did Professor Chittenden prove this to be the case in his own person, but he induced several of his fellow professors to pursue the same course and to reduce their diet, and carefully observed the results. In every single instance (five) the results agreed more or less exactly with that of Mr. Horace Fletcher. But further, to establish the correctness of the principle beyond doubt, and, at the same time, to show that a like reduction could be made in the cases of men leading a vigorous, active life, he instigated a prolonged series of experiments with thirteen volunteers from the Hospital Corps of the U. S. Army for subjects (who daily went through a regular drill—gymnastic work, etc.—of the army, *and other physical work in addition*); and with eight university students—trained in athletics—the results of which experiments form the bulk of the book. I cannot here attempt, of course, even a summary of these results—since the whole book is a mass of figures and calculations: suffice it to say that the fact was proved, most conclusively, that an equal proportionate reduction was possible in every case, that precisely the same conclusions were reached as in all the other cases mentioned: *i.e.*, that as soon as the attempt was once fairly made to see how far this reduction was possible, without harm resulting, the conclusion was reached that, in every case —man can not only live, but actually improve, physically and mentally, and show increased strength (p. 274), and an improved reaction time (pp. 442–5), on a diet that was, in proteid, but one-third as full and rich as is universally said to be necessary by physiologists, and as taught in all medical schools and colleges—while almost every man during that period, *stored* nitrogen, instead of losing it! (p. 223.) And, as before stated, there is hardly anyone who does not very greatly exceed even the amounts said to be necessary by the physiologists. How much greater, then, is the ingestion of food than the true requirements! Does it not become obvious—nay, certain—that the majority of persons are eating by far (probably four or five times) too much food? And how can this continued surplus be other than harmful?—crowding the digestive organs, choking the circulation, and necessitating a tremendous outlay of vital energy in order to effectually and finally dispose of it? It is quite impossible that it should be so; in fact, it *is* not.[1]

The whole question of the amount of food daily eaten is, in reality, purely one of habit. As Professor Chittenden so well said:[2]

" . . . The so-called cravings of appetite are purely the result of *habit.* A habit once acquired and persistently followed soon has us in its grasp, and then any deviation therefrom disturbs our physiological equilibrium. The system makes complaint and we experience a craving, it may be, for that to which the body has become accustomed, even though this something be, in the long run, distinctly injurious to the welfare of the body. There has thus come about a sentiment that the cravings of the appetite for food are to be fully satisfied, and this is merely obedience to Nature's laws. The idea, however, is fundamentally wrong. Anyone with a little persistence can change his or her habits of life, change the whole order of cravings, thus demonstrating that the latter are purely artificial, and that they have no necessary connection with the welfare or needs of the body. In other words, dietetic requirements are to be founded, not upon so-called instinct and craving, but upon reason and intelligence."

We thus see that persons are in the habit of guiding their food habits by what people *do* eat, and not by what they *should* eat. Everyone eats far too much; we thereby acquire false habits, and, as Doctor Lewis pointed out:[3]

[1] This agrees very well with what Mr. H. Irving Hancock has to tell us of the Japanese diet. In his "Japanese Physical Training," p. 17, he says: "A bowl of grain and a handful of fish is considered an ample meal for the coolie who is called upon to perform ten or twelve hours of hard manual toil in a day."

[2] *Century Magazine,* Oct., 1905, p. 860.

[3] "New Gymnastics," p. 239.

"If we give ourselves up to eating, the system soon learns the habit of receiving and disposing of a very large amount of food; but it does thus at the expense of brain and muscle."

It is a pretty safe maxim that "what makes the man sick is the thing which he never wants to relinquish." For measures that may be adopted to prevent over-eating with least discomfort to the patient, See *Appendix F*.

"But," it may be objected, "we must have a certain amount of food (fuel) to enable us to perform our daily work to the best advantage—or, indeed, at all. We may observe the analogy between the human body and the steam engine, in such cases. The engine must have sufficient fuel, otherwise the fires will burn low, and have to be built up again. And so it is with the human body; if we withdraw the food, the human fires (the energies) run low, and the system will again have to be built up and invigorated by augmented "coaling" later on. Hence it is obvious that withholding the food (fuel) from the body can do nothing but weaken and depress it, and can be of no possible assistance in any case—and may be the cause of much harm."

This, I take it, is the generally accepted position in this question, and the one usually assumed and defended whenever the question arises. That it is quite as erroneous in theory as in actual practice I shall show presently, in considerable detail (pp. 225–303); but, even granting for the moment (which I do not) that the body *does* resemble the steam engine in this respect, I would point out that the above comparison and supposed parallel is entirely erroneous for this reason. The cases are not parallel. The diseased body resembles, *not* the *properly* coaled engine, but the one that has been continually and vastly *over* coaled (if I may so express it): one in which the fire is clogged with an excess of combustible material (of good nutriment), and which only requires time, a forced draught (exercise), and to be "let alone," in order to burn up successfully this material, and set things to rights. If, however, during this period, we were to continue piling on the coal, we should, thereby, smother and altogether choke the fire; and for this reason it would "go out" even though there be a great abundance of the best and most combustible material heaped upon it. And so it is with the human organism. The body is clogged and overloaded with an excess of food material; of which it has been unable to successfully dispose—owing to the fact that more has been actually piled into the engine—ingested into the body—than it can successfully burn up, and in other ways dispose of.

Just in the same way that too great a force of coal gas will, when present, result in flare and waste, and will not produce so good and satisfactory a light as a lesser amount of gas would produce—just so, does too much food, ingested into the human economy, defeat its own object; it will fail to nourish, to properly sustain and supply the tissue with nutriment; and results merely in harmful waste, and frequently in disastrous results. This being so, how then are we to treat this condition? By continually adding *more* fuel—more food? Certainly not! We should stop all ingress of food—should *fast*, in fact—and stimulate the action of the excretory organs. Only in this manner can we hope for successful results—for a final cure. The fuel already *in* the body must be allowed to burn out before more is added; and the brighter the fire burns—the greater the heat and energy evolved—the cleaner is the system from all but utilizable fuel. As before stated, the analogy, in these cases, is the body to the *over* not the *properly* coaled steam engine.

There is then this one consideration which I should like to impress upon my reader with the utmost earnestness—asking him to let it sink into his consciousness and appreciate it in all its significance. The point is this: that *we are not nourished by the amount of food we eat, but by the amount we can properly use and assimilate.*[1]

If the system can only appropriate, and properly and beneficially utilize, as much food as can be placed in a thimble, *e.g.*, then that is all the food that should be eaten, and all the food that can possibly nourish, or do the patient any "good" whatever—all food over and above this must be expelled from the system through a useless expenditure of the vital forces; and further, food which the system cannot appropriate always undergoes a certain amount of decomposition and putrefaction

[1] See "Nutrition Investigations at the California Agricultural Experiment Station," by M. E. Jaffa, M.S., p. 28, etc.

in the digestive tract, and this toxic material is absorbed into the circulation, helping to poison the patient.[1] If the amount of food that can be properly assimilated is, in three test cases, 12 oz., 6 oz., and 2 oz. respectively, this weight of food is all that should be ingested, and the patient whose system is in a condition to assimilate but 2 oz. with benefit, will gain no more flesh and do himself no more "good" on the greater amount—the 8 oz. or the 12 oz.; but will, on the contrary, do himself an infinite amount of harm by swallowing the greater amount of food—the harm increasing in exact ratio to the amount ingested over and above the prescribed limit. This point is of the utmost importance. Now, the amount of food that can be used to advantage (assimilated by the system) depends upon the general bodily condition—the nervous vigor of the patient—and the ability of the digestive system to cope with, and properly assimilate, the food ingested. Properly interpreted, it is obvious that the ability of the digestive organs to utilize the food ingested depends absolutely upon, and is in direct proportion to, the needs of the system for nutriment. In cases of ill health the digestive system is obviously and certainly deranged throughout; the muscles refusing to properly perform their work, and the digestive juices being secreted in extremely small quantities throughout the alimentary canal (p. 504-5), their secretion must be *forced* to enable them to respond at all. And this brings us to another extremely important point—the importance of which, again, it is almost impossible to overestimate. The digestive fluids are throughout, secreted *not in proportion to the amount of food eaten, but in proportion to the amount of food required by the system.* As Doctor Page tersely put it:[2]

"In accordance with a universal law of nature—the conservation of energy—gastric juice, upon which digestion depends, 'is secreted from the blood by the glands of the stomach, in proportion to the needs of the organism for food, and not in proportion to the amount of food swallowed.' There is, therefore, a normal dyspepsia for whatever of excess is taken. Moreover, in such cases, none of the food is well digested."

[1] *Vide* "Aristocracy of Health," by Mary Foote Henderson, p. 710.
[2] "Natural Cure," p. 93.

Let me still further enforce this position by the following considerations. It must always be remembered that every particle of food we eat must be aërated in the lungs before it can be appropriated by the system, and used for building tisuse. No matter how much food we eat, if this aëration is not performed, this food must of necessity fail to nourish us. We only receive the benefit from as much food as has been aërated. And it must further be remembered that all food material not aërated merely clogs and chokes the organism, without nourishing it in the least degree. Says Dr. R. T. Trall:[1]

"Eating and breathing must correspond; that is to say, no one can in any way nor by any means, diminish the breathing capacity and increase the quantity of food with impunity. Every morsel of food requires a corresponding particle of air, or it can never be used. Else it becomes a burden, and must be thrown out of the organism as so much lumber or waste material."

And now if this be so, we can see that, if we habitually breathe impure air, and that shallowly and imperfectly, how are we to oxidize the mass of food material that is constantly ingested—in excess of organic needs—since the breathing is *less* than such needs? This constant disproportion must sooner or later have the gravest consequences: and precisely what the consequences are become manifest to us when we consider the millions of deaths annually from consumption and lung diseases generally. See *Appendix G.*

Now, the needs of the tissues will depend largely upon the amount of exercise taken, but more especially upon the freedom of the system from diseased conditions, and it will be noticed that, just in proportion to the needs of the system for food, is hunger present (p. 546-7)—and should be satisfied to that extent; but, in exact proportion to the *absence* of hunger, it is apparent that the tissues require no food—consequently any supplied them at this time would be unnatural and forced nutrition, which must either be stored as morbid or fatty tissue, or expelled from the system at a great loss of bodily and mental energy.

[1] "Digestion and Dyspepsia," p. 14.

That we do not gain flesh and weight in direct proportion to the weight of the food we eat is so obvious and readily observable that the mere mention of the fact here is barely necessitated. Do we not see, every day, the "fat" man, who eats comparatively little food; and the "thin" man, who eats as much as three men twice his weight? Are not these examples only too frequent? Many persons (and even physicians) seem to think that there is a certain *mystery* about such cases which cannot be explained—something, even, a little uncanny! Yet the explanation is simplicity itself. The fat man's digestive organs have not been impaired; he assimilates what he eats; and the excess of food taken, over and above his bodily needs, accumulates in the form of fatty tissue. The "thin" man, on the other hand, almost invariably suffers from dyspepsia;[1] from indigestion; from constipation, and from mal-assimilation in its many forms. Their digestive systems, being constantly overworked, and being weak naturally, have not vital vigor left for the digestion—the assimilation and elimination—of such quantities of food material, and consequently fail to perform their proper and allotted work *at all*, the consequence of which is that nearly all the food eaten passes out of such persons' systems without being digested or appropriated at all; it is a pure case of "starvation from overfeeding."

It is true that emaciation is largely (though not entirely) due to lack of nourishment; to the lack of food elements in one locality or to the body generally. But this is not due—as is generally supposed—to a lack of food supply, since the organism

[1] Nervous or "mental dyspepsia" is invariably considered a sign of purely mental influences, and, as such, is distinguished from the mucous variety, which is acknowledged to be due to physiological cause. My own view of the matter is somewhat different. Granting that the mental influences are the main contributory cause of this condition, I ask: what does this mean? Is it not tantamount to saying that the nervous influences or impulses to the stomach are too low in quality, or *insufficient in quantity, to properly deal with the amount of food-material that has been ingested?* And might we not argue that our best and quickest way of restoring the normal condition, would be to more directly proportion the nervous supply and the food-material; and as we cannot increase the former, we must accomplish our end by decreasing the latter? In other words, if the bulk of food ingested were less, would not the quantity and quality of the nervous influences to the stomach be sufficient to handle and dispose of this lesser amount? I think it most assuredly would. And, should *no* food be eaten, what would become of the dyspepsia—seeing that, at the return of natural hunger, a perfectly normal condition must of necessity be present?

is frequently overloaded with such elements, in a mal-assimilated form; but it is due to the inability of the blood to reach the anæmic parts—owing to the blocked and choked condition of the blood vessels—which, in turn, is due to the presence of effete material which should have been eliminated. Thus we see that emaciation results, not from an actual deficiency of nutriment, but from an excess! And the only way in which we can bring food to the starved tissues is by removing the *cause* of the obstruction, which prevents this nutriment from reaching the tissues involved. The blocking material must be removed, and this can be accomplished more safely, more quickly and easily by fasting than by any other method.

What such persons need, in order to gain flesh, is not more food, but a greater stock of vitality; an increased power of the digestive organs; and this can only be gained by giving them less to do—by *resting* them—and a rest is a fast! Paradoxical as it may seem, therefore, the only way in which thin persons may ever hope to gain healthy flesh and strength is by eating considerably *less*—giving the digestive organs a chance to assimilate more. It cannot be too strongly borne in mind that it is not the amount of food we eat, but the amount we successfully digest and assimilate, that does us good.

In certain cases of emaciation, exercise undoubtedly removes from the capillaries effete material—which has been obstructing and blocking these vessels, and preventing, consequently, the proper blood supply to these parts. This once removed, and the circulation restored, proper nutrition of these parts is again rendered possible. Thus we see that over-nutrition (by blocking of the peripheral blood vessels) causes actual starvation of these parts; a truth the importance of which it is impossible to overestimate.

Thus we see that fasting actually prevents starvation and increases nutrition! And it is because of a lack of knowledge of this great truth that many hundreds die of anæmia and other wasting diseases—starved to death by over-feeding. They starve because they are overfed to such an extent that they have impaired the organs of digestion so that no power remains to digest and assimilate food, however much or little may be swallowed. See *Appendix H*.

A word in this connection regarding cold hands and feet. This abnormal condition is due to the fact that the peripheral blood vessels are blocked with foreign material, and the only way to restore the animal heat to these parts is to restore the circulation. And this can only be done by ridding the blood vessels of the impurities they contain. This once done, a normal circulation and temperature will ensue; they will become as warm as the rest of the body, and of even temperature with it.[1]

And this brings us to a very highly important consideration. It may be contended—and probably will be—that fasting will only benefit fat individuals, and will be of no benefit to thin persons; but this is the greatest of errors. Thus, emaciated persons will receive an equal if not a greater benefit from the fast than do their more fleshy brethren; this being due, of course, to the fact that thin persons are thin because they are starving from overfeeding; that their emaciation is due to the choking of their smaller blood vessels with effete material. The benefit such patients will receive from fasting is very great.

We now see why it is that thin persons can invariably derive so much benefit from a fast. The fact that they are more or less emaciated does not by any means prove (as it is always supposed to prove) that such persons have had too little food; but is, on the contrary, disproved by the fact that many chronically thin persons have gained considerable weight on a greatly restricted diet (simply because the system could assimilate and appropriate the food ingested, which it could not do formerly); and also by the fact that fever patients, *e.g.*, continue to waste no matter how much food is eaten. Kuhne contended—rightly I think—that, so long as the "deposits" remained soft they were not dangerous, and were capable of being easily eliminated; but that if they were allowed to harden, shrink and contract, the condition was more or less serious, and the process of cure would be a long and tedious one.

In the thin person, something of this has doubtless taken place—the formerly normal and even fatty (soft) tissue having become obdurated and hardened—owing to the withdrawal of

[1] See Lahmann: "Natural Hygiene," pp. 108–10.

the watery juices normally present therein, and to the contraction of the muscle or flesh into a hardened, obstipated mass. The softening and vitalizing of this tissue is essential if health is to be restored; and this can only be accomplished by increasing the flow of blood and vital energy to those parts; and that can only be done by withdrawing—oxidizing, absorbing and eliminating—the material that blocks or prevents such flow, and by altering the chemical composition of the tissues; and this can only be done by fasting, since this absorbs and utilizes all such morbid, blocking material; alters the chemical composition of the body, and, in short, supplies all the requisite conditions for a successful cure. (See pp. 576–78.)

The fact of fundamental importance that must ever be kept in mind is that emaciation—the wasting of tissue—is due to the *wasting of disease, not to starvation consequent upon lack of sufficient nourishment.* It is not starvation from under-feeding, but over-feeding! Proof of this is found in those cases where the patient actually gains in weight by reducing the quantity of food eaten; and in cases of disease, where the patient wastes even more when food is given than when it is withheld. This conclusively proves that emaciation is due to lack of ability on the part of the organism to assimilate the food eaten, rather than to a lack of actual food supplied.

Since, then, the body can and successfully *does* nourish and sustain itself on this smaller quantity of food daily; the question arises—what happens with all the remainder of the food generally eaten—which, consequently must be excess? If this, at first sight, astonishingly small amount of food is all that is needed in order to successfully maintain the weight, the heat, the strength and the energy of the body, under the usually existing circumstances; if this amount of food supplies us with all that we need for the body's support and proper nourishment; if, on this amount of food, not only as much, but actually *more* energy and strength are available for the general purposes of life, and a greater degree of health and vitality be manifested from this restricted diet; if, in other words, this amount of food is all that the body actually needs for any purposes, or under any ordinary circumstances whatever; what effect does the rest of the food we habitually ingest have upon the system? If (and there is no disputing the fact that it actually does, *v.* pp. 113–14) 12 ounces of food are all the system requires for its proper nutrition and sustenance, and we habitually partake of 30 or 40 or 50 or even more ounces of food per day; what becomes of this balance? and what effect upon the organism does the unnecessary, and consequently useless, 12 or 22 or 32 or more ounces of food daily have? It must have *some* effect. It is quite impossible, as it is inconceivable, that exactly *equally* beneficial results should follow from both systems of diet! It is contrary to everything we know of this world; to all science, to philosophy, to logic, to reason. Different effects *must* follow the differing causes. The only question to decide is—what are the effects, and how great?

Now, all that we know of Nature and her workings force upon us the conviction that *economy* is the one thing sought—provided it be real, and not apparent, economy.[1] Whenever a thing may be done simply it is done so, rather than in any more complicated manner. If anything can be done by the expenditure of a small amount of energy it is so done. Nature will not expend a greater amount than is absolutely necessary in order to successfully perform what is required of her. And this law may be observed throughout the whole of creation. So, it is only natural to suppose that, provided certain results can be obtained by the ingestion of a certain quantity of food, just that amount will yield the best, the most healthful, and the most beneficial results. If the system can successfully perform its labors upon 12 ounces of food daily, only that amount should be eaten, and the digestion and enforced elimination of the remaining 20 or 30 or 40 or more ounces cannot be other than detrimental to the organism. It is superfluous; it is useless; it is unnecessary; it is an encumbrance; and as such must necessarily call for an undue and excessive expenditure of the vital forces, in order to dispose of this great bulk of food material, which is not needed. *Harm* must necessarily result! Not only are the vital energies wasted to an excessive degree—

[1] See "Technique of Rest," by Anna C. Brackett, pp. 29–30, where this distinction is made clear.

a degree which few appreciate or even dream of (*v.* pp. 104–5) but the eliminating organs become overtaxed; they become weakened and cease to properly perform their functions. Effete material begins to accumulate within the system. The process continues as the overfeeding continues. The system becomes more and more clogged, choked, and, by auto-infection, poisoned throughout by this corrupt, excrementous material.[1] *This process is the true cause of disease*—which we here see actively at work. All disease being traced to the one cause—the retention within the system of excrementous material—we are now enabled to see in and of what this material consists. *It is unduly retained, mal-assimilated food material, which we thus see to be the real and chief cause of all disease.* At last we have found the true, the all but universal, cause of disease; at last we have found the universally applicable means of cure! If not a panacea, we have at least come within an ace of finding it, in this simple method, for, like all Nature's methods, it is as simple as universal, when rightly understood.

It may be objected that I have, in the above argument, spoken of fat as though it were an altogether useless if not a positively harmful portion of the human economy, while it is almost universally taught, I shall be told, that a certain amount of fatty tissue is both normal and necessary—allowing for bodily variations and losses, and forming a certain store of readily assimilable food, in case of illness, when the body is incapable of utilizing food ingested in the regular manner. As may be surmised, perhaps, I do not agree with this position at all, but disagree in every important particular. Let us first of all discuss the point just raised—that a person lacking fatty tissue could not fast so long a time in illness, and so be less liable to recover than his stouter companion.

[1] See Crandall: "How to Keep Well," p. 455. This excess of food-material, passing into the blood, must either take the form of fatty tissue—more or less excretory matter lodged in the cellular tissue, or else it retains its crude, gross condition, floating at large throughout the blood—fermenting, decaying, putrefying, and poisoning the system. As Doctor Oswald remarked ("Fasting, Hydropathy and Exercise," p. 25); ". . . Not only the progress of digestion is thus interrupted (by overfeeding), not only that the body derives no strength from the inert mass, but that mass, by undergoing a putrid instead of a peptic decomposition, vitiates the humors of the system it was intended to nourish, irritates the sensitive membrane of the stomach, and gradually impairs the vigor of the whole digestive apparatus."

It is probable, I admit, that a lean man could not, *ceteris paribus*, fast so long as a fatter man, but *it would not be necessary for him to do sò*. The thinner man is already half free from the diseased condition from which the fatter man suffers, and consequently would not have to continue his fasting for so long a time, in order to obtain the same results. The fat man's fast is protracted largely on account of the very fact that he *is* fat; and all this his slimmer brother escapes; it is not necessary for him to fast for so long a period. Cornaro saw this, with his customary foresight, and wrote, *à propos* of this point:

"... He that leads the temperate life can never fall sick, or at least can do so very rarely; and his indisposition lasts but a very short time. For, by living temperately, he removes all the causes of illness; and, having removed these, he thereby removes the effects. So, the man who lives the orderly life should have no fear of sickness; for surely he has no reason to fear an effect, the cause of which is under his own control."[1]

Again, Doctor Graham wrote:[2]

"If the fat be designed for the nourishment of the body during protracted fasts, etc., then if a very fat man, in the enjoyment of what is ordinarily considered good health, and a lean man in good health, be shut up together, and condemned to die of starvation, the fat man ought to diminish in weight much more slowly, and to live considerably longer than the lean man; but directly the contrary of this is true. The lean man will lose in weight much more slowly, and live several days longer than the fat man, in spite of all the nourishment which the latter may derive from his adipose deposits."

It will be seen that Doctor Graham even denies that the fat man does live longer than the thin man, and I may state that that has been my own experience, precisely. I shall discuss this question later in some detail; see especially the chapter "On the Loss and Gain in Weight." But there are other authors who take the same stand on this question, as the result of their own experience—Doctor Trall being one of these. Finally it

[1] "The Art of Living Long," p. 61–2.
[2] "Science of Human Life," pp. 193–4.

must be remembered that a person may be quite fat, and yet die from starvation—while yet fat! Says Doctor Trall:[1]

" . . . Feed a dog on butter, starch, or sugar alone, and you will save in him the consumption of fat. But the dog will die of starvation. He will be plump, round, *embonpoint*, and yet die of inanition."

Doctor Pereira, M.D., F.R.S., etc., also asserts this to be the case; see his "Food and Diet," p. 85.

Now let us come to a consideration of the nature of fatty tissue, and its use in the vital economy. I shall take the stand that fatty tissue is invariably *diseased* tissue—and this, no matter in what locality it may be found.[2]

Says Dr. C. E. Page:[3]

"A fat person at whatever period of life, has not a sound tissue in his body; not only is the entire muscular system degenerated with the fatty particles, but the vital organs—heart, lungs, brain, kidneys, liver, etc.,—are likewise mottled throughout, like rust spots in a steel watch-spring, liable to fail at any moment. . Fat is a disease."

Doctor Yorke-Davies showed conclusively that fat persons are especially liable to diseases of all kinds.

The idea that fatty tissue is invariably diseased tissue may be somewhat disconcerting to the majority of my readers, and will doubtless be unwelcome news. We have been taught for so long to consider an increase of weight as a sign of returning health and strength that the news that this but indicates re-accumulation of disease will be received with incredulity.

And yet how obvious the fact is! And how readily it may be perceived by anyone understanding the true physiology—the *rationale*—of the process involved. Fatty tissue is, for all intents and purposes, *useless* tissue, and useless tissue has no place in a body which is intended for useful, energetic purposes. Proof of this (if such were needed) is to be found in the fact

[1] "Alcoholic Controversy," p. 101.

[2] In this I have the support of many eminent men; see Yorke-Davies: "Foods for the Fat," p. ix; Wm. Harvey: "Corpulence in Relation to Disease," p. 1; also the writings of Trall, Graham, Jackson, Nichols, etc.

[3] "Natural Cure," pp. 148–9.

that, when dogs and horses are trained for particular races or events requiring the greatest amount of energy and endurance, every ounce of this fatty tissue is purposely removed by hard work and by regulation of the diet. The same holds true with regard to athletes of all kinds—pugilists, *e.g.*, training down to the lowest possible weight—the remark being frequently heard: "He hasn't an ounce of superfluous flesh on him." And this is held to indicate the "ideal"; the perfection of health—by universal consent. Why this should be so in the case of animals, and even of *some* men, and fail to indicate a like condition in the remainder, is beyond the comprehension of the writer. The very fatty tissue which he would regard as a hindrance and a sign of "lack of condition" in the athlete, he considers a sign of improved health in the professional or business man! The very reduction in weight; the slim litheness of figure (so much admired in athletes, while in condition, and held to actually denote, in them, a condition of perfect physical health) we look upon as a sign of lost health when observed in ourselves and our neighbors! The pride with which we point out the fact that "every rib is showing" in our dog—and held to indicate his excellent physical condition—is turned to consternation when we observe a like condition in ourselves! And why? Is it possible to find any logical reason for such beliefs? Or are they not rather absurd delusions—absolutely unfounded, and illogical and irrational throughout?

But there are other weighty reasons for thinking that fatty tissue is diseased tissue. In the first place, we have the evidence afforded by illnesses of all kinds—where a considerable amount of flesh (weight) is lost—observable both by the scales and by the tape measure; yet, *coincidental with the loss, is health restored!* As Doctor Reinhold observed:[1]

"If a person at the age of 25 weighs 120 pounds, and at the age of 40 tips the scales at 150 pounds, this gain in weight usually means an increase of 30 pounds of corrupt matter. If the circumference of the abdomen at the age of 25 measures 30 inches, and at a later period 40 inches, the increase is due to the accumulation of abnormal material ..."

[1] "Pulmonary Consumption," p. 5.

Mr. Horace Fletcher, in speaking of his own case, said·

"I have had my weight reduced from 217 pounds to 130 pounds, and felt best when lightest."[1]

Doctor Higgins wrote to Mr. Fletcher in September, 1903:

"I have lost 104 pounds in weight and consider that I have gained very considerably in mental and physical fitness." (p. 228.)

This has been strongly confirmed by the recent researches of Professor Chittenden, of Yale.

And this brings us to a consideration of great importance. It is this: What is fatty tissue, and why and how does it accumulate? Without going too deeply into the matter, it may be said that it is material (food material) which has lodged in the tissues and been retained therein, *instead of being eliminated—as it should have been.* It is the result of over-nutrition, and always must be. If only sufficient food has been ingested at all times; just enough to balance the bodily expenditure, it would be impossible for fatty tissue to accumulate. The material that forms it would have been oxidized or eliminated, as soon as formed, instead of being retained within the system—clogging the blood vessels, and interfering with the functional activity throughout. The fact that health and strength invariably return, as fatty tissue is eliminated, should prove, to all sensible persons, that it is not only useless but harmful to us. In the ideal condition there is no fatty tissue whatever present. Its presence denotes a greater or lesser degree of disease—and this in direct proportion to its bulk. Instead of deploring the fact that weight is being lost, therefore, we should look upon it as a sign of returning health; instead of congratulating ourselves and others upon our fatter, sleeker appearance; instead of remarking: "Ah, Mr. Jones, how well you are looking! You were so thin when last I saw you, and now you are looking quite stout and hearty!" we should feel precisely opposite sentiments, and say: "Ah, Mr. Jones, I see you are considerably stouter than when I last saw you. You had better be careful in your habits, my friend, for you are surely accumulating some

[1] "Glutton or Epicure," p. 195.

form of disease that will manifest itself in one way or another before long—when you will attribute it to anything but the right cause. Take my advice, then, and work that tissue off again!" Such should be our thoughts—whether expressed or not! We have only to realize that fat is, strictly speaking, *retained excreta*, in order to appreciate the force of this position.

In this connection I cannot refrain from adding one or two reflections, suggested as the result of the above argument, whose practical importance seem to me very great. It has frequently been observed, *e.g.*, that women very frequently gain in weight, and "get stout" and plump soon after marriage, and this condition—the gain in weight—has been looked upon as highly beneficial, and "marriage" consequently recommended by many physicians, as the cure for such conditions as emaciation, anæmia, etc.—among others. The whole misconception arose out of the mistaken idea that fatty tissue is healthy tissue, and that gain in weight means a corresponding gain in health; whereas, more often than not (and although fatty tissue sometimes returns *together with* health), precisely the reverse of this is the case.

Bearing these facts in mind, let us consider, for a moment, the *rationale* of the increase of weight and flesh in the newly married woman—which, as may be expected, I look upon as altogether abnormal and injurious; and consequently seek the cause in some abnormal condition—dependent, in turn, upon some newly acquired, abnormal habit of life.

Of course the answer at once suggests itself. Sexual intercourse is that which is more or less directly accountable for the whole affair. And my tentative explanation of the *modus operandi* involved is as follows: Sexual intercourse lessens the vitality; that we may take as an established fact. Now, this loss of vitality would necessitate a lessened functioning of the various organs of the body—including the depurating organs. These organs, while under-functioning, allow the improper retention, in the system, of a certain amount of material that would normally have been eliminated; and this material accumulates in the body, and forms the fatty tissue—which is thus seen to be unduly retained excrementous material, here as elsewhere. And it will be seen why it is that I regard increase in weight as a sign of decreased, rather than increased health.

While many persons may see the force of the above reasoning, and consequently be willing to rid themselves of at least a very large proportion of their fat, in consequence, they yet do not know *how* to rid themselves of this superabundant material. They have recourse to anti-fat nostrums and other vile concoctions for this purpose—sometimes with the effect of removing a considerable proportion of this tissue (in an extremely harmful manner); sometimes with little or no appreciable effect at all. And yet all these persons *know* that, were they merely to abstain from all food for, from one to two months, this tissue would all be absorbed and oxidized or eliminated; and that they could remove just as much or as little of this fat as they desired, by the simple process of fasting for a greater or a lesser period! As Doctor Dewey said:[1]

"How simple! Only to fast, no matter if it costs a whole day, a whole week or a whole month, and with absolute safety. . . It is a process that you can push safely well on to the skeleton condition, if you cut the food down. You can determine in advance just what loss of weight is to be reached; for it is simply a problem of endurance and mathematics." (p. 205.)

Now, knowing all this, why has this method not been applied? Is it because the fear of death from starvation holds them back —the average person thinking that such would intervene long before the system is rid of this overplus of tissue? Or do they think it would be a difficult or a painful process? Or is it gluttony pure and simple which holds them back? I am very much afraid it is the latter consideration, almost altogether. As I have previously pointed out, the fasting cure, for this very reason, will never, probably, become a popular cure; people would rather eat and die than fast and live!

But to those few to whom this does not apply, it will be indeed welcome news to learn that the oxidation and elimination of their fatty tissue is not a more difficult or painful process than was its accumulation. And further, that it is a physiological

[1] "True Science of Living," p. 167.

impossibility for death to intervene before the skeleton condition is reached; in other words, until all this fatty tissue has been eliminated, and much more besides! Hunger will invariably return when the system is sufficiently clear of morbific material to render the ingestion of more food desirable; and, until this hunger appears, the fast may be continued in the confidence and knowledge that no harm can possibly result from such abstention; but, on the contrary, that increased health, strength and energy await the patient who has the moral courage to attempt and follow out this mode of treatment.

This habitual overfeeding, of which I have spoken above, extends unfortunately not only throughout the whole world of adults but to the babies and the aged as well. Doctor Dewey and Doctor Rabagliati repeatedly drew attention to this fact, in their writings; and Doctor Densmore reëmphasized the truth in his book "How Nature Cures," where he says (p. 54); "Infants almost always are fed too frequently." And again (p. 55):

"It is frequently, perhaps usually, said of this or that or the other babe that it is fretful or peevish. It is fretful because it is ill, and it is ill, usually, because of improper feeding. The same error that adult human beings make in regard to themselves is made in regard to the feeding of children—they are fed too often and too much."

I may add that practically every writer on the subject agrees with this view: see the writings of Wheeler, Holt, Jackson, Burney Yeo, Mendel, Chittenden, Trall, Crandell, etc.

But it remained for Doctor Page to show, with convincing fact and logic, the extent to which children, and especially babies, are overfed. In his very excellent book entitled "How to Feed the Baby," which I cannot too highly recommend to all mothers, Doctor Page proved conclusively that *three daily feedings*—of moderate quantity—(and none at night) are all that should be allowed the babe, from birth! (p. 54.)[1]

Doctor Page brought up his own—exceptionally healthy and robust—baby on *two* meals per day! (p. 55.) Yet to what

[1] Dr. B. F. Dawson strongly advocates fasting for babies in all diseased conditions, and mentions a case in which a week's fast completely cured a nursing baby of grievous stomach trouble.

extent is this exceeded! What outrages are not permitted in the feeding of the baby! To quote Doctor Page:

"During the nine months of fœtal growth the increase, except in cases of monstrosities, is about one-third of an ounce per day, or two and one-half ounces per week. Why it should be deemed rational for this ratio to be increased *six or seven hundred per cent.*, directly after birth, is beyond my comprehension. In spite, or because, of this hot-house forcing during the first few months the usual weight at, say, five years, is much less than if the rate of prenatal growth had been continued throughout these years!

"I consider that the excessive fat so generally regarded as the sign of the healthy babe, is simply a proof of the ability of the digestive organs to go on for a time digesting more food than is required for growth—the excess going to the production of fatty tissue, which, at any stage of life, after infancy, is, by universal consent, regarded as *disease*. I hold that it is no less disease in infancy, and tends to check the really normal growth; and that all excessively fat babies are only cured by either a considerable period of non-growth, or a violent sickness, which strips them of the fat, if not of life.

"The healthy born babe has the power to digest and assimilate easily and continuously an amount of food, sufficient to produce a normal growth. *This rate of growth can not be exceeded,*—however much food is taken. It can be checked, or stopped altogether, by either a deficiency, or an excess, of food, continued for any length of time. The increase in weight—the rolling on of fat—is a delusion and a snare."[1]

Doctor Page calculated (p. 23), that, were a man weighing 150 pounds to partake of as much milk, proportionately, as is quite commonly fed to babies, he would, during the twenty-four hours have disposed of no less than *twenty-two and one-half quarts!*[2] From this we may readily see to what an extent the youthful organism is abused; and how the seeds are laid, at that time, not only for its immediate consequent—disease; but also for a perverted appetite, and a deranged digestive system, which frequently accompanies us throughout life—never once permitting

[1] "How to Feed the Baby," pp. 33–4.

[2] This may seem exaggeration, but it may be readily seen that such is the case; see Virginia Levis: "Nursing," p. 42, where ten feedings *per diem* are recommended!

the call of "normal" hunger, or the healthful assimilation of a meal! See *Appendix I.*

What has been said about the overfeeding of babies and of adults applies also to the older members of the community; the same mistake is made here as is made in every other instance; too much food is eaten at too frequent meals. The idea that older persons should eat more food than the younger ones is a very grave error; and one which, I believe, has sent hundreds of men and women to a premature grave. In the older man (or woman) there is no longer the same active life as heretofore; but little tissue, comparatively speaking, calls for replacement; there is no actual *growth* to call for nutriment. In this very connection, I may quote the words of no less eminent an authority than Sir Henry Thompson, F.R.C.S., etc., who, in his "Diet in Relation to Age and Activity" (p. 39–40), thus expresses himself

"But as we increase in age—when we have spent, say, our first half century—less energy and activity remain, and less expenditure can be made; less power to eliminate is possible at fifty than at thirty, still less at sixty and upward. *Less* nutriment, therefore, must be taken in proportion as age advances, or rather, as activity diminishes, or the individual will suffer. If he continues to consume the same abundant breakfasts, substantial luncheons, and heavy dinners, which at the summit of his power he could dispose of almost with impunity, he will in time certainly either accumulate fat or become acquainted with gout or rheumatism, or show signs of unhealthy *deposit* of some kind in some part of the body—processes which must inevitably empoison, undermine, or shorten his remaining term of life. He must reduce his 'intake,' because a smaller expenditure is an enforced condition of existence. At seventy the man's power has further diminished, and the nutriment must correspond thereto, if he desires still another term of comfortable life. And why should he not? Then at eighty, with less activity, there must be still less 'support.'"

And again he says ("Food and Feeding," p. 64):

"I desire to point out that the system of 'supporting' aged persons, as it is termed, with increased quantities of food and stimulant, is an error of cardinal importance, and, without doubt, tends to shorten, or to embitter life."

CHAPTER IV

THE NO-BREAKFAST PLAN

"*Woe to thee, O land, when thy king is a child, and thy princes eat in the morning!*

"*Blessed art thou, O land, when thy king is the son of nobles, and thy princes eat in due season, for strength, and not for drunkenness!*"—Ecclesiastes, x., 16–17.

It is now all but universally admitted that we eat too much, even by those physicians and laymen who are opposed to absolute fasting as a cure for disease. Many individuals have accordingly tried (1) to lessen the amount of food eaten at each meal; and (2) to curtail the actual number of meals eaten—reducing the customary three or four meals *per diem* to two or one. I need hardly say that every step made in this direction is of inestimable benefit to the experimenter, as, in the vast majority of cases, the great object to be attained is to reduce the bulk of food eaten; and it does not matter by what method this end is attained—so long as it *is* attained. Consequently, no matter in what way the supply of food be lessened, nothing but good results will follow. The only danger to be feared is that, most persons experimenting upon themselves in this way, and not knowing what to expect, will find their appetite and general physical health and animal spirits so far improved after following the new régime for a longer or shorter period, that they counteract all the good effects of the more abstemious dietary by unbridled and promiscuous gluttony when food is eaten![1] For such cases, the only cure would be, of course, to

[1] I am now speaking, it must be remembered, of those persons who are but slightly, though probably, chronically diseased. For those patients who are seriously ill, and especially in all acute diseases, there must be no compromise; a strict and absolute fast for as long as may be necessary is the only course allowable.

restrain the patient's appetite until after this dangerous period has passed, when a normal appetite will invariably appear.

To those individuals, therefore, who are, by advice or voluntarily, restricting their diet by either of the above-mentioned methods, I have little to say; but as there must necessarily be some science and order in this, as in every other, branch of hygiene and dietary, I shall, in the present chapter, offer a few remarks that are intended to assist the would-be convert, and enable him to omit the minimum amount of food with the maximum amount of benefit to himself.

To do this, a very simple rule need be followed, *viz., omit the breakfast.*

A chorus of objections is at once raised by my readers—of that I am assured! Omit any other meal, yes, but breakfast, never! "I should be so faint all the morning I couldn't do anything," says the first. "I could do nothing without my morning meal; I have tried it, and was so hungry all the morning I could think of nothing but my stomach," says a second. "I should get a splitting headache if I omitted my breakfast," says a third, "it always affects me in that way."[1]

Those of my readers who have followed me thus far will readily perceive the fallacy and absurdity of such statements. Since, as we shall see, pp. 225–303, food does not give us strength or energy, but on the contrary detracts from both: and since, in addition, natural hunger does not appear in the stomach in any case (p. 549), it is obvious that all the untoward symptoms that manifest themselves during the morning's fast, are the results of (1) mental influences—expectancy, suggestion, etc.; (2) the sudden withdrawal of stimulation, and (3) the confusion into which the body is thrown as the result of (2) and of the general cleaning-up vital processes which are thus given free play, and the unaccustomed symptoms which are mistaken for

[1] To those individuals who claim they could do nothing without their morning *coffee*, I have merely this to say: that their craving for that stimulant is precisely on a par with the dram-drinker, who can "do nothing" before his glass of gin, and the appetite is, in my estimation, equally abnormal and depraved in both cases. *Stimulation* is the thing sought, and, while one intoxicates and the other does not, that difference is purely accidental. The disastrous effects on the nervous system is finally apparent in both cases. For both, too, the cure is the same—a removal of the cause of the desire for the drink. (pp. 110–11.)

hunger. All these unpleasant symptoms[1] may be greatly relieved, if not altogether removed, in every case, by drinking a glass of cool or hot water, and by resolutely refraining from thinking about one's stomach.

Regarding the third objection so far raised, *viz.*, that a more or less severe headache is occasionally induced, in some cases, by the sudden withdrawal of the morning meal, I must admit that this is frequently the case; but insist, in turn, that this is not by any means an unfavorable symptom, when judged from the proper standpoint. To be sure, a headache is an extremely unpleasant sensation at the time, to say the least. But here again we encounter the false teachings of the orthodox medical school, which sees in pain an enemy to life, and not the friendly action of the vital forces indicating the presence of obstructing material at that point, calling our attention to that part of the body, and clearly indicating that the cause of the pain should be removed—not that the pain itself should be subdued. (pp. 25-9.)

Now, in all those cases in which a headache is experienced, the thing to do is to abstain from all food until the headache is completely dissipated. I entirely agree with Mr. Macfadden when he says:[2]

"The mere fact that the omission of one meal causes a headache, is ample evidence that, instead of missing one meal, a dozen should be missed; for this headache is caused by the slime or the remains of fermented food and other impure matter that has collected in the stomach, or has remained there from the preceding meal, and as no food is introduced to excite the flow of gastric juice or to dilute this impure material, it finally flows out of the stomach and part of it is naturally absorbed by the circulatory system, and in the elimination of this foreign matter, one of the results noted is a headache. . All those who have tried the fasting cure for disease know that for a few days they will have a fever of more or less intensity, and nothing indicates more strongly that the purifying process is under way than this one symptom. It is one of the means adopted to burn up or eliminate the rank impurities of the body."

[1] Dr. George F. Pentecost, in his Introduction to Dewey's "True Science of Living," p. 10, aptly called them the "dying pains of a bad habit."

[2] *Physical Culture*, Vol. III., p. 132.

Eating a meal will frequently have the effect of temporarily relieving the headache, but almost invariably this returns with even greater severity than before, after an hour or two—showing that the pain was merely suppressed without the cause of the headache being removed. Undoubtedly, what really happened was this: Upon the ingestion of food, the blood which was until then in superabundance in the brain was drawn to the stomach for the purposes of digestion. This relieves the tension of the cerebral blood supply temporarily, but, after the meal is almost or quite digested, the blood returns to the head, carrying with it further nutrient material, and whatever toxic matter has been absorbed from the digestion of that meal, or is created within the system as the result of its ingestion. This, it will be seen, but aggravates the difficulty. The brain can derive no nutriment from food material when thus congested (practically diseased); its primary need is the removal of the superabundance of foreign material already present, and this can be more easily and quickly done in the absence of food material than when such material is being constantly forced upon the tissues—since these have no need for such excessive amounts of nutriment. It must be remembered that the excess of blood in the brain is due, in turn, to an excess of morbid matter which should have been absorbed and eliminated. Nature, in her attempts at cure, determines a greater supply of blood to the head in order to remove more quickly and effectually the foreign material present. Pain denotes here, as always, a diseased condition calling for removal or cure. And the only rational way to remove the pain is to remove its cause—the excess of impure material. Merely subduing the pain, without thus removing the cause, is quite worthless, and opposed to all true methods of cure.

Besides the foregoing objections, however, there are one or two others that might be raised to this theory of omitting the breakfast, which possess, at first sight, far more plausibility than those so far advanced—though they are, I conceive, based upon the same false theories of energy and nutrition. One such objection is the following: Instead of omitting the breakfast, would it not be better to omit the lunch—thus more evenly dividing the time between the two meals? Thus, instead of the periods of between-meal fasting being six and eighteen hours, they would be, at most, ten and fourteen hours, respectively. Would that not be more natural, and more evenly balance the work of the system?

A moment's reflection will, I believe, demonstrate the utter lack of plausibility, of reason, in this argument. The time division, in this case, is purely by the clock—not according to the dictates of the requirements of the organism. In one case, it will be seen, almost *all* the day's work is performed and energy expended, in the other, none. In one half of this arbitrary division, there is all the rest; all the repairing processes are carried on; there is all the accumulation of energy. In the other half, but little or no rest; a constant destruction and breaking down of the organic tissue, and all the expenditure of energy. And yet it is claimed that an equal amount of food is necessary to supply the loss in both instances!

No, the night must be altogether omitted from our calculations in this question and treated as if it did not exist; since no energy is expended during that period; no work is performed; no tissues destroyed; consequently, there is no need for any tissue replacement. As Doctor Dewey remarked:[1]

> " There is no natural hunger in the morning after a night of restful sleep, because there has been no such degree of cell-destruction as to create a demand for food at the ordinary hour of the American breakfast. Sleep is not a hunger-causing process."

The working day is the period in which all these destructive changes take place, and it is consequently to that period that we must confine ourselves, in making these time divisions for meals. Taking the hours of the working day, therefore, as a basis for calculation, we arrive at the conclusion that meals eaten at 11 A. M. and 6.30 P. M. would divide the day very evenly—judging from the time period, and also from the standpoint of energy expenditure.[2]

[1] "The True Science of Living," p. 161.

[2] This calculation is based upon the supposition that the patient rises at seven A.M., retires at eleven P.M., and spends an average of one hour at each meal. In one case, the interval would thus be six and a half hours, and in

Having thus disposed of the more obvious objections to the theory of the omission of breakfast, we must now consider the arguments *for* the practice, and understand the physiological reasons upon which are founded the system of dietary that omits this meal, in preference to any of the others.

Doctor Dewey has so well and so fully worked out the reasons in his published works that I cannot do better than to quote somewhat extensively from his "No-Breakfast Plan"—asking my readers to refer for further particulars to the books themselves. Only by quoting at length from any author can justice be done to his arguments, and any hope be entertained that the reader's opinions will change—especially in theories so novel as these:

"We rise in the morning," says Doctor Dewey, "with our brain recharged by sleep, and we go at once to our business. If we take a walk, or go to the gymnasium, we simply waste that much time and we also lessen the stored-up energy by whatever of effort is called out.[1] We can skip the dumb-bells and perform any other kind of exercise that is good for the health, and always with the certainty that we shall have more strength for the first half of the day if none is wasted in this way. . . For the highest possibilities, for a day of human service, there must be a night of sound sleep, and then one may work with muscle or with mind much longer without fatigue if no strength is wasted over untimely food in the stomach, no enforced means to develop health and strength.[2] When one has worked long enough, he becomes generally tired and there should be a period of rest, in order to regain power to digest what shall be so eaten as to cause the brain the least waste of its powers through failure to masticate. One need not always wait until noon to eat the first meal. Those in good health have found that they can easily go till noon before breaking the fast, but in proportion as one is weak or ailing the rule should

the other seven and a half hours—while the greater proportionate strain, mental and physical, which would be undertaken during the business hours of the day, as compared with the lighter tasks and frivolity of the evening, would amply repay and counterbalance the additional half-hour, which would be all that is required in order to render the time for the two meals absolutely periodic.

[1] See "The Noon-Breakfast Plan," by T. Owen, p. 7. "After a good night's sleep, the body is in the best possible condition for exertion, without the intervention of a meal."

[2] Physiologists have now just begun to recognize this fact. See Chittenden, "Physiological Economy in Nutrition," p. 20.

be; stop all work as soon as fatigue becomes marked and then rest until power to digest is restored. To eat when one is tired is to add a burden of labor to all the energies of life, and with the certainty that no wastes will be restored thereby.

"For the highest efforts of genius, or art, of the simplest labors of the hands, the forenoon with empty stomach and larger measure of stored-up energy of the brain, is by far the better half of the day, and more than this, it is equally the better for all the finer senses of the tastes, the finer emotions of soul-life. In addition to these—and what is vastly more important—it is by far the better half of the day for the display of that energy whereby disease is cured. (All this with no power lost in any special exercise for the health!)

"The time to stop the forenoon labor is when the need for rest has become clearly apparent, and there must be rest before eating to restore the energy for digestion. This always determines Nature's time when the first meal shall be taken and not the hour of the day.

"This is especially important to all who are constitutionally weak or have become disabled through ailings or disease. Disappointments have come to hundreds who have given up their breakfasts because of the mistaken idea that they must wait till noon before breaking the fast, and hence they become too tired to digest, and thus experience a loss rather than a gain, from the untimely noon meals.

"The desire for morning food is a matter of habit only. Morning hunger is a *disease under culture*, and they who feel the most need have the most reason to fast into higher health. They who claim that their breakfasts are their best meals, that they simply 'cannot do one thing' till they have eaten, are practically in line with those who must have their alcoholics before the wheels can be started.

"Now, it has been found by the experience of thousands that by wholly giving up the morning meal all desire for it in time disappears, which could hardly be the case if the laws of life were thereby violated—and the habit once fully eradicated is rarely resumed.

"To give up suddenly the use of alcoholics or of tobacco in any of its forms is to call out the loudest protests from the morbid voices that have been kept silent by those soothing powers—and yet no one would accept those loud voices as indicating an actual physiological need. The difficulties arising from giving up the morning meals—even as those from giving up the morning grog—are an exact measure of the need that they shall be given up in order that health, and not disease, shall be under culture. (pp. 98–101).

"The question is often asked me," says Doctor Dewey, again,[1] "whether it is safe for the old and infirm to abandon a lifelong eating habit for a method that requires that eating shall be regulated by the time of hunger, and not by the time of day. As well ask whether it is safe to abandon a lifelong habit of sin against a moral law by reason of age and infirmity. One can never get so old, never so infirm, as not to get an immediate change for the better, where there has been habitual sin against the Divine laws of digestion, and the older and the more infirm, so is the need more imperative."

The good effect which we receive from our breakfasts, then, are entirely due to *stimulation*—to the stimulating effects of the food, and to these only. And it becomes obvious also, that, when once the morbid cravings spoken of above have been subdued, and correct and favorable mental conditions substituted, mental and physical labor can both be performed with far greater ease than when a breakfast of any kind is eaten. A clearer head, greater nervous energy, increased vitality, and buoyancy of spirits, will be the invariable results of simply omitting this meal; theoretically this should be the case, and practically it is so in every one of the *scores* of cases I have known where this meal has been given up, either from choice or from necessity.[2] In every instance, too, has the person volunteered the remark that nothing could tempt him to return to the old practice of a hearty breakfast, or three meals a day. This in itself speaks volumes for the system, and the obvious benefits derived therefrom.

A most interesting point, in this connection, is the study of *instinct*. In healthy animals, especially, is this noticeable.

[1] "True Science of Living," pp. 317–18.

[2] Says Doctor Jackson ("Dyspepsia," pp. 8–9): "I have seen it (the two meal per day plan) tried by sick persons, *hundreds on hundreds*, and do not know of a single instance in which the customary method was preferred, after the new arrangement had become habitual." See also T. Owen's "How to Become Hale, Hearty, and Happy," p 3.

Thus Doctor Page cites the case of a foxhound in whom this instinct was very perfectly developed·[1]

"The old fellow, said the Captain, knows when I am going on a tramp, as well as my wife does—when I turn out for a hunt in the morning—and he won't touch a mouthful of food. I used to try and 'fool' him, by acting as if I wasn't going out at all, and sometimes I could get him to eat breakfast. But I never try that game now, for I noticed, after a while, that when he fixed himself, he did better work than when I managed to get breakfast into him."

In an article on "The Mystery of Migrations," printed in the *Saturday Evening Post* of August 22, 1903, it is stated that all migrating birds "let their last meal get thoroughly digested, that they may start on their long flight with empty stomach; that no power may be diverted to the digesting machinery of the stomach."

If the public would but recognize the fact that hunger must be invariably *earned* before it can normally appear, there would instantly disappear that prejudice against the omission of breakfast which is now prevalent and which is fostered and supported by medical teachings based on false theories as to the relations of food and energy. Were the principles outlined on pp. 225–303 fully recognized, there would be absolutely no excuse for the indulgence of this really depraved taste—except that of gluttony—disease under culture.[2]

We can now clearly see, for the first time, and in a rational light, the truth contained in the advice to "exercise on an empty stomach," *i.e.*, in the morning, before breakfast. Its object is to purposely and forcibly break down a certain amount of tissue which will call for replacement—in the shape of nutriment—thus creating an artificial call for food, and the possibility of digesting and utilizing it without actual damage done to the system. But would it not be far more normal and rational,

[1] "The Natural Cure," p. 199.

[2] Says Doctor Dewey ("True Science of Living," p. 170): "Most breakfasts are taken, not so much from any real want or pleasure, as to provide against a want before the ordinary time of the second meal—and so the hapless stomach is made the vehicle, and the very worst possible, for *carrying purposes* merely. No human stomach was ever made for a lunch pail to carry food in, before needed."

and at the same time save a vast amount of energy, to dispense with both the exercise and the meal—two excessive calls upon the bodily vitality? The usual practice necessitates the expenditure of a vast amount of energy, in order to digest the food material ingested; while the appetite and the ability to utilize this food have been artificially created by exercise—at the expense of more energy! Would it not be better, I ask, to wait until the normal activities of the day created a natural call for food—thus saving the energies which would otherwise be expended in two useless and even detrimental practices?

Thus far I have been considering the practice of two meals *per diem*, for the reason that this is the utmost amount of reform which we can hope to instigate, with any chance of meeting with general acceptance. The fact that it is a "physiological impossibility," as Mr. Haskell says,[1] for anyone to have this natural hunger more than twice a day;[2] the fact that the no-breakfast plan is now receiving a more ready acceptance than heretofore, and that its followers are now numbered by thousands—together with the fact that its physiology is unquestionable—all these reasons have led me, so far, to defend this system, and to take no note of the one-meal-a-day plan, which is receiving such wide acceptation.

Yet, the fact that a very large proportion of wild animals and very many domestic ones—eat but one hearty meal a day (or even more infrequently), would seem to indicate that man also might follow this course to advantage, could he but accustom himself to the change. In fact, a great many persons—some of them well known to the writer—are doing so continually. I myself live in that way half the time. "Few, in India especially, eat more than twice a day, and thousands only once," says Dr. Alice B. Stockham.[3]

"Two meals a day are enough," says Dr. Felix Oswald,[4] "perhaps more than enough, though we can accustom ourselves to swallow (not digest) five or six."

[1] "Perfect Health," p. 48.

[2] Says Doctor Page ("The Natural Cure," p. 118): "Conditions (of the organism) cannot obtain to the extent of rendering possible the digestion and absorption of three full meals a day." See also Rabagliati, "Aphorisms," etc., p. 31.

[3] "The Food of the Orient," p. 12.

[4] "Physical Education," p. 66.

There is little to choose between one hearty and two light meals a day, provided that approximately the same amount of food is eaten in both cases. On the two-meal system, the stomach is less liable to be filled to repletion, which might be the case on the one-meal plan; but, on the other hand, as Doctor Oswald and Mr. Macfadden have pointed out:[1]

"After a fast of twenty-two hours it is almost impossible to eat with relish more than the system can utilize in the course of a night and a day." "One meal a day is the life of an angel; two meals a day is the life of a man; three meals a day is the life of a beast."[2]

When really sick, of course, the amount eaten and the number of meals indulged in matter greatly; but, as before stated, there is little to choose between the above systems (the two- and the one-meal a day plan) provided there is a decided appetite for each meal, and the food is thoroughly masticated.

The objection is sometimes made that the one-meal plan would be less beneficial to the organism for the reason that it centers the work of the stomach too much at one time, while throughout the remainder of the day, it is virtually inactive. "Would it not be better," say these objectors, "to divide the work of this organ somewhat more evenly; giving the stomach a little more to do all the time—to "eat little and often"—rather than to force it to excessive labor at one period of the day, leaving it inactive for the remainder of the twenty-four hours?"

To this objection many hygienists have replied in forcible language. Says Doctor Dewey:[3]

"I would say at once that the idea was conspicuous for its ab sence of sound physiological knowledge of nutritive processes."

Doctor Rabagliati pointed out that meals taken near together allowed the digestion no rest,[4] which fact was insisted upon by Doctor Balbirnie[5] when he said:

[1] "Fasting, Hydropathy and Exercise," p. 24.
[2] "The Art of Living," by Ellen Goodell Smith, M.D., p. 16.
[3] "New Era for Woman," p. 235.
[4] "Aphorisms, Definitions, Reflections and Paradoxes," p. 234.
[5] "The Philosophy of the Water Cure," p. 76.

"The appetite is never natural, nor the digestion perfect, till the contents of the last meal are passed out of the stomach, and the ulterior stage of digestion is accomplished."

Doctor Pereira[1] stated that:

"It was found that when leopards and hyenas were fed with two meals daily they did not continue in equally good condition with those which had the same quantity of flesh food daily in one meal only"

In face of all this evidence, then, it can hardly be contended that the popular notion of eating "little and often" can be defended as having any true physiological basis for its practice, nor reason for its defense.

One more point must be touched upon, before closing this chapter. The last meal at night should invariably be light, and eaten at such an hour as to insure its perfect digestion before retiring. When the body is not in an erect posture the peristaltic motion in the stomach is not perfect, the dependent portions of the stomach being unduly affected by the weight of the food, from the force of gravity; moreover, in the lying posture, particularly during sleep, there is so little waste of tissue from cell destruction that there is very little if any need of food to replace the tissue-waste.

"Busch's experiments on a patient with fistula of the stomach demonstrated that the movements of the stomach and intestines were interrupted or more or less enfeebled during nocturnal sleep, while on the contrary they went on uninterruptedly if the patient slept in the course of the day."[2]

Dr. Dudley A. Sargent, also stated that:

"From the number of deaths that have resulted it has been found that it is an extremely hazardous thing to eat a very hearty meal just before retiring . . ."[3]

The fact that we should not work *this* muscle throughout the night, any more than any other muscle, should be so apparent as to need no further argument.

[1] "Food and Diet," p. 221.
[2] Virchow's "Archiv.," 1858, Bd. xlv. Quoted in M. de Manaceine's "Sleep," p. 17.
[3] "Health, Strength and Power," p. 151.

CHAPTER V

THEORY AND PHYSIOLOGY OF FASTING

We must now turn our attention from the facts supporting my theory to the theory itself, and discuss the philosophy of the system that seems to be so strongly borne out by the evidence so far examined. I propose to begin the discussion by a consideration of the normal processes of digestion, and what effects upon the system an excess of food material might be expected to have.

Our bodily tissues are made from the blood; the blood from the chyle; the chyle from the chyme; the chyme from the food (roughly speaking). At any stage in the process of digestion, therefore, if one of these becomes morbid or foul all become morbid and foul likewise. Similarly, if one of them is in excess, all are in excess, and grave results follow. A morbid excess of tissue in any part of the body must, therefore, depend directly for its formation, its nutrition and existence, upon the food eaten; and if this is unhealthful, or in excess, morbid tissues, excessive growths, etc., form—which are directly dependent for their existence, it will be seen, upon the bodily nutrition. We also see that, if only pure food were supplied, and only in sufficient quantity—just enough to exactly and evenly balance the bodily waste and repair—this morbid tissue, these excessive growths would be impossible; they are fed and sustained directly and solely by the excess of food ingested; by the overplus of food material within the system. We may now very readily see how it is that food taken in excess has the effect of directly *feeding the disease;* and conversely, it becomes apparent how, by fasting, we may thereby cure the disease (remove the cause) by withdrawing the nutriment upon which it has been dependent—by literally "starving it out."

Were there not, therefore, present within the organism an excessive amount of morbid, mal-assimilated food material, there could be no disease; all disease, rightly understood, being thus directly traceable to an abnormal and especially an excessive, alimentation. As Doctor Dewey so well said: "all disease originates in the digestive tract"—and indeed such is exactly the case.

Having previously arrived at the conclusion that the cause of every disease is the same—the retention within the organism of effete excrementous material that should have been eliminated—we are now in a position to see what this material is, and how it originates. *It is the excess of food material in a more or less advanced stage of putrefaction or decomposition!* How foul the system, then, which renders disease possible; how *disgraceful*, too, since gluttony, long and continuous, must have been practiced before any such condition be possible! Doctor Densmore made the remark that:

"Sickness and acute attacks of illness bear the same relation to diet that drunkenness bears to drink."[1]

And Doctor Dewey contended that:

"Every disease that afflicts mankind is a constitutional possibility developed into disease by more or less habitual eating in excess of the supply of gastric juice."[2]

Instead, therefore, of pitying those who suffer from disease, we should rather consider that they have brought such upon themselves, and we should rather *despise* them! Disease should be looked upon, not as an affliction, a "dispensation of Providence," but as a disgraceful thing, brought about by our own ignorance, or willful neglect of the fixed and unalterable laws of Nature. Doctor Rabagliati also takes this view; see his "Air, Food and Exercises," p. 335.

The whole trouble is that we are inclined to attribute to, and blame for our diseases, every conceivable *external* agency, rather than acknowledge that the cause of our diseased condition is violated natural law, which violations we ourselves have been guilty of; and consequently have brought upon ourselves

[1] "How Nature Cures," p. vii.
[2] "True Science of Living," p. 171.

the diseased condition present. We blame the weather, heredity, pre-natal influences, germs, insanitary surroundings, and, in fact, every conceivable external condition, that will enable us to escape the conclusion that we have ourselves to blame for our present condition, and ourselves only. It is an unpleasant truth we have to acknowledge; but, unfortunately for us, Nature clearly indicates that such is the case, by the constant infliction of disease and death—the results of violated law. The germ theory I have considered already. Insanitary surroundings are doubtless of very great moment, but I am persuaded that, if the body were kept in a normal, healthy condition, by proper management of the nutrition, living in the open air, etc., such surroundings would assume secondary, if not insignificant, proportions—as compared with the great question of internal cleanliness, or conditions. The application of these remarks to all *operations* may be obvious to the reader. The elaborate precautions at present in vogue would be largely unnecessary if the *internal* antiseptic condition of the body were better, and this receives indirect proof from the fact that those persons whose blood is in good condition recover more speedily and effectually from wounds, etc., than those whose blood is less pure. This was proved time and time again in the Russo-Turkish war, and lately, again, in the Russo-Japanese war. I hope to discuss this problem at greater length in another place. All this brings us to a highly important consideration. It is the question of the apparent causation of cancers and other malignant growths, by wounds, blows, bruises, etc., and the relation of the bodily condition thereto. I cannot stop to consider this question here; it will be found discussed in full in *Appendix J*.

Next let us consider this question of heredity, and its influence upon the health of the patient, and his freedom from disease. How willing we are to ascribe every evil to that little known factor in our lives; to blame every ill, every misery—which, by our transgressions of physiologic law, we have invariably brought upon ourselves—to heredity! Anything rather than acknowledge that we ourselves are to blame! Heredity has taken the place, in the public mind, which "a dispensation of Providence" held some years ago—and which is now rather out of date! Disease—the penalty of broken laws—is ascribed to heredity; the blame shifted to our parents, so that we ourselves may escape the just retribution of our own physiologic crimes. But Nature does not work in that way. No, it is exceedingly doubtful if disease, as such, is ever inherited—at least to any appreciable degree—save in some rare cases of blood poisoning. Doctor Rabagliati most forcibly combats this notion that disease is (as a rule, at any rate) transmitted, and, in his chapter on "Heredity," clearly demonstrated that such is very rarely the case. In Ribot's book on "Heredity," and works of a kindred nature, it is so far assumed that heredity of disease is a proved fact that 'it is hardly worth while discussing the question;' but that such is by no means the case can be seen by anyone looking at the question from another standpoint. I cannot stop to discuss that question now; I merely remark, in passing, that the solution of the difficulty is to be found, in practically every case, in the simple fact that like causes, acting on two or more individuals, produced like effects.

But even supposing that such *has* been the case; that disease —or the causes of disease—*have* been transmitted to the offspring; what then? We have seen that there is no such thing as an incurable disease (p. 67); all diseases are curable, if treated properly. What may be cured in the father may be cured in the son, therefore; especially since we know that *all disease has a tendency to decrease in virulence with every generation removed from the original infection.* It will always be far *easier*, therefore, for us to cure a case of hereditary disease than an original case; and since these (except in the very last states) can always be cured; hereditary disease can always be still more surely and rapidly cured. What, then, becomes of heredity, and its much dreaded dangers? Is this not only another medical bugaboo—serving merely to cover up and conceal our ignorance of the nature of disease, and of its cure?

There remains for our consideration only the effects of the weather. On this interesting subject I must here content myself with the following brief remarks.

Professor Dexter, in summarizing the results of his researches, thus speaks of the general weather influences on the health.

"Sickness and death are generally more prevalent during the winter and early spring months, though the latter (death) is tremendously increased by the intensely hot spells of the summer; sickness is aggravated by low temperatures, which do not much influence the death rate. The latter is, however, sent up by great heat; sickness is far above the normal during low barometrical conditions, and somewhat above for the other extreme. Both it and death show deficiencies for low humidities, with excess for high, though the effects are not very pronounced; both are above the normal for calms; below for moderate winds; and again above for greater velocities; both are excessive for cloudy, wet days."[1]

It is to be noted that the death rate is increased more during the hot spells of the summer than by any other influences. But I venture to think that Doctor Page had the right interpretation of this fact when he said:

"That the hot weather had much to do with this fearful slaughter of the innocents (babies) there can be no doubt, but, let us ask, does this more than express the simple fact, though in misleading terms, that *the excess of food that can be tolerated under the tonic and antiseptic influence of cold weather engenders disease during the heated term?*"[2]

Even in the hottest climates, such as India, it is acknowledged that overfeeding, rather than the actual temperature, is the cause (or at least the chief cause) of the diseases prevalent there. As Sir J. Fayrer, M.D., F.R.S., etc., said:[3]

"The power of tolerating climatic influence is great, if care be taken to observe simple hygienic rules. . . . As a general rule, people eat too much in India—more than they can assimilate, or is needed for nutrition. The consequence is derangements of digestion, faulty assimilation, disorganized liver, and engorged portal system, bowel complaints, and the presence of effete matter in excess in the blood. It is reported of an Irish soldier that he said, in reference to the evil effects of climate on his comrades—'They eat and they drink, and they drink and

[1] "Weather Influences," by Edwin G. Dexter, Ph.D., p. 197.
[2] "How to Feed the Baby," p. 47.
[3] "On Preservation of Health in India," p. 21.

they eat, and they write home and say it was the climate that killed them.' The soldier was not so far wrong in his estimate of the part climate plays, though he put it *more hibernico.*" (p. 10).

As for climatic influences, it is doubtful, I think, if they, as a rule, ever influence anyone to the extent that is commonly supposed. For, as Mr. I. P. Noyes pointed out:[1]

"If 'Low' remained in one place for months or even weeks there might be some reason for believing it to be the cause of disease; but 'Low' is ever on the move—not remaining long in one locality—passing over well-known healthy localities as well as over localities said not to be healthy, and instead of being a non-healthy agent, or a generator of disease, it is the agent that purifies the air by keeping it ever in motion, thereby preventing it from becoming impure and hurtful to us."

The truth of the matter is this: Climatic changes and conditions alter or influence us, but *only to the extent that the body is susceptible to such influence;* that is, the climatic changes merely modify an organism which has been brought into its present condition by its food and other habits. The organism is there —the result of its previous habits of life, and among them, and most important of all, are the food habits. The modifications such a body may receive from the climatic changes are only slight and are *inciters* rather than true causes. As Doctor Trall put it:[2]

"Sudden and extreme changes of weather are the exciting causes of many diseases; but they would be comparatively harmless did not the predisposition to disease exist as the consequence of our erroneous habits of living"

With this I dismiss that portion of the subject.

We are now free to discuss the question of the causation or evolution of disease. Doctor Dewey states the position clearly, in his "No-Breakfast Plan," pp. 70–3, and I quote from that book, omitting part of the passage in question:

"It is my impression that, with rare exceptions, people are born with actual structural weaknesses, local or general, that

[1] "How to be Weather Wise," p. 13. [2] "Popular Physiology," p. 214.

may be called ancestral legacies. These are known as constitutional tendencies to disease. In parts structurally weak at birth the blood vessels, because of thin and weak walls, are larger than in the normal parts, and because of dilation the blood circulates slower. There is an undue pressure upon all between-vessel structures—a pressure that must lessen the nutrient supply more or less, according to its degree. The death of parts in boils and abscesses is due, I believe, to strangulation of the nerve supply. The blood vessels are elastic, and capable of contraction and dilation, a matter regulated by the brain.

"Now, in these weaknesses always lie the possibilities of disease; they may be supposed the weak links in the constitutional chain, and can no more be made stronger than the constitutional design than can the body as a whole. By whatever means brain-power is lessened, abnormality is incited in the weak parts; hence gradually from the original weakness there is a summing-up as a bronchial or nasal catarrh, or other acute or chronic local or general disease.

"The first step in any disease is the impression that lessens brain power; the slightest depressing emotion, the slightest sense of discomfort, lessens brain power, and to a like degree, the tone of all the blood vessels; hence, dilatation in degree. That the stomach, as the most abused organ of the body, plays the largest part in over-drafts upon the brain is not a matter of doubt."

Says Dr. Shew:

"The principle on which the hunger cure acts is one on which all physiologists are agreed, and one which is readily explained and understood. We know that in animal bodies, the law of nature is for the effete, and worn out, and least vitalized matter first to be cast off. We see this upon the cuticle, nails, hair, and in the snake casting off his old skin. Now, in wasting or famishing from want of food, this process of elimination, and purification, goes on in a much more rapid manner than ordinarily, and the vital force which would otherwise be expended in digesting the food taken, acts now in expelling from the vital domain whatever morbific matters it may contain. This, then, is a beautiful idea in regard to the hunger-cure; *that whenever a meal of food is omitted, the body purifies itself thus much from its disease,* and it becomes apparent in the subsequent amendment both as regards bodily feelings and strength. It is proved also in the fact that during the prevalence of epidemics those who have been obliged to live almost in a state of starvation, have been free from attacks while the well-fed have been cut off in numbers by the merciless disease."[1]

We are now able to appreciate the value of the fasting cure. By depriving the body for a time of the supply of food material it has been continually receiving in excess, we give the eliminating organs a chance to "catch up," so to speak; to expel, unhampered, the overload of superfluous impurities the body contains. It is merely the process of purification, and, as such, is a true, a quick and an effectual method of cure.

Doctor Oswald and Mr. Macfadden supply us with a very simple statement of the facts that take place, during the fast, as follows:

"Denutrition, or the temporary deprivation of food, exercises an astringent influence as part of its general conservative effect. The organism, stinted in its supply of vital resources, soon begins to curtail its current expenditure. The movements of the respiratory process decrease; the temperature of the body sinks; the secretion of bile and uric acid is diminished, and before long the retrenchment of the assimilative functions reacts on the intestinal organs; the colon contracts and the smaller intestine retains all but the most irritating ingesta."

As will be seen later, my own observations do not altogether agree with these of our authors.

We thus reach the point at which we are capable of appreciating two grand truths; *first*, that, during a fast, the energy which was previously utilized in the digestion of food material is now set at liberty, and may be used, to cure the body; and, *second*, that during a fast the useless, the dead, the excrementous matter is always *first* eliminated—leaving the healthy tissue *in statu quo*—freed, moreover, from the presence of the effete, disease-producing material. "*Take away food from a sick man's stomach*," says Doctor Dewey, "*and you have begun, not to starve the sick man, but the disease*."[2] Or, as Hippocrates put it: "the more you nourish a diseased body, the worse you make it."

[1] "The Hydropathic Family Physician," p. 797.
[2] "True Science of Living," p. 5.

I shall now proceed to prove this a little more in detail, and to show that fasting is beneficial, and nothing but beneficial, in its effects upon the organism; that by striking at the root, the real cause, of the disease; by giving the eliminating organs a chance to expel the overload of impurities the body contains; we thereby remove the *cause* of the disease and hence effect a true and lasting cure. We purify the blood, and we thereby cleanse every tissue and fiber of the body. We purify it throughout, and, as Doctor Trall well said: "Purification is the one thing needed." Further, I shall endeavor to prove that the body invariably loses in time of sickness not healthy, but morbid, tissue; and when nothing but healthful tissue is left, hunger returns; the fast is ended; the disease is cured.[1]

In a most readable article on "The Fasting Cure," in *Good Health*, for January, 1905, pp. 1–5, Dr. J. H. Kellogg draws an interesting parallel between the body, during a fast, and a furnace run short of fuel, and shows, most clearly, that in both cases it is the *useless* material that is consumed, or burned up, before the more useful (the healthy tissue in the latter case), is attacked. He says in part:

"If there should be a fuel famine, the first thing you would do would be to rake over the ash heap and take out all the cinders that had been carelessly thrown there. The next thing would be to look round for waste papers, old boxes, and other useless things; all the odds and ends you could find would be put into the furnace to keep the fire going. If the famine should continue, you might be forced to burn up some of the furniture. One of our Arctic explorers burned up part of the ship's staterooms in order to keep warm in a very long winter. This sort of thing is just what happens when a person fasts. When he does not have his regular meals, he soon begins to feed upon himself. After a day or two, he no longer feels hungry. The body says, metaphorically, it is of no use to call for food, for none is supplied, I will seize on something else, close at hand.

"The body draws from its stored resources; every particle of fat will be utilized; then all the cinders—the half-burned fuel

[1] For a fuller discussion and elaboration of these difficult and much misunderstood points, see Chapter "When and How to Break the Fast," pp. 540–71.

that has accumulated in the body. Food that has come into the body partially digested, imperfectly burned, and left as cinders is seized upon and utilized.

"Uric acid, a product of proteid metabolism, is the body's cinders.[1] A man can consume, profitably, only an ounce and a half of proteids per day, but ordinarily from three to five ounces per day are eaten. All the books say that three or four ounces are necessary to keep a man healthy. The army rations supplv four or five ounces, which is a great excess. The majority of people are eating two or three times as much as they need, and the consequence is that they cannot utilize it all, and it accumulates in the

[1] This question of uric acid is now attracting a great deal of attention—owing, largely, to the laborious and persistent work of Dr. Alexander Haig, in whose "Uric Acid in the Causation of Disease," is to be found much interesting material as well as in his smaller books, "Food and Diet," and "Uric Acid: An Epitome." Doctor Haig showed conclusively the disastrous effects of excessive uric acid in the system, and the fact that excessive meat eating was the principal cause of such acidity. He also proved that (strange as it may appear) one great means of ridding the system of the acid is by the drinking of large quantities of lemonade! ("Food and Diet," p. 58.)

It is possible, however, that this uric acid idea has been pushed too far of late. Dr. H. Lahmann ("Natural Hygiene," p. 76), pointed out that: "Recent researches show that uric acid arises from the decay of cell nuclei. That portion of uric acid which has its origin in the digestive organs is, like other alloxanic bases, changed into urea, or rather should be. But a diseased liver, or a healthy one which is overworked owing to an excessive ingestion of food containing cell nuclei and therefore an excessive amount of uric acid, is unable to transform all the uric acid formed into urea."

This uric acid question is well summed up by Doctor Rabagliati in his "Air, Food and Exercises," pp. 309–10, when he says:

"Neither the muscles nor their sheaths will work smoothly or easily, and the sensation of fatigue is really caused mainly because the muscles are loaded with bad blood containing ptomaines and other unassimilated materials. The blood is said to contain uric acid. No doubt it often does, but it is very unlikely that uric acid is the only poison carried by the blood to the tissues in such circumstances. No doubt other materials besides uric acid are present, some of them known to chemists as *e.g.*, lactic acid, and very probably others as yet unknown. In fact, uric acid stands mainly as a symbol or sign of imperfectly oxidized and imperfectly assimilated products of digestion, and it is these in their totality or aggregate which poison and fatigue the muscles and the whole locomotor mechanism."

There is one most significant fact in this connection, which strongly supports the view taken. I quote the following from Doctor Haig's "Etiology, Prevention, and Treatment of a Common Cold," pp. 5–6; the significance of the facts will be appreciated by all those who have grasped the philosophy of the treatment, by fasting, as outlined in this book. It is: ". . . The other important solvent of uric acid which acts in the same way is alkali, and we all know that the old treatment of rheumatism before salicylates were known was that of alkali. Here there is one physiological fact which we must bear in mind, and that is, that *a low diet is equivalent to a dose of alkali*, because diminishing food diminishes the acidity of the urine, and the alkalinity of the blood is at the same time increased, for diminishing food diminishes the formation of acid products in the body; hence diminished food is equivalent to a dose of alkali, and conversely, it is quite useless to give small doses of alkali while feeding the patient up on full diet."

body as half-burned material—just as cinders will collect from the furnace until you cannot get air through the grate. You have to remove them before you can get a good bright fire burning. Fasting gives the body a chance to clear up all the unnecessary material, which it will do before it will begin to consume the vital tissues. It is exactly the same principle that you follow in your house when you have a coal famine; before you burn up the bric-a-brac and the furniture, you get rid of all the rubbish and unnecessary things. . . . There is really only one benefit that is gained by fasting and that is getting rid of the cinders, the uric acid, the proteid waste of the body."

Doctor Graham, so long ago as 1843, wrote:[1]

"It is a general law of the vital economy, that when, by any means, the general function of decomposition exceeds that of composition or nutrition, the decomposing absorbents always first lay hold of and remove those substances which are of least use to the economy; and hence, all morbid accumulations, such as wens, tumors, abscesses, etc., are rapidly diminished and often wholly removed under severe and protracted abstinence and fasting. The eliminating organs of the system will first be employed in removing the adipose matter, in order to restore the system to the most perfectly healthy condition.

"The accumulation of adipose matter in the human body, therefore, always evinces more or less diseased action in the general function of nutrition, and can only be carried to a very limited extent without degenerating into serious disease, terminating either in morbid obesity, dropsy, or apoplexy, or reacting with violence on some of the organs belonging to the digestive apparatus."

This is a much misunderstood question, and these facts—their vast and far-reaching significance and applicability—have never been fully appreciated before; but that they *are* facts, I shall endeavor to prove, more abundantly, as we proceed—though direct experiment would soon settle the question beyond controversy.

From the facts and arguments I have presented, we are enabled to grasp one very important idea—one that many persons

[1] "Science of Human Life," pp. 194-5.

overlook and even doubt. It is that fasting is a great deal more complicated than is commonly supposed; than is involved in the mere idea of "going without food." It must be remembered that there is a *science* of fasting (as I shall hereinafter endeavor to prove), which we are just now beginning to realize. Fasting rightly applied is an extremely potent and far-reaching method of cure; of its therapeutic value I cannot, indeed, see the limit, while its dangers are so slight, so insignificant—as compared with any other method of cure—as to be altogether unworthy of consideration. But fasting should be applied by skilled hands; or rather, practiced only under the close supervision and observation of one skilled in this method of cure; one who thoroughly understands the *philosophy* of the treatment, and who has unlimited faith in its effectiveness. The average physician is no more qualified to undertake the supervision of a protracted fast than is any other man who has a good working knowledge of physiology; the theories involved are as new to him as to the merest layman—and I cannot, consequently, too strongly advise anyone who contemplates undertaking a fast of any length to do so only under the supervision of some reputable *hygienic* physician, and moreover, one who is thoroughly familiar with the theory and phenomena of fasting. For, as above stated, fasting is far more than merely "going without food"; many more factors must be taken into consideration than this one. The amount of daily exercise to be undertaken; the question of water drinking; of enemas; of bathing, breathing, and a hundred and one minor—but highly important—factors must be reckoned with—if the fast is to be conducted easily and satisfactorily. Such information this book will set forth at length and, I believe, for the first time—since no work has heretofore appeared which contains this information in anything like a connected and practical form. I venture to hope that this knowledge will be of considerable benefit to the human race; for, having the faith I have in this system of medication, I cannot but believe that benefit will follow from its practice—whenever or wherever adopted.

Doctor Dewey thus relates the incidents that led up to his discovery of the fasting cure—one that will shortly be recognized, I believe, as the greatest of modern times, but which may be looked upon, it will be seen, as almost accidental. Thus, after relating one or two most interesting cases of health having been restored by *in*voluntary fasting (that is, cases in which fasting was rendered necessary by the condition of the patient), and of his growing interest in such cases, together with his increasing conviction that here was a most important, though all but unrecognized physiological law in operation, which must, if true, ultimately revolutionize the care of the sick, Doctor Dewey goes on to say:[1]

"As the months and years went on, it so happened that all my fatalities were of a character as not to involve in the least any suggestion of starvation, while the recoveries were a series of demonstrations, as clear as anything in mathematics, of evolving strength of all the muscles, of all the senses and faculties, as the disease declined. No physician whose practice has been extensive has failed to have had cases in which the same changes occurred, and in which the amount of food taken did not explain this general increase of strength.

"Believing that I had made a most important discovery in physiology—one that would revolutionize the dietetic treatment of the sick, if not ultimately abolish it, my visits to the sick became of unsurpassed interest. I watched every possible change as an unfolding of new life, seeing the physical changes only as I would see the swelling buds evolve into the leaves or flowers—reading the soul- and mind-changes in the more radiant lines of expression.

"I saw all these things with the naked eye, and more and more marvelled at the bulk of our materia medicas; the size of our drug stores, and the space given to healing powers in all public and medical prints.

"For years I saw my patients grow into the strength of health without the slightest clue to the mystery until I chanced to open a new edition of Yeo's "Physiology" at the page where I found this table of the estimated losses that occur in death after starvation:[2]

Fat............................	97%
Muscle..........................	30%

[1] "No-Breakfast Plan," pp. 31–33.

[2] This table agrees exactly with the figures given by other authorities; see, *e.g.*, Wesley Mills, "Animal Physiology," p. 451.

Liver. 56%
Spleen. 63%
Blood. 17%
Nerve centers. . . . . .0 !!!

"And light came as if the sun had suddenly appeared in the zenith at midnight. Instantly I saw in human bodies a vast reserve of predigested food, with the brain in possession of power so to absorb and to maintain structural integrity in the absence of food, or power to digest it. This eliminated the brain entirely as an organ that needs to be fed or that *can* be fed, from the light-diet kitchens, in times of acute sickness. Only in this self-feeding power of the brain is found the explanation of its functional clearness where bodies have become skeletons.

"I could now go into the rooms of the sick with a formula that explained all the mysteries of the maintenance and support of vital diseases that was of practical avail. *I now knew that there could be no death from starvation until the body was reduced to the skeleton condition,*[1] that, therefore, for structural integrity, for functional clearness, the brain has no need of food when disease has abolished the desire for it. Is there any other way to explain the power to make wills with whispering lips in the very hour of death—even in the last moments of life, that the law recognizes as valid?

"I could now know that to die of starvation is a matter, not of days, but of weeks and months—certainly a period far beyond the average time of recovery from acute disease."

Before proceeding, one or two points in the above argument might call for some elaboration and addition. The point here made, that is is *physiologically impossible* to starve to death until the skeleton is reached (and by this is meant the mere weight of the skeleton and viscera), is one of the very greatest, but as yet least understood, truths before the world to-day.

The objection will be made, perhaps, that cases are on record in which persons *have* starved to death long before this skeleton condition has been reached; while there was still considerable flesh on the body, and, indeed, within a few days—which would seem at first sight to disprove the theory. Upon actual investi-

[1] "It has been estimated that strong adults die when they lose four-tenths of the body weight," Mills: "Animal Physiology," p. 452.

gation, however, it will be found that such cases are extremely few and far between; are very rare exceptions, rather than the rule. I have myself tried for many months to discover one such case, that rested upon respectable evidence, without success. But, did such cases actually exist, they might, I think, be easily accounted for. In such cases, it is not the fasting, but the *mental conditions*—fear, etc.—which have killed the patient. It might be objected that this is practically an impossibility; is at least highly improbable. I ask, why so? Have not individuals, through grief, fear, etc., worried themselves into the grave, within a few days—even under normal conditions? Aye, do we not know cases in which instantaneous death has resulted from the mere reading of a telegram? There is no assignable limit to the powers of the mind on such occasions.

Doctor Schofield, in his book, "The Unconscious Mind," (pp. 360–2), has recorded a number of cases in which severe illness and even death has resulted—in some cases instantaneously—from mental shock. In the *Lancet*, 1867, is the case of a woman who died in a fit when her daughter, whom she supposed had been killed in a wreck, walked in upon her suddenly. Doctor Sweetser tells of a lady who, feeling a living frog fall into her bosom, from the clutches of a bird, was seized with such profuse hæmotysis that she lived only a few minutes. Doctor Lys tells us of a man suffering from angina, who dropped down dead in a fit of anger at St. George's Hospital. Many other cases of a similar character are to be found in the works of Hack Tuke, W. B. Carpenter, etc. On the other hand, there are cases of remarkable *cures* having been performed; notably the various "miraculous" cures, etc. I have discussed these at some length elsewhere, however. Camille Flammarion quotes several cases in which rheumatism, and other diseases have been cured as the result of a flash of lightning. Cases of paralysis have also been cured in this manner. See his "Thunder and Lightning," p. 118.

Now as to the fasting cases. I have long contended that a patient might starve to death in a certain number of days, if he only thought he might do so; and fast with benefit an equal number of days, if he but understood the theory of fasting, and was not afraid of starving to death. Recently I have come across a proof of this view in the case of Miss Marie Davenport Vickers, who fasted forty-two days, into health (April 19—June 1, 1904), and, in writing of her fast, and her experiences at other times while fasting, she volunteered the following interesting and significant remarks:

"We hear so much of people starving to death after only two or three days abstinence from food, that the impression is given the public that one is liable to starve to death during a prolonged fast. The latter is not possible while the former is, for starving and fasting are not the same, and the action of the mind in these two conditions is entirely different. To prove my assertion, I am tempted to give a bit of personal experience that came into my life before I ever heard of fasting, except that mentioned in the Bible: twice I was forced to go hungry for some days owing to lack of funds with which to purchase food, *and I did almost starve to death.* The mind was so oppressed that I could see no way out of the difficulty, and felt sure I never would have anything again; still, tenacity to life, the incentive to 'hold on' in spite of hardship, kept me from going to pieces until things could take another turn. Of course, this was long before we knew anything of breathing, or that one could survive for weeks, even months without food. During a voluntary fast the mind is at rest. The bare fact that we know there are 'no strings on us,' that, if we feel we can not carry out the fast, we can go and eat, relieves the mind of all tension. And I know of no other time when one is so rested, mentally and physically."[1]

So that I am surely justified in my contention that the cause of death, in such cases of fasting as those narrated, is mental; both for the above reasons, and because we have seen, and shall more abundantly prove, that actual starvation within so short a time is a *physiological impossibility.*

Proof that the brain does not become starved, or shrunken, one iota, during a fast of however long duration, is to be found in the following quotation from the "New Era for Women," pp. 37–87. Says Dr. Dewey:

"(*a*) In all post-mortems, no matter how wasted the body, the brain is found to fill the cranial cavity when not itself diseased.

[1] *The Mazdaznan*, February, 1906, p. 28.

"(*b*) The mind is often clear to the last moment of life, even when the body has become emaciated to the skeleton degree. This could not be if the brain had become emaciated.

"(*c*) The tissues do disappear during sickness and what becomes of them, if they are not used to feed the brain and perhaps also the heart and lungs—for these never reveal any appreciable loss during disease, when they themselves are not diseased?

"(*d*) For eighteen years, while in continuous attendance on the acutely sick, I have in every case permitted the brain to feed itself in its own way, and in not a single case where death was not beyond all question inevitable did it fail to do itself ample justice, and in some cases for four, five, six weeks, and even longer!

"(*e*) And in strong support of the conception of this wonderful power of the brain has been the fact that as disease declined, mental, moral and physical energy *increased.* What better feeding of the sick can a rational human being ask for than the feeding that Nature prescribes; and that it should be such, it has placed a sentinel at the danger point in the garb of a food-loather, to shield the reparative processes while the battle with disease is going on."

Professor Mosso completely confirms and agrees with this statement. Thus, in his "Fatigue," p. 285, he writes:

"When the body is receiving no nutriment, the less important are sacrificed to the more important tissues in the combustion which must finally destroy life. To the very last moment as long as there is any possibility of life being saved, all the organs give of their substance, save the heart and the brain; and even when the heart has been reduced by hunger to desperate straits, and the temperature of the blood has fallen to 30 degrees, the cardiac contractions having become both weaker and less frequent, even then this organ, which was the first to give any sign of life, will continue faithful to its duty to the end, and will collect the last remains of energy from the wasted organs, to transmit them to the brain. And the final transference, the final cession of living material from the body to the brain will be made with the final systole of the heart. Marvelous example of an arrangement in which the supremacy of the intellect is respected and maintained to the last in the midst of that most terrible of destructions—death by starvation!"

To proceed with the argument: Let it be granted that the brain and nervous system do not, and cannot, shrink or lose weight during a fast of however long duration, and consequently that their functional capacity is unimpaired; also that they possess the ability, as they most obviously do and must, to feed themselves at the expense of the rest of the organism—the less necessary and vital parts, and the question at once arises: what can we feed? In health and under normal conditions our chief (or as I claim—*v.* pp. 248–9 our *only*) need for food is to supply tissue that has been broken down by exercise—the wastes of the general activities—and, as Doctor Dewey points out:

"This is a process in the order of Nature that actually tires the entire brain system, or, in a common phase, the whole body, unless the stomach has powers not derived from the brain system." (p. 38).

Again, he says ("True Science of Living," p. 95):

"If Nature were able to support vital power unaided in so severe and prostrating a disease as typhoid fever, (a case had just been given) why should she not be able to do the same in other, in all other, severe diseases?"

But how much activity is there as a rule during disease? Practically none at all! In many cases the patient is even too weak to move hand or foot, to turn over in bed; and yet the daily feedings are continued as though the patient were still performing a hard day's work! Should it not be obvious that this cannot be other than injurious in its effects upon the system? The most respected medical writer in England, upon the question of diet—Sir Henry Thompson—in his two books "Food and Feeding" and "Diet in Relation to Age and Activity"—was particular to point out, over and over again, and to insist upon the truth of the statement that the "income" should be exactly proportionate to the "outgo"—*i.e.*, that the amount of food daily consumed should be exactly proportional to the amount of daily exercise. As that is increased, the food may be increased, and *vice versa*.

And this fact (that the income should always be proportioned to the outgo) is one of cardinal importance—one whose importance it would be impossible to overestimate. If the exercise is abundant, a considerable bulk of food is necessary, in order to replace the tissue destroyed; if but a moderate amount is indulged in, only a moderate quantity of food should be eaten daily; and if but a very small amount of exercise be taken daily (the case with most of us), then only a very small quantity indeed is required to replace the almost insignificant amount of tissue destroyed. (It must always be remembered that a *little* tissue is destroyed in the very process of living.) If people once realized that they should gauge the bulk of food daily consumed by the amount of tissue broken down, and then realize what a very little that really is, they would surely appreciate the enormous extent to which everyone of us overeats, and that habitually. It should be doubly clear, also, that in all cases of sickness, where the vital energies (and consequently the powers of digestion) are low, the amount of tissue destroved is practically *nil.*

Yet how seldom do we find that great rule obeyed! Indeed, we almost invariably find the person of sedentary habits has the most voracious and abnormally excessive appetite (as judged from the standards of the amount the body actually requires), while the active outdoor worker is content with a comparatively far less amount of food than the former. This is because the latter's appetite is more normal and true to his instincts, whereas the former's is more perverted and unnatural.

And do we not constantly see patients fed even *more* during disease than their customary amount?—in order to "keep up the strength"—quite ignoring the great, far-reaching truth, that "*disease, in proportion to its severity, means the loss of digestive conditions and of digestive power.*" The stomach cannot digest, the intestines cannot convert, the glands cannot absorb this excessive amount of food material. Yet something must be done with it, or we die! At the expense of the whole of our bodily energies, then, this mass of ingesta is actually forced along, and out of, the intestinal canal, now rendered quite incapable of successfully handling or receiving benefit or nutriment from this mass of worse than useless material. Doctor Latson has so well described the conditions that do and must prevail under such circumstances, that I cannot do better than to quote the not very edifying picture he draws; as follows:

"Imagine the complex mass of solid and liquid matter, comprising an average meal, undigested, fermenting, putrefying, passing slowly down the digestive tube thirty feet long at the rate of perhaps two feet in an hour. As it passes along, growing constantly more and more offensive and poisonous, the walls of the tube, true to their function, absorb, absorb—not food, mind you, which they ought to get; which the body needs for its maintenance—not food but the poisons resulting from the decomposition going on in the mass. Thus in the dyspeptic, the body is at once starved and poisoned.

"Even more, it is overworked, for it is only by the greatest activity of the liver, and other organs, in antidoting the deadly effects of the absorbed poisons that life is preserved. Sometimes, owing to weakness or fatigue, those organs cannot counteract that effect of the absorbed poison. Death is then the result. 'The man who came home tired and ate a hearty meal of ham, bread and butter, pickles and several glasses of milk, died—died because his tired organs could not fight the poisons formed within his body. The cause of this man's death was given as 'heart failure.' The term 'heart failure' is too often merely a scapegoat. The heart fails because the nervous system which actuates it fails, and the nervous system fails because it is poisoned through the absorption into the blood of the toxic matters formed in the alimentary tube."[1]

As Doctor Bellows said:[2]

"We may not be able perfectly to understand the cause of all these different difficulties or diseases of the heart; but they are all undoubtedly connected with erroneous diet or erroneous habits, for other animals in their native conditions have none of these troubles or diseases, although the circulation is affected by the same mechanical arrangement."

That this is the true explanation of many cases of heart failure there can be no doubt. It may be thought that a poison would not act in this manner, but we have the very positive evidence that it does in cases of "tobacco heart"; where the

[1] "Common Disorders," by W. R. C. Latson, M.D., pp. 119-20.
[2] "Philosophy of Eating," p. 401.

effects of the nicotine poisoning are extremely noticeable, and even generally acknowledged. The parallel in these cases is very striking—both resulting from the long-continued abuse of the organism in the form of a daily, but miniature addition to the poisons collected in the system. And this accumulation may go on till death results. Says Dr. J. D. Malcolm:[1]

"It is conceivable that death may be produced almost with the suddenness of shock. In accordance with this view we know that, in scarlet fever, *e.g.*, a fatal result is sometimes brought about by the poison before any pathognomonic signs of the disease show themselves, while the cold state of cholera may develop and prove fatal within a very short time."

The fact that "Japanese vital statistics will show that heart disease and nervous prostration are almost unknown as causes of death,"[2] where the diet is so simple and abstemious strongly confirms this view.

It will thus be seen—and I wish my readers to particularly remember this far-reaching and fundamentally important point—that food, eaten during diseased conditions, *does not nourish the patient*, but that it does, on the contrary, have the directly opposite effect—of *starving, poisoning and weakening him.*

Says Doctor Page:[3]

"From the observation of a number of cases I came to the conclusion that languor and faintness of which many patients complain . . . is due to the products of digestion of breakfast and lunch. The only chance for the patient's possible recovery, therefore, and for a return of his health and strength, is a withdrawal of the cause of these abnormal conditions, of the excess of food present in the system, giving rise to such disease-provoking conditions, and this can best be done, of course, by fasting. The term 'starvation cure' is both misleading and disheartening to the patient; in fact, he is both starved and poisoned by eating when the hope of digestion and assimilation is prohibited, as is in great measure the case in all acute attacks, and more especially when there is nausea or lack of appetite;

[1] "Physiology of Death from Traumatic Fever," p. 127.
[2] "Japanese Physical Training," p. 56.
[3] "Natural Cure," p 60.

and he can only escape from the danger by abstaining temporarily."

The one great truth upon which depends my argument, very largely, and which the medical profession, as well as the world at large, has failed to grasp, is that, as the body is only as strong at its weakest link; if it is weakened and devitalized by disease, *so is every organ and function weakened and devitalized to precisely the same extent.*

Each organ becomes weakened and incapable of performing its legitimate duties, just in proportion to the general lack of vitality, of tone, and the extent of the diseased condition of the organism. The more diseased the organism, the weaker must be the functioning power of each and every organ, and as the diseased organ or part should be made the standard of the ability of the system, the less work should it be called upon to perform—until healthy, normal conditions be restored. There can be no escaping the legitimacy of this conclusion.

Now, the stomach, is one very important organ, and that as "the stomach is but part of a man . . . and that while he suffers with it, it suffers with him";[1] and is, as we have already seen (pp. 102–4), a machine which must be run at a great expenditure of nervous energy, we must consider it as very intimately connected with the rest of the organism and its functionings. Why, therefore, coax or force this organ to perform its unusual duties, as when in the best of health?—aye, even forcing it to perform far *more* than is required of it in health (in feeding up the patient, in order to increase his strength)? Is it not most certain that this organ should be given its legitimate and much-earned rest, just as every other organ is permitted to rest—until normal conditions ensue? It should be apparent that this is the very worst time possible to practice enforced feeding, since the organ is weaker, and less capable of assimilating the food material ingested than at any other time. Yet this is the occasion selected for forced and artificial feeding, for extra meals—for richer foods! The stomach's prime need, at such a time, is *rest*—rest complete and absolute—for as many days *or*

[1] "How Can I Cure My Indigestion?" by A. K. Bond, M.D., p. 96

weeks as may be necessary for it to recover its lost tone and strength, and the capacity for properly assimilating food.[1]

A further analogy—which may help to make my meaning still clearer—is this. Whenever a machine of any kind is "out of order" and needs repairing, the first thing to do is, invariably, to *stop the machine.* Now, the human body is a machine, pure and simple (on its purely physiological side), and, in disease, it is out of order. What is more rational, therefore, than that we stop the machine (or stop it from working as much as we possibly can, at any rate) while the process of repair is progressing? The process of repair is the healing process; and one of the most important, all-involving and greatest taxes, or modes of work, which the human system ever undertakes, is the digestion and elimination of food material. Is it not obvious, there fore, that *this* work, this vital tax, should be stopped, as far as possible, while the process of cure is proceeding? Does not every analogy compel us to answer this in the affirmative?

Many persons refuse to enter upon a fast for the reason that they are, they assert, afraid of thus "experimenting" upon themselves—to "try such dangerous experiments," etc. Granting its possible utility in some cases, and that it is sound in its philosophy, they are still afraid to experiment upon themselves! This attitude strikes one as extremely ludicrous, because they are, all unknown to themselves, *continually* experimenting upon their own health in their daily lives; their modes of life being one incessant experiment upon their vitality and health! As Doctor Graham wrote, with his usual illumination:[2]

" It seems as if the grand experiment of mankind had ever been to ascertain how far they can transgress the laws of life, how nearly they can approach to the very point of death, and yet not die, at least so suddenly and violently as to be compelled to know that they have destroyed themselves."

[1] It must be distinctly understood that all stimulants of the appetite are bad—no matter how good these may be *per se.* Even sea bathing, *e.g.*, perhaps the best, is open to objection, since, as Dr. Ghislani Durant pointed out ("Sea Bathing," p. 43): "All who have practiced sea bathing know that one of the first effects is to increase the appetite; but, unfortunately, the digestive organs are not strengthened in the same proportion. . . . The stimulation produced by the sea air and the baths, on the stomach, does not augment the power of digestion in the same ratio as the appetite is provoked." (P. 58.)

[2] "Science of Human Life," p. 254.

And yet people are afraid to "experiment" with themselves, in trying this system of cure, which is philosophical from beginning to end, most common sense, and based on the exactest of physiology!

Doctor Keith in his chapter on "Natural Cravings and Dis likes"[1] writes as follows:

"A natural and sometimes extreme craving by the sick for some special food or means of relief is not uncommon, and it is usually looked upon as absurd and is disregarded."

He then gives several cases of remarkable cures having been effected by gratifying the desires of the patient no matter how whimsical they may have appeared, and indirectly states his conviction that such desires always express some organic need. This, I believe, is becoming to be more and more recognized and accepted. The cravings indicate some peculiar state of the body which the substance or the thing craved will satisfy or appease—just as water satisfies this craving in cases of fever. This is, as I say, coming to be generally recognized, but the *converse* of this is by no means seen or appreciated. Let me again quote Doctor Keith, where he says:

"If I am not much mistaken, a wider and more important subject is the converse of this craving for some specific means of relief. I mean the dislikes of the sick, especially of the food, but also to noise, motion, light or close air. In all these matters the invalid is, when it is possible, allowed to have his own way, except in the case of the most important of them all—his dislike for food. Here he is very much at the mercy of his doctors and his friends, and unless he has a very strong will, he must obey. He may, indeed, be a willing victim, so far as he can resist his natural antipathy, and supposed duty may induce him to take what he would much rather avoid. I have the strongest conviction, and that after more than forty years' experience, that the forced giving of food when it is not wanted is the cause of more misery, more aggravation of disease and greater shortening of life, than all other causes put together. This doctrine I have held absolutely for very many years—almost, indeed, from the beginning of my medical career."

[1] "Fads of an Old Physician," pp. 130–3.

Doctor Burney Yeo admits this aversion points to the inability of the patient to take food with profit.[1] Yet even this cannot be seen by many men, so perverted have their views become on this diet question. Thus, Dr. H. Partsch, in his "Sea Sickness" (p. 184), writes: "Man will eat from obvious necessity when food is repugnant . . ." Why must he do so, any more than any other animal? Is this not the result of the silly superstition that the stomach must not have a minute's peace, and that man will starve to death in a few days if food is withdrawn? It may be said, however, that all writers on this subject do not agree with this statement. Dr. Thomas Dutton, *e.g.*, says:[2]

"Strange to say, the officers and stewardesses, although they have had much experience in seasickness, generally make their passengers worse, and even undo the little good the surgeon may have done, by advising them to eat a good meal, bringing them this and that, persuading them to take a little. . . . I think there is nothing more disgusting as to persuade anyone to eat food, knowing that the same will be vomited immediately; and it does not require much common sense to know that Nature, by rejecting food, plainly shows she can not digest it."

As Doctor Shew so well remarked:

"Almost all persons are benefited by this affection. (Being really seasick) But how comes this benefit? It is by the beneficial power of fasting that the benefit of seasickness is caused. It is the law of Nature that when the body is wasted for a time, by want of food, it grows more pure. Nor does abstinence cause disease, as many suppose. A person who dies by starvation dies of *debility*, and not of disease. It is the purification of the system, then, that causes the benefit in seasickness; and this could be accomplished by suitable fasting, better without the reaching and vomiting than with them. But so good and useful are abstinence and fasting, it will repay one to take a voyage at sea, if he can be certain of becoming really sick, so that he will be compelled for a time to abstain wholly from food."[3] See *Appendix K*.

[1] "Food in Health and Disease," p. 303.
[2] "Sea Sickness," pp. 22–23.
[3] "Family Physician," pp. 300–301.

Many persons may have the idea that they will never become hungry, no matter how long they go without food. And to this Mr. Macfadden replies:

"You need not worry one moment about this. Fast from one to seven days, and there will not be the slightest doubt that your appetite will be resurrected in all its youthful intensity, and with this appetite will come renewed enjoyment of everything in life."[1]

Kneipp said: "Never urge a patient to eat."[2]

An objection often raised to this plan of frequently omitting a meal is that, if one meal is altogether omitted, the person so omitting it will get "so hungry" before the next. How dreadful! One would think that getting hungry was some frightful pestilence to be avoided, whereas this is exactly what we *should* experience before food is eaten—ever! Moreover, it is practically certain that in all such cases it is not hunger that is experienced at all, but a form of morbid irritation. (pp. 549–54). The practice of eating "a little something" to prevent the return of hunger cannot be too strongly deprecated. It is unphysiological and unhygienic in the last degree. It is, moreover, disease producing.

How simple it all is. Merely to wait till an appetite returns —knowing that it eventually will return and that, until it does so, the system does not require food and is much better off without it. There is no danger, no harm, practically no discomfort; while we know that, when hunger does return, it is a positive indication that food is needed and will be digested; moreover, the system is now in a condition of health.

Of course, as soon as any person is inclined to omit a meal, his friends or relatives at once endeavor to persuade him to change his mind—to "eat a little something" in order to "keep up his strength." (To keep himself weak and ill, in reality, if people once realized that truth!) "I am worried about so-and-so," one constantly hears, "he won't eat his meals at all; he has no appetite." Surely that is a clear indication that no food is needed! Listen to the voice of Nature! Meals eaten under such circumstances *do not nourish.* Let that fact be well

[1] "Virile Powers of Superb Manhood," p. 150.
[2] "My Water Cure," p. 352.

understood. On the contrary, food eaten at such a time does incalculable harm. As Doctor Oswald stated the case·[1]

"The overfed organism is under-nourished to a degree that reveals itself in the rapid emaciation of the patient."

What one should do, under such circumstances is simply to wait till Nature does call for food; omit a meal; two meals, three, a dozen, a score, if necessary; hunger will always come in time—when Nature demands her proper supply of food. There can be no risk, no danger, in such a wait; nothing but benefit can possibly result. Nature does not work against, but for, the welfare of the race, and it is always safe to heed her voice of counsel.

Take, for example, the following case, mentioned by Doctor Dewey, and quoted by Doctor Keith:[2]

"A boy of five had lost his appetite a year previously. All means were used for his relief by regular and homœopathic doctors, but he got worse and his food was regularly ejected shortly after it was eaten. All hope of recovery was lost, and, as a last resort, his father was carrying him to a consultation of several doctors. On the way a friend met him who had been cured after a much longer illness by Doctor Dewey, and he urged the father, weak as the boy was, to give him nothing till a desire for solid food returned. The doctor had faith in his friend, took his boy home, and gave him no food for four days. A beefsteak was now asked for and digested, and soon the boy was in the best of health, in which Doctor Dewey saw him five months later. 'This boy,' he remarked, 'had suffered a living death; week after week, month after month, and yet always within four days of a beefsteak appetite!'—a very natural remark, says Doctor Keith, but what a reflection on our science of medicine! Had the poor boy been let alone at first, till the dislike for food was changed into a natural desire for it—what an amount of suffering for him and anxiety for his parents, would have been prevented!"

The *rationale* of all this is simple enough. We know that as the body is enfeebled by disease, the digestive system must suffer proportionately, and become enfeebled also. As the nerve energy lessens—owing to the presence of diseased condi-

[1] "Household Remedies," p. 57.
[2] "Fads of an Old Physician," pp. 134–5.

tions, so does digestion become impossible; and, as the digestive juices are secreted in proportion to the needs of the organism, and not according to the amount of food ingested, food eaten under these circumstances is not and cannot be digested, and consequently cannot and does not nourish the organism. On the contrary, this food is mostly disposed of by decomposition—not digestion—and the pushing of this foul material through thirty feet of bowel must and does involve such a tremendous tax upon the vital powers that the patient unknowingly keeps himself worn out and emaciated—a clear example of the process of "starvation from overfeeding."

Says Doctor Keith:[1]

"In a very large proportion of cases they lose more or less their power of digesting food at all, or they do it in a very imperfect manner. Even when there is no structural change to be noted, the nervous force necessary to perfect digestion is wanting, and to take any food into the stomach can only do harm." "There can be no doubt that a simple and short case is often converted into a severe and long one by giving food when it is not wanted, and when it can be of no use." (p. 41.)

It will thus be seen how utterly fallacious is the idea that the strength is or can be in any way dependent upon the food eaten; at any rate, in anything like a proportionate degree. Food eaten under such circumstances *does not increase the strength*, and it certainly is not required for the maintenance of the bodily *heat*—since in all such cases a feverish condition is frequently, if not always, present.

"This (the giving of food in great quantities to the sick) they do on the false idea that it will 'support his strength,' and enable him to throw off the disease, whatever this may mean; or that it will at least retard the waste of the body. I have known for many years that there is no truth whatever in these ideas, and that on the contrary nothing causes more discomfort and weakness than taking food which cannot be digested, and which only adds to the matters which the system is busied in getting rid of."[2]

In an acute illness, enforced feeding is frequently resorted to because of the patient's loss of appetite, and in order to "keep

[1] "Plea for a Simpler Life," p. 35. [2] "Fads of an Old Physician," p. 150.

up his strength."[1] In such cases, the unwilling stomach often rejects the meal immediately it is swallowed; yet the feeding is continued in spite of such obvious protests; the fear of leaving the patient alone—in Nature's hands—counteracts every other consideration. The feeding is continued; the patient shows no signs of becoming stronger, in spite of (really, on account of) this continued feeding. But, by-and-bye, a meal is retained. Ah! Now the patient is on the road to rapid recovery. His stomach has grown strong enough to retain the food; nourishment must ensue; strength will return; and a rapid recovery is hoped for. But, strange to relate, a *relapse* shortly follows; the patient rapidly sinks; loses strength, and dies—a victim of the false notions and medical philosophy of the day.

Since we know that the food does in no case furnish strength to the body (pp. 225–303), what is the signification of the above fact—that the stomach finally retained the food forced upon it after continually vomiting it up for so long a period? That "it has now gained sufficient strength to retain it" is the universal belief, whereas exactly the reverse of this is true! What has really come about is this. In the early stage of the disease Nature vehemently protested—indicating her needs and desires by forcibly ejecting whatever food was introduced into the stomach—thus clearly showing to all sensible persons that no food was needed, at that time. But the feeding *is* continued; and what is the result? The stomach gradually but steadily loses its vital vigor, and becomes weaker and weaker, as the vitality lessens, until it finally becomes so weak as to be incapable of ejecting the food, as it should, and the food is thus retained merely because of the lack of vitality—the amount being insufficient to eject it. The fact that the food is "kept down" then, indicates the very reverse of what it is generally supposed to prove—a great reduction of, and not an addition to, the vital powers; not that "the stomach is strong enough to retain it," but that it is too weak to eject it—a vast difference. The cart has been again placed before the horse. On the above theory, the "relapses," "collapses" and "complications," and other

[1] See, *e.g.*, "The Surgical Complications and Sequels of the Continued Fevers," by Wm. Keen, M.D., p. 45.

startling developments of the "improvement" become at once explicable and their reason obvious enough.

As a further illustration of my meaning, let me place before the reader the following considerations on the much misunderstood question of "acclimatization." When a person moves from a healthful and invigorating climate to an unhealthful and debilitating one, certain changes or modifications of the organism invariably become manifest. Instead of the healthy cheek, the buoyant tread, emaciation and disease ensue; the patient becomes feverish, the vitality gradually diminishes, and the patient subsides into a more or less chronically ill, devitalized condition. By-and-bye, however, he seems a little better—able to "cast off the disease" (so it is said) and finally he goes about his daily business no longer incapacitated, but free from the previously ever-present fever. He is now said to be "acclimated," and impervious to the attacks of fever, to which he was formerly subject.

Now, what does this really mean? To call it a question of "temperament," as some authors have done, explains nothing. It is usually supposed that by becoming acclimated the person's system is rendered immune by reason of the fact that it has passed into a peculiar condition which rendered it unfit for the habitation of that form of disease—just as a house might be unfit for the tenant! But, as disease is not a *thing*, and consequently cannot inhabit, exist in, or attack any person whatever, it is certain that we must seek the explanation elsewhere. What, then, is the condition called acclimation in reality? It is simply this: When first such a climate is entered the vitality is high, and reacts against the unhealthful surroundings and conditions; but, after having lived in that climate for some time the vital powers gradually become lessened, the quick and effective response of the organism is no longer possible; a condition of "toleration" is present; and *this toleration is acclimation.* It is due simply to the fact that the vital powers are so hopelessly lowered that reaction is no longer possible· and depression and premature death are the inevitable consequences of such a condition.

In the previous argument it has been shown that food

eaten when the body is diseased, cannot nourish it—cannot supply it with heat, or energy; nor nourish its tissues in any degree. Now, if heat and energy are not furnished by the food eaten, what is supplied? Why, under such circumstances, do we eat? Taking all the facts into consideration, we are thus forced to the conclusion that our *only* need for food is to supply the wastes of the general activities; to replace the tissues that have been broken down by exercise or by the bodily muscular functioning—internal or external. But, as before pointed out, how much is this in disease? Practically nothing at all! If the question of energy production be left out of consideration for the time being (and I must ask my readers to put this objection quite out of their minds *pro tem*, as I shall consider that phase of the subject at considerable length presently), of what value is the feeding of tissue in disease—since the nutriment digested cannot be converted into healthy tissue, owing to diseased and debilitated condition of the digestive organs? Of what physiological *use* is the food? What can it feed or supply with nutriment? What organs need to be fed under such circumstances, in order to maintain their structural integrity? We have seen that the most important part of us, the nervous system, does not waste during a fast at all. It has the capacity for feeding itself indefinitely on the body, at the expense of the other tissues; and as we need not, cannot, feed the brain in time of sickness, what can we feed? In all diseases in which there are a high pulse and temperature, pain or discomfort, aversion to food, a foul, dry mouth and tongue, thirst, etc., wasting of the body goes on, no matter what the feeding, until a clean, moist tongue, and mouth, and hunger mark the close of the disease, when food can be taken with relish, and digested. This makes it clearly evident that we cannot save the muscles and fat by feeding under these adverse conditions.

And if the muscles and fat cannot be saved from wasting, surely no part of the bodily organism can be saved, for nothing should be more easily preserved than they! So far as the mere physical body is concerned, therefore, it is not only useless but worse than useless, to attempt to nourish it at such a time, since the waste will proceed all the more quickly as the result of feeding—due to added obstruction, to consequent auto-infection, in addition to the loss of vital energy, in needless attempts at digestion.

For purely "body reasons," therefore, a fast cannot fail to be in every way beneficial; enforced feeding correspondingly harmful.

And it must not be forgotten, in this connection, that, if improper food be eaten, *i.e.*, food lacking in the requisite elements for sustaining the bodily integrity—starvation will result, no matter how much of this food be eaten. Twice the mere *bulk* of food will not sustain the body any better than the proper amount, while the brain and nervous system continue to be taxed in getting rid of the increase of food material. In other words, the body is at once starved and exhausted—the food being incapable of nourishing the body—no matter in what quantities it mav be eaten, while still requiring digestion—and its accompanying nervous tax.

Indeed, it is known that, in certain wasting diseases, the emaciation goes on no matter how much food is eaten, and in spite of (or perhaps on account of) the presence of a most marked appetite. Says Doctor Trall:[1]

" . . . This wasting of the body is usually attended with a craving, and often quite voracious appetite; in some cases the craving is insatiable, and the patient wants to eat constantly."

The results of this Doctor Trall clearly points out in his "Throat and Lungs," p. 34, where he writes:

"In these low diatheses and malignant forms of disease all the powers of the constitution are struggling with all their energies to throw out the morbid matter. If they succeed, the patient will recover; but if this effort is unsuccessful, the patient must die. He has no ability, until this struggle is decided, to digest food; and to cram his stomach with it, or to irritate the digestive organs with tonics and stimulants, is merely adding fuel to the fire; it is adding another to the great burden the vital powers are obliged to sustain, and thus lessening the chances for Nature to effect a cure."

[1] "Sexual Abuses," p. 68.

But the greatest objection to fasting has yet to be considered. Granting that all the above argument be sound—what about sustaining the bodily *energies* during this period? A fast might do all that has been claimed for it; might cleanse and purify the bodv thoroughly; yet, if the patient were to almost or quite die of weakness meanwhile, its therapeutic value would be somewhat doubtful! Since the energy of the body is supposed to be derived from the food we eat, what will be the effects of withholding this food? Will not the patient be weakened and depleted to an alarming extent? And if not, why not? Such are a few of the all-important questions we shall have to consider; and that I propose to discuss at length in Book III., Chapter I. It will first be necessary, however, before passing on to this aspect of the problem, to give a collection of a number of cases that have actually been cured by the method suggested—they forming a tangible and practical proof of the correctness of the theory of disease which I have outlined in the foregoing chapters, and the physiology and philosophy of fasting defended in this volume.

CHAPTER VI

CASES CURED BY THIS METHOD

IN THE present chapter I shall give in outline a number of cases of patients treated by the fasting method, and who have had health restored by that means—generally, when all other methods have been tried and have been found to fail. I shall not give, in this place, the actual details in all these cases for several reasons; partly because such detailed records were not kept—in some cases; partly because the details are of comparative unimportance, and not worthy of the space their narration would necessitate; but chiefly because such details as are of especial note are recorded in Book V., which is devoted entirely to this side of the question, and where such facts will be found in their necessary fullness. The first twenty-one cases I have given at some length; because in these cases I had the opportunity either of watching the cases from day to day, while the fast was in progress, and so of forming a first-hand opinion —and having in that manner an opportunity to make all the necessary observations, which I have embodied in Book V.; or because I have had subsequently, the opportunity to cross-examine the patients, since their fast; or in other ways to gain first-hand and accurate accounts of the case. In this way I am enabled to offer a number of cases that are in every way well authenticated, and for the accuracy of which I can vouch. The *length of time* that many of these cases have fasted but illustrates the point made in the next chapter—that we do not and cannot derive our strength and energy from the daily food; while the *variety* of diseases (so-called) that have been cured, and which the following cases illustrate, but demonstrate the truth of the theory of fasting, elaborated in the last chapter. That such a variety of diseases can be cured by this one method may strike the reader all the more forcibly when he comes to read the cases—even though he may be prepared more or less to acknowledge the possibility of such cures after reading the chapters that have preceded this one. Still, the *modus operandi* may appear more or less mysterious to him, when actually applied and seen in operation. That paralysis, *e.g.*, should be cured is, to some, most extraordinary; yet the explanation of how fasting effects this result is, in most cases, perfectly simple. That paralysis frequently results from an undue pressure upon certain nerves is now acknowledged to be a *vera causa*—tumors; engorged blood vessels; an unduly contracted or rigid muscle; as well as mechanical obstruction—all these are recognized as frequent causes of paralysis. Now I contend that there is in addition to these, another cause—a potent and a frequent cause, too. *It is the pressure over the nerves of unduly retained effete material.* When the system is heavily encumbered throughout, this pressure upon certain nerve fibers or ganglia is certainly going on to a greater or lesser degree—dulling the sensibility, and rendering life, in its fullest and completest sense, impossible. After reaching a certain point, then, paralysis results, as a natural consequent. As Doctor Rabagliati expressed it:[1]

> " There is always a cause or causes, such as pressure on nerve centers or degeneration of some kind, on which the paralysis depends."

It can readily be seen, therefore, that fasting, by removing the cause, by absorption, and elimination, would of necessity remove the effect also; *i.e*, relieve the paralysis.

It is unnecessary for me to trace out in detail the causation of every disease, and to show how it is that every one of them is caused by overeating; it would be an easy task, and one that I hope to perform some future day. The general theory must suffice in a book of this character; and it is, I trust, sufficiently clear to enable any student of nutrition problems to work out the details of each case for himself. An outline of the cases and their cure is all that can be attempted here, and this I

[1] "Classification and Nomenclature of Diseases," p. 57.

shall now proceed to give, following the cases given in detail by a number of other cases, to which a brief mention only will be made—since I have not verified these cases at first hand. They will, however, serve to show the medical world the extent to which cures of this kind are now being performed, and the great influence over the public mind which this method of cure is beginning to have. If the medical world is wise, it will take the initiative, and educate the people in the hygienic system of medication, and the true nature of disease and its cure, instead of waiting for the public to leave them behind and to shift for themselves, regardless of the medical men—which recent developments would seem to indicate.

I now turn to an account of the cases themselves; and I shall begin with a case of *paralysis*, since we have just discussed that affliction—its possible causation and cure.

George E. Davis,[1] age 61, fasted for fifty days—which fast presented many symptoms of unusual interest. For one thing it was possible to watch the *daily* improvement in the patient's condition more easily than in any other case that I have ever observed. At no time was the patient in any way seriously distressed, or rendered incapable of enjoying life as much as his then crippled condition enabled him to enjoy it. Perhaps I cannot do better than to reproduce first a copy of a letter Mr. Davis circulated among his friends shortly after his fast was broken, and epitomizing the case for the general reader—giving him a condensed view of what actually occurred. The letter is as follows, copied practically *verbatim:*

"January 15, 1903.

"My Dear Friend:

"I take this unusual method of communication because of the long list of people to whom I owe letters, and the almost utter impossibility of writing so long a letter as this to each. You must regard it as no less personal because of its peculiarity, however.

[1] This was the case referred to by Doctor Dewey, in his "Experiences of the No-Breakfast Plan," etc., p. 31. Doctor Dewey had, however, confused the facts of this case with that of Mr. Tuthill, given on pp. 189–91, and the case as given in his book is, consequently, erroneous. In this book are to be found the facts of both cases—I having supplied these facts to Doctor Dewey by letter.

I have passed through a remarkable experience, a mere outline of which follows.

"I reverently give thanks for my recovery to God, the Source of all Good. I am sixty-one years of age. My entire right side was completely paralyzed July 1, 1901. I immediately commenced recovery, but improvement was substantially at a standstill when cold weather came in the fall. A temporary advancement came and ceased with the unusual warm weather of the early spring of 1902, followed by a relapse to about the previous condition, which continued without material change to August 15th of last year. I was totally incapacitated for active manual labor of any kind, living in dread of a second stroke, with a strange, unnatural depression throughout upon slight over-exertion, accompanied by great drowsiness. On these occasions I would sleep thirty to thirty-six hours, almost without intermission. My mentality was impaired, my eyesight not fully recovered, and my speech impeded. My right hand and arm were clumsy and weak. At this stage all ordinary human aid was powerless. I commenced a preliminary or partial FAST on August 15th last, eating two light meals daily until the 20th, when I ate one light meal only. On August 20th I commenced a full fast, and from that time until September 29th—FORTY FULL DAYS AND SEVEN HOURS—I took no nutriment whatever, liquid or solid, and no drugs. During the next three days I had very little nourishment, and then began a supplemental full fast of one week, making in all FIFTY DAYS.

"Contrary to my expectations, to the general belief, and to some experiences, I had no hunger from the third day to the fortieth. (See Matthew, 4:2.) To affirm that there was no inconvenience, however, would be untrue, for by every avenue of elimination most offensive impurities were thrown off, being at times unbearable, had the object been lost sight of.

"My weight before the fast was 228 pounds, and my stomach girth 45 inches. At the close of my fast (October 9th.), my weight was 174 pounds and my girth 38½ inches. November 26th my weight was 184 pounds and my girth 39 inches. At this writing (Januarv 15th) I weigh about the same as at last date.

"I am cured of paralysis. My mentality is clear and normal; my entire digestive system is apparently perfect; my vision is better than for years; my hand and arm are strong; I have no dread of a second stroke; I have no sleepy spells; I feel lighter all over; and when I am weary I am quite refreshed and ready for further exertion after a short rest, which is always, as is my food, simply delicious; I feel much younger, and my neighbors say I "look it." I have been working in St. Paul, ten miles distant, over a month, traveling to and from that city daily, and am in every way more robust than I have been since boyhood.

"My dear friends, who regard human physical ailments as proper subjects of miraculous interposition only, are referred to Matthew, 9:12; read, also, Matthew 17:21.

"I know you will rejoice with me, my friend, at the great change. Tell other friends and acquaintances: and if you or they know of one afflicted as I was, let him read this. I would be glad to correspond with such. I hope to have a good, long letter from you soon.

"Very sincerely yours,

"GEO. E. DAVIS."

Many interesting phenomena occurred during the fast, in the case under discussion. One such phenomenon was that throughout the fast the patient was troubled with a very bad "taste in the mouth"—the saliva being highly offensive in character, and at times almost nauseating the patient. This continued for almost the entire period of the fast—certainly for thirty or more days. This beautifully illustrates how Nature. utilizes every possible avenue for elimination, during a fast; how superhuman are her efforts to right the wrong, and how excessive and grievous must have been that wrong! Such a case well illustrates in as clear a manner as possible, also, that Nature herself will determine when the fast should be broken; and that it should not have been broken before the thirtieth day, *at least*—since the signs of active elimination continued up to or beyond that date. As a matter of fact, the signal for breaking the fast (hunger) was not given until the fiftieth day, as we have seen.

This case was remarkable also because of the fact that—though enemas were taken daily for the entire period of fifty days, quantities of fecal matter were removed on almost every occasion—the result of each enema surprising both the patient and the physician watching the case, and proving conclusively what an enormous quantity of fecal matter may be retained for so long—without showing signs of its presence, and never being eliminated! On the thirty-eighth day, even, a large quantity of fecal matter was removed—though enemas had been taken daily for the preceding thirty-seven days! For a discussion of such cases, see the chapter on "The Enema."

Mrs. I. Matthews, age 45. This patient had suffered for many years from chronic catarrh, which caused her the greatest inconvenience. A bad "cold" seemed to have settled on her chest, for many days past, and showed no signs of abating. She was, on the other hand, threatened with worse and graver consequences. The patient began her fast weighing 150 pounds, and fasted twenty-two days—breaking it (somewhat prematurely, I think) when weighing 123 pounds—having lost twenty-seven pounds. Throughout the fast, the patient felt well and strong, and, with the exception of feeling a little "cold" occasionally —experienced no unusual symptoms whatever. Especially after the tenth day did she improve—feeling markedly stronger than for some time past—her senses being rendered more acute; while the catarrh completely disappeared; and, so far as I have been enabled to learn, never returned.

Rev. N. J. Löhre, age 35, had suffered from alternate consti pation and diarrhœa, and from insomnia, for many months past, (more than a year) and had taken innumerable drugs to improve his condition—without the least benefit. The patient entered upon a fast, which lasted ten days. He exercised regularly and attended to his usual business affairs throughout that period. His bowels gave no hint of their presence, save on one occasion—when he moved them artificially by means of a glass of Hunyadi water. During this period, the patient reduced his weight from 178 pounds to 165 pounds—a loss of thirteen pounds. The net result, in this case, was a complete and revolutionary cure; the insomnia disappearing about the third day of the fast; while, when feeding was resumed, it was found that the bowels continued to act in a perfectly normal manner. Several months later, Mr. Löhre told me he had had no return of the former distressing symptoms.

Professor F. W., sometime vocal instructor in one of the largest churches in Minneapolis, Minn., age 46, fasted twenty days, to a practically complete cure for incipient diabetes. Added to this, a heavy "cold" had settled on the patient's chest, practically incapacitating him from taking any part in the services of the church, while it was most essential that he should. His voice was temporarily ruined by the cold, which had lasted in its present state for several weeks, and showed no signs of abating. The patient was weak; headaches were constantly present, as well as a cough—accompanied by the frequent spitting of phlegm; the body was in a puffy, bloated condition; the mentality impaired; pain in the kidneys was experienced; constipation was present; and difficulty was experienced in urinating—the urine itself, of course, containing the characteristic sugar of diabetes mellitus.[1]

Shortly before entering upon the fast, the patient sent a sample of his urine to an expert for examination—his report confirming that of the local physician. Diabetic symptoms were undoubtedly present.

The patient entered upon the fast with scant hopes of recovery, and no faith whatever in the treatment prescribed. His weight at the commencement of the fast was 182 pounds, and at its close 158 pounds—a loss of twenty-four pounds in twenty days. Within five days all traces of the "cold" had disappeared; the headaches had vanished also; while the hearing, the mentality, and the voice were again practically normal. As the fast progressed, the patient continued to improve, until toward the end (on the seventeenth day) the patient made the remark that he felt better and more active, physically, and clearer mentally, than he had in many months—his only trouble being more or less lassitude. The fast was broken before natural hunger had returned; but the patient was apparently well in

[1] It is now beginning to be recognized that diabetes is a disease of the *blood* rather than of the kidneys. Says Dr. Floyd B. Crandall ("How to Keep Well," p. 431): "Diabetes is a constitutional disease in which sugar accumulates in the blood and is excreted in the urine. It is not a disease of the kidneys, as it is frequently believed. The kidneys act only in removing the sugar from the blood, as they do other foreign substances." A most interesting case of the cure of this disease by fasting is recorded by Mr. C. C Haskell, in his "Perfect Health," pp. 37–9. It is easy to see how it is that fasting is enabled to effect a cure, in such cases.

every way for some days past—hunger only being absent. The patient continued free from all his lesser symptoms as long as I knew him; but he moved away within a couple of months from the time of breaking the fast, and I have since lost trace of him.

Now, the most interesting point in connection with this case is the fact that the diabetes mellitus was completely cured! As the fast progressed, the symptoms of the disease gradually grew less and less; the condition of the patient continued to improve steadily, until, when the fast was broken, not a trace of the former condition remained. The disease had been *cured*—just as any other diseased condition would have been cured. These facts—the results of the fast—are beyond all question. On the tenth day of the fast, a rather dramatic incident occurred. A sample of urine was taken, and sent "East" for examination by the same expert who had made the examination on the day before the fast was entered upon. So great was the difference in the composition of the urine, and the amount of sugar it contained, that the expert refused to believe that they were passed from the same man—and probably remains a disbeliever to this day! (The samples were only ten days apart, be it remembered.) I cite this merely to show the marvelous improvement that can result within so short a time, when this potent method of treatment is utilized—even after every other method has been tried in vain. The diabetes was cured in this case; of that there can be no doubt.

J. B., age 45, fasted twenty-three days. The patient had suffered from chronic catarrh for many months past; also disordered liver, and the many symptoms to which this gave rise. For twelve years Mr. B. had tried everything known to medical science, in order to (if possible) effect a cure, or alleviate his sufferings in some degree. The patient had no appetite (clearly indicating that food was not needed), and suffered severe pain in the right side—over the ascending colon. The patient's weight at the commencement of the fast was 165 pounds, and at its close 154 pounds—a loss of only eleven pounds. This case is noteworthy for one reason, at least. No inconvenience was experienced by the patient until the eighteenth day, when a slight nausea was experienced; and, on the following day, a vomiting spell occurred, causing considerable alarm. Thence forward, such vomiting spells were experienced daily, and for this reason the patient broke the fast on the twenty-third day —though hunger had not, in reality, made its appearance. Still, the patient had become alarmed over his condition, and broke the fast, contrary to advice, on the twenty-third day. Fortunately, no ill results followed this rash procedure (prematurely breaking the fast), but, when broken, a good appetite and a sense of general well-being at once manifested themselves; while it was noticed that the pain in the right side had all but entirely disappeared. Unfortunately, I lost sight of this patient soon after his fast was completed, and am unable to state the ultimate outcome. The great benefits he derived from the fast at the time were apparent to all, however.

Mrs. B., wife of Mr. B., whose case is given above, age 31, fasted eight days for continued headaches, and a chronic "cold in the head" for which she had tried "everything" in vain. Her hearing had become defective, and her appetite had practically disappeared entirely. This condition had been more or less constant for nine years, and the patient had well-nigh given up hope of a cure that would prove permanent.

The patient entered upon a fast, weighing 135 pounds, ending it at 127 pounds—a loss of eight pounds—or exactly one pound *per diem*. At the termination of the fast, a good, normal appetite was experienced; the hearing was rendered normal; while the chronic "cold" had entirely disappeared. In a great variety of ways the patient was very greatly benefited, and, like all persons who really undertake the fasting cure, her faith in the method of treatment had grown to be unlimited. The doubts, the sneers and the jests are, as usual, found only in the mouths of those who have never actually experimented upon themselves—have never tried the method of treatment here advocated—and who, consequently, can know nothing whatever about it.

George W. Tuthill, formerly of Minneapolis, Minn., age 47, undertook a fast which was one of the most interesting I have ever had the opportunity to observe. Up to the year 1892, Mr. T. was nearly always well and apparently in good health—but at that time he was suddenly seized with convulsive spasms, which rendered him unconscious—in which condition he remained, on this first occasion, for about half an hour. These attacks continued to occur at intervals, until he was forced to seek medical advice, which he did, and was heavily dosed with bromide of potassium, and other drugs. The symptoms gradually lessened under this treatment; the "fits" occurred at somewhat rarer intervals, and, after about two years, Mr. Tuthill was enabled to undertake some kind of work—which he did—going on the road in the capacity of a road salesman for a large wholesale house. During the next few months, a few slight attacks occurred, and the drugging was continued. In 1895, the patient went "East," and suffered a very severe attack in Baltimore—and, no relief being found from local physicians, he went to Philadelphia, and entered the Orthopœdic Institute, and Infirmary for Nervous Diseases, where he was treated by Dr. S. W-M. and others for three months. During this period, several severe and many lighter attacks occurred —but no permanent relief was obtained. The diagnosis was organic brain disease, and it was stated that the only possible means of relief was an operation for the removal of the growth on the brain. It was decided, however, that the patient was too low and weak to stand such an operation, at that time, and the patient was discharged—uncured.

After this he continued at business for several years, his condition, at times, necessitating his remaining in bed, and incapacitating him from all active work. In 1901, however, some improvement was noted, and Mr. Tuthill again took to the road —but, largely through worry and overwork, he suffered a relapse the following spring, 1902, which again incapacitated him from any active occupation. The patient could, at this time, write only with the very greatest difficulty; his vision was greatly impaired; his speech considerably affected; wracking headaches were constantly present; partial paralysis of the right side (hemiphlegia) ensued, and it was necessary to assist him at all times; and the patient was in an all-round miserable and extremely low condition. He was fully persuaded that to enter a hospital and demand that an operation be performed at once was his last desperate chance. It might terminate fatally—but life, under the existing conditions, was unbearable; the patient was in a truly dejected and well-nigh hopeless condition.

Just at this juncture, and largely through an accident, Mr. Tuthill heard of Doctor Dewey and of the wonderful cures that had been effected by his system of treatment—by fasting. The common sense aspect of the theory at once struck him; he purchased Doctor Dewey's "No-Breakfast Plan" and immediately determined to enter upon a fast of indefinite length—or until death should intervene, or a cure be effected. Accordingly, he wrote to Doctor Dewey, and entered upon a fast, which lasted a few hours over twenty days. During the early part of this fast, he was without any guidance whatever, but later came under the observation and direction of Doctor B. and myself. In consequence, the latter part of the fast was attended with far better results than the former—owing to the fact that enemas, water drinking, etc., were not neglected, as they were before; and the patient also received daily, an osteopathic (stimulative) treatment. The patient's weight declined, meanwhile, from 114 pounds to ninety-eight pounds—a decrease of sixteen pounds. But this loss (marvelous coincidence!) was attended only with increased health and vigor! During this period of twenty days, the most remarkable changes in the patient's condition were effected; the benefits derived from so short a period of treatment (to be compared, it must be remembered, with *more than ten years* unsuccessful treatment, by regular physicians and specialists) would seem well-nigh miraculous. For see! *Within ten days* the patient's paralysis had almost entirely disappeared—and he was enabled to walk about, almost as well and as freely as ever! His hearing and vision became practically normal. His headaches left him, never to return—and, at the end of the twenty days, the patient was enabled to resume his business, practically a well man—all this without any drugs being administered at any time—within three weeks—as opposed to ten years' ineffectual treatment—

while health and strength returned, and were enjoyed as they had not been in many years.

Under such circumstances, the patient and his previously skeptical friends could hardly think but that the fast had been a great success—nor indeed did they.

Most unfortunately, however, the benefits derived did not last indefinitely owing to the fact that the patient lived most carelessly, and in such a manner as to invite if not to induce a second attack. Buoyed up with health and good spirits, the patient had quite disregarded hygienic—and especially dietetic—precautions; and ate as much as a morbid appetite craved of anything desired. A relapse to something of the former condition resulted during the next few months; but this was easily accounted for—the reason for the relapse being palpable and obvious. The relapse does not in any way detract from the benefits derived from the former fast—since the benefits were patent and were recognized and acknowledged by all at that time. As I have previously stated, any man can make himself sick—very easily; and no matter how well he may be. All he has to do is to continue to live contrary to Nature's laws for a sufficiently long period of time, and the "desired" ill results will follow! And so the fact that Mr. Tuthill again became ill is no reason for stating that the former fast did not benefit or cure the patient, for we have proof that it did: all it proves is that riotous living can make a healthy man ill—a statement hardly necessary to prove. Another reason for this relapse is to be found, I believe, in the fact that the patient broke the first fast before it was quite ready to be broken—before natural hunger had really returned. This was a very great pity, and its effects were undoubtedly noticed by the patient later on. The patient accordingly determined to undertake a second fast of indefinite duration—incidentally showing, by the way, the great faith in the efficacy of fasting which every patient feels who has actually tried it—and has not been content to scoff and sneer at the practice without knowing anything about it—theoretically or practically. He accordingly commenced the second fast when weighing but ninety-eight pounds (clothed) and continued it without break of any kind for forty-one days.

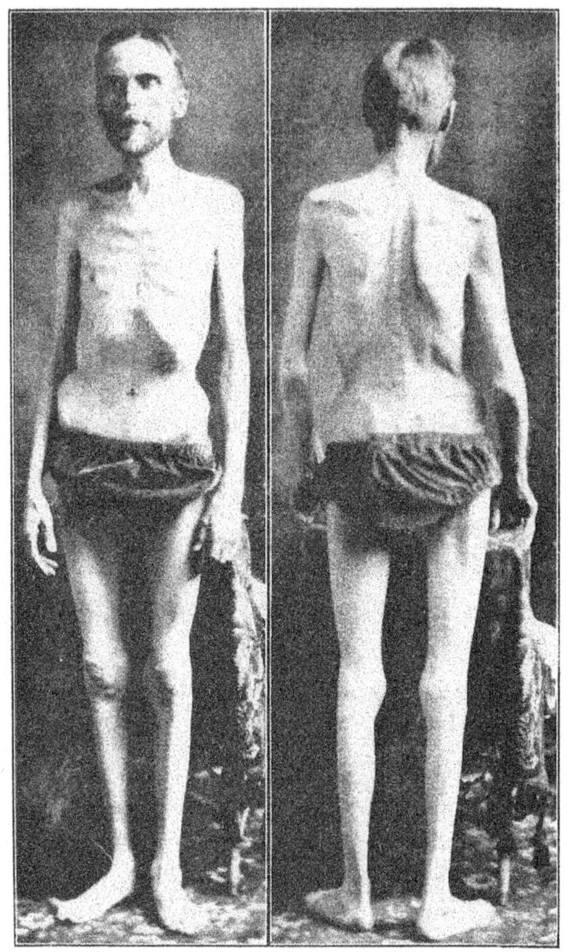

FIG. 1. FIG. 2.

Taken on the last day of his forty-one day fast. I helped the patient to undress and dress, though he could easily have done this himself.

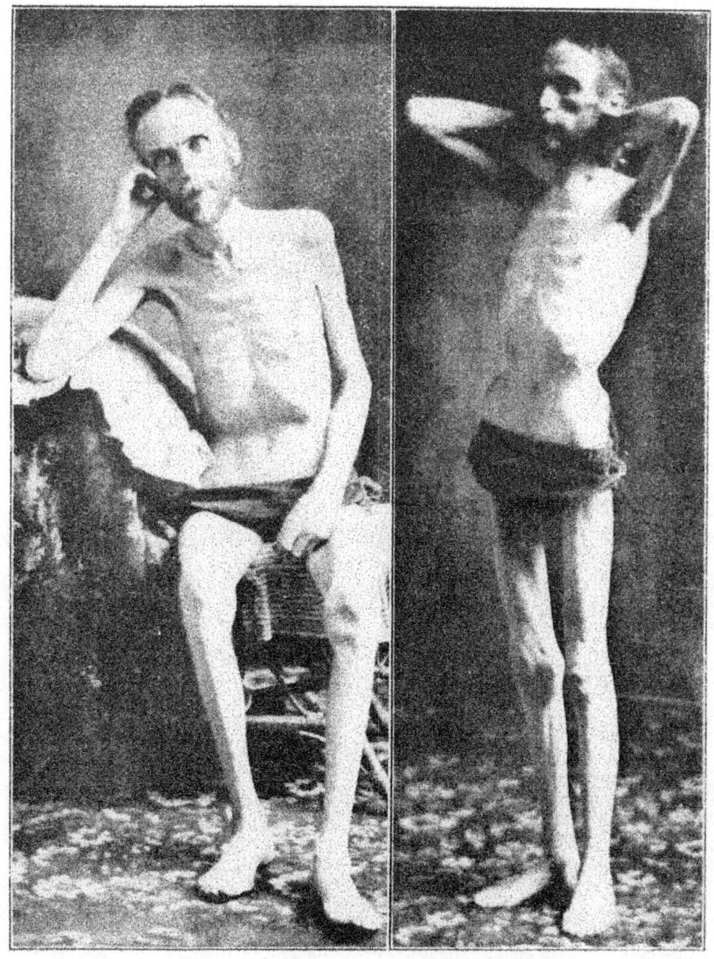

Fig 3. Fig 4.

It will be noted that the skeleton condition has been nearly reached this being particularly noticeable in the thighs and arms. (v. Fig. 4.)

During this fast, many interesting phenomena presented themselves for observation. The patient was "cold" almost the entire time, and a gnawing feeling—commonly supposed to be hunger (p. 549), was experienced throughout. The senses were again rendered more acute, and the paralysis was almost entirely relieved. At the close of the fast, the patient weighed (stripped) but seventy-two and one-half pounds—demonstrating once again the extent to which the body may be reduced without detriment—and, indeed, with nothing but continued benefit. The accompanying photographs will illustrate the patient's condition at this time—showing that the skeleton condition has been nearly reached. (Figs. 1, 2, 3, 4.)

I, for one, was now persuaded that the trouble was organic, not functional; and that a complete cure could never be effected by any hygienic measures alone; that it was, in fact, one of those *very rare* cases in which a surgical operation was the only chance for the patient's recovery; the trouble was obviously not functional. In the first fast the growth or clot, or in whatever form the obstruction may have been present, was evidently partially "absorbed as brain food," as Doctor Dewey wrote; or in some manner utilized or eliminated. And, in the second fast, it may have been that the growth was again increased—after the fast was broken, and during the intermediate period of overfeeding—and had become more fixed or deep set—more malignant, perhaps—an organic defect now past relief by hygienic agencies, though it might have been so relieved at the time of the former fast. The facts seem to confirm this theory as the correct one; but, however it may have been, although the general health of the patient was improved remarkably, the fast was not entirely successful on this occasion. Unfortunately I have lost sight of this patient—owing to the fact that he moved from his former home—and I cannot now state what the ultimate outcome of the fasting was in this case. I have included the case largely because of the interesting points it contains, rather than as an ideal example of the curative powers of fasting—though, it may be added, the patient's faith in fasting remained unbroken—even after the termination of the second fast. He realized that he had not recovered because recovery was impossible; and would, *even then*, have been the very first to have defended the theory and the practice of fasting, in cases of acute and chronic disease. I ask my reader to compare this confidence with the lack of faith almost invariably present in patients that have failed to be cured by the present systems of treatment.

Mrs. J. F. C., age 47, weight 127 pounds, mother of five children, had been ailing for six years from bronchial trouble and there were indications that this was rapidly degenerating into pulmonary consumption. Four of the most expert physicians in the city had treated her; but to no avail. The patient had made two trips to Florida and one to California, and had tried every conceivable treatment with no apparent benefit. The coughing had increased in violence, and the patient showed signs of rapid breaking up and emaciation. At this time—and at the suggestion of one of her attendant physicians—the patient, now considered practically a hopeless case—undertook a fast which was to last until a cure was effected or until symptoms developed which would indicate the advisability of breaking the fast. The patient first of all omitted breakfast for one week, and then lived on one meal a day for one week—losing nine pounds during these two weeks, with great improvement, however, in general health. On October 20, 1902, the patient, who now weighed 127 pounds, began a strict fast, in which nothing but water was taken, and fasted for twenty-eight days—breaking it on November 16, 1902—and weighing at that time (clothed), only 103 pounds—showing a loss of twenty-four pounds. In a word, it may be said that the result in this case, was a complete cure—the patient's lungs at its conclusion showing no traces of any diseased condition. The eyes were bright, the spirits cheerful, the mentality clear, and a perfect state of health was present—which state was maintained during the months following the fast—no relapse ever occurring.

In observing this case, one could almost *see* the effects of the fast becoming daily more manifest. Every day the patient became stronger and stronger, in spite of the fact that flesh was being constantly lost—and the wasting was progressing more rapidly than ever. The curative power of the fast cure had never been more manifest. Thus, on October 22nd, the patient reported that she had not coughed at all the preceding night—the first night in *six years* which had been free from coughing spells! Thus, as the result of only two days' fast (preceded by two weeks of abstemious dieting) the patient had improved more than during six years of doctoring! On Oct. 25th, the patient reported that the soreness, which had always been present, was leaving the throat, but that phlegm was occasionally coughed up, and expectorated. The pulse at this time was somewhat above normal, 82. The patient continued to improve steadily until Nov. 14th, when the first signs of nausea appeared—the patient felt "sick at the stomach" and "gagging" frequently took place. The next day (15th), the symptoms had somewhat abated, though the patient still felt sick and ill at ease. The next morning, however (16th), the symptoms had entirely disappeared, and the patient felt well and strong. Toward noon—the call for food was experienced, and the fast was broken—on the 28th day—the patient being cured.

Only liquid food was permitted, however, for the next six days; but at the end of that time (Nov. 22nd), the patient weighed 113 pounds—a clear gain of ten pounds since the breaking of the fast. This was on liquid food only (*v.* p. 479). The patient was at that time feeling greatly elated, both in body and mind—and no trace of the old trouble existed. The case was a most wonderful cure. A brief account of the case was published in the Minneapolis *Tribune*, Nov. 18, 1902.

Mrs. T. A., age 50, fasted thirty-four days, for indigestion and severe liver trouble. The weight, at commencement of the fast, was 117 pounds; at its conclusion, ninety-two pounds—showing a loss of twenty-five pounds. The comparatively small loss was due to the somewhat emaciated condition of the patient. It is to be observed that, in spite of the fact that the patient was already under-weight, and although she weighed only ninety-two pounds (clothed), at the conclusion of the fast—health was gained simultaneously with this loss. (p. 129.)

As previously stated, this patient suffered from a complication of ills, the chief of which were chronic indigestion, headaches, and a painful and imperfectly functioning liver. The patient was emaciated, the skin sallow, the whites of the eyes yellow, the spirits depressed. Headaches were frequent, and there was a tendency toward melancholia. Extreme constipation was also present. The temperature was continually low, 94° F., and very frequently even less.

These troubles had extended over a period of thirty years, they constantly increasing in intensity. It had become impossible for the patient to eat anything at all—the food immediately fermenting in the stomach, and constant use had to be made of the stomach-pump.

The patient commenced her fast; and most interesting phenomena resulted almost immediately. The bile, the decomposing food, which had been collecting for so many weeks and months, was suddenly thrown into the blood-stream (Nature's attempt at rapid elimination) and extraordinary results followed. I have referred to these phenomena at greater length in the chapters on "The Temperature" and "Crises" and shall not discuss them at any length here, in consequence. Suffice it to say that, for the first few days, the patient became desperately ill; the skin grew parched, and dark yellow; the whites of the eyes became yellow also. Sickness of the stomach was experienced, and a quantity of bile and mal-assimilated food was vomited. Masses of evil-smelling feces were passed; and, more than all, she became practically *insane* for several days; she became delirious and her temperature rose to the fever point. Had not her friends possessed supreme confidence in the fasting cure, she would doubtless have been forced to break the fast at this point, and the consequences would have been, if not fatal, at least disastrous. As it was, she continued the fast. These symptoms were all due to the forcible and rapid elimination of morbid material that was going on within the system, and should by no means have been interfered with. As it was, the temperature soon sank again to its former level—below the normal—and only rose again to normal toward the close of the fast. The vomiting and the discharges from the bowels gradually ceased; the eyes and the skin assumed their normal color and appearance; and the patient returned to her normal state of mind. She was delirious only forty-eight hours. The crisis had been passed. (p. 520.) From that hour, until the fast was broken, on the thirty-fourth day, the patient continued to improve steadily, without a single serious relapse, mentally or physically; and, when the fast was broken, the patient was practically a well woman. The headaches, the liver-aches, and the stomach-aches had all vanished; and thenceforward the patient enjoyed better health than she had been enabled to enjoy for several years past. I lost sight of the case soon after, and cannot state the present condition of the patient; but as to her condition immediately after breaking the fast, there can be no doubt.

Robert B., age 29 years, fasted seventeen days, for deafness and catarrh. His weight at the beginning was 135 pounds, decreasing to 118 pounds—a loss of seventeen pounds, or exactly one pound *per diem.* The patient was totally blind in both eyes; deaf in one ear and partially so in the other, and spoke defectively. The senses of taste and smell were also affected. All this was the result of a dynamite explosion that had occurred eight years previously. Both eyes were blinded and the left ear made deaf immediately, as the result; but the right ear—though defective, retained a certain amount of sensation for nearly three years—only becoming totally deaf about fifteen months before the fasting treatment. The patient had been examined several times by competent specialists, and the deafness pronounced incurable—beyond repair. (Of course, any attempt to restore the eyesight was out of the question, since the organs themselves had been blown out at the time.) The patient had been treated for his hearing on several occasions, but with no lasting benefit. The fact that the patient was totally blind makes his fast of especial interest, since the patient was alone all the time, his sister only coming for him once a day, to take him to the office for treatment. Under such conditions, a fast must have been a trying ordeal indeed; but for all that, the plucky patient never wavered, and, at the end, stated he was willing to undertake another fast, if he thought his hearing could be still further benefited by that means! Such a case should shame those patients who are afraid of fasting, when surrounded by every comfort, having their faculties perfect, and when under the supervision of an expert in the fasting cure!

But to return. The patient began fasting on Sept. 28, 1902, and fasted seventeen days, breaking it Oct. 15th, at noon. During the early days of the fast, the hearing grew perceptibly worse (p. 520), and continued to grow worse for several days. About the tenth day, however, the hearing in the right ear became more acute, and the sense of hearing in the left ear became manifest to some degree, also. It must be remembered that the patient had never heard a sound with this ear since the accident, eight years before, and this ear had been pronounced incurable—hopelessly deaf. Manipulation of the ear was resorted to, and a quantity of pus was discharged from the ear, after which the hearing still further improved; the head was clearer, and the catarrh almost entirely disappeared. A general feeling of elation, of well-being, also became manifest. The patient could now hear words and sounds at a distance of several feet. This had been impossible for several years.[1] The fast was broken before natural hunger appeared, owing to the fact that the patient had to return to his home in another city, and so the fast was really broken (most unfortunately) prematurely, and before its full curative effects were realized. This was a great pity, as it would have been most interesting to watch the final effects of the fast, in this particular case. However, the results that were achieved were most astonishing, and afforded a complete vindication of the soundness of this method of cure—extraordinary benefits having been derived from its adoption. I lost trace of the patient, and have never heard whether a second fast was undertaken or not.

Miss Louise W. Kops. The following account was sent me by Miss Kops immediately after the fast was completed, and contains several items of interest. I give the account *verbatim*, and hope it may stimulate others to keep accounts of their fasts with as much detail and precision as this one is recorded.

[1] Dr. James C. Jackson remarked that: "A majority of the deaf are so by reason of their gluttony." "The Gluttony Plague," p. 20.

A Sixteen Days' Fast

"Thursday, June 20th, 1907.—Coffee and rolls, and one saucer of berries at 10 A. M. Weight, 128 pounds. Had a very strenuous day, seeing people, transacting business, etc. The day was a very hot one, and my head was throbbing all the afternoon. At night it was impossible for me to hold up my head, and had to go to bed at 6 P. M. Walked about two miles.

"Friday, June 21st.—Up at 7 A. M. Headache better. Had a glass of hot lemonade. Another very busy day; giving scalp treatment, and other hard work. In the evening went to the theater, feeling the same as usual. Bed, 11.30 P. M. Had one glass of lemonade and about two and one-half quarts of water. Had no desire for food all day. Walked one mile.

"Saturday, June 22d.—Up at 7 A. M. Out, interviewing people all day. Have been feeling languid all day, but not hungry. Head and shoulder ached badly; went to bed, 10 P. M. Drank three quarts of water and one glass of lemonade. On my feet all day. Walked three and one-quarter miles.

"Sunday, June 23d.—Up at 9 A. M. Head better but shoulder and neck aching. Worked hard at fixing up my rooms from 11 A. M. till 4 P. M. Had a steam cabinet bath. Spine and shoulder ached severely; cried with pain.[1] After bathing them in hot water felt relief. Went out and walked one and one-half miles briskly. Felt better than for some time past. Drank three quarts of water. Bed at 10 P. M.—quite tired.

"Monday, June 24th.—Up at 8 A. M. Feeling languid. Had a busy day, seeing people regarding business. Very hot day. Had one glass of lemonade. Feel better between the hours of 10 A. M. and 4 P. M., then felt very weak and tired, and went home and lay down for an hour. Then got up and gave treatment. Took enema; then felt better for a couple of hours. Bed, 8.30 P. M. Weak feeling down legs; head feeling very drawn and a tight feeling at the back of the neck and along spine. Did not walk very much. Urine very dark in color. Drank usual three quarts of water.

"Tuesday, June 25th.—Up at 7.30 A. M.—Did not sleep very well—I think owing to stuffy room. Awoke not feeling very well; felt better after I got out into the air. Gave treatment, and

[1] It was largely because of the severe pain experienced in the neck and shoulder—due to no assignable cause—that the fast was undertaken.

received one from osteopathic physician. Felt better; did a lot of walking and saw many people regarding business. 5 P. M. returned home, and found little woman in the next flat very ill and feverish—she having had a baby six weeks ago. Took her in hand; gave sponge bath, enema, etc., and got her feeling better in two hours. Also bathed baby. It slept through the night quietly—the first time since it was born! Had a pain on her left side about the end of heart during the night; felt like a pres sure. Went to bed at 12 o'clock, midnight. Feeling quite well. Drank usual water. Weighed 125 pounds—a loss of three pounds. Took high enema, removing a great deal of fecal matter.

"Wednesday, June 26.—Up, 7 A.M. Feeling fine. Slept well. Spent a very busy day. Saw little woman again; she very well. Hot day. Severe pain across small of back and under lungs toward evening, and get spells as though legs did not want to move. Head is perfectly clear. Drank a lemonade druggist made for me—with soda by mistake. Drank it and had a bad attack of hiccoughs. Drank hot water, and felt better. Gave a treatment in evening. High enema; hardly any feces. Weight, 125 pounds.

"Thursday, June 27th.—Up, 7 A. M. Feeling fair. Pain on left side during night, but in morning across small of back and down thighs. Head better; no pain and clear. Better later. Pain along spine left toward end of the day. Mucous rises up in throat quite a great deal, in hard lumps of greenish yellow color—every few minutes during the day—and very easily; tongue clear of the greenish colors it had some days ago. It is now whitish. The breath has had no bad odor at all. Food looked interesting to me to-day. Two glasses of lemonade. Felt very strong. Urine very dark color, and a great deal passes away at a time and often; the breath bad once. Had quite rosy cheeks to-day; legs a little weak. Walked two miles in evening. Temperature at 12 M., 96° F. Just normally tired.

"Friday, June 28th.—Awake early; up at 7 A. M. Feel strong. Pain in back not quite so bad; just a sore spot at right side of spine under shoulder. Another busy day. Low enema; some feces. Did a lot of walking. Feeling well all day. Bowels moved freely at 6 P. M. The water was retained all day from morning enema. People will not believe I am fasting. Weight, 123 pounds. Do not show my loss in weight. My face does not look drawn and thin, as it has for months back. Theater in evening; feeling very well. Temperature 8 A. M., 96.1° F.; 3 P. M., 100° F.; 11 P. M., 98° F. To bed 11.30 P. M. Urine still very dark.

"Saturday, June 29th.—Up, 8 A.M. Not feeling brisk; blame the room; not enough air. Went to a doctor and had urine examined; he said it contained uric acid and some albumen. Also had spine and shoulder examined. He could find nothing wrong. If my back did not ache I should feel very strong. Pulse good. Look well. Urine dark. Temperature, 9 A. M., 98° F.; 3 P. M., 98° F.; 11 P. M., 97½° F. Weight, 122 pounds.

"Sunday, June 30th.—Awake very early; brain very clear. Up, 8.30 A.M. Slept well. Not feeling brisk. Took steam bath and enema. Quantity of feces passed away; bad odor; felt better afterwards. Back not quite so bad. Bed, 1.30 A. M. Temperature, 8.30 A. M., 98° F.; 5 P. M., 97° F.; 1 A. M. (after steam bath), 96.3° F.

"Monday, July 1st.—Up, 7.30. Slept well. Legs feel a bit stronger. Strenuous day, getting house in order, etc. Tired in evening. Juice of one-quarter of an orange. Less than usual amount of water. One lemonade. Temperature, 8 A. M., 96.1°F.; 6 P. M., 99° F.; 11 P. M., 96° F.

"Tuesday, July 2d.—Up, 7.30 A. M. Busy day again, till 9 P. M. Then read two hours; feeling well. Bowels moved, rather loosely. Juice of one-half of an orange. Tongue quite clear. Urine clearer. Mucous still rises up every day; this morning it contained a tinge of blood. Feverish about noon. Weight, 119 pounds. Temperature, 8 A. M., 96° F.; 9.30 P. M., 97° F. Bed, 12 M., feeling better. Neck not aching; back better; legs stronger.

"Wednesday, July 3d.—Up, 7 A. M. Feeling well. Busy day again. Tongue quite clear. Felt fine all day. Two lemonades; usual water. Low enema; no feces. Very thirsty. Bed, 10 P. M. Temperature, 7.30 A. M., 96.2° F.; 7.30 P. M., 97.3° F.; 1 A. M., 96.2° F.

"Thursday, July 4th.—Up, 6 A. M. Head very clear. Very busy day again. Running up and down stairs all day. Lemonade; legs tired at night. Slight headache at night. Bed, 11.30 P. M. Temperature, 6.30 A. M., 96.4° F.; 11 P. M., 98° F. Urine clear.

"Friday, July 5th.—Up, 7 A. M. Feeling strong. Hunger coming on. Urine slightly darker. Bed, 12 M. Weight, 117 pounds. Juice of two oranges. Feeling well. Temperature, 7.30 A. M., 96.4° F.; 8.30 P. M., 98° F.; 11 P. M., 97° F.

"Saturday, July 6th.—Up, 7.30 A. M. Not feeling so well. Had wine-glass of grape juice 3.15 P. M. Feeling like eating. Juice of two oranges. Walked one and one-half miles. Very hungry in evening. Ate yolk of egg and two whole wheat crackers. Temperature, 3.30 P. M., 99° F.; 12.30 P. M., 98° F. Weight, 117¼ pounds. Urine light. Feeling very well."

Mrs. G. Y. I give a full account of this case for the reason that it presents certain phenomena of great interest to the student of fasting cases, though the case itself does not afford an example of the benefits derivable from the system; the patient dying soon after breaking the fast. Her death was, however, as we shall presently see, unavoidable; and hence no proof that the fasting cure was in any way the real cause of the death, or that the treatment was other than beneficial, so far as it went, as in all other cases. This was the only case of death with which I have ever personally come in contact, in spite of the fact that I have seen many scores of patients fasting—at various times, for various troubles. In every other case was a cure effected. I have discussed this question of death during fasting on pp. 537–9, to which passage I would refer the reader. However, I must not anticipate; but return to my case.

Mrs. G. Y. came to the office on the First of October, 1902, partially paralyzed on the right side. She stated that she had heard of the numerous successful cases that had recently been reported in the papers, and stated that she had determined to try the method for herself. I believe she met Mr. George E. Davis and one or two other patients who had been cured by this method, in the office; but I am not sure of the details now. She stated that the paralysis from which she suffered was "the only thing the matter with her," and made no mention of any other complaint or complication. She was taken *as a paralytic case*, and as such only.

The patient began treatment on Oct 3d, lessening the amount of food, and commenced fasting early in October (exact date uncertain, since the patient did not state the truth about the day on which the fast was commenced). The fast probably lasted from thirty to forty days.

The progress of the fast was interesting to watch. On Oct. 11th, the patient developed a severe cold—one of Nature's curing processes. On the next day this had entirely disappeared, and the patient felt greatly relieved and improved in every way.[1] On the 16th, the improvement was more marked; still more so on the 19th. The paralysis was fast leaving the patient, who could now walk up and down stairs, and move about in a manner she had not been enabled to in several years. This steady improvement continued until Oct. 27th, when the patient commenced vomiting bile, etc., and this vomiting continued, incessantly, from that day until Nov. 12th—a period of sixteen days—during which time the patient emaciated rapidly, and became exceedingly weak. Many efforts were made to stop the vomiting, but to no avail. For long the patient would not hear of food being administered; but when it was finally given, after several days vomiting, it was promptly ejected, and the vomiting continued as before. Evidently Nature did not wish for food, and consequently no more was administered. It was well that this was the method adopted, for, on Nov. 13th, the vomiting ceased of its own accord—leaving the patient very weak, and, she asserted, *blind*. She could see nothing! The next day (Nov. 14th), this blindness continued; the urine was retained and a catheter had to be used. The weakness was as great as ever; the temperature was low, but the pulse exceedingly rapid. The patient constantly turned the head to one side, whenever she was placed on her back, and stated that it caused her pain to lie on the back of the head. The next day these symptoms continued; the temperature continued very low, but the pulsation ran up to 120 beats a minute. The weakness continued and the patient could talk only with great difficulty. The breath was foul and the tongue heavily *cankered*. The alarming symptoms continued to increase—the temperaature constantly falling—and the pulse running up to 140 beats a minute. Evidently, life could not be long maintained under

[1] Note how *quickly* a cold disappeared during the fasting cure; it did not "hang on all winter" in *this* case, but practically disappeared in one day.

these circumstances. Food was administered, and retained on this day, and on the two following days, but made no change in the patient; and was only administered to prove to the friends of the patient that starvation was not the real cause of the death, should such occur. On Nov. 16th, in spite of the greatest care, the patient died—only in her last moments revealing the secret of her life, and confessing to the hidden disease lurking within her, which was the real *cause* of her death (and as the result of which, and its subsequent mal-treatment, she really died, and not from the fast). The patient was tainted—with syphilis!

I have purposely omitted mention of this side of the case, while discussing it, for the reason that the real cause of the trouble did not develop until the fast was well under way—nor was the patient's confession wrung from her until the very end. It had been noticed on several occasions that the mouth was cankered, but no significance was attached to that fact, since the mouths of fasting patients frequently coat and canker more or less in this manner. But the truth was finally revealed. The patient was syphilitic! Her paralysis was merely the result of this disease, which had been suppressed (not cured) long since; and, in the fast this condition, so long latent, had come to the surface, and become manifest. (pp. 521–23.)

At the time of Mrs. G. Y.'s death, the newspapers were full of accounts of the patient who had been "starved to death"; and I quote by way of reply to these reports a part of an article we contributed to *The Liberator* (Dec. 1902, pp. 71–3), defending our position, and giving the exact facts in the case. In part, the statement ran as follows:

" . . . The patient reduced her three daily meals to two· and the next week she took but one; thus taking two full weeks to get down to actual fasting. The result of these two weeks was that the patient was enabled to move at will the toes on the foot of the affected side—which she had not been able to do since her 'stroke,' two years and one month previously! She then commenced a total fast, *during which time her paralysis entirely disappeared.* No trace of her former condition remained. . The food given Mrs. G. Y. was retained in the stomach and assimilated in a perfectly normal manner; and this, and the fact that she weighed 105 pounds at death, conclusively prove that she had not starved to death—seeing that one patient fasted down to 72½ pounds without injury. These two facts, together with the other points . . . that she was suffering from an incurable blood disease, and that a clot or growth had formed on her brain, (on the motor area of the sinistro-cerebral hemisphere)—all these facts indicate, in fact, conclusively prove, that Mrs. G. Y. died from a complication of bodily disorders, of the worst kind, brought on primarily by the disease from which she suffered."

As previously stated, this case is given merely on account of the points of interest it contains for the student of fasting cases, and not by way of vindication of the method itself. As death was inevitable in any case, it could not be contended that the fast had in any way *caused* the death; but only that it had, perhaps, hastened the end. For a discussion of this difficult point, however, see pp. 537–39.

J. Austin Shaw. I now give in outline a case which is, in many ways, the most wonderful case on record, and the importance of which, from a theoretical and philosophic—no less than from a practical—standpoint it would be hard to overestimate. This case is that of my friend, Mr. J. Austin Shaw, who fasted for a period of forty-five days, into complete health, without losing (even apparently) any strength whatever; but, on the contrary, gaining it; and working constantly every day throughout the fast. I shall contend, in the chapter on "Vitality" that, if my theory be correct, no vitality should be lost during a fast, but on the contrary much should be conserved or gained, and I shall try to show why it is that this energy does not become manifest to us, as such; but why, on the contrary, the patient, in most cases, appears to become weaker instead of stronger—whereas they are not so in reality. If that theory be true, we should be enabled to find cases here and there which exemplify the theory defended—in which no energy is even apparently lost; and any such cases, if found, would at least go far toward disproving the theories held to-day—that food is the source of the bodily heat and energy—and that, upon their withdrawal, the latter must of necessity sink, and sink rapidly (and it would be quite impossible for them to *increase*). And if such a case or such cases were found, they would, as stated, go far toward disproving the theories held to-day. The force of these remarks will become more apparent when we come to the chapter on "Vitality," Book III., Chap. I.

In the case I am about to describe, Mr. Shaw not only fasted for forty-five days, into perfect health, but actually increased in strength throughout. And I contend that such a case as this must cause us to stop and readjust our ideas of vitality and its causation by food; and if the current theories are shown to be erroneous, then a great step will have been made toward the correct interpretation of vital phenomena. For this reason, this case and others of a similar nature should be considered as highly important, scientifically.

Mr. Shaw's case is given at length in his own book, "The Best Thing in the World," to which I would refer the reader. I must very briefly summarize the case here. Mr. Shaw, through previous overeating for a long period, had become diseased in more than one direction; his mental and physical powers had become impaired; his eyesight affected—while his weight was far in excess of what it should have been—200 pounds. (At the conclusion of the fast, Mr. Shaw weighed just 175 pounds—a loss of only twenty-five pounds, in forty-five days. This is exceptionally little, *v.* p. 468). In fact, Mr. Shaw was on the verge of becoming dropsical. He was, moreover, threatened with Bright's disease.

The fast was begun on April 9, 1905, and continued for forty-five days, ending May 24, 1905, at 11 P.M. Mr. Shaw worked throughout the fast from twelve to eighteen hours a day. (p. 36.) I quote from Mr. Shaw's own book, as follows:

On the fifth day Mr. Shaw writes:

"I have no diminution of strength, no drowsiness, no weariness, no disinclination to work. Every sense is alert, and every hope and ambition intensified."

On the ninth day:

"I positively can detect no change, since my fast started, to indicate anything out of the ordinary, unless it be lightness and

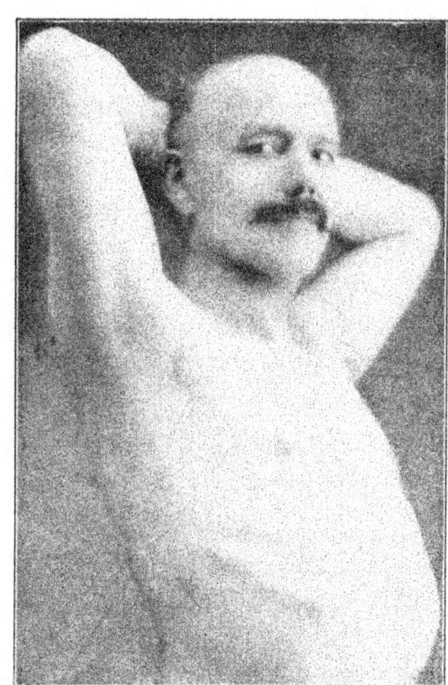

FIG. 5.

MR. J. AUSTIN SHAW.

Taken on the fortieth day of his forty-five day fast. It will be seen that Mr. Shaw's body is still well covered with flesh, though he had at the time fasted as long as Mr. Tuthill. (See Figs. 1, 2, 3, 4.) A comparison of these photographs will be of interest, illustrating the effects of fasting upon two organically differentiated individuals.

ease in climbing the elevated stairs, and more restful sleep than I have had for many a day; less drowsiness, a greater desire and willingness to work, and an alertness that makes doing something a necessity."

On the tenth day:

"I feel better this morning than any time since my fast began."

On the twenty-fifth day:

"I detect no weakness; no lack of enthusiasm in my work; no desire for food, nor need of it."

On the thirtieth day:

"This, the thirtieth day, which I had intended to make the last of my fast, finds me as strong as ever, full of energy, and with so much to do and so many calls to make, and so perfectly contented with my condition, that it may seem a duty to continue the fast a little longer."

On the thirty-first day:

"The days pass as they would if I were not fasting; only I accomplish more than usual without weariness, and a sense of lightness and elation constantly inspires me."

On the thirty-third day·

"I feel stronger, rather than weaker, as my fast goes on."

On the fortieth day:

"Until now at midnight no trace of fear or weakness exists."

On the forty-first day:

"Not a sign of weakness or nervousness appears."

On the forty-second day:

"I am better than any morning since my fast began."

On the forty-fourth day:

"No hunger, nor weakness, and it is evident that Nature is in no special hurry, or has forgotten me."

On the forty-fifth day (the last):

"If anything, I find my strength greater this morning than on any of the forty-five days, which close at six to-night, when I have concluded it best the fast should end."

Such a case as this cannot fail to carry conviction to any intelligent mind; and certainly seems to overthrow the current theory that strength is derived totally from the food we eat—and from no other source.

Mrs. E., age 65, mother of Professor W., whose case is given on p. 187–8, suffered a stroke of partial paralysis (hemiphlegia) affecting the right side. She fasted one week, on one occasion, and two weeks on another, deriving great benefit and relief from the fast on both occasions—not only in her general health, but because of relief from the paralvsis. As an example of this, I may state that the patient, who could not, under any circumstances, climb the stairs that led to the second floor of the house before the fast, did so at its completion with ease and with a firm tread.

In both cases, the fast was broken before true hunger appeared; and the patient quite realized and acknowledged that if she were to continue the fast, a complete cure would probably result. But she did not relish the idea of fasting the necessary time—being so little hampered with the paralysis that she considered it "not worth while." A vast improvement was, however, noticed on both occasions during the fast, and for some time after its completion.

Doctor B.'s case was most interesting, in some respects. An experimental fast of four days, on one occasion, resulted in the loss of eight and one-half pounds during that period, which may be attributed, perhaps, to the fact that Doctor B. continued to give vigorous osteopathic treatments almost hourly, during that period—a severe tax, at any time, upon muscular and vital strength. The subsequent gain in weight was no less interesting. Within two days, upon three extremely light meals (certainly averaging less than twelve ounces of solid food each), a total gain of eight pounds resulted—being another example of that interesting class of cases in which far more weight is gained by the patient than is contained in the food eaten. (pp. 478–81.) Greatly increased strength and vigor was noted, as the result of the fast.

Mrs. T. J., age 47 years. This patient had suffered for several years from various stomach and bowel troubles—a variety of abnormal symptoms indicating a generally diseased condition of these organs. The patient had tried all the regular methods of cure, and even tried the water cure without receiving material benefit. Her condition had gradually become worse; she continned to increase in weight, until, when the fast was undertaken, she weighed 250 pounds. A three week's fast brought her down to 175 pounds, a decrease of seventy-five pounds, in twenty-one days—or an average of three and one-half pounds *per diem!* This unusually great loss was undoubtedly due to the fact that the patient's body was loaded with easily assimilable fatty tissue. The fast was broken (contrary to advice) on the twenty-first day; but, as a result, a complete cure was effected, and the patient continued to enjoy the best of health. None of the abnormal symptoms had returned at the expiration of one year.

Mrs. A. E. R., Minneapolis, Minn., and one of the most incessantly active women for her age I have ever seen, is a living example of the benefits to be derived from fasting. For more than thirty years, Mrs. R. had suffered from more or less chronic colds, bronchial troubles, diarrhœa alternating with constipation, and general dejection—together with an abnormal rigidity of the knee joints; suffering, moreover, from varicose veins. During the years preceding the treatment, the patient had taken several trips to California and the South in search of health, and had tried three different and well-known physicians, as well as two osteopathic physicians, but all to no avail. Her condition failed to improve, and, at the time the patient undertook the fast, she was suffering considerably, her ankles being constantly encased in elastic stockings, without which she was unable to stand or to walk about.

When the fast was undertaken, the patient was 69 years of age, and weighed 225 pounds. The patient decided to fast in this manner; to fast entirely for three days—eating, on the fourth day, one very light meal, consisting of milk and rice, or fruit and lemonade, etc. This plan was followed for a little more than three weeks, during which time the patient's weight dropped to 185 pounds—a decrease of about forty pounds. During the fasting period, the patient was continually on her feet, attending to her business as usual, and in every way living her normal life. For a woman of her age, I consider this most remarkable.

During the fast, the patient was careful to follow all advice relative to water drinking, enemas, etc., and took an osteopathic treatment daily. The elastic stockings were discarded when ever the patient was not actually upon her feet—cold water bandages being substituted. These were applied thrice daily, and the bandages changed several times at each application. Toward the end of the second week, the elastic supports were discarded entirely—cold wet cloths being worn instead. These she was still wearing when last I heard from her. In all other respects a complete cure had been effected—no diarrhœa, no headaches, no colds, no bronchial troubles remained. The patient fairly personified good health, while her capacity for work seemed unlimited. The results of the fast were beneficial, almost to the point of being miraculous.

Mrs. R. T., age 32, had suffered for several years from head aches, nausea, complete loss of appetite, and an unaccountable pain in the right side (high up, on the ascending colon, apparently) which occasionally caused the patient great pain. What the real cause of this pain was we never distinctly ascertained (and now probably never shall); but that it was a growth of some kind upon or in the bowel seemed indicated by a number of facts it would take too long to detail here. Many of the symptoms indicated this, and this only. But, whatever the cause, the prime object was to remove it! Mrs. T. had heard of Doctor Dewey, through an interested friend; had procured his book, and she proceeded to put his theories to the test!

Unfortunately, Mrs. T. had no one to guide her through her fast, and consequently neglected her enemas, her water drinking, and other important auxiliaries, which should have been attended to, and which, had she known of them, would have helped her greatly. The benefits she derived from the fast were, without doubt, largely negatived by the omission of these important hygienic aids.

Let me say here that Mrs. T. weighed, at the commencement of her (eighteen-day) fast but ninety-eight pounds, clothed! Her fast continued for eighteen days, and from every day's abstinence did she derive benefit. She unfortunately neglected to be weighed at the close of the fast, but her weight must have been very low, as the patient lost a good deal of flesh during the fast. It conclusively disproves the notion that only *fat* persons derive benefit from fasting. (p. 123–4.)

In this case, the patient was extremely emaciated when she commenced her fast, and yet she derived benefit from it every day notwithstanding. She was upon her feet, and actively exercising the entire time.

The net result, to be brief, was that the patient's health became excellent; she was apparently quite normal in every way —save that a slight pain still lingered in the right side—showing that the work of cure was not yet quite completed, which, I think, could hardly be expected, seeing that enemas, water drinking, etc., had been neglected, and that she had been treated for years unsuccessfully; above all, that the fast had been broken prematurely, and before the return of natural hunger. However, the patient followed up the fast by living carefully and abstemiously, on two meals *per diem*, taking plenty of exercise—particularly those strengthening the muscles around the waist line. Bv following these instructions, the patient continued to improve, and, within three months, the pain had entirely disappeared, and has never returned. Whatever the cause of the pain—whether a growth or not—it was evidently removed by fasting and the subsequent, abstemious life. The ultimate results of the treatment cannot possibly be doubted; since, so far as can be seen, a complete cure had been effected.

G. W. S. This case is perhaps one of the most remarkable I have to record—not because I can furnish minute details of the case, for I regret that I cannot—nor can I tell the ultimate results—not being present during the latter part of the fast, but only during the opening days. But, if for no other reason, this case deserves mention simply because of its *length*—demonstrating, as it does, the length of time that it is possible for man to go without nourishment of any kind—and with no ill effects, but on the contrary, with continued gain and improvement.

Mr. S., age 45, had been completely bedridden for more than nine years—paralysis of the entire body being present, together with a degree of partial anæsthesia. Though the mentality was, all this time bright and clear, the trunk (from the neck down) was completely useless—it being impossible for the patient to move even a finger or a muscle in any part of his body. Everything had been tried in vain. During this whole period, however (nine years), three meals had been daily ingested, and no diminution in the bulk of the food eaten had ever been suggested or even thought of by the doctors and attendants present during all that long period! And the fact that this mass of food, throughout that period of complete inaction, had been disposed of by the system without serious disease of any kind resulting, is, I think, one of the most remarkable examples of the extent to which the system can be abused without showing such abuse, and of the extraordinary recuperative powers of the human body. One other fact of interest is the illustration of how perfectly the vegetable functions of life may be conducted without guidance, and while the voluntary muscular system is completely paralyzed and useless.

I can only state, in connection with this case, that the patient entered upon a fast, while in this condition—and having been about the same for the length of time specified—and that, before the fast terminated, the patient had so far recovered as to be able to use both arms slightly—the right arm with comparative freedom—and that he was enabled to sit up in bed and to move, at will, the toes on both feet, and even the legs themselves slightly. His health had meanwhile improved marvelously. I regret that I cannot record the final outcome of this fast, or how the patient ultimately fared—I leaving the city about the third week of the fast—and losing trace of him altogether shortly after the fast was finally broken. A complete cure was not, of course, ever effected in this case; but that is not the point I wish to illustrate in citing it. It is this: The patient fasted the extraordinary length of time of *seventy-nine days*—and this, it must be remembered, with only added health and increased strength! I ask, how, if our energy is derived from our daily food, are we to explain such a case as this?

C. G. Patterson, age 69½ years, is, perhaps, one of the most interesting fasts I have to record—partly because of the ad vanced age of the patient, and partly for the reason that a diary was kept—extracts from which I offer below. That a man of Mr. Patterson's age should enter upon a fast of thirty-one days and derive from it the benefit he did, speaks volumes for the treatment advocated; while the gradual increase in strength throughout the fast clearly shows that the energies were in some way independent of the food supply. The sudden weakening at the end of the fast is very clearly traceable to the purgative and the Turkish Bath then most foolishly taken, and cannot be said to be due to the lack of food.

For the first few days of the fast the patient noticed no especial symptoms worth recording. His strength and general health and spirits seemed to remain about as usual—as, indeed, they did throughout the fast. The following is a brief résumé of the case—partly in Mr. Patterson's own words. The case was sent to Mrs. Dewey, soon after Dr. Dewey's death, and by her sent to me for perusal. The extracts are, therefore, copied from the diary kept at the time.

The patient was treated by Dr. R. H. W. of New York City; also by Dr. G. W. C. of Washington, D.C.—altogether for seventeen years. Excessive nasal discharge was present—apparently catarrhal in character, but I could not very well tell from the report I was permitted to read—and other minor troubles. Fasted thirty-one days; slept well and restfully throughout, except occasionally. Drank a considerable amount of water during the fast. Noticed no particular alteration in strength during the fast. (N. B. In a man of nearly seventy years of age.) The fast commenced August 4th, and a diary was kept throughout, from which I have copied the following notes, and been enabled to summarize the case.

On August 9th, Mr. Patterson writes:

"At this moment I could not define any particular change in my physical condition since the fast began five days ago.

"August 12th.—The changes in my condition that I am able to discover are, a clearer complexion, steadier nerves, the absence of gas in the stomach; and, it seems, a lessening of mucous discharge from my nose. The disagreeable stickiness of my mouth and eyelids is undiminished. . . . I have no desire for food, but continue to drink water freely.

"August 13th.—Soon after rising I went down town as far as Twenty-third Street on an errand, and returned to the hotel at 9.30 A. M. Upon investigation I was surprised to find my tongue showing at the end, and extending up perhaps half an inch, and of clearer appearance than usual. For more than twenty-five years it has been thickly coated, and I have taken into my stomach unknown quantities of medicine to remedy this condition, administered by skillful physicans, but all to no purpose.

"August 15th.—For the first time since beginning this fast I perceived that the nauseating smell so long characterizing my urine was considerably lessened; it is now of a natural color, clear and almost odorless."

Mr. Patterson was examined by physicians several times during his fast; and was advised not to eat any food until he was hungry, "which," he adds, "I certainly am not." He writes, Aug. 19th:

"I have noticed recently that, instead of proverbially cold feet I have warm ones now; they are never uncomfortable of late.

"August 20th.—At 4 P. M. took a warm bath, and weighed 113½ pounds—a *gain* of 1½ pounds for the week. (*v.* pp. 469–70.) Within a few days I have observed that my finger nails have grown very much harder than usual, and the cuticle seems dried and tough. The nails have not lengthened as has been customary; these changes are pronounced, and easily discoverable. I cannot be mistaken."

The pulse, when examined, was always found improved and more nearly normal.

"August 22d.—I find, since beginning this fast, that my nerves have improved immensely. I can now write with a steady, confident hand; this has not been the case before in several years.

"August 24th.—My skin has been clearer, and my complexion never had a healthier glow. . I think my sight is improved; the vision is clearer and steadier . . . I have no desire for food."

Aug. 26th. On this day a little "medicine" was taken, and the next day (27th), Mr. Patterson noticed he had grown weaker! (Precisely what we should expect.) On the 27th, the patient writes:

"I notice especially my finger-nails. They seem to have become hard, almost like shells, and grow but very little; the cuticle does not appear to extend a particle over the nails. . . . There is marked change for the better in my mouth.

"August 30th.—There has been no loss of strength to-day; on the contrary, I think I feel rather more aggressive than for some time past.

"September 1st.—Took two little black pills, to be taken two hours apart, and followed three hours later by a glass of Hunyadi water.

"September 2d.—My strength remains without perceptible change, and I have no craving for food.

"September 3d.—Arose, feeling fatigued. Took a Turkish bath. Felt much weaker. Next day, again weak and was persuaded (on 31st day) to break my fast."

It will be observed that the patient was not really hungry, and he should have fasted longer. The patient took two meals daily, after breaking the fast, and, four weeks later wrote:

"My weight has increased from 102¾ pounds, on September 3d., to 114 pounds to-day. My skin has a healthy glow; my vision is certainly clearer; my ability to endure physical exercise is greater than for several years past, and, generally, my health is good. Nasal discharge not quite cured—due to belladonna taken in quantities, having dried and thickened the mucous membrane of the nose. My hands and feet are now the same temperature as the rest of the body."

From many points of view, I consider this a most interesting case.

The following case was reported in the *St. Louis Republic*, June 30, 1907, and contains Doctor Eales' own account of his case. It is therefore authentic, and presents many points of great interest.

Dr. I. J. Eales, of Belleville, whose experiment in the nature of dietary reform by abstaining from food thirty days has aroused widespread attention throughout the medical fraternity of the Middle West, will complete his self-imposed task at noon to-day. On the stroke of 12 he will break his fast for the first time in a month by partaking of a glass of malted milk. At noon Monday he will take another glass of malted milk, and will then begin the series of physiological experiments to learn the effect on his body of various foods.

Doctor Eales celebrated the last day of his fast yesterday by testing his strength. He went to the butcher shop of Hugo Heinemann, in the public market, where he has made a daily record of his weight, and, in the presence of half a dozen witnesses, lifted Mr. Heinemann, who weighs 242 pounds, grasping him under the armpits. He sustained Mr. Heinemann's weight for approximately five seconds without extraordinary effort. The test was satisfactory to the spectators and particularly so to the doctor.

After this exhibition Doctor Eales went on the scales. He weighed 164 pounds. When he began his fast, May 31, he weighed 192 pounds. The loss of twenty-eight pounds in nearly thirty days was suffered, Doctor Eales says, with a minimum depreciation of physical strength, and no appreciable discomfort of body or mind. In fact, he declares that the conclusion of his thirty-day regimen of air and water has left him in better physical and mental condition than when he commenced his experiment.

Doctor Eales said he would embody the data, which he has obtained as a result of his observations and experiences in this fast, together with the additional facts he expects to glean from his experimenting with foods later on, in a work which he expects to publish later on, dealing with the subject of dietary reform, and the value of fasting in health and disease.

Doctor Eales' Statement.

"Now that my long fast is ended, and as so many interviews have appeared in the different papers, some of them inadvertently misquoting me, it seems but proper that the public be informed correctly regarding my experiments and what value there is in fasting.

"In all ages fasting has been practiced for various purposes. The meek and lowly Nazarene set us an example by fasting in the wilderness of Judea for forty days and forty nights. How many Christian people are there who follow His example one day a week? All nations had their religious fasts and feasts. Fasting comes as near being a panacea for human ills as anything can be. By fasting we subdue the baser nature and illuminate the spiritual part of our nature. By fasting we rest every organ of the body, and while they are resting the body is being renovated, rejuvenated, the blood purified, all the senses rendered more acute, the brain becomes clear, every cell of the body, in fact, is cleansed.

"Up to about twelve years ago I was a heavy eater. I weighed 235 pounds, had an abdominal circumference of 47 inches, had an irritated stomach and was threatened with acute albuminuria and functional disease of the heart. I realized that something must be done to remove the mountain of adipose tissue I had accumulated, or I might drop off with heart failure at any moment. What was I to do? I knew that drugs could not help me. I realized that I must get back to normal weight, give my vital organs a rest and stop the manufacture of fat. I knew of no other way to do this but to stop eating, and stop eating I did.

"I had read of Doctor Tanner's fasts—one of forty and one of forty-two days—and decided I would try a few days of his medicine. The result was I reduced myself by a few short fasts to 180 pounds; my kidneys were cured, my heart trouble vanished, my stomach was normal; I felt physically regenerated and my waist measure was reduced to 42 inches—in fact, I was well. Since that date I have indulged in periodical fasts whenever my weight increased to 190 pounds, always feeling rejuvenated at the expi ration of the fast. It was a revelation to me, and I began using it in my practice, with the result that acute and chronic troubles that defied the usual methods of medication yielded in some instances like magic as soon as a rest was given to the stomach, and consequently to the entire organism. I began to study.

"I found others who were using the system with the same results as myself. I wondered why I could retain my strength and not eat. About the year 1901 a work on diet reform, written by Doctor Dewey, came to my notice, and I discovered that Doctor

Dewey had been in the same quandary as myself, but the secret was revealed to him by a table found in "Yeo's Physiology," which gives the estimated loss of the different tissues of the body in starvation of animals as follows:

"Fat, 97 per cent.; spleen, 63; liver, 56; muscle, 30; blood, 17; nerve centers, 0.

"I found a table of Professor Chossat and one by Professor Voit, which practically agree with that of Professor Yeo.

"These tables prove that during a fast the nervous system is fed by the adipose tissue, muscles and glands, and consequently does not suffer, and so long as the nervous system is fed there is no danger of starvation and the strength is kept at par. Animals do not eat when sick. They keep a clean alimentary canal, and while the vital organs are resting, nature, the vital force, cures the disease.

"The standard weight in proportion to height and lung capacity is about as follows in males: (In females the lung capacity is three-tenths less and weight five to eight pounds less than males of same height.)

Height		Weight, Pounds	Lung Capacity, Cubic Inches
Feet	Inches		
5	0		
5	1		
5	2		
5	3		
5	4		
5	5		
5	6		
5	7		
5	8		
5	9		
5	10		
5	11		
6	0		
6	1		
6	2		
6	3		

"When people become fleshy they should breathe more to supply the extra cells with oxygen, as every cell in the body requires about 20 per cent. oxygen, but the fact is, as we become heavier we breathe less. The vital organs are surrounded with fat. Fatty infiltration takes place and we suffer for want of oxygen. During my fast my lung capacity increased from 290 to 305 cubic inches. When I weighed 235 pounds my lung capacity was 250 cubic inches. I now weigh 164 pounds and my lung capacity is 305 cubic inches. We should eat less and breathe more.

"A great many are dying slowly from autointoxication and food poisoning, from overeating and underbreathing. Many people to-day are eating themselves into the grave. It is time that some simple truths were taught in the public schools about the care of the human body. Every child should be taught first how to live to attain a ripe old age, and the knowledge afterwards gained would be of some benefit; whereas at the present time we find our children on the verge of nervous prostration before they graduate, and many die before the prime of life. Over 90 per cent. of disease is caused by errors in diet—eating too much food, too large a quantity of either the proteids, fats or carbohydrates, or the wrong combinations of food.

"In regard to my own fast, hunger left me on the third day, and from that day to the time of breaking my fast I never knew what hunger was. I worked eleven and twelve hours each day at my profession. I felt very energetic during the time; drank freely of distilled water during the day, and had it not been for the publicity given by the paper, one would hardly have known I was fasting. My reasons for the fast were to reduce my weight, and to make some scientific tests and demonstrations which will in due time be given to the public in a work I shall publish on dietetics, dietary reform and the value of fasting.

"I have disproved some of the theories taught for years in some of our standard text books. I have tested my strength and endurance almost daily, and at the end of a thirty-day fast I was able to lift and hold a man of 250 pounds weight by grasping him under the arms.

"My pulse has been normal during the entire period, and my blood normal on the twenty-first day, when last examined. It is true I have been severely criticised by some of my medical brethren, but science answers important questions by investigation, not by epithet. I have not sought notoriety. I have no need to advertise in any way, have all the work and more than I can attend to, and steadily increasing.

"These facts furnish food for thought, and, although I had much preferred that my long fast had not been made public, still, if by being commented upon I have in any way stimulated thought and investigation so that the value of fasting and dietary reform may be brought forcibly to the notice of suffering humanity, I shall be perfectly satisfied with the knowledge that the fact has helped others besides myself. Yours for humanity and in perfect health,

I. J. Eales, M.D., D.O."

Van R. Wilcox. This case is, in many ways, also very interesting. Mr. Wilcox has written a little book, entitled "Correct Living," in which he states his own case in outline; and from this booklet I draw the facts of the case, as here given. For fuller information, I refer the reader to the book itself. In brief, the case is this.

Some twenty-five years ago, Mr. Wilcox informs us, he was a well and healthy man. Through constant overfeeding, however, he gradually became more and more disabled and diseased —suffering from a variety of ills. Boils, eczema, hemorrhoids, partial paralysis, defective eyesight, baldness, rheumatism, kidney disease, constipation alternating with diarrhœa were only some of the ills that made life a burden and kept him constantly "doctoring"—with no ultimate good effects.

In June, 1904, however, Mr. Wilcox started a fast (when excessively emaciated, as his photograph, taken at the time, indicates), which lasted for sixty days. No solid food was taken for seventy days, (p. 15), but the author took, in several of the opening and closing days, milk and water, or farinaceous water. The fast was broken March 27, 1904—a shredded wheat biscuit being the first article of solid food eaten.

The result of this fast was that Mr. Wilcox was completely cured of every one of his many infirmities. In so fine a physical condition was he, indeed—such a high state of health had he attained—that he set about walking across the American continent—from New York to San Francisco—a distance of some three thousand six hundred miles, as walked—which remarkable feat Mr. Wilcox performed in 167 days—an average (taking into account the fact that Mr. Wilcox could not walk as the "crow flies") of slightly more than twenty-two miles *per diem*—he carrying, throughout, from twenty to thirty pounds of baggage! (p. 95.) During this period, Mr. Wilcox was exposed to dangers and hardships galore; the temperature being at times 125° F. in the sun; at others 13° F. below zero. During all this time, though the physical exertion was as great as it was, *not once did he eat a breakfast.*

"On no day during that entire tramp did I partake of more than two meals. The breakfast was always omitted. Further, on a few occasions, I went two days at a time without any food—not even a glass of milk." (p. 59.)

Surely this should explode once and for all the fallacy that a hearty breakfast is required by those doing hard muscular labor—since there is no exercise more taxing than walking, or one that arouses more keenly the appetite.

Mr. Wilcox summarizes the results of his own case as follows:

"What do you think of the two pictures? My physical man of three years ago, and of to-day, with my dropsical symptoms all gone; my rheumatism all gone; the weariness on my left side—all gone. Most of my time now is being spent in reading and writing, with little inconvenience to my eyes. The top of my head is getting a new growth of hair. No boils or pimples. Hemorrhoids or piles about gone. There is no re-appearance of that troublesome skin eruption present for more than a year. Two years ago I weighed about 105 pounds—now 160. Muscular development good." (p. 96.)

Theoretically, of course, Mr. Wilcox should have died from inanition and vital exhaustion about the twentieth day of his fast—if the current theories of vitality be true. I leave the results to speak for themselves, and to tell their own tale.

I shall now mention, briefly, a few of the many cases that have been brought more or less directly to my attention; giving an idea, as they do, of the wide *range* of diseases that have been cured by this method, and how large a portion of the intellectual persons in America and other countries are being drawn to this method—of how widespread a following the system has. Some of these cases are quite as remarkable as those that I have given, if not more so; but, for the reason that they have been published before, or because of the fact that I had not the opportunity of cross-examining the patients, I have only briefly mentioned them; trusting that the cases given in more detail will serve as examples and illustrations of the method of cure by fasting—since too constant repetition of details would only prove tedious. With this I pass on to enumerate the cases themselves:

E. A. P.—Cured of paralysis; fasted thirty days.

Mrs. John B.—Cured of "liver and stomach trouble"; twenty-six days.

Mrs. George F. B.—"Nervous troubles" cured; twenty-one days.

Mrs. Nina H.—"Liver and stomach troubles"; eighteen days.

William F.—Nervous prostration; thirty days.

Rev. I. G. A.—Congested liver; ten days.

Mrs. N. A. M.—Consumption; twenty-seven days.

Mrs. Harriet M. Closz.—Rheumatism; forty-five days.

M. Christ. Mortensen.—Rheumatism; fifty-two days. (Case reported in *The Liberator;* August, 1906, pp. 115–16.)

Edward R. Taylor.—Obesity; thirty days. (I interviewed this patient personally.)

Andrew Alexson.—Consumption; twelve days. (Case reported in *Physical Culture;* Volume V., pp. 150–2.)

Mrs. C. Cole.—Rheumatism; thirty-one days. (Case reported in *Physical Culture;* Volume VI., pp. 109–10, 163.)

George Propheter.—Experimental fast; fifty-one days. (Case reported in *Physical Culture.* Volume VII., pp. 70–3.)

Thomas Morin.—Dyspepsia; forty days.

Ambrose Taylor.—Rheumatism; twenty-three days.

Mrs. Judith Sampson.—Dyspepsia; seventeen days.

James D. Wren.—"Stomach trouble"; twenty-three days.

Cora Brown.—Nervousness; twenty-seven days.

Edgar Wallace Conable.—Loss of appetite; fifteen days.

J. M. Chaffee.—Eczema, boils, etc.; (Case given in Haskell's *Perfect Health,* pp. 143–5.)

Charles T. Potter.—Asthma; forty days.

"A Missionary."—Malaria; twenty-eight days.

Mr. Henry Ritter, an enthusiast on the fasting theory, stated several years ago, that he "had brought more than twenty cases to a successful conclusion"—which number I do not doubt is greatly increased by now. "I have directed over twenty cases," he writes, "the longest fifty days—two of forty-five days—and two of forty-two days—and others running, in the majority of cases, from twenty-five to forty days."

In addition to all these cases, there are those given by Doctor Dewey, in his "No-Breakfast Plan"; notable among them being the following:

C. C. H. Cowen.—Catarrh; forty-two days.
Milton Rathbun.—Obesity; twenty-eight days.
Milton Rathbun.—(second fast) thirty-six days.
Miss Estella Kuenzel.—Insanity; forty-five days.
Leonard Thress.—Dropsy; fifty days.
Miss Elizabeth W. A. Westing; forty days.
Rev. C. H. Dalrymple; forty days.

Taken in conjunction with the other cases that have been given in this book, and are given in the other books to which reference is made in the text, I think that the above cases are representative enough and forcible enough to place this system of treatment upon a secure and firm footing—one that will necessitate a thorough investigation of fasting cases by scientific men, who are in a far better position than the writer to observe and record facts obtained in this manner. Many other such cases could be given, but it is hardly necessary. The points of interest should be apparent to the student; and especially after reading the chapters dealing with the study of the cases in Book V. I should by all means advise my reader to go back and read again this chapter of cases when he has finished the book, for he will find a new light is thrown upon them by the additional arguments, facts and theories advanced in the latter portion of this volume; the cases will then be found to illustrate many points brought forward and discussed in the text, and will be found to sustain the theory of vital energy advanced in this book far more strongly than a first casual reading would indicate. Having thus given a brief account of the cases themselves; we must turn to a consideration of the theory of vitality which these cases seem to establish; and to a theoretical discussion of their meaning and significance. To this aspect of the problem

I shall devote Book III., reserving Books IV. and V. for a detailed discussion of the fasts from a therapeutic and physiological point of view. In both directions I think we shall find that they are of supreme importance; in the one case to philosophy and philosophical science; in the other to practical and clinical medicine.

BOOK III

VITALITY SLEEP, DEATH, BODILY HEAT

BOOK III

CHAPTER I

VITALITY[1]

§ 1. *Present Theory of the Causation of Vital Energy by Food*

WE NOW come to a consideration of this question of vitality—its relation to the daily food supply and its supposed causation by it. This theoretical side of the discussion is of the very greatest importance, necessitating, as it does, a reconstruction of our views of the law of the Conservation of Energy, and the relative significance of life.

Of the *essence* of vitality we, of course, know absolutely nothing. Its nature and the problems of its origin and destiny are equally the problems of the origin and destiny of life, with which it is inseparably united (if, indeed, it is not the same thing) and to this latter question modern science has, as yet, but one answer to make—*ignoramus*. Certain theories have, it is true, been advanced from time to time by scientists, one or two of which I shall quote as they have a more or less direct bearing on the discussion, as we shall see later on. Doctor Reinhold, *e.g.*, stated a position frequently occupied when he said:[2]

"It would appear that each being is supplied with a definite fund or capital of vital power at birth, to which no art of ours can add, but on which we subsist; and, gradually thus exhausting the stock, we finally die when it expires. But it appears that we

[1] In the present volume, I shall not even attempt to distinguish between such terms as vitality, vital force, energy (as applied to the organism), life force, vital energy, etc.—using these terms as more or less interchangeable and, for all practical purposes, meaning the same thing. I shall consequently use them throughout the present chapter in that manner, and without implying any of the subtler, finer distinctions which might, theoretically, be possible; and I must ask my reader to distinctly remember that I have done so throughout this discussion.

[2] "Nature *versus* Drugs," p. 39.

have the power to economize this fund, and so spin out our existence to a longer period than if the vitality were wasted in wrong living. Its working may be compared to the spring of a watch. The action of this is strongest just after being wound up, and grows weaker and weaker as time goes on, till it finally runs down."

But to this idea there are many objections, as Doctor Evans points out:[1]

"In many diseases how often is the sunbeam of life nearly extinguished, known to recover, and shine again, perhaps more brilliantly than before! If we ask its source, can parents, whose supply of vitality is decreasing, give more than they possess to their offspring, and yet keep a portion to themselves?"

Doctor Taylor[2] and A. Dastre[3] have also some very interesting theories to offer, but we cannot stop to consider them now.

All that we know of vital force, then, is that it is lost through excessive exertion, bodily or mental; through sexual excitement;[4] through overeating (see pp. 104–5); through nerve tension, such as in resistance to cold weather;[5] and, generally, through all unphysiological habits; and that it is increased, on the contrary, by the adaptation of all wholesome, hygienic

[1] "How to Prolong Life," p. 28–9.

[2] "Massage," p. 14.

[3] "The Theory of Energy and the Living World," p. 534.

[4] "Vital Force," by E. P. Miller, M.D.

[5] In cold weather this continuous muscle contraction is often very marked almost causing pain, in the intensity of the contraction. The *object* of this contraction is doubtless to prevent such a free circulation of blood at the periphery, as would normally occur—this preventing too rapid cooling of the body. The nerve force is thus constantly expended. We thus readily see how, in the winter months, our vitality is used up in "resisting" the cold. This offers, perhaps, a solution of one other well-recognized fact. It is commonly stated that the passions are at their height in the spring-time, and observation of the animal world would seem to confirm this statement. The reason is, I venture to think, this: Throughout the winter months, we have been expending, daily, a considerable amount of energy in "resisting" the cold, and when this resistance is no longer called for and necessitated that amount of energy is available for other purposes; and, if not expended in active exercise, may be, I suggest, the source of the sexual excitement noted at this time. It has also been noticed that all animal organisms both function and grow more rapidly in the warm weather than they do in the cold. ("Temperature and Life," by Henry De Varigny, p. 423. "Weather Influences," by Edwin G. Dexter, Ph.D., pp. 75, 117.) I suggest that this phenomenon is also due to the same cause—the energy, formerly expended in "resisting the cold," is now set at liberty and utilized for purposes of development and growth.

or physiological habits[1]; but, beyond this, we are at present unable to go; its essence, its origin, its connection with and intimate relation to the body, are problems which we are absolutely unable to solve; phenomena which we can merely observe. We must record the facts in the case, in so far as we can discern them, and leave the further, more detailed and deeper discussion for some future generations, who will doubtless have collected more *data* than we at present possess.

In order to make perfectly clear my position in the discussion that follows it will be necessary for me to go into the question in considerable detail, and to discuss not only the outline of the theory, but its *minutiæ*, since that is necessitated in such a case as the present, where I am attempting to combat and to overthrow one of the fundamental postulates, both of physiology and of physics, and, at first sight, even the law of the conservation of energy itself—though we shall presently see that this law, in so far as it relates to the physical world, has been in no wise contradicted. I should like to state, however, that I cannot possibly discuss this problem, and all the difficulties and objections involved, at the length it should be discussed, for the reason that that would require an extensive volume alone. For the present, then, I must confine myself to the space available, and my arguments to the principal aspects of the problem. I shall in the first place, therefore, briefly state what is the position of the scientific world, as such, upon this question of the relations of food and human vitality; of the causation of the latter by the former; and of the further inter-relation of the vital or life forces with the other forces or energies in the universe; and in doing so I shall, in every case, quote unquestionable authority, in order that it may not be said that I am perverting or mis interpreting the facts, or the attitude of the scientific world, in this question.

In the first place, then, I must presume that all my readers are thoroughly conversant with the law of the conservation of energy—of the law, *i.e.*, that all the forces in the universe—light, heat, motion, chemical affinity, gravitation, electricity, magnetism, etc., are in some manner inter-related, and are

[1] "The Building of Vital Power," by Bernarr Macfadden.

transmutable, the one into the other. Thus, a certain amount of (say) motion may, under appropriate conditions, be transformed or transmuted into a certain amount of (say) heat; and further, that the quantity of this heat would exactly correspond to the quantity of motion destroyed; the amount of the two forces would exactly counterbalance one another; and this law holds good throughout the whole of the physical world; the sum-total of all the forces in the universe remains unchanged and eternal, throughout their transformations. All change in nature amounts to this; that force can change its form and locality without its quantity ever being affected.

Now this law, so far, is pretty clearly and certainly established, and I have no desire to enter the lists in order to challenge this statement of the case as it stands. Indeed, I believe it to be essentially true. My contention is that *life*, or vital force, which is commonly held to be also inter-related and transmutable into one or other of these energies, is placed wrongly in the list; that it is not transformable or transmutable into any of the other forces or energies whatsoever, but that it is absolutely alone, separate, distinct, *per se*. My attempt will be to show that it is not interchangeable with, or derivable from, any other force whatever; that its origin is not what it is generally supposed to be, *viz.*, the food ingested, but that it is due to an altogether different source. Loosely speaking, my position might be termed that of a Vitalist, though I shall presently endeavor to show that it is very different from the crude form of vitalism formerly held by a large number of thinkers, but now all but given up, save by some few conservative scientists.[1]

I am well aware that the position I assume is indeed revolutionary; is, in fact, practically unprecedented, and that I shall challenge the law of the conservation of energy in a way it has never been challenged since its general acceptance; but I hope to make good my position, and hope to establish the correctness of my contention, before I conclude this volume. As to that, however, I must leave the reader to judge for himself.

I have stated that vital force is regarded, by the scientific world, as only one special form of energy, which may, under

[1] See "The Riddle of the Universe," by Ernst Haeckel, pp. 262–3.

certain conditions, be transmutable into, and in turn derivable from, certain other physical forces or energies. A terse and concise statement of the position generally accepted is the following—the opening sentence of Professor LeConte's "Correlation of Vital with Chemical and Physical Forces," contained in Balfour Stewart's "Conservation of Energy." There he says (p. 171):

"Vital force: whence is it derived? What is its relation to the other forces of Nature? The answer of modern Science to these questions is: It is derived from the lower forces of Nature; it is related to the other forces much as these are related to each other—it is correlated with chemical and physical forces."

So much is definite and precise. Just *how* it is related; the *nature* of its relation; above all, the source of vital energy is, perhaps, well and clearly stated in the following extract from Prof. Robert Mayer's "Organic Movement in its Relations to the Mutations of Matter."

"The sun is, so far as human knowledge goes, an inexhaustible store of physical energy. The stream of this energy which pours forth upon our earth is the everlasting spring which maintains the activity of everything which moves upon the globe. The surface of the earth would in a short time be covered by the ice of death if the great quantity of energy which is continually dissipated into space, in the form of undulatory movement, were not continually restored to it by the sun.

"Nature has set herself the problem of clipping the wings of the light which arrives upon the earth, and of storing in a fixed form the most mobile of all the forces. To attain this end, she has clothed the earth's surface with organisms which, in living, collect the light of the sun. These organisms are the *plants.* The vegetable kingdom is a reservoir in which the rays emanating from the sun are fixed and accumulated in order that they may be utilized again; a providential arrangement upon which depends the existence of the human species, and which excites in us an instinctive feeling of pleasure every time our eyes fall upon rich vegetation.

"Plants receive a force—light, and from it produce another chemical change. The physical force accumulated by the activity of the plants comes to the service of another class of creatures who make it their prey, and use it for their own benefit. These creatures are the *animals*.

"The living animal constantly takes from the vegetable kingdom oxidizable foods to combine them afresh with oxygen from the atmosphere. Parallel with this result is manifested the characteristic feature of animal life; the production of mechanical work, the production of movement, the raising of weights.

"The chemical force contained in the ingested foods and in the inspired oxygen is the source of two manifestations of energy, namely, movement and heat, and the sum of the physical energy produced by an animal is equal to the corresponding and simultaneous chemical processes."[1]

It may be said, in short, that the statement, as above outlined, indicates the position of practically all physicians and physiologists to-day, and it has been their position for the past fifty or more years; it is the theory taught in all text books, in all medical colleges, and by all scientific men, so that I am certainly fully aware of the immensity of the task before me in attempting to refute the theory. Nevertheless, I shall endeavor to do so, feeling that I have arguments and facts in my possession which undoubtedly overthrow and render untenable their position.

The claim put forward is that the latent energy of the food exactly corresponds to the amount of mechanical work done, or heat evolved, *i.e.*, the two added together. Professor Atwater, *e.g.*, in his "Principles of Nutrition and Nutritive Value of Food" (p. 11), says:

"These experiments have shown that the material which is oxidized yields the same amount of energy as it would if burned with oxygen outside the body, *e.g.*, in the bomb calorimeter. The experiments show also that when a man does no muscular work (save, of course, the internal work of respiration, circulation, etc.), all the energy leaves his body *as heat;* but when he does muscular work, as in lifting weights or driving a bicycle, part of the energy appears in the external work thus done, and the rest

[1] See also: Stewart: "Conservation of Energy," p. 145, 163: Grant Allen: "Force and Energy," p. 51; Carpenter: "The Correlation and Conservation of Forces," pp. 401–33; Kirke: "Physiology," p. 516; Bastian, "Nature and Origin of Living Matter"; while the instructions issued by the Japanese Government to their soldiers contain this same statement. "Real Triumph of Japan," p. 168, etc.

is given off from the body as heat. The most interesting result of all is that the energy given off from the body as heat when the man is at rest or as heat and mechanical work together when he is working, exactly equals the latent energy of the material burned in the body. This is in accordance with the law of the conservation of energy. It thus appears that the body actually obeys, as we should expect it to obey, this great law which dominates the physical universe."

§ 2. *Weaknesses In and Objections To that Theory*

Now, if this statement were true; if it could be definitely proved (which, *un*fortunately for my argument, is not the case), that the total bodily heat and measurable muscular work exactly corresponded to the amount of latent energy in the food, then I think my contention would be definitely proved, and the theory I am combating definitely and finally refuted. Contradictory as this may appear, it may easily be shown to be the correct interpretation of the case. And, in order to prove the correctness of this statement, I think it is only necessary to ask ourselves this question. How about our *mental* life, and the operations of consciousness? Do they, then, require no energy at all for their successful operation? If they do *not*, then they lie outside the law of conservation, and materialism is refuted; but if they *do*, (and we know that they not only do require energy, but far *more* energy, proportionally, than muscular work of any kind),[1] then the position just stated becomes quite untenable; and not only that but, in reality, rank nonsense. Professor Atwater himself, indeed, writes on the very next page to the paragraph above quoted:

"We have been considering food as a source of heat and muscular power. There is no doubt that intellectual activity, also, is somehow dependent upon the consumption of material which the brain has obtained from the food; but just what substances are consumed to produce brain and nerve force, and how much of each is required for a given quantity of intellectual labor, are questions which the physiological chemist has not yet answered." (pp. 12–13.)

[1] Mosso: "Fatigue," p. 121.

This, it appears to me, completely negatives and disproves his former statements. For, either the operations of consciousness require a constant expenditure of energy or they do not. All physiologists would be the very last men on earth to contend that they do not, and Professor Atwater is not an exception to this rule. But if they do, then the amount of this expenditure must be measured and added to the amount expended by the voluntary and involuntary muscular activities. But, since we have but the very vaguest notion of the amount of energy the internal and involuntary muscular work necessitates, and practically no notion at all of what the operations of thought and consciousness necessitate (by Professor Atwater's own showing), and by the admission of practically every physiologist now living,[1] except to know that these are enormous, I ask, how are any calculations to be made from such *data?* How can we know that the amount of energy expended during the day equals the latent energy in the food, when we have not even the vaguest idea of what the former is? And I must insist, if Professor Atwater's point is made; if he could, by any means, prove his statement that the amount of heat and muscular work exactly equals the amount of latent energy in the food, and so his point be apparently proved, it would, in my estimation, completely *dis*prove it, because we should then *know for certain* that our energy is not all derivable from our food, for the reason that the expenditure of energy occasioned by the internal muscular work and by the operations of thought and consciousness would then have to be added to this calculated amount of energy, with the result that the total would far surpass the theoretical amount the food contains, and so (since the less cannot contain the greater), could not possibly be derived from it. The position would thus be refuted, instead of established. Unless a part can equal its whole, there can be no escape from this conclusion. And the fact that attempts have been made to fit the figures to the theory is no proof whatever of anything beyond the fact that such attempts have invariably ended in disastrous failure,

[1] Kirke: "Physiology," pp. 517–18; Thurston: "The Animal as a Prime Mover," p. 325. It is here admitted that the figures generally advanced as representing the internal muscular and mental work are "little better than guesses."

and that, in all such cases, the figures have obviously been *made to conform* to the theory, and in no wise prove it.

I would point out, in the next place, that these experiments are absolutely unscientific for the reason that we do not and cannot possibly know what the actual, potential energy of food is. Says Professor Atwater:[1]

"We have neither the means for measuring potential energy, as such, nor a unit for expressing such measurements if they were made."

The only possible way in which we can test the question is to artificially digest or oxidize the food material outside the body—assuming that the heat and energy given off is the same *in* the body. But what proof is there of this? The two sets of conditions are so entirely dissimilar that it is in reality nothing more than a monstrous assumption to assert that the results are exactly the same in both cases—especially since we know that experiments conducted along these lines have given very differing results.

Conceding this point to my adversary, however, I would point out that, in many cases, it has been shown mathematically that the theoretical amount of energy supplied by the food is not even enough to account for the external muscular work of the body—let alone the tremendous amount required for the internal muscular work, and to say nothing of the operations of thought and consciousness![2]

Doctor Austin Flint, for example, in discussing the case of Weston's remarkable walk, so carefully studied by himself, said:

"The actual work performed is more than ten times the estimated force-value of the nitrogenized food and muscle consumed, deducting that used in the 'internal operations'; and, estimating for the weight of clothing carried, it is even more than the total force-value of food and muscle consumed, taking no account of the force used in circulation, respiration, etc. There

[1] "Experiments on the Metabolism of Matter and Energy in the Human Body," 1898–1900, p. 145.

[2] See "The Effect of Severe and Prolonged Muscular Work on Food Consumption, Digestion, and Metabolism," by W. O. Atwater, Ph.D., and H. C. Sherman, Ph.D., pp. 9–10.

must be some fatal error in the basis of calculations the results of which appear to be so far removed from the actual facts."

Adopting the method of Doctor Pavy, and basing his calculations on the reports of the cases of Perkins, Weston, etc., he estimated the amount of muscular work accomplished for each day in foot tons. He then calculated the force value in foot-tons of nitrogenous matter equivalent to the nitrogen eliminated in excess of the average during rest. The result of this calculation was to show that:

"The force obtainable from the nitrogenous matter disintegrated is totally inadequate to supply the power for the work performed. In every case the force-matter of the nitrogenous matter standing in excess of that disintegrated according to the average for the days of rest, and representing, it may be considered, the effect of the exercise, falls very far short of the power expended in walking. Upon only four occasions does it amount to more than half, and upon two, it is less than a third. Even in five out of the twelve days the force-matter of the total nitrogenous matter disintegrated is below the force employed."[1]

To Doctor Flint's mind, these calculations were so conclusive that he wrote:[2]

"I have gone thus elaborately into a discussion of the application of what we know concerning the force-value of nitrogenized food, as calculated from the heat-units, to muscular power, for the reason that the application of the known laws of dynamics to physiological processes has lately become an important element in the study of physiology. It is to be feared, however, that physiologists are often reasoning in advance of the experimental development of facts, and theorizing upon the basis of formulæ so inaccurate, that, when they come to the consideration of millions of foot-pounds, the variations between the facts and their

[1] *The Lancet*, London, December 16, 1876, pp. 849–850. It is interesting to note, in this connection, that it is no longer believed that energy is derived from nitrogenous matter at all! Professor Chittenden, in his "Physiological Economy in Nutrition," writes (P. 327): "There is more reason for believing that the energy of muscular contraction comes primarily from the oxidation of non-nitrogenous matter. The energy of muscular contraction does not come in any large degree from the breaking down of proteid matter." (P. 328.)

[2] "The Source of Muscular Power," by Austin Flint, M.D., Professor of Physiology and Physiological Anatomy in the Bellevue Hospital Medical College, New York, etc., pp. 68–9.

calculations become enormous. If such a method of study be accurate, the advantage of its application to physiology are almost incalculable. If it be shown that it is grossly erroneous, it should be abandoned until our *data* are more complete and definite. I can not see how we can avoid banishing, for the present at least, these uncertain and erroneous processes from physiological research as applied to the theories of muscular action and the source of muscular power . . . Purely physical laws can not as yet be applied absolutely to the operations of the living organism." (p. 74).

And just here I must protest that brain work, and the operation of consciousness do require a very great deal more energy than has been allowed them by the physiologists. Indeed, it seems to me that they have in these cases, simply calculated the output of energy, voluntary and involuntary, as nearly as possible, and then agreed to simply "throw in" the remainder as mental work—since they have no means whatever of proving how much this is. The amount allowed—twelve to fourteen per cent.[1]—is absurdly and ridiculously small, and is distinctly disproved, it would seem to me, by the fact that a man can sit still all day and think, and yet be as fatigued—or even more so—at the end of the day, as the man who has taken an abundance of physical exercise, where the difference in the output should be immense (unless the energy did not depend altogether upon the nervous system, when it becomes intelligible). Moreover, Professor Mosso distinctly proved,[2] that the operations of consciousness and of the mind are comparatively far more exhausting *ceteris paribus*, than are the bodily activities. We require sleep more in order to restore our brains than our bodies; and to allow the small per cent. of energy now allowed for the operations of consciousness seems to me not only the height of absurdity, but absolutely disproved by the facts of everyday experience.

In order now to avoid misunderstanding, let me once more state the present position of the scientific world in this matter, in as few words as possible. Says Professor Bain:[3]

[1] "The Animal as a Prime Mover," by R. H. Thurston, p. 326.
[2] "Fatigue," p. 121.
[3] "The Conservation of Energy," by Balfour Stewart, F.R.S., etc., pp. 206–7.

"As applied to living bodies, the following are the usual positions. In the growth of plants, the forces of the solar ray—heat and light—are expended in decomposing (or deoxidizing) carbonic acid and water, and in building up the living tissues from the liberated carbon and the other elements; all which force is given up when these tissues are consumed, either as fuel in ordinary combustion, or as food in animal combustion. It is this animal combustion of the matter of plants, and of animals (fed on plants) —namely, the reoxidation of carbon, hydrogen, etc.—that yields all the manifestations of power in the human frame. And, in particular, it maintains (1) a certain warmth or temperature of the whole mass, against the cooling power of surrounding space; it maintains (2) mechanical energy, as muscular power; and it maintains (3) nervous power, or a certain flow of the influence circulating through the nerves, which circulation of influence, besides reacting on the other animal processes—muscular, glandular, etc.—has for its distinguishing concomitant the *Mind*."

I flatly deny, and shall endeavor to disprove, all three of the above statements.

In the present volume, I shall not attempt to adduce any philosophical, metaphysical or other kindred objections to the generally held theory—valuable and valid as some of these objections are; but shall treat the problem from the purely physiological or physical standpoint. But even here, the position generally assumed can, it seems to me, be completely refuted both by argument and by facts, as I shall now attempt to show in some detail.

In the first place, then, it appears to me that the position might be completely and immediately refuted by the following consideration alone. Let us ask ourselves how, on the accepted theories, the vital force might be augmented or increased? The position is this; if vitality depends upon the combustion of food elements, as it is asserted, then it should be positively certain that the same degree of combustion of the same amount of food would, in all cases, produce precisely the same amount or equivalent of energy—for otherwise there would be no "law" of conservation or equivalence about it. We should have to allow for a "personal element" in the case, and this we cannot possibly do when we are supposedly dealing with mechanical and physical forces, and with them only. The oxidation of a certain amount of food, then, "produces"—it is claimed—a certain equivalent amount of vitality; and from this the conclusion is obvious that, in order to produce or create *more* vitality, we should ingest and oxidize *more* food. Such a conclusion is unavoidable, if the premises are correct. If the theory is, at basis, true, this is the only logical conclusion to reach—one it is quite impossible to avoid. Nor, indeed, does Professor Bain try to avoid it. With the true courage of his convictions, he asks and answers this question as follows:[1]

"There is nothing incompatible with the principle in allowing the possibility of combining, under certain favorable conditions, both physical and mental exertion in considerable amount. In fact, the principle teaches us exactly how the thing may be done. Improve the quality and increase the quantity of the food; increase the supply of oxygen by healthy residence; let the habitual muscular exertion be such as to strengthen and not impair the functions; abate as much as possible all excesses and irregularities, bodily and mental; add the enormous economy of an educated disposal of the forces, and you will develop a higher being, a greater *aggregate* of power."

Now, on a first careless reading, this statement may carry some degree of conviction, but it assuredly will not stand the test of closer scrutiny. Let us see. The first two sentences I purposely pass over for the moment; I shall consider them in some detail presently. "Let the habitual muscular exertion be such as to strengthen and not impair the functions." What does this really mean? Does it mean that exercise should be indulged in to the point of fatigue, but never after that point has been reached? If so, then it is good hygienic advice to be sure, and sound, but what does Professor Bain hope to prove by this statement of a universally accepted fact? Does it help to explain why or how energy is thereby increased? or how an expenditure of energy, in exercise, can add to the system's store of vitality *more* energy than was expended, without turning the human organism into a perpetual motion machine?

[1] "Conservation of Energy," pp. 224–5.

"Abate, as much as possible, all excesses and irregularities, bodily and mental; add the enormous economy of an educated disposal of the forces, and you will develop a higher being, a greater aggregate of power."

Now I must protest in the strongest manner possible that this is a mere shift and evasion, a begging of the question. It does not tell us how to *add to* the body's store of vitality, but how to *prevent the loss of* that store. That is a very different thing. It tells us how to save energy—not how to make it. To be sure the ultimate, physiological effects might be the same, but the theoretical difference is absolute. It is no explanation of the *cause* of vitality whatever, or of how or what to do to increase it. Were you, *e.g.*, to pay five dollars for the secret of how to make money, and you were told (as once happened) to "work like the devil and don't spend a cent," you might feel the advice to be correct, but you would doubtless feel highly indignant at such an explanation being offered as the true "secret" of the method that must be followed. Professor Bain's remark is precisely on a par with this one, it seems to me, and is no more satisfactory or explicit; indeed, I might say less so, since the above piece of advice at least gave the positive directions of what to do, as well as the negative ones of what not to do, which Professor Bain's does not. The knowledge of how to *make* money is not the same thing as the knowledge of how to *save* it; and the explanation of the one is by no means the explanation of the other. Whatever the practical, ultimate effects may be, the theoretical, explanatorv difference is immense, and if we try to build a world theory upon such loose and slovenly statements as these —ignoring plain differences—such a writer's position becomes little less than grotesque.

We come, therefore, to a consideration of the main part of the contention, which is, that, by increasing the food supply, and by oxidizing this greater amount of material, at the same time, by deeper breathing, more exercise, etc., we thereby directly add to the store of the patient's bodily vitality. That is the *crux* of the whole position. But it appears to me that this contention may be completely refuted by the following considerations.

In the vast majority of cases, when the vital powers are feeble and low, and in need of this augmentation if ever, such a method of treatment would still further prostrate the patient, even to the point of causing his death, from complete weakness and debility. Should we force the weak and sickly patient to ingest large quantities of food and then force him to take vigorous and prolonged exercise in order to oxidize it off, it is almost certain, I contend, that practically every patient so treated would die from vital or nervous exhaustion.[1] But yet, theoretically, this is precisely the course that should be pursued. If not, why not? I cannot see any loophole of escape by which this conclusion is to be avoided; it is, in fact, merely a statement of the case as it is supposed to stand; and that doctors, as a matter of fact, *do not* so treat their patients is simply because they have found, from practical, bitter experience, that they would die if they were so treated; but the theory says, none the less, that this should have been the course pursued. The practice and the theory do not agree; in fact, they are as antagonistic to one another as possible.

On the contrary, it has been found, by repeated experiment, that greater energy, more vitality, results, in almost all cases, from the giving of *less* food (pp. 114-15), and from taking less exercise, and by resting more; and this is directly opposed to the theory which states that our vitality is proportioned to the

[1] It may have been noted by the acute reader that the current theory, carried to its logical conclusion, leads to sheer nonsense. Thus, if, by increasing the food supply, we could add to the bodily vitality, it might quite reasonably be argued that we need only increase the food supply *enough* in order to supply too great an amount of energy, and this surplus energy might lead to disastrous consequences, since this added energy, having no natural outlet, in the majority of cases, might have to be "worked off" as crime—just as an abundance of energy in a child becomes manifest in an added show of naughtiness! Such a statement may appear far-fetched and ridiculous (which indeed it is) but that it is not the logical outcome of the theory held, I challenge anyone to show, and to prove this I quote the following passage from an address before the American Academy of Political and Social Science (if you please), entitled "Overnutrition and Its Social Consequences," on p. 34 of which the following passage occurs:

"If an organism enters an improved environment or increases its power to assimilate food, additional motor energy is generated that must find an outlet. If this organism is already well fed, more motor energy will be generated than can be carried over the motor nerves to the muscles. Overnutrition thus creates a plethora of nervous energy which must be used up in some way. . . ." Of course, the results of overnutrition are—not added nervous power—but disease and death, as we have seen.

amount of food we successfully oxidize off. By oxidizing less we should certainly have less energy, whereas it is found, by simple observation, that we have more. This is directly contrary to the theory; theory and practice are once more in direct opposition.

Finally, I shall adduce evidence, in this book, that will show that energy is not lost, but on the contrary, actually *gained* during a fast, when *no food at all* is eaten, and when, theoretically, the energies should, and in fact must, sink and wane and die out altogether in the absence of the necessary food supply, the supposed source of our energy.

This aspect of the problem is entirely new, and one that has, as yet, never been even mentioned. And for a very good reason. The observations upon which such a statement could be founded have never as yet been made. The phenomena of fasting, which I shall presently discuss at length, have never been the subject of careful study; but, having once been so studied they will be found, I am convinced, to completely revolutionize our ideas as to the source of our energy, and to completely disprove the idea that the bodily energies are derived from the daily food, through the process of oxidation. For, if the theory held to-day be correct, is it not obvious that a complete withdrawal of the bodily fuel—the food—the sole source of the energies—would and must result in the gradual diminution and final complete extinction of the vital energies; the source of the energy is withdrawn, and consequently the energies (since they are being constantly expended) must, in a short time, be themselves completely exhausted, when death will ensue?

This, I believe, is the position generally assumed, and the majority of thinking persons—both medical and lay—will assert that it is both correct and logical. "See," they will say, "how, when a person starves to death, the body becomes emaciated; how the mind is impaired; how all the bodily and vital powers are gradually lessened, weakened, and finally exhausted altogether; how prostration, more and more complete, follows upon the withdrawal of food from the organism; and, how, finally, complete prostration and death ensue—the body shrivelled and emaciated, the mind gone, the vital energies totally dissipated!

How, in the face of such evidence, can you say that our general theory is incorrect, or that the withdrawal of food does not necessitate and frequently correspond to an equal withdrawal and extinction of the vital powers; and even that they are increased by such withdrawal? Your position is obviously absurd and erroneous!"

I have a very simple answer to such objections. Such "facts" do not occur at all; the "evidence" is non-existent; the facts and the evidence, in cases of fasting (as distinguished from starvation, pp. 563–4), are all the other way. The foregoing "argument" is really a dogmatic and altogether erroneous statement, based upon what people *think would* occur, if a fast were instigated and persisted in for a long enough period. Had they settled down and studied the actual facts in the case; had they observed fasting patients, or experimented upon themselves; or if they once realized the vast difference between fasting and starving (pp. 563–4), they would have found that none of these supposed occurrences really do take place. They exist (like our canine teeth!) only in the imaginations of the medical fraternity and the lay public. They have no foundation whatever in fact. I have given this special subject my very closest attention and the best of my thoughts for some eight years; I have watched dozens and scores of patients during their protracted fasts—some of them lasting forty, fifty, or more days; I have experimented repeatedly upon myself; I have induced some of my friends to experiment upon themselves likewise; I think I may claim to have read everything written bearing either directly or indirectly upon this question; and I can honestly say that, as a result of this work, and in spite of, or rather, in consequence of, my observations and repeated experiments, not one iota of evidence has ever been forthcoming that our energies are in any way dependent upon our food, or that they lessen upon its withdrawal; or that the present, generally accepted theory of the relations of food and energy is anything but absurdly and demonstrably untrue; that the vital energies, so far from being lessened, invariably increase, as the fast progresses (no matter what the *feelings* of weakness may seem to indicate); that the mind is never affected by the fast, in any manner whatever, or in any other way than beneficially, being rendered more acute and clearer (pp. 516–17); and that emaciation does not ensue to anything like the extent generally supposed—being even then due to other causes than the withdrawal of the food (p. 124); and, if the fast be terminated at the return of natural hunger (p. 549), the reduction noticed will be only that from a diseased to a normal condition; and, finally, that the theory that the vital energies—bodily and mental—are completely prostrated and dissipated in consequence of the withdrawal of food is a pure myth—existent only in the minds of those persons who think that this must be the case (and, indeed, it must be if the theory held to-day is correct), but having no foundation whatever in actual fact.

These are broad and sweeping statements, but I can and will substantiate every one of them before I conclude this volume. For the present, suffice it to say that, to my mind, these facts completely refute the general doctrine of the dependence of our vital force upon the combustion of our food, and prove, conclusively, that such a theory is as outrageously false in practice as it is truly absurd in theory.

For consider. Were the theory generally held true it would only be necessary, when tired, to go first to the dining-room, and then to the gymnasium in order to recuperate our strength and energies. We should ingest more food, then oxidize it off, and the process of its internal combustion would add more energy to the system; and so on, *ad infinitum.*[1] A truly pretty theory, but unfortunately (for it) we all know, from actual, practical experience that we must, when weary, retire to bed, and not to the dining-room, in order to recuperate our energies; and there comes a time when we can sustain ourselves no longer, but must seek rest and sleep, or die; and this, no matter how much food we may have eaten, or how industriously we may have exercised and breathed in order to oxidize it off. As a matter of fact, we know that it is exceedingly unhygienic and unwholesome to eat at all when exhausted by the labors of the day; and that exercise at such a time is most doubtfully beneficial, and

[1] It must always be remembered that, were the generally accepted theories true, the process is a purely *mechanical* one, and cannot in any way be affected by any vital or nervous, or "personal" conditions whatever.

that no amount of deep breathing will succeed in indefinitely postponing the oncoming of fatigue, exhaustion and sleep. Yet, according to the theory now held, such should be the case. But most certainly it *is* not! What then is wrong? Obviously the theory. And the more we consider the matter the more certain does this fact become. No matter how careful we are in our habits; no matter how deeply we breathe, how much exercise we take, or how much food we eat, there comes a time when we must retire to the bedroom and not to the dining-room in order to regain our energies. This is most undeniably the case. At the conclusion of a long day's march, let us say, does the tired soldier seek, as a first impulse, food or rest? Sometimes it is food, I admit, but this is purely habit training, and, if the exhaustion be very complete, food will not be given a thought. Such a soldier's sole aim and thought is rest, rest. Rest and sleep! Yet, if the generally accepted theory were true, we should say to our hypothetical soldier: "What, the vital energies exhausted? Then here, eat this beefsteak, and then exercise thoroughly in the open air; oxidize it in your body and—since we can calculate exactly how much energy this will yield[1]—it will yield or 'give' you 683 calories of energy! Up! Up! Why do you lie there? That cannot add to your energies, since it in no wise assists in the oxidation of food material!"

How ludicrous! How absolutely absurd the theory appears when carried to its logical and legitimate conclusion! And why is it not logical and legitimate? Professor Bain made no mention whatever of rest or sleep in his statement of how to recuperate and add to the bodily store of energy. And, indeed, it is hard to see just how this phenomenon of recuperation during sleep and rest is related to the theory of the causation of vitality through the combustion of food; how, indeed, it is not actually opposed to it in every sense of the term. For, as we see daily, there is invariably a point at which rest and sleep become an imperative necessity, and nothing else will take its place—nor food, nor exercise, nor breathing—absolutely nothing. And

[1] "Using the proper factors, we may approximately determine the value of any food as a source of energy by measuring its heat of combustion." "Bread and the Principles of Bread Making," by Helen W. Atwater. (U. S. *Dept. of Agriculture Bulletin*, No. 112.)

yet sleep is a state of absolute quiescence in which all the bodily functions are reduced to the lowest ebb, and where, theoretically, the combustion of food would be at its lowest point also. Indeed, this is now a pretty generally accepted fact. Says Dr. Frank Horridge:[1]

"As to general character of sleep, there can be very little doubt. The decrease in the amount of carbonic acid produced shows that it is essentially a period of diminished oxidation."

And further, indirect, proof is afforded by the fact that no more N. is excreted during periods of extreme muscular exertion than when there is no such exertion.[2]

Now, how are we to explain these facts? I contend that, if the generally accepted theories are true, they cannot be explained at all—they are inexplicable. Sleep and rest have accordingly, and because of this difficulty, been altogether left out of account by our scientists and omitted from their considerations in consequence. And it is easy to see why this should be the case. The restoration of strength and vitality through their means is not explicable by the mechanical theory of energy—in fact, is opposed to it. For, by that theory, we are supposed to gain our energy through the combustion of food—just as a steam engine gains its energy through the combustion of fuel; and it is contended that the parallel is, in the two cases, almost exact. But, unfortunately for the theory, the parallel is not exact in just this way; the human engine (the body) reaches a point where it refuses to evolve energy, no matter how much fuel (food) is forced into it, and no matter how full a "draught" is turned on (exercise and deep breathing taken). The engine does not recuperate and restore itself, during its periods of rest, and the body does; the engine continues to wear out, and can never replace its own parts by new ones, and the body can. Indeed:

"In the case of the locomotive the fuel does not build up the substance and structure of the machine, but in time destroys it."[3]

[1] "Dynamic Aspects of Nutrition and Heredity," p. 41.

[2] "Experiments on the Effect of Muscular Work upon the Digestibility of Food and the Metabolism of Nitrogen," by Charles E. Wait, Ph.D., F.C.S., etc. (U. S. *Dept. of Agriculture Bulletin*, pp. 43, 64, 76.)

[3] "How to Gain Health and a Long Life," by P. M. Hanney, p. 12.

But the main point is that the body does, in time, arrive at a condition in which it cannot possibly evolve or give out more energy, no matter how much food is eaten, and the engine (being an engine) can. Thus, the great difference between them is that one is self-recuperative and human, and needs sleep in order to effect this; and the other is not self-recuperative, and needs no rest, so long as it works at all; and, in spite of this most obvious and all-important difference (since sleep is the greatest restorer of vital energy, as daily observation shows), and merely to bolster up the absurd attempt to include vital force in the law of conservation; and in spite of the most every-day and obvious proofs to the contrary, the scientific world has continued to ignore this question of sleep altogether, and to treat this matter of the renewal of the vital force by food as a proved fact, instead of a mere theory, open to these very objections, and a most monstrous absurdity because of them. In short, the plain differences between the human body and the steam engine have been completely ignored, and treated as if they were non-existent—merely because they were impossible to dovetail into the present materialistic theory. To me, it is amazing that this very plain and obvious untruth should have gone so long unchallenged.

How absurd is this endeavor to ignore the vital importance of sleep is made clear when we remember that it has been proved, by actual experiment, that animals can live longer without food than without sleep![1] My researches in the phenomena of fasting have confirmed and much extended this view. Without sleep we can live and retain all our bodily and mental faculties but a few days at most (and the greater portion of that time would doubtless be spent in the greatest physical agony and mental imbecility); in fasting cases we know that patients can and do under favorable circumstances, live two months or even longer—and this without the slightest physical or mental disturbance, but, on the contrary, with only heightened powers![2]

[1] "Sleep," by Marie de Manaceine; *Contemp. Sci. Ser.*, p. 65.

[2] "For while a man, fasting, may go 30 or 40 days, and under some circumstances even longer without any sort of nourishment, the utmost limits of sleeplessness that can be endured seem to be within ten days." "Sleep and Dreams," by Dr. Friedrich Scholz, Director of the Bremen Insane Asylum, p. 89.

And yet it is claimed that the food is the source of our energy, and sleep so insignificant an affair as to be altogether overlooked. So long as such plain and patent differences are ignored, we can hardly hope for any true progress along these lines of investigation, as at present pursued.

Let me cite one illustrative and instructive case. Weston, in his remarkable walk, continued to eat highly nitrogenous food, yet on the fourth day, he "completely broke down." He had had practically no sleep till then. But "on the fifth day, after nine hours and twenty-six minutes of sleep, the system reacted completely and Weston walked forty and a half miles." "If Weston," says Doctor Flint,[1] "had been able to supply his waste of tissue by food, this collapse of muscular power might not have occurred."

Again, were the combustion of food the source of our energy, it would require a considerable *time*—several hours, certainly—in which to evolve sufficient energy to accomplish a task which was impossible at the commencement of that period. We know, on the contrary, that this is not the case; that, in fact, four or five minutes' rest, if taken properly, will sufficiently energize and invigorate us to enable us to accomplish, with comparative ease, what was impossible immediately before the period of rest, and though no food whatever has been eaten during that period. Can this be explained on the current theories? Says F. W. H. Myers:[2]

"It is a fully admitted, although an absolutely unexplained fact that the regenerative quality of healthy sleep is something *sui generis*, which no completeness of waking quiescence can rival or approach. A few moments of sleep—a mere blur across the field of consciousness—will sometimes bring a renovation which hours of lying down in darkness and silence would not yield. A mere bowing of the head on the breast, if consciousness ceases for a second or two, may change a man's outlook on the world. At such moments—and many persons, like myself, can vouch for their reality—one feels that what has occurred in one's organism—alteration of blood pressure, or whatever it may be—has been in some sense discontinuous; that there has been a

[1] "The Source of Muscular Power," p. 86.
[2] "Human Personality and Its Survival of Bodily Death," Vol I., p. 123.

break in the inward *régime*, amounting to much more than a mere brief ignoring of stimuli from without. The break of consciousness is associated in some way with a potent physiological change. That is to say, even in the case of a moment of ordinary sleep we already note the appearance of the special recuperative energy which is familiar in longer periods of sleep, and which, as we shall presently see, reaches a still higher level in hypnotic trance."

And these same objections that have been raised to the theory of creating the bodily energy by means of more abundant food and exercise, apply also the theory, held by many, that vitality is introduced into the system by means of deep breathing. The Yogis of India and their followers, *e.g.*, contend that our bodily energy is derived from the air we breathe, rather than from our food and drink, and consequently practice and highly indorse deep breathing as the great energizer. Thus we read:[1]

"Prana is found in its freest state in the atmospheric air, which, when fresh, is fairly charged with it, and we draw it to us more easily from the air than from any other source. . . . The oxygen in the air is appropriated by the blood and is made use of by the circulatory system. The prana in the air is appropriated by the nervous system, and is used in its work."

On p. 154 of this author's "Hatha Yoga" the prana is stated to be the "active principle of what we call vitality." The position, then, is plain.

But there is, it appears to me, one great objection to this theory, which may readily be seen when pointed out, and which vitiates the whole argument; and consequently I cannot accept it as conclusive, even though it has much more in its favor than the theory advanced by our own scientists. It is this: Were we to carry this argument to its legitimate conclusion, we should be able, theoretically, to do away with sleep altogether, and substitute deep breathing exercises for it—whereas we know that this is not and cannot be the case. For, if we derive our energy from the "prana" breathed together with the air, it must be seen that, so long as the air is pure enough, and the breathing is

[1] "Yogi Science of Breath," by Yogi Ramacharaka, pp. 18–19.

deep and continuous enough, exhaustion should be impossible, since we should only have to take a few breathing exercises, out of doors, in order to completely restore our energy, and consequently need never retire to bed and to sleep. While sleep may undoubtedly be postponed for a considerable period by this practice, we know from experience that we cannot continue indefinitely without sleep—which we should be enabled to do, were this theory true. In other words, all the objections that were raised to the theory of deriving or gaining our strength and energy from food, apply with equal force to this theory also.

§ 3. *Author's Theory of Its Causation*

Before we proceed further, therefore, and in order to avoid misunderstanding, I shall now state my own position in this question, and the theory I propose to defend. The general position is, of course, that food has three main functions. (1) Replacement of tissue, that has been broken down by the daily activities. (2) That it is the source of our bodily and mental energies—of the human vitality; and (3) that it is the source of our bodily heat—the latter two being derived from it by the chemical processes of combustion. Now the stand I shall take is that food has but *one* function in the human economy—the replacement of tissue, and that it supplies no heat and no energy whatever. The replacement of tissue is its sole and only function. This being so, the question might be raised: Why do we need more of it while performing active muscular work than when this work is not being performed? The answer to this is readily found. All exercise breaks down tissue; and this tissue must always be replaced; food is the material from which tissue is formed. Food, therefore, merely supplies the body with material from which it draws in active exercise; and consequently the greater the amount of exercise taken, the greater must be the amount of food eaten to replace this waste of tissue. The greater the one, the greater the need of the other, and *vice versa*. But the observed fact does not in any way prove that the food supplied more vitality in the latter case, as we shall presently see.

I contend, then, that we do not (all prevalent opinions notwithstanding) at any time, or under any circumstances, derive any part of our bodily or mental energy from the food we eat; that vital force is in no wise inter-related or transmutable into any other forces whatever; that it is innate, inherent in the living tissue, distinct, a force absolutely *per se*;[1] that it is the governing and controlling force of the organism so long as that may be termed *live*, and leaving it at death (pp. 330–1), when *chemical* action, or decomposition begins; that it is expended in every thought, will, emotion, conscious or unconscious muscular action; in sexual excitement, and in purely vital action (such as digestion, secretion, assimilation, etc.) throughout the organism; that we have the will to expend, but never to make or "manufacture" this energy by any means in our power. I contend, further, that the body is not an exact parallel, in its action, to the steam engine, as has heretofore been contended, but is rather that of the *electric motor*[2] which has the power of recharging itself with life or vital energy, just as the motor of the electrician receives its energy from some external source—the brain and nervous system being that part of us which is thus recharged, and constituting the motor of the human body; that this recharging process takes place during the hours of rest, and particularly of sleep, and at such times only—all activity denoting merely an expenditure or waste of this vital force

[1] This, of course, has always been the contention of the school of much-despised vitalists. Professor Beale, *e.g.*, frequently insisted upon the absolute distinctions between the vital and the physical forces in such passages, *e.g.*, as the following: "The phenomena which I have described as characteristic of every kind of living matter in Nature, and which are known only in connection with living matter, I must ask you to regard as purely *vital* actions, due to the operation of a force or power capable of controlling matter and its forces, but neither originating in them, nor formed by or from them, nor capable of being converted into them—a power which we cannot isolate or physically examine, but the effects of the action of which we may study." ("On Life and Vital Action in Health and Disease," etc., by Lionel S. Beale, M.B., F.R.S., etc., pp. 59–60.) See also this author's "Vitality: An Appeal to the Fellows of the Royal Society," p. 92; "Vitality: Its Bearing on Natural Religion," Chapter IX., §31, etc.

[2] Mr. Horace Fletcher devoted several pages in his "New Glutton or Epicure" (pp. 136–41), to showing the exact parallel between the body and the electric dynamo, but failed to grasp the central idea that our energy is not derived from our food. Dr. Albert J. Atkins, of San Francisco, and Prof. Edgar L. Larkin have both performed a number of experiments, if reports speak truly, that go to prove that Life and electricity are closely related, and that the body is closely akin to the electric motor. I am unaware that their researches were ever followed up.

(p. 41); that we can thus only *allow* or *permit* vitality to flow into us, as it were, in this recharging process—such coming from the universal, all-pervading, cosmic energy, with which we are surrounded, and which our nervous systems (and bodies) merely transmit or transform[1] into the external work of the world, acting merely as *channels through which* the all-pervading energy may find personal expression; channels through which it may individually manifest. Such, in brief outline, is my theory.

To put it more plainly: My idea is that energy can flow into the organism from some external source[2] rather than that it is manufactured or secreted within the organism, by the combustion of food, or by any other means whatever. We cannot ever *make* energy; it is something over which we have no possible control; we can allow it to flow into us, by becoming passive, and by this means only; the instant we attempt to make it, or in any way to *force* it into ourselves, so to speak, we at once commence—not to gain energy, but to expend it, to lose it—and this is the prime, basic, and most fundamentally important aspect of the problem. Vitality we can never make; we can only allow it to enter our bodies by becoming passive; and the degree to which the vitality will then enter or flow into us will depend, *ceteris paribus*, upon the body's physical condition from diseased states; the mental attitude, perhaps; and the degree of relaxation attained. Only by such means is our vitality replenished, and we can no more restore it through the ingestion

[1] It is interesting to note how near to my theory many writers have already come—without absolutely conceiving it. Thus, R. H. Thurston, on p. 336 of his "Animal as a Prime Mover" (Smithsonian Report), calls the body an "energy transforming machine"—accepting the theory, however, that our energies are derived from our food. "Joule, as long ago as 1846, working with Captain Scoresby, concluded that the animal motor 'more closely resembles an electro-magnetic machine than a heat engine,' and this is reaffirmed by Tait, in our own day. (See his "History of Thermo-Dynamics.") Sir William Thomson, now Lord Kelvin, in his papers of about 1850, adopts the idea of Joule."

[2] I do not pretend to say what this source is, and do not feel I am called upon to explain this any more than I am the essence of vitality. Both must be, in a sense, accepted without explanation, like the connection of mind and matter. I need only say that, to the physicist, the theory should have no objections on that ground, since the fact that such an all-pervading energy exists is becoming more and more manifest. Says Mr. Thurston ("The Animal as a Prime Mover," p. 334): "All space is pervaded by heat, light, electricity and magnetism; why not with vital and spiritual energies?"

and oxidation of food (both *active* measures, and so necessarily merely means for its expenditure) than we can by any other active or wasteful processes whatever. It is merely because both are stimulating—and so give the *feeling* of increased strength—that they can be even thought to do so for an instant.

It must be understood that the degree of energy present in any organism depends altogether upon the degree of receptivity of that organism, not upon the fact that more food is being oxidized in that body than in any other—a truly absurd notion, it seems to me. The amount of this energy (itself limitless) is limited, in its individual, bodily manifestation, solely by the condition of the organism through which it manifests. The idea we must conceive to ourselves is that the body is like, not the steam engine, but the electric *motor*, capable of recharging itself during the hours of sleep and rest.[1] New strength, new energy, is infused into the body during rest and sleep, and at that time only—since it is only then that the human motor—the nervous system—is in the condition that renders this recharging process possible. During the day, this recharging process practically ceases; but the expenditure continues unabated. Hence the exhaustion we notice at the end of the day. No matter how careful we are in our habits; no matter how much food we consume and successfully oxidize off, exhaustion will eventually result in every case; the fact that we are tired and that this feeling can only be satisfied by sleep, will dawn upon us more and more. No matter how great the amount of nourishment that has been taken and assimilated, loss of strength—of energy and vitality—is bound to result, as the day proceeds, and it becomes more and more obvious to us that we must retire to bed and not to the dining-room, in order to repair lost strength and energy.

I have stated above that the influx of energy, during sleep, is exactly proportional to the degree of receptivity of the organism. In other words, energy flows through us, or is transmitted

[1] Since the perfection of wireless telegraphy, this conception of recharging the body (or rather nervous system) by cosmic energy, from some external source, becomes much more readily conceivable, since, in these cases also, the instrument receives its energy wirelessly, and is not physically connected with any recharging apparatus—formerly necessary.

or transformed by us, in the same ratio that the bodily organism is free from disease—is *clean.* All that we have to do, therefore, in order to insure that the greatest amount of energy shall be available for our active, daily purposes, is to keep the body clean and free from disease—bright and clear—a good transmitter.

Just as a storage battery may be charged more rapidly and forcibly at certain times than at others—depending upon the circumstances in the case—so, I conceive, may our bodily (nervous) organism be recharged more rapidly and effectually under one certain set of conditions than under another set. The principal reason for variation is, I believe, the condition of the body at the time—whether it be receptive or not—and this depends upon various, previously mentioned conditions—the state of the blood; the amount of physical and mental labor indulged in the previous day;[1] whether the stomach is at rest or enforcedly active, all these and other considerations[2] must be taken into account, as well as the degree of relaxation attained by the patient, during this period of rest. If this latter is not complete and thorough we cannot expect the best results from our period of repose; and, as Miss Annie Payson Call pointed out, in her excellent little book "Power Through Repose" (p. 16), many persons do not *ever* rest and relax properly and in a thorough and sufficient manner—even during sleep! The baneful effects of this constant muscular tension upon the mental life is well illustrated by Prof. William James; see his "Talks on Psychology," etc., p. 211.

There is another factor that must be taken into consideration, in this problem, *viz.*, the mental influences. We all know that a "guilty conscience" is a great preventive of healthful and refreshing sleep, while fear, anger, jealousy, and many other mental states also affect the character of the sleep, and its resultant benefits. I consider it quite possible that if we *understood* this problem (which we do not) we might, eventually, be enabled to concentrate and enforce this recharging process, so

[1] "How to Gain Health and a Long Life," by P. M. Hanney, p. 108.

[2] It seems to me that Just's experience that added energy is gained by sleeping on the ground might be explained by some such means. "Return to Nature," p. 87.

to speak; thereby regaining as much energy in a few hours, or even minutes, as we now obtain in a whole night's sleep. As M. Berrier pointed out[1] we have only to learn the law, and we should be enabled to draw upon this great store to any extent we please. Indeed, the hypnotic trance may be one such condition, artificially induced, which renders this possible; a state which borders, apparently, very closely on this peculiar and much-sought-for condition, and, consequently, may be of great assistance in restoring the energy, and consequently the health, of the debilitated and the sick. Its therapeutic advantages, in such cases, would be most marked.[2]

Now, this theory is, it seems to me, supported by every analogy from the vegetable world. The veriest tyro knows that we cannot force plants to grow with greater rapidity or more beautiful, by supplying them with an excess of nutriment; all we can do is to supply the *conditions* (heat, moisture, sunlight, and the *proper* amount of nutriment—so that the plant may draw upon them for its growth; we cannot force its nutrition, its power of absorption, be it remembered) that are most favorable for the growth of the plant. The conditions being supplied, growth becomes more easily possible; but it will be observed we are not actually adding to the life force of the plant, but merely supplying the conditions that render the outward manifestations of this life force more favorable. The force, the energy of growth, is inherent, and the absurdity of trying to force or "manufacture" this energy should be apparent.

My whole contention hinges on the fact that, contrary to all accepted teachings, Vitality is not a thing that can be made or manufactured at will. It is present, inherent, in every living organism, and the most we can do to favor its influx is to supply the proper conditions that make its manifestation possible. The more perfect, the better these conditions, the greater the influx of vital force, and *vice versa*. We must see that all the electrodes and avenues and channels are bright and clear, so that there shall be as little hindrance as possible to either the

[1] "Personal Magnetism," p. 14.

[2] See F. W. H. Myers' address before the British Ass'n., "Proceedings of the Society for Psychical Research," Vol. XIV., pp. 100-8.

inflow of energy in the form of power, or to its outflow in the form of work done.[1]

"In a normal condition we receive the vibration and rhythm of the great ocean of life, and respond to it, but at times the mouth of the inlet seems choked up with *débris*, and we fail to receive the impulse from Mother Ocean, and inharmony mani fests within us." ("The Science of Breath," by Yogi Ramacharaka, p. 52.)

This much we may claim is certain. Now what are the conditions? Turning again to the vegetable world for guidance, we find that *cleanliness* is the all-important factor—the prime requisite—for successful and healthful growth. Cleansing the soil, freeing it from the growing vegetable matter, from destructive insects, animalculæ, etc., paving the way for its growth, this is all that can be done in agriculture—the vital force of the plant does the actual *growing*. "Man cannot make power, but he can supply the conditions which utilize the power."[2] And so it is in the human body. All that we can do in order to insure rapid and healthful growth is to supply the proper conditions, and among them cleanliness. Only by keeping the body clean, pure, and free from disease, from grossness and encumbering material, can we attain the highest amount of force—the greatest influx of vital energy—the most elevated conception of life and its possibilities. The old saying that "Cleanliness is next to Godliness" assumes a new and vital interest in connection with these truths. But what folly to endeavor to increase the body's energy and life by forcing excessive and uncalled-for nutriment into an already clogged and diseased organism! The effect must, of necessity, be the very opposite of that sought.

And it is, I think, quite possible that this energy, which is thus shown to be a far more immaterial and intangible thing than is generally supposed, may be *transmitted*, under certain conditions, from one organism to another—provided that the organisms of the two persons are in the proper condition for this

[1] In this connection it is most interesting and significant that "the only way yet discovered of influencing the output of energy by radium is simply to increase the activity of the material by purifying it. " "Radium Explained," by Dr. W. Hampson, p. 64.

[2] "The Exact Science of Health," by Robert Walter, M.D., Vol. I., p. 59.

transmission to take place; that one is in a motive, the other in a receptive, attitude. Thus we have a ready explanation of the effects of "magnetic healing," of the "laying on of hands," and of kindred phenomena—all illustrating the method of transference of energy from one organism to another. In such cases, I conceive, the operator merely acts as a go-between—a channel through which the universal energy can more easily flow, and so reach the patient—than is possible under normal existing circumstances. The energy is, in such cases, transmitted through another organism, and so reaches the patient "second hand," as it were. While this method may be extremely valuable in some cases, where, by a constitutional peculiarity, the patient's organism may be rendered unreceptive to direct inflow, it is needless to say that the other, more normal method is by far the better, and much to be preferred, if possible.

Now it will be seen that, if this theory be true (its correctness I shall presently proceed to prove in considerable detail) vitality must continue to flow into and through us so long as life is present, and quite independent of whether ingested food is or is not being oxidized in the body; whether combustion in the tissues is taking place or not. So long as life lasts, just so long is vitality present, and is in no way dependent upon the food being oxidized for its presence. It is innate, inherent, as much a part of—as inseparably connected with all living tissue as is gravitation with matter and "wetness" with water. It is inseparably united with it; bound up with each atom of living tissue is its accompanying vital force—more intimate in its connection with the living tissue, more associated or connected with it, than is "wetness" with water. As well might we try to add to a body's store of gravity as to add to its vitality—aye, more so, since we have in electricity and the modern theories of matter some slight inkling of the *modus operandi* of gravitation —however slight that idea may be[1]—and it is certainly more easily conceivable (to me, at least), than is the idea of creating or adding to the bodily store of vitality or life force, which is far more innate, more *per se* than is gravity; for here we have absolutely no analogy whatever to guide us—no similar phenom-

[1] M. Sage, "Theory of Gravitation," etc. (*Smithsonian Reports*)

ena with which we can compare the life force. And, this being the case, it is obvious that, no matter whether the body be, at the time, digesting food or fasting, the vitality is present and active, and must necessarily be until death severs the hitherto indissoluble tie, and the "twain are one" no longer!

§ 4. *Objections to the Theory and Replies Thereto*

Now, to the acceptance of this theory, I know there are many objections. In the first place, it may be objected that this theory would seem to imply that there must always be present the *same amount* of vital force, since we see, at first sight, no means for its regulation, so to speak, whereas we know that this is most certainly not the case. But, all more subtle objections aside, there is the apparently plain and obvious truth that *we do get weak*, as a rule, during a fast; that we have less energy to expend than formerly, and that death from starvation will ultimately and certainly result, provided that food is withheld for a sufficiently long period of time. Such, it may be claimed, are hard and certain facts which cannot be gainsaid, nor evaded by any amount of fine theorizing.

I quite agree with this main contention, nor shall I attempt in any way to deny the facts themselves—simply because I believe them to be facts. But the inferences drawn from the observations I believe to be erroneous; the facts themselves are true—the deductions wrong.

I shall first consider these objections, coming first to that which says that death from starvation would soon result (and on any theory whatever, therefore, the vital energies come to an abrupt termination) were a fast persisted in long enough. I have discussed this question at some length on pp. 326–9, and again on pp. 537–9, and I must for the present beg my reader to dismiss this aspect of the problem from his mind, and altogether cease to consider it, until it is there discussed in the light of the further *data* accumulated, both in fact and argument.

Reverting, then, to the other objections, I must admit that they are the most serious that my theory has to encounter. The fact that the majority of us do, apparently "get weak"; that we have less energy to expend during a fast than at ordinary times; that greater bodily weakness is temporarily experienced in many cases—all this I admit. I shall return to a discussion of this difficult problem a little later on. But first I must digress to say that if our energy were entirely dependent upon our food combustion for its presence, it would, of course, immediately begin to decrease in its absence and upon its withdrawal, and this result could not possibly be evaded by any means whatever. Yet, as a matter of fact, this result does not follow as an invariable consequent—as it must follow if the generally accepted theories were true. Though a more or less temporary weakness and lassitude may occur in the majority of cases, it certainly does not occur in *all* cases, as it would certainly have to, were the prevailing theory true. There are numerous instances on record where no loss of strength whatever (I mean even no apparent loss) was noticeable during a fast of twenty, thirty, forty, and even more days. Mr. J. A. Shaw's extraordinary case, quoted on pp. 205–8, is a remarkable instance of this; and so is that of the Rev. C. W. Dalrymple[1] in which this gentleman fasted thirty-nine and one-half days into complete health, leaving on record the statement:

"I gained strength beyond all question about three weeks before my appetite returned. I would work all day long finally."

In the case of Mr. Leonard Thress, again, who fasted fifty days,[2] and Miss Estella F. Kuenzel (forty-five days)[3] and others that might easily be added to this list, there was no loss of vitality at any time during the fast (not even any feeling of weakness)—nothing but added health and strength. The flesh and the weight decreased, to be sure, but the energies increased, in spite of—or, as I think, on account of—that fact, and apparently in direct ratio to the amount of flesh lost. Now I ask, how are such cases as these to be accounted for, if the present theory of the dependence of vitality upon food combustion be true? Unless we deliberately impugn the good faith of both the patients and the narrators, which we have not the least right

[1] "No-Breakfast Plan," etc., pp. 154–5.
[2] *Op. cit.*, p. 148–53.
[3] *Op. cit.*, p. 136–47.

to do (and, in fact, we should, by so doing, simply display our ignorance of the phenomena of fasting, since, as I shall show on pp. 446–7, that it is a physical impossibility for the patient to deceive the skilled observer as to the fact of the fast; *i.e.*, whether or no he is really fasting) I cannot see any possible loophole by which we can avoid the conclusion that—frequently, at least, no loss of energy is even apparently or temporarily experienced, but that gain and nothing but gain of energy and vitality is manifest, in spite of the fact that the food—the supposed source of the vitality—has been entirely withdrawn.

And this distinct and uninterrupted gain of energy is most marked and steady where the greatest degree of prostration and weakness is observed, and where, if anywhere, we should expect to find collapse follow upon the total withdrawal of all food. Again I ask, how are these facts to be explained upon the theory of vitality in vogue?

And now I come to a consideration of the difficult question: why some patients do (apparently, at least) become weak at all during a fast—since, or rather if, vitality is not dependent upon the daily food for its maintenance? This is a very difficult and complex problem indeed, the solution to which cost me many months' mental effort to solve.

If my theory be correct, we should apparently never experience any sense of weakness at all, during a fast, but should, on the contrary, become stronger and more energetic as the fast progresses, while we know, on the contrary, that this is frequently not the case, and that extreme weakness, even to temporary prostration, may be experienced by patients undergoing a fast. This argument seems conclusive, at first, and is seemingly calculated to silence all opposition. The fallacy in the argument, however, can easily be seen when once it has been pointed out, and this I shall endeavor to do. The fundamental error is that the significance of the fact observed has been misinterpreted; not that the fact itself is wrong, but that the deductions drawn therefrom are erroneous.

First, I would point out that this weakness observed is not real weakness, in the ordinarily accepted sense of the term, *i.e.*, of strength altogether gone out of the system. It is weakness of altogether another kind. That we feel weak very frequently I do not for a moment deny; but I shall endeavor to show that this feeling is deceptive. That it is not real weakness can be easily seen by anyone thoroughly conversant with fasting and its phenomena. If such were the case, strength would and could not return to the patient as the fast progressed, and before food was eaten, as invariably is the case. Were this weakness real, and due to the withdrawal of food, as is commonly supposed, we should surely be justified in maintaining (and the vast majority of persons would maintain) that the longer the food is withheld, the greater the consequent weakness; the greater the cause, the greater and the more noticeable the effects. Such a position is, in truth, the only logical one to assume, and, were the premises correct—that food "makes" strength—would be quite incontrovertible.

The fact, then, that such is not the case proves that the premises are wrong. Food does not furnish our strength, our energy. On the contrary, the withdrawal of food places more energy at the body's disposal, for the reason that all the energy that was heretofore expended upon digestion, may now be utilized for other purposes. (pp. 174–5.) This theory is further supported by the fact that, though immediate, temporary weakness may result from the withdrawal of food, strength will sooner or later return to the patient, if the fast be persisted in, and though no food whatever be ingested during that period. Under the generally accepted theories this would be quite impossible; but it is a fact nevertheless, which may be readily demonstrated by direct experiment. In cases which are already weakened by disease, and consequently where the vitality is already at a very low ebb, this increase of energy, consequent upon the withdrawal of food, is always most readily seen and most marked.

Theoretically, of course, the complete withdrawal of food, in such cases, should have the effect of causing the speedy death of the patient, for the reason that the last source of the bodily energy has now been withdrawn. But, in actual practice, we find that the very opposite is in fact the case, and that the patient's strength and energy return and continue to accumulate during this period of fasting. And, I ask, how is the fact to be explained? On the generally accepted theories of vitality, it must remain inexplicable—a paradox—and the only course open to its defendants is to deny the fact, and this I challenge them to do. But, if the above-elaborated theory be true, the solution is easy to find—the explanation complete. We no longer use the precious vitality remaining in us to digest and eliminate food material, which, consequently, can now be reserved and utilized for other and more immediately important purposes. A consequent increase of vitality follows. In such cases, then, where the vitality is already low, we see, more easily, the effects of fasting upon the organism, and such cases, I contend, indirectly vindicate my position. The actual increase of energy afforded by fasting is not noticed, to a like extent, in those who are comparatively well and strong for the reason that such increase is more than counterbalanced by the lack of customary stimulation, which is first noted, and which temporarily overshadows the effects of fasting, for the reason that these effects are more immediate and intense. For that reason, the first few days of a fast are always the most trying. These once passed, it is invariably noticed that strength and energy return and continue to increase as the fast progresses. Needless to say, this would be quite impossible were the theories commonly held correct.

Let us now consider this paradoxical question from a slightly different point of view. While it is true that abstinence from food will at first produce a species of alertness and awareness and activity, it will, if persisted in, gradually weaken the patient (apparently)—this weakness continuing to increase, moreover, as the fast progresses. This would seem to disprove my contention that the energy increases and never decreases with the continuation of the fast; but when further inquired into, I think it will be found, not to contradict but to confirm it. And in order to prove this contention, I must ask my reader to consider, with me, the *rationale* of the apparent strength and of the weakness here observed.

The elation of spirits noticeable, as the result of a few hours fast, is simply due to the fact that the bodily energies are conserved just in so far as they have not been called upon to digest and eliminate the mass of food material ordinarily ingested—this energy being available for expenditure, and consequently noticeable in the daily life. But it may be urged that this energy should be more and more noticeable as the fast progressed, were this the case, for the reason that more and more energy would thus be conserved, whereas we know that this is not the case—weakness (at least apparent) resulting, in the great majority of cases, if the fast be persisted in, and not increased strength and energy.

The whole difficulty is just here. The energies *are* increased as the fast progresses, gaining strength daily because of the fact that no food is eaten calling for digestion, but these energies are not noticed by us after the first few hours of fasting for the reason that, if food is not supplied, *they are turned or directed into other channels*—cleansing the body of its diseased condition, *e.g.*—hence they are not noticed by us *as energy*, for the reason that they are no longer being forcibly expended, but are turned into an unnoticed field of operation—we noticing energy in its expenditure, never in its accumulation, as I have so often pointed out and insisted upon. The reason for the observed weakness, therefore, is that the energies are now directed into unnoticed channels, and are accumulating; not that they are lessened or decreased by the fast, for such is certainly not the case.

We are now in a better position to answer the question: Why is the feeling of weakness experienced at the commencement of a fast? If energy is not lessened, but commences to increase the instant the fast is entered upon, and continues to accumulate throughout the entire period, why should weakness and lassitude be experienced, when we should expect added strength and energy?

The answer is this: Strength is not actually lost, during this period; weakness does not result from the withdrawal of the accustomed food; only the *feeling* of such weakness—a very different matter. Our senses are deceived, just as they are deceived when we see the sun "rise" in the east and "set" in the west. We know the sun neither rises nor sets; yet the illusion is perfect. Our senses are deceived most readily, and the true reason that we experience this feeling of loss of energy (not actual loss, be it observed) is that we have suddenly withdrawn a regular and customary stimulant, and the withdrawal of all stimulants will have precisely this effect. As Doctor Trall so well expressed it, when writing on stimulation:

"All persons know how they feel; but all do not apprehend the true sources of their good or bad feelings, and the majority mistake the sense of mere stimulation for the condition of actual strength; they do not distinguish between the feeling of strength and vital power; they do not consider that strength or power is only shown in its waste or expenditure, not in its accumulation or possession."

And the whole *crux* of the matter is just here. *Food is a stimulant;* its apparently "strengthening" effects and qualities are, in reality, due to the fact that we no longer call forth force to digest food that may have been eaten. It must be remembered, always, that we invariably notice energy in its expenditure, never in its accumulation (p. 41). Food, then, instead of adding force to the body, merely acts as the occasion for its expenditure. All food calls forth force from the body, but does not add it to the body. The vital forces, being no longer expended upon what I may call "external" things (the digestion of food, *e.g.*—it being noticed by us at the time as "strength" —energy expended, in reality) turn and concentrate their attention upon the inner man—to internal work—where they are not, to any such great extent, noticed by us. The outlay has become less; consequently we notice it less. But has the actual strength been reduced, in the sense that it has been absolutely withdrawn and dissipated? By no means; it is being augmented; but, since we never notice energy in its accumulation, but always in its expenditure (p. 41), we cannot appreciate the fact that we are becoming stronger and regaining lost energy, because we temporarily *feel* otherwise. And if it be thought that this argument is not sound, I ask—why so? Consider the opposite aspect of the case. It must be maintained, if my theory is

[1] "Hydropathic Encyclopædia," Vol. I., p. 418.

wrong, that sleep is an extremely depleting process, since, in that case, strength and vitality are totally absent and unnoticeable! We know, on the contrary, that for that very reason we are gaining energy and becoming stronger. And it is precisely the same in the case of fasting when the daily food is withdrawn, and the vital energies are seemingly greatly reduced. In both cases, the vital energies are being gained when they are apparently at their lowest ebb.

But it may be objected that we frequently receive benefit from a meal—we feel decidedly "better" for it—and consequently it must be strengthening us, for how, otherwise, would these effects become apparent? Now I contend that this feeling is not strength, but stimulation; and this may be readily perceived, it seems to me, when we realize that, even according to the accepted theories, food must be assimilated and digested before it can impart any energy to the system, and this process requires considerable time. Obviously, therefore, the immediate effects of food must be due to its stimulating, not to its "strengthening" quality.

It may be contended, on the other hand, that we frequently experience a feeling of depression after a meal, followed, later, by a feeling of added strength, and this is taken to denote the strength derived from the food, after the tax of digestion is over. But the facts can be accounted for on my theory just as easily. When we experience the increased feeling of strength and rejuvenation, following the period of depression, what has really happened is simply this. In *starting* the digestive machinery into active work, under such extremely adverse circumstances as the ingestion of a superabundance of food necessitates, an enormous amount of energy is required; so much so that every other part of the body is rendered almost totally torpid and inactive—this being the feeling experienced soon after the ingestion of the meal. This we directly notice. But every machine, when once started, runs far more easily and necessitates the expenditure of far less energy than is required in starting it; the carriage runs smoothly, without any noticeable strain upon the energy of the horse pulling it; the engine runs some distance simply by reason of its impetus. But in starting the carriage or the engine, a very great amount of energy was required. And so it is with our digestion, and the digestive energies. Until digestion is fairly started all the energies of the body are focused and concentrated upon the task of commencing this process of digestion with all possible expediency; but, when once fairly started the energies are, in part, released, and it is possible to utilize them for other purposes. Thus, we apparently add to the system's total of force, while, as a matter of fact, we are simply releasing a part of the energy we had previously stored within us, ready for use—it being used in the process of digestion. Had we eaten nothing, *all* of the energy would have been available, of course; but we feel so much stronger even regaining a part of our rightful strength—as compared to the previous feeling of almost complete prostration—that we believe strength has been added to us! As a matter of fact, we have merely had restored to us a part of our rightful stock of energy, which should have been ours *in toto*. Again, we see how utterly illusory and unreliable are our senses and feelings—so far as the bodily energy is concerned.

Perhaps a deeper and more mystical interpretation of the causation of vitality by food might be advanced by those physicians who are somewhat less materialistic than the average in their view-point, yet who would still contend that our food is, *in some sense*, the source of our bodily energy. Such, *e.g.*, is the position—or rather the suggestion—of Prof. John Uri Lloyd, who, in his ingenious book "Etidorhpa" (pp. 125–7), pointed out that food is not matter, merely the "carrier of food"; sunshine is the real food, which is bound up with the food; "the flesh of animals, the food, of living creatures, are simply carriers of sunshine energy." "Food and drink are only carriers of bits of assimilable sunshine." But even granting all this to be true, it is obvious that the problem is unchanged for our present purposes. For, if we withdraw the food, the energy it carries would not enter the body either, and consequently the body would weaken and become devitalized, just in the same way as it would if the current theories were correct. But that even this interpretation of the phenomena is incorrect is proved by observations in the phenomena of fasting, which show that the energies do not decrease, but, on the contrary, invariably *in* crease, as the fast progresses. (pp. 257-8.)

One very important consideration springs into view, however, as the result of this discussion; and that is that some food seems to be much more "live" than other food. And that this property of "liveness" accompanies all uncooked foods is insisted upon by many writers upon dietetics. And we can very readily see that, in the cooking process, this property of liveness is destroyed, to a very large extent, at least—the process of cooking leaving nothing but dead, inert ashes—*minus* some of the most important properties of the foods, and having had these abstracted in the very processes of cooking; and this is a contention that food reformers (at least those who advocate the raw-food diet) have long been urging and insistently pointed out. Viewed in this light, it finds a scientific explanation.

There remains one and only one valid objection to my theory (that the bodily energies are not derivable from the food we eat) which is this: That the bodily tissues are themselves drawn upon during a fast, and are thus absorbed and oxidized and utilized by the system as food—they yielding energy to the system, during the process, just as all other food material would; and consequently that there is no evidence tending to prove that our energies are not derived from food, since such food would be supplied by the tissues so long as they would last; and this is the position, I take it, of the scientific world to-day.

Now, at first sight, this position is quite plausible, to say the least, and the difficulty of completely disproving it is, I admit, verv great. I do think, however, that the position can be shown to be untenable in the last analysis, and my reasons for thinking so are, briefly, as follows:

In the first place, I would ask: Why is it that we become stronger and more invigorated so long as we continue to *fast*, but immediately *starvation* begins, weakness and debility at once become manifest, and continue to increase until death puts an end to all life manifestation? I ask, why is this so? Tissue is being absorbed and oxidized, during the period of starvation just as it is during a fast—as is evidenced by the continued decrease of flesh and weight—and we should expect *more* energy to be gained from the oxidation of this tissue, it seems to me, for the reason that this tissue is more normal and healthful and highly vitalized than the formerly oxidized tissue—which was more or less morbid—whereas we know that precisely the reverse of this is, in fact, the case, though the reason is far from obvious. Tissue is absorbed and oxidized, during starvation, just as it is oxidized during a fast, and, this being so, why is it that energy is sustained (apparently given off) in the one case and not in the other? I cannot see any clear reason for this. And, during the latter days of a fast, when we are averaging the loss of one-half a pound a day or less, as against the one and one-half pounds or more, at the commencement of the fast—how is it that we derive *more* energy from the one-half pound of tissue at the close of the fast than we do from the one and one-half pounds of tissue at its commencement? If we accept my theory—that weakness is, in the first place, due to disease, and that, with its removal, health and strength return—all this becomes readily intelligible; but on the generally accepted theories, I venture to think that such facts flatly contradict the theory at a point where it is essential that such contradictions should not be forthcoming.

But there is another aspect of the problem that must be taken into consideration—one that has been generally overlooked, though it is highly important in considering this question, and has a practical bearing upon the treatment of the sick, as I shall try to make clear. Even were we to grant—for the sake of argument—that our energies are derived from the oxidation of our own tissues, during a fast—our energies being sustained in this manner—why is it that, if this were so, the medical profession should insist upon our partaking of food so regularly, and in so great quantities—in order that we should "keep up our strength"—while, by their own showing, the strength can be maintained and preserved, for some considerable time, at least, by the oxidation of the tissues and food already in the body? If this is possible, as they have just been contending it is (and if they do not grant this, then our energy is certainly derived from some other source than our food) if, I say, this is possible, then why should they insist on the regular and enforced feedings of the patient by other food—when his energies can be maintained by the oxidation of food and tissue already in the body, and when we know that all digestion calls for a certain amount of wasted energy in digestion tax? And if it be argued that, though energy is doubtless imparted to the body as the result of the oxidation of food and tissue already in it, still, *not so much* energy is gained or given off to the body as in the case where the daily food is oxidized—and this is the only logical ground to take—then I may answer that this is directly opposed to the facts in the case, which show that *more* energy is gained, as the fast progresses, and less food is oxidized, presumably, than before—and not less, which should be the case, were the present-day theories correct. It is, in fact, simply another aspect of or repetition of Professor LeConte's statement, when he said that, in order to gain more energy, we must ingest and oxidize more food; while I have tried to show that all true philosophy—no less than the actual facts in the case—show this to be incorrect and flatly disproved by the evidence. If we conceive, on the other hand, that the energies increase in direct ratio to the return of health and physiological cleanliness, all falls naturally into place, and becomes readily explicable.

§ 5. *Facts Supporting This Theory*

That my theory is correct may be shown in a number of ways. Let us take the drunkard, *e.g.*, who is accustomed to his habitual stimulation. Let this be withdrawn and what is the result? Prostration and weakness, absolute. Since we know that stimulants do not and cannot really impart strength to the organism, but only occasion its expenditure (p. 41), it is obvious that the parallel is exact. A withdrawal of stimulation does, in both cases, result in weakness and apparent loss of energy; but in both cases is the weakness illusory—resulting from a withdrawal of the cause of vital expenditure; the resultant weakness being exactly proportioned to the amount of the previous stimulation, and just as much as it is missed, just so much is a fast necessary—since the greater the stimulation, the more necessary is the fast, in order to restore the health and wasted energies—since the more abnormal the condition of the organism. In both cases is the apparent "weakness" necessary and beneficial, indicating that the energies are being gained and that a real cure is being effected.

Another line of proof, which is really subsidiary to the above, is based upon the fact that the more stimulating the food, the more is the fasting noticed—and, of course, the greater the immediate weakness. Those who live simple, abstemious lives, and whose diet is largely fruitarian, can undergo a fast of several days without any consequent depression and lassitude worth remarking; while those who are in the habit of eating bountifully, and of stimulating foods, meats, etc., notice any such deprivation exceedingly.

Dr. Graham, many years ago, noticed the same thing, writing:[1]

"This peculiar condition of the stomach (the feeling of ab normal hunger) will pass away much sooner and with less uncom fortableness of feeling in the pure vegetable eater of regular habits, when the ordinary meal is omitted, than in the flesh eater; and he who makes a free use of stimulating condiments with his food, experiences still more inconvenience and distress at the loss of a meal, than he who eats flesh simply and plainly prepared. Hence, the pure vegetable-eater loses a meal with great indifference, fasts twenty-four hours with little inconvenience or diminution of strength, and goes without food several days in succession without suffering anything like intolerable distress from hunger. The flesh-eater always suffers much more from fasting, and experiences a more rapid decline of muscular power; and he who seasons his food highly with stimulating condiments, feels the loss of a single day severely; a fast of twenty-four hours almost unmans him; and three or four days abstinence from food completely prostrates him, if he is cut off from all stimulants as well as aliment."

Dr. John Smith remarked:[2]

"The more stimulating the food, the sooner does the demand for it return."

And Doctor Trall stated that:

"I have often noticed, in conducting a water-cure establishment, containing more than a hundred inmates on the average,

[1] "Science of Human Life," p. 559.
[2] "Fruits and Farinacea," etc., p. 173.

about half of whom were either vegetarians in principle, or were restricted to an exclusively vegetable diet by special prescription, that such patients can bear fasting for a time much better than the flesh-eaters; and they suffer but little; in comparison with those who enjoy a mixed diet, from the 'craving' sensation of the stomach, on the approach of dinner or supper hour. To this rule I have never known one exception."

Thus we see that the apparent "strength" resultant from the ingestion of food is due, in reality, to its stimulating effects upon the organism—such effects being noticeable in direct proportion to the degree of stimulation produced by the food ingested. Now, if such be really the case, we should look to find little or no stimulation—and consequently very little feeling of imparted strength—if we could find food that was practically free from stimulating properties. Indeed, since the digestion of all food is a tax upon our vital energies, we should expect to find an actual feeling of depression following the ingestion of such food, if absolutely free from stimulating properties. But, as a matter of fact, such a food does not exist. In any case, the mere *ingestion* of food acts as a stimulant, more or less, and this feeling at least counterbalances the depressing effects of the tax of digestion. But over and above this slight stimulation, all feeling of added strength must be due to an increased degree of stimulation, *i.e.*, to a *waste* of vital force. "Added energy" is thus merely added waste of energy—stimulation necessarily implying consequent reaction, and hence less strength in the long run.

But, if the commonly accepted theories were true, the reverse of this ought to be the case. Those persons who were the "strongest"—as a result of their "generous" diet—should be enabled to withstand the supposed "weakening" effects of the fast better than those who are already "half-starved" and debilitated. Their energy should last longer; they should notice the fast last and least. But, since the reverse of this is actually the case, it clearly demonstrates that it is stimulation, not strength—or the cause of strength—that has been withdrawn.

The weakness present during the fast may further be explained in this manner. We know that fasting is a curing process—a process of purification,—and, as such must necessarily expend an extraordinary amount of vital energy in this process of cure or purification. It must be remembered that, since disease is a curing process, fasting is—in one sense of the term—a disease, artificially and purposely produced! We aggravate the symptoms, in exciting the expulsive effort, in order to bring about, the more rapidly, an effective and actual cure. (p. 61.) We must remember that *weakness always results from the presence of disease*—or the causes of disease—its presence necessitating and implying a certain lack of vital force.[1] The process of elimination—itself necessitating an exceptional expenditure of vital energy—must also be decidedly weakening, since all the available energies of the body are now turned into that channel or direction. When, however, the body is once freed from disease—or its causes—the energies are again at liberty to resume the business of daily life, and then the greater strength and energy we experience fully convince us that no energy was lost by reason of the fast; but, on the contrary, that greater strength and energy are present than at its commencement, *i.e.*, that there has resulted from the fast an appreciable *gain*.

Again, it may be contended that, in many instances (shipwrecked sailors, *e.g.*, who have been exposed in an open boat for a considerable length of time) extreme weakness, even to complete collapse, has been observed in those undergoing such compulsory privation. This I do not deny, but I object to the conclusions drawn from the observation (that the weakness resulted because of the withdrawal of food). I believe that the weakness and prostration in such cases can be traced to other causes. First, we have to take into consideration the mental condition of the subjects in such cases. The anxious suspense; the alternate extremes of tense excitement and uncontrollable despair; the depression; the uncertainty of life—such potent influences might well exhaust and sap the vitality of the most

[1] Says Doctor Dewey ("New Era for Women," p. 154–5): "It is disease that prostrates vital power and not the loss of two or three digested daily meals; hence, as disease loses its grasp with its generally prostrating effect on the mind as well as on the muscles, so must there be increase of strength, since the brain is being duly supported."

healthy, the "best fed," even under normal conditions. We must by no means leave such important factors out of our account. Again, we must take into consideration the actual, physical trial of the experience that has been endured; the exposure to cold or heat; the buffet of the elements; the sleepless and anxious nights; the hardships; the toils and privations of the journey. These, in themselves, are, surely, enough to waste and exhaust the strength, the energy of the most robust and hardened adventurer, if long experienced. Add to all this the effects of the mental stórm through which such persons must surely pass, and I believe that the exhaustion, the lack of vitality noticeable in such cases may readily be explained—to seek no further for the cause. But such a contention is not, fortunately, necessary in order to establish my contention; another cause may readily be seen to exist by those who understand and appreciate the true *rationale* of the fasting cure. For, let us consider the situation. Suppose that our shipwrecked sailors (a typical case) have been practically without provisions for (say) four weeks, at the time of their rescue. Now, living the healthy, active life that most seamen live, I do not think we are justified in asserting that any of them would be sufficiently diseased to require a longer fast than from two to three weeks, in order to restore them to perfect health (I think from one to two weeks would be nearer the truth, but I give my opponents all the latitude possible in the argument) that is, from two to three weeks, as we would fast under normal conditions. But, in the fresh, bracing sea air, which they constantly inhale, exposed to the fury of the elements, and, frequently, the continued and great exertion of rowing, we can readily see that a fast, under such circumstances, would be terminated much more speedily than under the comparatively quiet, tranquil mental and physical conditions surrounding an average fast, conducted in the seclusion of the home. The certain effect of this would be to shorten the fast—making it necessary to fast only a week or so, before hunger returns, and the normal fast be terminated. From that moment—when normal hunger returns —starvation begins (p. 564), and with it consequent weakness and emaciation. For the last three weeks of the experience, therefore, these men were truly starving (not fasting), which, as I have frequently insisted upon, is a purely abnormal process, and one that I should deprecate and discourage as much as any man living. Fasting is a very different thing from starving, and where the one ends, the other begins. The effects of starvation would doubtless be enervating and depleting to the last degree; and this is the process that has been weakening our supposed subjects for a full three weeks before their rescue! I think we can now fully and easily understand why, in such cases, extreme weakness is present; it is the result of starvation, not of fasting, and the results could not well have been otherwise.

Is it asserted, then, that vitality is *in no way* connected with the digestion of food; that the two are absolutely distinct, and in no wise related to one another? By no means! There is a connection, but it is not such a connection as is generally supposed; in fact it is precisely and exactly the opposite. For, although we do not derive the least particle of energy from our food, at any time, the digestion of every atom of food necessitates the outlay—the expenditure—of a tremendous amount of vital force! All digestion calls for and necessitates this outlay, and must necessarily do so. As Doctor Dewey so well remarked:[1]

"There is no movement so slight, no thought or motion so trivial, that it does not cost brain-power in its action—and this is true of even the slightest exercise of energy evolved in digestion."

Every morsel of food digested must, therefore, occasion the expenditure of a certain amount of energy, and it is this expenditure which we feel as strength (p. 41), and think it is energy being added to the system, while it is, in reality, being abstracted from it; and necessarily so, for the very reason that we *do* feel it! Food digestion, then, merely occasions this expenditure of energy, and that is the reason we apparently feel the added strength, consequent upon its ingestion.

It may be objected to this that, were we to pursue this line of argument to its legitimate conclusion, we should be forced into the position of admitting that the greater the amount of exercise

[1] "The No-Breakfast Plan," etc., p. 38.

taken, the less should be the amount of food eaten—since exercise and digestion both call for an expenditure of energy; less should be expended in one direction if more is being expended in another. Logical as this may sound on first reading, it is nevertheless a fallacy, and the argument does not lead to any such conclusion if the theory be properly and thoroughly understood. Such objectors have lost sight of the fundamental principle that normal hunger is the expressed demand of the tissues for nutriment. When hunger is experienced, therefore, it follows that the tissues are craving for food material[1] and this material should consequently be supplied; it follows, also, that *there is sufficient vitality present to digest the food eaten*, for otherwise there would be no hunger. The fact that exercise may be freely indulged in, during a fast (in some cases), without reviving hunger and a call for food, conclusively proves this to my mind. Hunger is manifest in direct ratio to the need of the tissues for food; and the strength of this call (and consequently the degree of vitality present) is always directly proportioned to the organic needs. The call of hunger, therefore, denotes, incidentally, the presence of a certain degree of vital energy, sufficient in amount, to digest the required amount of food (which is all that should be eaten at any time and under any circumstances). All the above, of course, applies only to *true* hunger (p. 549)—for morbid cravings there is no rule—save that food should be withheld absolutely until it disappears and true hunger follows.

Now, exercise destroys tissue; consequently an urgent demand is present for material with which to replace this tissue—the hunger is "keen." But exercise, having also purified the body to a certain extent, by reason of its stimulating effects upon the various depurating organs, etc., renders possible a greater inflow of energy; and in health this more than counterbalances the energy expended in the exercise. Were this not so, exercise would ultimately deplete and weaken, instead of strengthen and invigorate us. We can thus perceive why exercise should, in its ultimate effects, strengthen us, and also why extra bodily exertion calls for more, not less, food—an answer to the original objection.

[1] It must not be forgotten, in this connection, that, during long periods of work, water is craved more than food, though we derive no nutriment or "strength" from water, as we are supposed to do from the food.

And this theoretical argument is still further enforced by the very practical fact, of daily observation, that it is decidedly unhygienic and most prostrating to the vital powers to eat at all, when tired—at which time food should be more necessary than at any other period, if we derived our strength and energy from its assimilation and combustion. Indeed, it might certainly—and most rationally—be claimed that, if food has the power, the ability to keep up and support the strength, there should not be so much strength lost in the general activities; indeed, it would seem that fatigue should be practically an impossibility. But as Doctor Dewey so well pointed out:[1]

"The fact remains that from the first wink in the morning to the last at night there is a gradual decline of strength, no matter how much food is taken, nor how ample the powers of digestion, and that there comes a time when all must go to bed, and not to the dining room, to recover lost strength. The loss of a night of sleep is never made up by any kind of care in eating on the following day, and none are so stupid as not to know that rest is the only means to recover from the exhaustion of excessive physical activity."

The digestion of all food, therefore, must necessitate an expenditure of, and never an addition to, the vital forces.

I now pass on to consider one or two other apparent objections to my theory. First, it may be contended that certain classes or kinds of foods obviously "supply" more energy than do foods of other kinds or classes, since we can perform a greater amount of physical and mental labor while eating one class of foods than when eating the other. So it is claimed that we derive more energy for work from one class of foods than from the other class.

At first sight, this might appear quite logical—if not conclusive—but as a matter of fact it is entirely erroneous, and the facts may be accounted for upon my theory just as readily as upon the other theory. Let us look at the question from this other standpoint.

The problem is simply this: we eat certain foods, and we have a certain amount of energy to expend; we eat certain other

[1] "No-Breakfast Plan," etc., p. 37.

foods, and we have (say) less energy to expend. Does this prove—as it is universally held to prove—that the former food "supplied" us with more energy than the latter? It might be so, certainly, but as certainly it does not prove it. The facts may be readily and philosophically accounted for as follows: Since all food requires an expenditure of energy for its digestion; and since some foods are more readily and easily assimilable than others, it follows that certain foods require, for their digestion, the expenditure of less energy than do others—leaving more energy available for the practical affairs and business of life; for mental work, and for expenditure in various other ways. We thus see that, instead of some foods supplying more energy than others, the cart has again been placed before the horse, and the real truth of the matter is that some foods call for a lesser outlay of vital force for their digestion; consequently, in such cases, the vital energies are the sooner relieved of their burdensome task, and are more ready and available, as well as more powerful, for the performance of other work. The extent to which food "furnishes" force, therefore, is in reality merely the degree to which the vital force is economized during its digestion.

The elation which we feel some time after the ingestion of a meal is not, therefore, due to the strength or energy which that meal has furnished, but is due to the fact that the vital powers which had, until then, been almost entirely utilized in the digestion of the meal are now freed from this labor and set at liberty, being then usable for the general organic purposes—muscular and mental effort, etc.—and should be utilizable for those purposes; and, if we conserved them, we should be enabled to so utilize them. But as soon as we begin to feel the elation resulting from the liberation of the vital powers—they having largely completed the digestion of the former meal—we at once divert them again into the active, wasteful processes of digestion, and so uselessly expend all that might be otherwise so usefully employed by us for other and better work.[1]

[1] This is tacitly admitted by physicians when they administer "easily digested" foods. It must be borne in mind, however, that easily digested foods are not always the *best* foods—ultimately—far from it. I hope to discuss this important question at some length in another volume.

Again, I ask, if the mere mechanical process of oxidizing food material were all that was necessary in order to furnish the system with a definite amount of energy, then how comes it that the oxidation of a certain volume of food in the body of an athlete builds the athlete's body, and not only that but supplies it with the energy for its constant and enormous output; while the *same* bulk of precisely the *same* food material will build the weakling's body; and, further, supply no more vital energy to *it* than we observe to be present in his puny frame, and never apparently adds or supplies one iota of vital vigor, or in any way strengthens him as the same food strengthens the athlete? As Dr. Austin Flint pointed out:[1]

> "A man may take a certain quantity and kind of food, and still, without training, be able to perform only a certain amount of work. After proper training, with precisely the same food, he can develop greatlv increased power."

Now I repeat, why is this? On the generally accepted theories, can this be explained? If the process of supplying the body with vitality were a purely mechanical one, then such contradictory results as the above should never appear. The fact that we do not increase the vitality by increasing the bulk of food has already been considered and disproved. (pp. 236–7.) Obviously, there is somewhere a defect in the theory. To my mind, the explanation of this problem cannot be found so long as we cling to the theories of energy at present in vogue. If so, how? There is only one possible way of even attempting an explanation of the fact just mentioned, and that is to assert that, in the athlete's body, the food ingested was more completely and perfectly oxidized (owing to the greater amount of exercise indulged in and the more perfect lung action) than in the other case.

At first sight, this objection has a certain amount of plausibility, but I immediately ask: If this is the case, then why do you insist on giving the thin, weak, emaciated man more food, in order to "make him stronger," when it is, by your own show-

[1] "The Source of Muscular Power," p. 30.

ing, due to the very fact that he is not properly aërating and utilizing the quantity of food he *does* eat, that he is so thin, weak, and emaciated? If this is not so, then your reasoning is self-contradictory and absurd. If it is, then your practice is founded upon totally erroneous principles—being, in fact, a direct inversion of the truth. Thus we see that we should give such a man *less* food in order for him to aërate and properly assimilate and get the benefit from *more* of it—a fact I have been continually emphasizing throughout this book. But if it be agreed that we can thus increase the vital energies by the taking of less food into the system, then we are in direct opposition to the actually held theory, as stated by Professor Bain on p. 237, where he asserted that we can only increase it by taking more food—and, in fact, if the theory as at present defended be true, this must be the case. So that we are driven into this dilemna; either of rejecting the correctness of the theory as it now stands, and as it is universally accepted; or of shutting our eyes and ears to very definite and certain and numerous facts and arguments which completely disprove the correctness of such theory. On the horns of this dilemma, I leave my reader to choose the one on which to impale himself.

Only on the theory outlined above can we explain, it seems to me, the tremendous difference in individuals, all of whom live more or less on the same food, and about the same amount of it. If the prevailing theory were true, these various persons should have, as nearly as possible, the same amount of physical strength—or at least some should not have two or three or even ten times the strength of others—and that, too, on even less food than the weaker man daily consumes. It seems to me that such cases conclusively disprove the theories held to-day. But if we can conceive, on the contrary, that the greater output of energy, in the case of the stronger men, necessitated and conditioned, in turn, a larger *draught* upon the unlimited cosmic energy, which flows into his organism according to the amount of its output—its physiological needs—then we have, I think, a conceivable basis of explanation for such remarkable cases as these. And it follows from this that the greatest degree of life—living in the highest sense—will be realized only by those whose daily output and inflow of the cosmic energy is the greatest. As Doctor Trall so well said:[1]

"The heart of him who creeps through the world languidly and mincingly is small and weak in its power to circulate the blood, while the man who rushes into active business earnestly, and uses his muscles vigorously, his heart is called upon for energetic action in sending the blood copiously to all parts of the system, and the consequence is an increase in the size and strength of that important organ."

§ 6. *Fatigue: Its True Nature*

One other very forcible objection to my theory remains, which will doubtless be raised by some acute critic. The objection is that fatigue is due—not so much to nervous exhaustion as to the manufacture and retention within the system of poisonous compounds, which more or less poison the tissues and are the true cause, in fact, of what we term "fatigue." This may be all very true, and I do not doubt that, so far as these observations go, they are correct, but the conclusions drawn from these observations are, I am persuaded, incorrect; the facts are misinterpreted.

Professor Mosso, in his excellent book on "Fatigue," thus describes the phenomena observed:[2]

"Fatigue is a chemical process. . . . The lack of energy in the movements of a weary man depends . . . upon the fact that the muscles, during work, produce noxious substances which, little by little, interfere with contraction. . . . If these waste products accumulate in the blood, we feel fatigued; when their amount passes the physiological limit, we become ill." (p. 118.)

See also the remarks on this subject in Pyle's "Hygiene," pp. 323–7.

Now, it seems to me that there is positive proof that the fatigue we experience at the end of the day is not due to these poisons collected within the system, but to the exhaustion of and the need for recharging the human motor—of replenishing

[1] "The Family Gymnasium," etc., p. 65.
[2] "Fatigue," by A. Mosso, Professor of Physiology in the University of Turin, etc., pp. 104–5.

our nervous systems with vital energy. For, were the fatigue experienced due solely to this retention of poisons, the surest way to vitalize, or reënergize the body would be to rid it of these poisons, and this we can do more effectively and more rapidly by *e.g.*, deep breathing, colon flushing, Turkish baths, etc., than by any other method—certainly far more rapidly and easily and more effectually than by the mere process of resting quietly, for a short time—often in a badly ventilated room, too! Yet we know that deep breathing, while of inestimable benefit to the organism in every way, will by no means postpone indefinitely exhaustion, fatigue and sleep (p. 247–8), while we know that a Turkish bath is frequently a most debilitating process! (p. 368).[1]

How, then, are we to explain these results—so contradictory—upon the accepted theories? For, if the fatigue generally experienced be due to the retention of poisonous compounds, the elimination of these poisons must be practically all that is necessary in order to restore the bodily vitality and energy. But we know that this is not the case. However carefully we eliminate the poisons from the system, fatigue—lack of energy—ultimately ensues, and energy must be replaced by sleep and by sleep alone.[2] That energy can be replaced in no other manner is our daily—or rather hourly—experience. All this finds a ready explanation provided my theory is the true one—that fatigue is not caused, as imagined, by toxins, but that the poisons generated merely render the body incapable of transforming the energy into work. True fatigue is really nervous

[1] We must be careful to distinguish, always, true sleepiness from the exhaustion of tissue-poisoning—produced by decomposing food material. This is most important. Thus, after a full meal, we frequently feel exhausted for some hours, this being due to nerve-poisoning. Bad combinations of food decompose, forming gases, which are absorbed by the system, and act upon the nervous tissue. But later on, we seem to recover our strength and energy. This, while largely due to the causes mentioned above, is also due to the fact that the created poisons have been mostly eliminated, and hence we experience the feeling of added fitness and energy, which we put down to the food we have eaten. But this exhaustion is entirely distinct from *real* exhaustion, which is not self-recuperative in this manner. True fatigue is ever present, in increasing degrees, when once originated.

[2] It is true that the bodily energies may be apparently and temporarily increased by baths, very often. Thus Mr. Purinton writes ("Philosophy of Fasting," p. 39): "I found repeatedly that what seemed to be fatigue was only some remnant of undigested food still lurking in my system. A few eliminative measures quite refreshed me." This may be very true, but, by reaction, rest is called for, and, as I stated, fatigue ultimately ensues, and energy must invariably be replaced by sleep and sleep alone.

exhaustion; it is that and that only. Fatigue is not due to the presence of poisons within the system, because fatigue can only originate in the nervous system. The inability to perform a certain task with the muscles is due to the inability of the muscle to properly convey and transform the nervous impulse it receives, owing to its poisoned condition. This is the state brought about by tissue poisoning, and will be superseded, in time, by a feeling of refreshment, when this period has passed. This I would distinguish from true fatigue. The *impulse itself* may be there, in such cases, as strong as ever, but the poisoned muscle cannot transform or turn into work this energy received. The lack of power lies in the process of transformation—not initiation; and is purely of peripheral—not central—origin. The exhaustion of nerve cells is the true cause of fatigue; this is what we experience at the end of the day, when the body is normal, and this fatigue can only be replaced by rest and sleep, and by no other means or process.

Indeed, this is the position which Professor Mosso is driven to assume, though the significance of the admission did not, it would seem, appear to him in its full force. Thus, on pp. 243–4 of his "Fatigue," he remarks:

"The nervous system is the sole source of energy. . . . The conclusion to which we are led by my experiments is that there exists only one kind of fatigue, namely, nervous fatigue; this is the preponderating phenomenon, and muscular fatigue also is at bottom an exhaustion of the nervous system."

Or, as Doctor Pyle put it·[1]

" When the fatigue is pushed so far that it is no longer possible by a voluntary effort to cause the finger to lift the weight, it is the nerve cells, and not the muscular fibers, which first give out. For at this moment direct stimulation of the muscle by an electric current will generally cause it to contract and raise the weight."

But, after all, the feeling of fatigue, of lassitude, is very largely a *mental* thing—a part of our psychic, and not of our physiological life. We can only *feel* tired in the brain; and the simple idea

[1] "Personal Hygiene," etc., pp. 324–5.

"I am tired" is as purely a mental state as "I am joyous," or "I am bored." To be sure, such a mental condition accurately corresponds to the state of the organism at the time. As such, it represents a real condition of the organism, and should certainly be heeded; but the feeling of "tiredness" is, I contend, purely a mental, not a physical state. No matter how that mental state arose; no matter what it corresponds to, it is purely mental, none the less. We may easily prove this by simple observation. Thus: a person is extremely fatigued; sleep is about to overcome him, when, suddenly, something happens which terrifies him exceedingly. Away with sleep! Away flies all feeling of "tiredness." The patient is awake, active, vigorous, and even *less* tired than he has been all the preceding day! Now, if fatigue were purely a physical or chemical process, this would be an impossibility; but depending, as it does, upon the nervous system, and so upon the mind, we can readily see that the fatigue we experience is, after all, purely a mental state—not a physical thing.[1]

Another proof that fatigue is purely a mental state is afforded by cases of secondary and multiple personality; in which cases the patient is fatigued, or even paralyzed or bedridden, in one state; but, with the change of personality, he instantaneously regains his strength and vigor, and presents none of the symptoms of disease or of fatigue. One of the most remarkable and significant of these cases is that recorded by Dr. Morton Prince:[2] when he says·

"Not the least interesting of the curious phenomena manifested, are the different degrees of health enjoyed by the different personalities. One would imagine that if ill health were always

[1] Incidentally, I may remark that Professor Mosso's experiments seeming to show that the energy for work is increased after injections of sugar, are quite valueless for the reason, (1) that the sugar would act as a stimulant, and hence bring forth a greater amount of energy from the body, merely (p. 41); and (2), the possibilities of suggestion were never eliminated. Says Miss Abel ("Sugar as Food," by Mary Hinman Abel, U. S. *Dept. of Agriculture Bulletin*, p. 15): "The ergograph, which recorded the amount of work done, was concealed from the person using it, in order that he might not unconsciously influence the result, a caution not observed in Mosso's laboratory. Doctor Langemeyer obtained only negative results as to the effect of sugar on muscle work; an increase of muscle power occurred as often when no sugar was taken, or after a short rest, or after taking a drink of water."

[2] In his "Dissociation of a Personality," pp. 17, 287.

based on physical alterations, each personality must have the same ailments; but such is not the case. The person known as B I has the poorest health; B IV is more robust, and is capable of mental and physical exertion without ill effects, which would be beyond the powers of B I; while B III is a stranger to an ache or pain. She does not know what illness means."

How can such cases be accounted for on purely chemical theories?

§ 7. *Additional Arguments Supporting the Author's Theory*

My theory further explains the loss of vitality due to sexual and other stimulation. It is now known that the exhaustive effects of sexual excitement are due, not to loss of semen, as was formerly supposed, but to the peculiar and prolonged excitement of the nervous system. Says Doctor Graham:[1]

" nor is there the least evidence that the mere loss of the semen, apart from the concomitant excitement, irritation, functional disturbance, and expenditure of vital power, is the source of any considerable injury to the human system. But it is perfectly clear, on the other hand, that all the evils resulting from the abuse of the genital organs, occur, in their very worst and most incorrigible forms, where there is no secretion and voluntary emission of semen."

This may be seen more readily when we consider that, when sexual excitement takes place, *even though the crisis be not reached,* an exhaustion follows, almost or quite equal to that which would follow were the act completed. We know also, that continued erotic and abnormal *thoughts* will tend to deplete the vitality of the person only in a lesser degree than the actual commission of the act; while, further, we know that, in the female, there is, of course, no seminal discharge whatever. Again, in seminal emissions (nocturnal) in the male there is practically no loss of energy whatever. It is obvious, therefore, for these and other reasons, that the prostration following sexual excitement is due solely to its effect upon the nervous system.

[1] "Chastity," by Sylvester Graham, M.D., p. 7. See also p. 56 of Dr. John B. Newman's "Philosophy of Generation"; Dr. James C. Jackson's "Hints on the Reproductive Organs," etc.

The explanation is easily found, I think, in view of the above elaborated theory. If the vitality depends altogether upon the nervous system, the solution of this problem is self-evident.

Again, I ask, why is it that *pain* so weakens us—so wastes the energies and lowers the vitality—so much, indeed, as to completely prostrate the strongest man in a few days or even hours? If our vitality were so easily and mechanically replaced (and so infallibly too, of necessity), surely it should be impossible for us so completely to lose our energies, in so short a space of time. And they cannot (strange to say!) be replaced at such a time by any amount of food that we may ingest and oxidize. On the contrary, we know that we are, as a rule, almost completely incapacitated from taking any food at all at such times—our instincts indicating that none is needed, that none can be utilized, and that, if much is eaten, it will in no wise add to the bodily energies, but rather detract from them. And yet we are supposed to be able to replace this lost energy through food alone!

It may be urged, again, "is not the stronger man (the man with the bigger muscles) stronger because the muscle itself is bigger, and evolves more energy because of the greater combustion taking place within it?" Apart from the objection to this theory raised on pp. 245–6, I think an explanation may be found by assuming (as we have every right to do) that the stronger man's body, being larger, affords the opportunity for the transmission of a greater volume of vital energy than does the weaker man's body; it is capable of transforming into active work a greater amount of the cosmic energy than is the smaller frame —which is precisely what we should expect. As Doctor Walter expressed it:[1]

> "Increased development of body and brain does not necessarily mean increased power possessed by the individual, but rather increased capacity to expend the power."

The bigger, stronger, more muscular man possesses more energy and needs more food than his slimmer brother simply because there is a greater bulk of tissue calling for replacement, and also because more of it is broken down by the daily activities

[1] "The Exact Science of Health," etc., p. 8.

than in the latter case—a greater amount of exercise invariably being taken. But this does not prove that the greater bulk of food ingested has made or created the greater muscular power, in the former case; not at all. The larger man is stronger—has more energy—for the reason that his larger frame, or its superior physical condition, affords a better or wider channel (so to speak) through which the cosmic energy might flow and manifest more abundantly. The larger frame affords the means for such increased inflow, while his better or cleaner or less clogged physical condition renders such inflow more easily possible. But the thinner man, provided his body is equally clean, can allow an equal proportionate amount of energy to flow through it—the amount being proportioned to the size of the bodies in each case. The greater strength of the larger-muscled man is thus due to the fact that his larger and (generally) better conditioned frame affords a larger and better *channel through which* the all-pervading energy can flow; and, I think, to this cause only.

To this I would add a remark first made by Dr. T. L. Nichols, which strikes me as highly suggestive and most true. He says:[1]

"The truth is, that the amount of food said to be eaten by navvies and other strong men is not the cause of their strength, but it is their strength which enables them to digest and dispose of such quantities of food. Weak men would break down under the burden."

True, most true! And this is proved by the fact that when these same strong men are enfeebled by disease, they, too, break down under the strain—and on account of it.

§ 8. *The Origin of Life: Criticism of Recent Attempts at Creation*

In considering the theory of vitality generally held, one most important factor is, so far as I can see, almost entirely overlooked, *viz.*, the *origin* of life or vitality. The ideas as to the origin of life at present held seem to me little short of ludicrous. First, the idea of spontaneous generation (at least a thinkable

[1] "The Diet Cure," p. 21.

hypothesis, and one which does, indeed, find champions in a host of scientific men—Professor Haeckel, of Jena, being, probably, the most famous living exponent and defender of the theory) has never received and is not to-day receiving, and as I shall presently try to show, *can never* receive definite proof, for the reasons I there enumerate. Then there is the theory, first advanced by a French writer, Count de Salles-Guyon, and defended by F. Cohn, H. Richter, Helmholtz and Lord Kelvin (being, in fact, made known to the English-speaking world by the last-mentioned scientist, and the idea commonly credited to him, though this is a mistake) that life never had any "beginning" *on our planet:*

"It was transported to the earth from another world, or from the cosmic environment, under the form of cosmic germs, or cosmozoans, more or less comparable to the living cells with which we are acquainted. They have made the journey either included in meteorites or floating in space in the form of cosmic dust."[1]

But M. Verworn considers the hypothesis of cosmic germs as inconsistent with the laws of evolution, and L. Errera pointed out that the necessary conditions for life were lacking in interplanetary bodies.

Du Bois-Reymond's theory of cosmic *panspermia* is one very similar to the above, and needs no separate statement of its position. The same objection applies to both, *viz.*, that it is really no "explanation" at all, since it merely pushes back our inquiry one step, and, if we were to ask: "What was the origin of the life on the planet or in the space from which such germs came, supposedly? we should obviously be in as great a quandary as ever. So superficial a hypothesis is not only not explanatory, but absurd. Realizing such objections, W. Preyer was forced to admit that "Life . . . must have subsisted from all time, even when the globe was an incandescent mass." This position—apart from its inherent absurdity—practically admits that life was and is as eternal and persistent as matter and energy; and this is the position which all true scientists will, I think, some day be forced to admit.

[1] "The Life of Matter," by A. Dastre, p. 401.

If my theory of vitality were proved to be true, we should have no difficulty with this perplexing question. For, if true, we see that life never had any beginning, nor need it have such; it is just as persistent and continuous as matter or force, and exists, equally with them, without end and without beginning. Life has been capable of manifesting through a material body at certain times and under certain circumstances; but its actual existence is as eternal as matter or force (perhaps more so) and to ascribe immortality to two out of the three supposed realities, and to deny it to the third is certainly illogical and unwarranted.

But it may be contended that this theory of the eternal persistence of life has been lately—if not actually disproved—at least thrown under a strong cloud of suspicion by the experiments recently conducted by Professors Loeb,[1] Butler Burke,[2] Bastian,[3] LeDantec,[4] and others—which seem to prove that life can be generated or created in its lowest forms from inorganic matter; and consequently that vital force may, under suitable and appropriate conditions, be derived from and manufactured by chemical and other physical forces in conjunction with the matter upon which they operate—since life is, it is claimed, actually generated or created in such cases, and consequently cannot be so innate as I have contended. And further, that the life force can thus, under certain appropriate conditions, obviously be derived from inorganic matter; and this would seem to disprove the position I have throughout defended, *viz.*, that life or vital force is a thing *per se*, and in no way related to, or derivable from, the other physical forces, with which it is nevertheless connected in some mysterious manner, during the individual's organic life. In other words, the recent experiments in "spontaneous generation" or the creation of organic out of inorganic matter, might be held up as discrediting and disproving my theory. I do not myself think so; I do not think that these experiments will or can ever prove the creation of the living from the non-living, and for the three following reasons:

First, we have the antecedent improbability of any such thing

[1] "The Dynamics of Living Matter," etc.
[2] "The Origin of Life."
[3] "The Nature and Origin of Living Matter."
[4] "The Origin and Nature of Life."

—this doubt being legitimate inasmuch as it is founded on past experiments and not *à priori* speculation. It is admitted by practically every scientist (*pace* Professor Bastian) that life only springs from antecedent life. And yet we have men seriously defending the position that life can spring—not even from inorganic matter, but from decomposition! Says Professor LeConte:[1]

"In all cases, vital force is produced by decomposition."

And on p. 188:

"Whence do animals derive their vital force? I answer, from the decomposition of their food and the decomposition of their tissues."

The statement seems inherently absurd. However, we can afford to set aside such speculations, and come to the main objection to these experiments, which is this: It is exceedingly doubtful whether the supposed forms of life created, in these experiments, are such in reality, or only physico-chemical compounds, having many of the appearances of life. Doctor Burke, indeed, admits that:

"We can not claim that in all our observations there is the slightest evidence of anything which is the same as natural life."[2]

Professor Burke discredits the results of Doctor Bastian's experiments (who also discredits his) so that the whole series of experiments can hardly be said to prove anything decisive. Doctor Walter clearly shows the fallacy of Professor Loeb's experiments in his "Exact Science of Health," pp. 115–18.

Secondly, it would be next to an impossibility to demonstrate, to a scientific certainty, that the experiments conducted have not merely quickened or brought into active being, life already present—and this no matter how perfect, theoretically, the sterilization and all the conditions of the experiment were shown to be. The skeptic might always insist (and there would be no way of rendering his position untenable) that life was somewhere

[1] "Conservation of Energy," etc., p. 175.
[2] "Origin of Life," p. 87.

in the substance treated—having escaped all attempts at sterilization, etc.—and that the experiments conducted merely quickened and rendered active this life, already present.[1] He could, at least, boldly assert that the improbability of creation having been effected was certainly greater than the alternative—that the experiment was in some way defective, and that, however incredible his own position, the alternative was certainly equally incredible—if not more so; and this position can hardly ever be distinctly disproved.

But, aside from such objection—which, after all, might be rather begging the question, the real and valid (third) objection remains. I mean by this that, *even granting the conditions were theoretically perfect,* and that no life whatever was present that was merely quickened into being by the experiment, still, I contend, such experiment would not and never could prove the creation of life from the non-living, and for the following reason.

I have, throughout this chapter, been contending that life is a thing *per se,* distinct from every other physical force, which forces it merely *directs* during its connection with the organism, and that it utilizes during that period—the natural body through which it manifests. Now, for this manifestation, it requires a certain material body—a certain arrangement, that is, of inorganic matter and physical forces which are necessary for its manifestation; and, without this arrangement, there could be no manifestation, and consequently no life. It must be distinctly understood that, in order for life to manifest, it must have this certain very intricate and most delicate arrangement of matter and force, and that unless this arrangement is present, and absolutely perfect in every detail, life cannot utilize such a combination of matter and force, or use it to manifest through.[2]

[1] Professor Burke himself admitted this ("Origin of Life," p. 194). He says: "How can it be ascertained that all forms of life have been destroyed? Most assuredly it can be asserted that in certain circumstances organic forms can be destroyed, but it cannot be shown that ultra-microscopic or even ultra-atomic types of organic or inorganic life do not still remain."

[2] That life is not the mere resultant or product of this combination could be shown in detail, had I the time and space. I would only say here that the vital element is outside of the physical forces present as the result of this combination. This is indirectly proved by the very distinction between organic and inorganic bodies; one is alive and the other not—though they

This much being granted, we can readily see that, in all experiments so far conducted, with the object of creating life, this *exact* combination and arrangement was not obtained—some little defect or flaw was present, sufficient to prevent the manifestation of life through the material utilized for the experiment. But now, suppose we meet with an experiment that has been successful; where life has, apparently, been created from the inorganic material used; does this in reality prove that this life had actually been made or brought into being by the inorganic matter, or any particular combination of it? By no means! It simply proves that the experimenters have at last succeeded in arranging their material in exactly the right quantities, qualities and relations—have, in fact, formed exactly the correct material body *through which* the life force can manifest; *i.e.*, they have finally succeeded in so arranging their material basis as to render possible the manifestation of life force through it. And for this reason I do not see how such experiments as those now being conducted can ever prove the generation of life from non-living matter, for the very reason that this other alternative explanation of the facts would always be open and could be employed by anyone who cared to do so—thus rendering forever impossible this supposed proof of the creation of organic form from inorganic matter—of life from no life—and so doing away with this objection to my hypothesis, since it is thus shown to be no valid objection at all.

It is interesting to note that the above was written, in substance, before the appearance of Sir Oliver Lodge's "Life and Matter." On pp. 172–3 of that book occurs the following passage, which I consider a remarkable coincidence of thought. Speaking of such experiments as I have been criticizing above, Doctor Lodge writes:

"But suppose it (the experiment) was successful; what then? We should then be reproducing in the laboratory a process that

are both composed of the same chemical elements. Why is this? A striking example is found in this fact; bread and strychnine are composed of precisely the same chemical elements, C. H. N. O.—arranged in slightly different combinations. In one case it is a deadly poison; in the other nutritious gluten. Can any purely chemical theory explain such facts? and is the theory of the different arrangement and grouping of the molecules any real explanation at all? ("Occult Science in Medicine," by Franz Hartmann, M.D., p. 56)

must at some past age have occurred on the earth; for at one time the earth was certainly hot and molten and inorganic, whereas now it swarms with life. Does that show that the earth generated the life? By no means; no more than it does that the earth necessarily has generated all the gases of its atmosphere, or the meteoric dust which lies upon its snows."

I conclude this part of the discussion by quoting the following most significant passage from Sir Benjamin Ward Richardson's "Ministry of Health" (pp. 151–5), in which the relations of vitality and the material body are touched upon in as masterly a fashion as it has ever been my good fortune to see. After discussing the possible nature of vitality—its essence, comparing it to light, emanations, etc., and discussing its possible source, our author goes on:

"But this mere physical element of vitality does not prompt us to motion. As the steam engine is motionless till the hand of the engineer outside the mechanism sets the motion free and in order, according to the build of the machine; so we, while our purely physical organism is in motion, are moved by some influences or impressions from without, which pass through our senses, which traverse our nervous cords when they permit it, and which are ever in manifold activity whether we are present or not to be influenced; which existed before we were, and exist after we are dead. If this be the true reading—and it is the reading which many years of special study of the phenomena has impressed most seriously on me—then vitality is, even from a physical point of view, a compound of two processes; a mechanical and—there is no better word—a spiritual. The mechanical part, perfect when it is natural, but destructible and destined to run only a given course limited by time: the spiritual indestructible, moulding the physical to its uses, and, to our present senses, incorporeal; acting sometimes by one wave or impulse through masses of living beings; acting always in some measure through masses, in so far as the general outline of the living things permit; but acting also individually, through and by reason of the physical peculiarities of the individual. What, then, we should abstractly call vitality is universal, and in persistent operation in inanimate matter, constituted to be animated. What we call life is the manifestation of this persistent and all-pervading principle of

Nature in properly organized substance. What we call death, or devitalization, is the reduction of matter to the sway of other forces, which do not destroy it, but which change its mode of motion from the concrete to the diffuse, and, after a time, render it altogether incapable of manifesting vital action until it be re-cast in the vital mould. We are at this moment ignorant of the time when vitality ceases to act on matter that has been vitalized. Presuming that an organism can be arrested in its living in such manner that its parts shall not be injured to the extent of actual destruction of tissue, or to change of organic form, the vital wave seems ever ready to pour into the body again so soon as the conditions for its action are reëstablished. Thus, in some of my experiments for suspending the conditions essential for the visible manifestations of life in cold-blooded animals, I have succeeded in reëstablishing the condition under which the vital vibrations will influence, after a lapse not of hours, but even of days; and for my part I know no limitation to such re-manifestation, except from the simple ignorance of us who inquire into the subject."

I need hardly point out the extreme suggestiveness of these remarks, and their relation to a possible explanation of historical cases of "raising the dead" by those who, perhaps, understood the operations of the law of süspension here hinted at. See *Appendix L.*

I am aware that my theory will probably be attacked upon the ground that crystals (notably) present very many of the phenomena of animal life, or rather of primitive vital action—forming, in fact, a sort of bridge across the gulf that separates the living from the non-living world.[1] The similarities are doubtless many and striking, being well summed up in M. Dastre's "Life of Matter," pp. 417–29, and are too well known to need restatement. Still, it might reasonably be contended that the differences so far outweigh the similarities as to render the assertion that they are identical most unjustifiable and unwarranted. Professor Beale takes this stand, and, throughout his writings has contended that this attempt to identify the vital and the chemical forces because of the phenomena observed in the crystal is pure assumption, and in no wise a scientifically proved

[1] Nageli "Mechanico-Physiological Theory of Organic Evolution," p.

fact. He pointed out the fact that the growth of the crystal is by *accretion*, and not the result of any process of *metabolism*, and always from the *same* materials from which their bodies are built, while animals build their bodies from materials *different* from that of their own bodies. (See Burke's "Origin of Life," pp. 27, 102.) But as Doctor Burke, on p. 139, states that "only when there is metabolism there is life"—this would seem to shut out the crystal from the same sort of life that the animal enjoys. Or as he says on p. 60: "They (crystals) have everything in common with microbes except the principle of vitality!" And M. Dastre himself admits that "there seems to be a complete opposition between the crystal and the living being as regards their manner of nutrition and growth." ("Life of Matter," p. 422.)[1] How scientists can continue to urge the close similarity of living beings and crystals in face of such facts is a mystery.

But even were it shown that a sort of life or vital force manifests itself in crystals, would that prove that all life is thus semi-crystal (so to speak) and so related to the physical world in some intricate manner? Most certainly it would not. It would merely prove that the crystal is just so constructed as to render possible the manifestation, through it, of a certain kind or character of life—a certain degree of mentality—which could thus manifest through it to just the extent to which the structure of the crystal rendered such manifestation possible.

> "If the material encasement be coarse and simple, as in the lower organisms, it permits only a little intelligence to permeate through it; if it is delicate and complex, it leaves more pores and exits, as it were, for the manifestations of consciousness."[2]

And so I do not consider that the objections to my theory drawn from observations of crystals are any real objections at all, and I shall consequently refuse to consider them further.

Nor is the objection valid which seeks to identify vital or life force with the physical forces because of the fact that the vital force of certain creatures seems to be transposed into *light*—in the cases of those "living machines" (fireflies, etc.) where such

[1] See also Doctor Moore's "Matter, Life and Mind," pp. 92–125.
[2] F. C. S. Schiller: "Riddles of the Sphinx," p. 294.

light is observed—at first sight, seeming to identify the light-production with the vital forces. As M. Raphael Dubois expressed it,[1] it is merely the power or property "possessed by certain organisms of radiating into space, as luminous vibrations, a part of the energy that animates them." This does not disprove my theory of vitality, then, because no one doubts that there are operative within the organism physical and chemical forces of all kinds, but this does not show that the vital forces—the life of the creature—has been utilized in its production; we have no proof whatever that this is the case. In fact, all the arguments advanced go to show that such is not the case.

It may be objected that this is a return to Vitalism, and that the facts in the case disprove that idea. I reply; not so. I do not deny that the forces operative in the production of this light may be purely physical or chemical, but this does not identify it with the vital or life force of the creature in whose organism it is apparent, nevertheless. Let me make my meaning clearer by the following quotation from the late Claud Bernard's writings—illustrating a position with which I wholly concur.

"Arrived at the termination of our studies, we see that they lead us to a very general conclusion, the result of experiment; namely, that between the two schools, one holding that vital phenomena are absolutely distinct from physico-chemical phenomena, the other, that they are wholly identical with them, there is place for a third doctrine, that of physical vitalism, which takes account of what there is peculiar in the manifestations of life, and what there is that conforms to the action of general forces; the ultimate element of the phenomenon is physical, the arrangement is vital."[2]

I have throughout admitted the intimate relations of life and matter, though denying that the former was in any way *created* by the latter. I have no very definite theory of my own to offer *re* this question of their connection—what it may be or how possible—save to say that the connection is, during life, the most intimate possible or conceivable, and that the energy does in some inscrutable way issue from some central spot or point,

[1] "Physiological Light," p. 413.
[2] "Leçons sur les phénomènes de la vie," Paris, p. 521.

vitalizing the matter in its immediate neighborhood. Professor Burke's recent researches should go far to prove this; his chapter on "The Nucleus as a Source of Energy" defending this view, and saying, in part:

" The ultimate nucleus (is) the fountain, so to speak, of the vital energy, that sets and maintains the whole mass going. This energy would seem to spring from some immaterial source. . . . "[1]

Surely, here is a practical acknowledgement of the view that vitality is a force, distinct from other physical forces, though, strange as it may seem, Professor Burke is, throughout his book, contending that this is not the case! But our interest is doubtless stimulated, by such conjectures, to inquire into what actually takes place in this *n-th*, or final nucleus. To that question, science has, as yet, no final answer: we can but speculate and theorize, being aided by such facts as are known to occur. The most ingenious speculations of this kind, and probably the nearest correct of any so far advanced, are those of Professor Beale, from whose "Vitality: An Appeal to the Royal Society," p. 100, I quote the following interesting passage:

"It seems to be in these inmost centers that life is ever being communicated to the non-living matter as it is made to flow toward them: so that those powers by which the formation of every tissue can only be effected, and all other wonderful powers are conferred upon matter by vitality, manifest everywhere in the living world, and which are not only communicated without loss, but which may be renewed generation after generation with increasing vigor, as life succeeds life—powers of no ordinary kind, but ever characteristic of the whole world of life, and caused by vitality—welling up, as it were, from centers that seem inexhaustible, illimitable, undemonstrable. . . We get but an imperfect glimpse of the vital phenomena in minute structureless centers—too central to be ever reached by mortal eye—where matter, as I believe, is certainly beyond the operation of all ordinary physical laws—where movements are free and incessant, and in a direction *from* each center, thereby ensuring a flow of fluid in which lifeless matter is dissolved, in the opposite direction —*inward*, *toward* the center."

[1] "The Origin of Life," pp. 146–8.

§ 9. *Practical Results and Theoretical Considerations*

And now, as the net result of all the above chain of argument and theoretical reasoning, we reach a conclusion of cardinal and of immediate and practical importance. Briefly, it is this. If my theory be correct, what must be the effects of going without a certain quantity of food, on any one occasion? Obviously, it cannot be loss of energy, since we have seen that no energy is ever lost, as the result of omitting food, at any time. If this is so, and if, on the other hand, all digestion necessitates the expenditure of vital energy—as we have seen it does and must—then the conclusion to which we are driven is this. The omission of any one meal, or any number of meals, merely adds to the body's general store of vitality just as much energy as would necessarily be expended in digesting, assimilating and eliminating that meal or series of meals. In other words, we should invariably increase, instead of decreasing, the stock of vitality, by the fast; we should invariably add to it, and never subtract from it. Startling and, indeed, revolutionary as this statement may seem to my readers, it is the logical outcome of my theory, and one which the facts in the case conclusively prove to be true.

In many ways, it is now *practically* recognized that food does not furnish our strength and energy—at least, to anything like the proportionate degree to the amount of food ingested. Business men realize this fact, and for that reason they eat the lightest of lunches when a heavy afternoon's work is in sight—which means, of course, that the nearer they approach an actual fast, the more energy they will have for their bodily and mental labor for the rest of the day. But if food supplies the energy, exactly the reverse of this should hold good; the greater the amount of work necessitated, the more food should be eaten. This is the logical outcome of the theory, and the only conclusion we can possibly reach—provided we are logical. Seeing that such is not the case, it is evident that the theory must be wrong, and that our strength and energy cannot be derived from the food we eat, but is, on the contrary, the one great cause of its expenditure and waste. Those physicians who counsel fasting, or even a reduction in the diet, for the purpose (obviously) of increasing the energy, do so in direct opposition to their theory. They have found, from bitter experience, that this is the true and the rational method of treatment, and that benefit invariably results from its application; it is, however, in direct opposition to their theory, which says precisely the opposite. Theory and practice are hopelessly opposed; while, if the other theory be correct, they are in the strictest harmony, and agree in the minutest detail.

Now, as a matter of fact, we find that when food is completely withheld, during a fast, the energy does actually increase, and continues to do so—noticeably after the stimulation from the daily food and the reaction from such stimulation has worn off. After this period has once been passed, the strength constantly and visibly increases, as we have seen (pp. 256–63). Theoretically, on this view, this should be the case; actually it is so: the theory and the practice, in this instance, are in precise accord.

Proof that the energy is not lowered and that the general tone, both of the skin and the whole system, is improved, is afforded by those cases in which the ability is present to take cold baths, *e.g.*, when this has never been possible before, owing to the poor reaction on the part of the patient. Now we know that the ability to react, after a cold bath, is due solely to the degree of vitality present—being proportional, *ceteris paribus*, to the extent of the reaction. If, consequently, the ability to react thoroughly be greater during a fast, it is evident that more vitality is present and available for this purpose than at other (ordinary) times. It would certainly be impossible if vitality had been decreased. A notable case, in this respect, is that of my friend, Maurice V. Samuels, the playwright, whose fast, undertaken at my suggestion (with most satisfactory results) presented a clear demonstration of this principle. In this case, cold baths were taken daily, during the fast, and almost enjoyed, whereas the patient had *never in his life* been enabled to take a cold bath without suffering the greatest bodily discomfort—due to lack of reaction—as well as mental aversion. In such cases, the increase of energy derivable from the fast is clearly demonstrated.

Scientists may fail to accept this theory because it recognizes vitality as a thing *per se*, and as not capable of being transformed or transmuted into one or other of the physical forces. I shall be told that it violates the law of the conservation of energy. It all depends, I answer, upon how we regard this all-embracing law. If we limit it, as we should, to the physical world, then, I say, this theory does not contradict it in any way. But—while I am willing to admit that some such unification of energy as that suggested by Doctor Bryant[1] might be quite possible, theoretically, at all events—I must insist that if we try to include in the circle of transmutable and transformable forces, *life*—vitality and energy—as is now universally done, then I say; yes, it does violate it. And I shall take mv stand upon this ground, whatever the consequences. I believe my arguments and the facts I have brought and shall bring forward completely disprove this dogma, and render the usual position untenable. If my arguments and facts violate the theory, then so much the worse for the theory! I shall certainly not withdraw my facts and arguments simply because they threaten to overthrow and disprove an altogether stupid and never logically demonstrated theory; that I do not by any means intend to do.

The fundamental laws of the indestructibility of matter and the conservation of energy may be perfectly true and valid, so far as they go, but it does not need much insight to perceive that neither of these include the phenomena of human vitality and life, which seem to be quite distinct and separate; and I say this without being influenced by any religious or theological considerations whatever (for I am a frank agnostic) but because I believe it is borne out by facts—and facts are stubborn things! The eternal change of matter, from the inorganic, dead matter to living tissue (p. 294), and again, this organized tissue being resolved, at death, back to its original chemical elements—all this may be very true; the laws governing it may be as fixed and unalterable as you please, but it must be remembered that this concerns only the *material* of the body; and the thinking, willing, and active life forces are distinct and separate always. Life *utilizes* the body for its various purposes; it guides and controls it throughout its life history; but it does not spring from it, and above all, is not made by it! The most dense should

[1] "The World Energy," etc., p. 268.

appreciate that fact—so obvious is it, even in our present state of knowledge.

But if, on the other hand, we exempt life from the circle of forces, admitting it to be a thing apart, *per se*, separate and distinct from all other physical forces—to which it is in no wise related—a theory which is altogether logical and to which every fact points—then I say: No, my theory does not violate the law of conservation of energy, for I am as firm a believer in the operation of that law as the most conservative scientist. That portion of the law which ever had any real support is as true to-day as it ever was. It is only that portion which was always intrinsically absurd, but which materialistic scientists simply assumed and accepted, without ever properly criticizing—merely because it *was* a materialistic, and so an "easy," though obviously erroneous, interpretation—which is here combated.

Even before my arguments and facts were in the field it must be distinctly remembered that there was no evidence whatever tending to show that we derived our strength *directly* from our food, or from anything we ate, drank or inhaled. It was always contended by one school of medical philosophers that the sole purpose of food was to furnish bodily tissue, and the tissue, force; *i.e.*, when once the food substance had been transformed into living tissue, the destruction or breaking down of that tissue was that which created or liberated the force; and that, consequently, no energy could possibly be furnished or supplied to the organism at all unless that food material were capable of first forming healthy tissue; and this at once barred out all poisons, and all inappropriable material (such as alcohol, *e.g.*), since they could not form bodily tissue in the first place—not being foods. (pp. 36–8.) And thus we see there never was any definite and altogether accepted proof that we derived our strength directly from any material whatever—it being apparently incapable of imparting it in that manner. It must first have formed the tissue, and the tissue supplied the strength. But we have seen that even this theory can no longer be maintained—no strength whatever coming from the food, either directly or indirectly.

§ 10. *Philosophical Conclusions*

And now I must bring this lengthy chapter to a close, though I must first make one or two remarks on particular aspects of my theory, and the deductions that may be drawn from it, if correct. I have endeavored to devote this chapter strictly to the physiological aspects of the problem, but must add one or two words on the important philosophical conclusions to be drawn from the facts, if established, and the manner in which a number of hitherto sporadic and disconnected facts find a connected and logical explanation. By way of illustration, let us consider the phenomena of so-called "miraculous cures"—of cases of mental healing, *i.e.*, where almost instantaneous cures of grave affections are asserted (on good authority) to have taken place. Now I submit that, upon the theory of energy outlined above, the connection between mental and physical phenomena, and such cases of miraculous healing, become much more intelligible to us. For, if our energy be dependent upon, not the oxidation of food material, but the inrush of external energy, which inrush is limited only by the degree of receptivity of the organism at the time, we can readily perceive that, should the condition of the organism be, in some manner, so modified as to permit a greatly increased influx of this energy (owing to some obstacle being removed or condition modified) most extraordinary results might follow—since we know that tissue growth and tissue replacement are largely due to and determined by the extent of the available energy for those purposes. Should this, then, be temporarily almost *unlimited* in amount, we can conceive that this process of tissue growth, tissue replacement, etc., might proceed at an almost indefinitely rapid rate. Granted, then, that this degree of receptivity is once established (in some unknown way) and the consequent inrush of energy follows, and we can see how, on this theory, these "miraculous" cures are wrought. On the commonly accepted theories, I contend, any explanation is at present quite impossible and practically inconceivable.[1]

[1] As an interesting parallel, compare "How to Be a Yogi," by Swami Abhedananda, pp. 139–41. I had not read this book when I wrote the above passage, but it serves to illustrate the close similarity of Eastern and Western thought, when working on philosophical problems.

It is not the province of this book to touch upon the wider problems of world philosophy or metaphysics, but I cannot refrain from adding one or two remarks upon what I conceive to be the logical philosophic import of my theory. For I can see in it far more than a mere scheme of vitality; more than a mere speculation as to its nature and its relation to the human organism and to the intake of food; more than its revolutionary effect upon medical practice—important as these should be. It is more than all these. It is an answer, if not an absolute refutation, of the present, generally accepted materialistic doctrine of the universe, and its influence upon our conceptions of the origin and destiny of the human soul. Without further ado, let me illustrate the great importance of the theory in its application to the phenomena of mind, and the world-old question of the immortality of the soul.

I have endeavored to show, in the preceding pages, that the life or vital force is in no way inter-related, transformable and transmutable into any one or other of the physical forces known to us; that it seems to stand absolutely *per se*, in this respect, and that, in fact, its laws and actions are, apparently, totally different from—if not actually opposed to—the other forces, in its action and laws. It is in no way related to them, and that the nervous or life energies are different, *toto cœlo*, from all other forces or energies whatsoever. But if this is the case, we must most certainly revise our ideas and beliefs with regard to the supposed impossibility of the soul's immortality; for that problem at once assumes a different and a new meaning in the light of these newer facts.

Let me better illustrate my meaning by first quoting from Professor Shaler's excellent book, "The Individual" (pp. 301–2), the following paragraph, which tersely states the argument of the materialistic philosopher and well illustrates the position assumed by the majority of physicians, psychologists, biologists, physicists, and in fact by most scientific men to-day. It is this:

" . The functions of the body are but modes of expression of the energy which it obtains through the appropriation of food. As regards their origin, these functions may be compared to the force which drives the steam engine, being essentially no more mysterious than other mechanical processes. Now, the mind is but one of the functions of the body, a very specialized work of the parts known as the nervous system. We can trace the development of this mind in a tolerably continuous series from the lowest stages of the nervous processes, such as we find in the *Monera* or kindred *Protozoa* to man. Thus it is argued that, though the mental work of our kind is indefinitely more advanced than that of the primitive animals, there is no good reason to believe that it is other than a function of the body; that it is more than a peculiar manifestation of the same forces which guide digestion, contract muscles, or repair a wound. Furthermore, as is well known, at death all the functions of the organic body fall away together in the same manner and at essentially the same time, so there is in fine no more reason to believe that the functions of the brain persist than that a like persistence occurs in the digestive function or in the blood-impelling power of the heart. All this, and much more, can be said to show that the phenomenon of death appears to possess us altogether when we come to die."

Now this position is, to my mind, perfectly logical. The conclusion arrived at is, indeed, the only one to which we can possibly come—is, in fact, the actual "truth" if the premises are correct. No! Provided that these are true, I can see no possible loophole of escape for the logical mind; the conclusion is inevitable. Professor Shaler's attempts to abstract himself from the position into which he has been led, and which he so well and plainly stated, are to me pathetically futile; it is a hopeless failure; his arguments would, I think, prove quite inconclusive to the critical, scientific thinker; and, in any case, philosophic and metaphysical speculations have no place whatever in a purely scientific argument of this kind—which should deal with facts and facts only.[1]

[1] Prof. John Fiske, indeed, tried to surmount this difficulty—here presented—in his writings, and I select the following passage as illustrative of his argument. He says ("Life Everlasting," pp. 77–9): ". . . if we could trace in detail the metamorphosis of motions within the body, from the sense organs to the brain, and thence onward to the muscular system, would be somewhat as follows: the inward motion, carrying the message into the brain, would perish in giving place to the vibration which accompanies the conscious state; and this vibration in turn would perish in giving place to the outward motion, carrying the mandate out to the muscles. If we had the means of measurement we could prove the equivalence from step to step.

No: provided that the premises are correct, the conclusion stated by Professor Shaler is not only legitimate, but absolutely incontrovertible, and the conclusion we are driven to adopt if the premises of the argument are sound.

And now we perceive the great significance of my theory in its relation to the problem of immortality, and of its revolutionary effects upon the present-world philosophy. It is not only anti-materialistic or negative, but pro-vital and positive in its attitude. It is not destructive, but constructive; not devolutionary, but evolutionary. For we now perceive that this great argument against immortality crumbles to dust; it is worse than useless. The premises are not correct; for, as we have seen, nervous or vital force is not dependent upon food combustion at any time, nor under any circumstances whatever; and consequently mental energy—one form of nervous energy—is not dependent upon this physiological process either; it is altogether independent of it; mental energy, together with all other bodily activities, are quite separate and distinct from, and independent of, this process; so that, when the process itself ceases, it is no proof whatever—and there is not even a presumption in favor of the argument—that mental life ceases at the death of the physical organism. In fact, the presumption is all the other way. So that this main, oft-quoted and central argument against survival is no valid objection at all. Provided

But where would the conscious state, the thought or feeling, come into this circuit? Why, nowhere. The physical circuit of motions is complete in itself; the state of consciousness is accessible only to its possessor. To him it is the subjective equivalent of the vibration within the brain, whereof it is neither the producer nor the offspring, but simply the concomitant. In other words the natural history of the mass of activities that are perpetually being concentrated within our bodies, to be presently once more disintegrated and diffused, shows us a closed circle which is entirely physical, and in which one segment belongs to the nervous system. As for our conscious life, that forms no part of the closed circle but stands entirely outside of it, concentric with the segment which belongs to the nervous system." (See also, in this connection, "The Parallelism of Mind and Body," by Arthur K. Rogers, Ph.D., pp. 3–4; Sir Oliver Lodge: "Life and Matter," p. 116, etc.) This theory is defective, it seems to me, in that it takes no account of ordinary thinking, but only of sensations; and we know that a man may sit still at his desk all day and think, and yet be as tired as though he had exercised vigorously, and even more so. Or he may exercise half a day and think half a day, and be as tired as though he had done either one or other the whole day. Obviously, then, thinking *does* use up vital energy; and, inasmuch as this energy is derived from our food—so it is claimed—the mental life must be directly or indirectly dependent upon the food supply and the energy derived from it.

my theory be true, it proves to have no foundation in fact. The possibility of conscious survival of death is thus left quite an open question—capable of scientific investigation or of philosophic dispute;[1] but the grand, negative physiological argument vanishes. And it is because of this fact that I think my theory not only of practical importance to the physician, but of theoretical importance in its bearing upon human thought; upon current scientific and religious opinion; upon the morals and the ethics of the race.

[1] I would point out in this connection that, if this theory of vitality be true, there can be no valid objection to the actual existence—far less the investigation of—psychic phenomena, because the objections to a future life would thus be cleared away, and the field left open for facts. Such facts psychic phenomena apparently are; and at least there can be no objection to their study any longer. I would also point out that the old, materialistic notion, which compared the body to a lamp, vitality and life to the flame, which simply ceased to exist with the extinction of the lamp, is thus shown to be invalid, and based upon an incorrect interpretation of the facts. Life is not the result of any process of combustion or oxidation whatever, but on the contrary, the guiding, controlling principle—the real entity, for whose manifestation the body was brought into being.

CHAPTER II

SLEEP

§ 1. *Current Theories of Sleep—Their Unsatisfactory Nature*

THE theory of vitality outlined above enables us to arrive at what is a new, and I believe a correct explanation of the causation and the nature of, and the necessity for, sleep. Hitherto, theories as to its nature and its causation have been almost as erratic as numerous. Some have taken the purely spiritual standpoint, and asserted, as does Mr. Bigelow, in his "Mystery of Sleep" (p. 144):

"That it (the soul) has been emancipated from the restrictions of its prison house and set free to do, be, or become whatever it has been prepared for becoming during its earthly confinement."

This may be very fine sounding, but it does not in the least explain the nature of fatigue; its connection with sleep; the question of the renewal of vitality, or in fact any of the real physiological aspects of the case at all. So, for the present, we must altogether refuse to consider it. Then we have had the innumerable materialistic theories of sleep; the localizing theories; the chemical theories; the histological theories; the psycho-physiological theories—to mention only the principal ones in the list. Each of these theories is open to very grave objections, as Doctor de Manaceine and others have proved conclusively. Thus: The theory that sleep is caused by the abnormal functioning of some organ or gland—generally the thyroid gland—is refuted by the fact that, in cases where the thyroid gland is altogether removed, sleep occurred the same as usual; the same was true when the gland atrophied. Osborne's theory that sleep is due to excessive functioning of the arachnoid plexus is practically the same thing as the cerebral hyperæmia theory to be mentioned immediately. Doctors Cappie, Langlet, Blumroder, and others regard sleep as possible when the brain is in a state of venous stasis; while Doctors Cabanis, Marshall Hall, Macnish, W. B. Carpenter, G. H. Lewes, Holland, Sieveking, and others defended the theory of cerebral congestion or hyperæmia, which was afterward completely disproved by the experiments of Durham, Mosso, Fleming, Corning, Weir Mitchell, W A. Hammond, and Tarchanoff—which showed that precisely the reverse condition—cerebral *an*æmia—is present during sleep. As this would necessarily *follow* decreased nervous action, however, it proved nothing as to the real causation of sleep.[1]

Then there came the innumerable chemical theories. Sommer attempted to prove that sleep is caused by impoverishment of oxygen in the brain, appearing as soon as the reserve of oxygen in the tissue and blood is exhausted. This found some support from the experiments of Pettenkoffer and Voit. Preyer believed that sleep is the direct consequence of fatigue, or rather, of the fatigue products of the blood, these being easily oxidizable substances which absorb the oxygen required by the brain, and consequently that the artificial injection of lactic acid and similar bodies causes sleep. Unfortunately, experiments in this direction have yielded contradictory results. (Preyer, Fisher, L. Meyer, etc.) Pfluger held somewhat similar views. Professor Leo Errera, of Brussels, regards sleep as essentially a process of physiological intoxication—a theory supported by many facts, but refuted by many others—notably the power we possess of postponing sleep, or of awaking at a fixed hour.

Of recent years, Professors Rabl Ruckardt, Lepine, Duval, Ramon y Cajal, Howell, and others have advanced ingenious histological theories; but, as they do not seem ever to have

[1] Sleep is not, it must be remembered, *due* to cerebral anæmia, but its *cause; i.e.*, the anæmia follows the lessened nervous action, and does not cause it, which is the mistaken idea held by many materialistic minds. See, *e.g.*, Wm. A. Hammond's "Sleep and Sleeplessness," p. 35. Prof. William James most emphatically insisted upon this fact when he wrote ("Principles of Psychology," Vol. I., p. 99): "I need hardly say that the activity of the nervous matter is the primary phenomenon, and the afflux of blood its secondary consequence. Many popular writers talk as if it were the other way about, and as if mental activity were due to the afflux of blood. But, as Prof. H. N. Martin has well said: 'That belief has no physiological foundation whatever; it is even directly opposed to all that we know of cell life.'" Professor Mosso proved this later by direct experiment; see his "Fatigue," p. 195.

gained much general acceptance, it would be hardly worth our while to summarize or criticize them here. In any case, as Wundt pointed out, practically all the theories of sleep possess the common defect in that they neglect its fundamental and direct cause. This will become more apparent as we proceed. The chemical theory of sleep is refuted by the fact that mere boredom or monotony is sufficient to cause sleep, and so is hypnotic suggestion, though fatigue is not present in any degree. See my discussion under "Fatigue."

As the result of considerations such as the above, Dr. M. de Manaceine was driven to reject all the current theories of sleep, and in her own book on the subject, asserts that the only real definition we can give of sleep is that "sleep is the resting time of consciousness."[1] This may be—undoubtedly is—very true; but it can hardly be called an *explanation* in the strict sense of the term. It is merely a statement of a condition—*one* condition—accompanying sleep. It is no explanation at all of the real causes of sleep, or of the conditions that necessitate it, or what sleep actually does, or in what manner it restores the bodily energy, or the altered brain conditions which render possible the unimpeded renewal of consciousness on the following day. It does none of these things, nor does any other theory at present extant.

It must be remembered that sleep is, in a sense, a positive process, as well as a negative one; that it is, as Dr. J. R. Tillinghast pointed out:[2] "not a passive process, but an active repair of tissue." Or as Dr. Wesley Mills says:

"Can the molecular machinery of life entirely stop, and yet be set in motion again? We know that cold-blooded animals may be frozen and completely restored to a natural condition. This and the encysted condition of protozoa are suggestive of such a possibility. Yet in insects a condition of perfect quiescence is accompanied by the most wonderful changes. The worm-like caterpillar becomes within it's cocoon the butterfly, with locomotive powers immeasurably greater."[3]

[1] "Sleep: Its Physiology, Pathology, Hygiene and Psychology," p. 59.
[2] "How Can I Cure My Catarrh?" p. 50.
[3] "Animal Intelligence," p. 111.

Says E. A. Fletcher:[1]

"Only in moments of quiescence do we give the soul a chance to inaugurate its recuperative work; to send its vital influences of regeneration through the complex systems of nerves, veins, and arteries of the body."

It will be obvious from the above that we cannot merely state that sleep is a negative quality—present only when the organism is too poisoned to retain its waking faculties—but is a positive condition, and one in which the most vital organic and important changes take place. It is a period of great recuperation; and to assert that this state is merely the result of poisons formed within the body is simply nonsense.

I should like to enter into a discussion of this question of the true causation of sleep in considerable detail, but my space does not permit. On some other occasion, I hope to do so, as the question is as interesting theoretically, as it is important practically. But for the present I must content myself with merely stating—and that briefly—my own theory of the nature and causes of sleep, and to showing how it accounts for every one of the phenomena observed—physiological and psychological.

§ 2. *Author's Theory of Sleep*

It is now, I presume, generally acknowledged that all forms of bodily energy—muscular, functional, etc.—are but aspects or modes of expression of the general stock of vitality; but so many varied channels through which it is expended while doing the internal (organic or bodily) work—and the external (muscular or "world") work. And just here let me state most emphatically, in order to avoid misunderstanding, that I regard these two forms of energy as most certainly but faces of the same underlying cause; but differing modes of expression of the same energy. The internal and the external work are both dependent upon the same energy—and are both derivable, ultimately, from the same source; and, since one of them is certainly not due to food combustion, neither is the other. Just as consciousness resides in every cell throughout the living body, but is only

[1] "Philosophy of Rest," pp. 36-7.

manifest to us, as consciousness, when particularly connected with the nervous system, and the cerebrum especially; so, I conceive, is vitality or life inherent in every cell throughout the body, but only becomes manifest to us when operating through the nervous mechanism. The two—internal and external, work—are but differing ways or modes of the expenditure of the same causal energy—the same vital force—and any attempt to distinguish them, and to show that the one is dependent upon the food and the other not, is altogether unjustifiable and unwarranted by the facts; they are but modes of expression of the same energy, and have the same source. And since this is not the food in the one case, it is not and cannot be, in the other.[1]

But, further, it is now generally accepted by science, that the *mental* energy is also but one aspect of this vital force. The mental life is closely related to the activity of the brain cells (whatever theory we hold) and we all know that mental work is as much or more exhausting than is physical labor. (Mosso: "Fatigue," p. 121.) But it is unnecessary to dwell upon this point. It is now accepted as an axiom of science, and as I do not propose to dispute it, we will pass on without further comment.

All forms of bodily or mental activity, then, are dependent upon the same source for their renewal. I have, I trust, proved in the preceding pages that the source is not the daily food, as it has universally been contended—or rather taken for granted, since no one has produced any respectable evidence for such dependence, or inter-relation.

But, if this is so, the question arises, what is the source? Through what means and channel is this energy derived? The answer to this is certain and obvious; through *sleep*, and through sleep alone is this renewal of the vital forces effected. This being granted, my position becomes clear, and I may tersely state my

[1] Doctor Rabagliati, in his address before the Bradford Medico-Chirurgical Society, on November 15, 1904, in which he tentatively advanced this idea, as a result of my communicating the outline of my theory to him ("Record of a Case of Tubercular Synovitis of the Right Knee Joint," etc., p. 6), took this position of attempting to differentiate the two—the internal and external work; but, in response to a letter of mine, criticizing this attitude, and pointing out what I conceived to be its inconsistency, Doctor Rabagliati wrote me, on June 25, 1905, withdrawing from his own previous position, which he then saw to be inconsistent and untenable, and renounced his former conviction.

theory of the necessity for, and the causation of sleep somewhat as follows. Granting that the bodily activities are quiescent, and that the expenditure of vitality has consequently ceased; also that consciousness is absent or "at rest"—*sleep is that physiological condition of the organism in which the nervous system of the individual* (in precisely the same manner as the electric storage battery) *is being recharged from without, by the external, all-pervading cosmic energy,* in which we are bathed, and in which we live and move and have our being. The purpose of sleep, therefore, is to recharge the human motor; to replenish, in it, the stock of energy which it had expended in the previous day's bodily and mental exertion—to restore and fit it for the next day's work. This, and only this, is the cause of, and the necessity for, sleep—to repair the vital waste of the previous day.[1]

Revolutionary as this theory may be, it is, it seems to me, a very simple one, and one that is verified, moreover, in everyday life and experience; and which has the additional advantage of explaining all the facts—which certainly is not the case on any other theory whatever. And there are, on the contrary, many facts which seem to point to it as the correct theory. Says Dr. M. de Manaceine:[2] "The dynamometer showed a steady decrease in strength of both grip and pull, regained after sleep." It was noted also that the sleep was deeper after a certain amount of sleep had been lost, and the patient was "catching up" the necessary sleep, so to speak. This theory also agrees with the fact, pointed out by Dr. William H. Thomson,[3] that "only those parts and those organs which consciousness has been employing and dominating grow weary and worn and cry for rest." We can also understand why it is that "the first two or three hours of sleep are the most important, for it is during these hours that sleep reaches its culminating point."[4] During the early period,

[1] A somewhat similar theory has been advanced by Dr. George Black ("Brain Work and Overwork," p. 113), also by Percival Lowell ("Occult Japan," p. 333), and by Robert Dale Owen ("Footfalls on the Boundary of Another World," pp. 132–5). The similarity of thought is quite striking, in these passages, but no one of the authors seems to have followed the idea out to its logical conclusion.

[2] "Sleep," etc., p. 68.

[3] "Materialism and Modern Physiology of the Nervous System," pp. 87–8; "Brain and Personality," pp. 297–8.

[4] "Sleep," etc., by M. de Manaceine, p. 32.

the "vital reservoir" is emptiest, so to speak, and the recharging process would be most rapid and effective. It also explains why "the depth and amount of sleep are in inverse proportion to energy of consciousness." (p. 223.) Thus we have for the first time a satisfactory theory of sleep—its necessity, causes and phenomena, which can be found to answer completely all the facts that have been noted.

It is interesting to observe the close parallel between my theory of sleep and that of Mr. F. W. H. Myers—who worked out the problem from the psychological standpoint, while my argument has been entirely physiological. Yet the conclusions are strikingly similar. Thus, he says:[1]

"In subliminal states—trance and the like—the supraliminal processes are inhibited, and the lower organic centers are retained more directly under the spirit's control. As you get into the profounder part of man's being, you get nearer to the source of his human vitality. You thus get into a region of essentially greater responsiveness to spiritual appeal than is offered by the superficial stratum which has been shaped and hardened by external needs into a definite adaptation to the earthly environment.
If our individual spirits and organisms live by dint of this spiritual energy, underlying the chemical energy by which the organic change is carried on, then we must presumably renew and replenish the spiritual energy as continuously as the chemical. To keep our chemical energy at work, we live in a warm environment, and from time to time take food. By analogy, in order to keep the spiritual energy at work, we should live in a spiritual environment, and possibly from time to time absorb some special influx of spiritual life."

§ 3. *Objections to the Theory and Replies Thereto*

I am well aware that there may be—doubtless will be—many objections raised to this theory of sleep, and I regret that I cannot stop to consider any such objections here at any length. But, if for no other reason, at least to escape the charge of short-sightedness to the obvious, I must answer one or two of the (apparently) most serious objections to this theory—those which, at first sight, actually disprove it, that is. The first of

[1] "Human Personality," Vol. I., pp. 217–18.

these objections is that we frequently (especially when somewhat indisposed) feel exceedingly weak in the morning, instead of stronger—so much so, in fact, that it is an effort for us to rise, to move, to think. But, as the day progresses, we feel stronger and stronger; our bodily activities are performed with more and more ease, and, apparently, with more vim and vital power behind them as the day proceeds; our thinking becomes clearer; our senses more acute; our social and benevolent selves become more expanded; until, finally, we feel stronger, better, more keen and active and alert at the end of the day—at bedtime—than we do at its beginning. Now, if we accept the current theories, all this is quite intelligible, and clear enough. In the morning, after the night's protracted fast (l) the body is naturally weakened; its energies are at their lowest ebb; and it is only when we increase the bodily energies by the oxidation of food ingested, that more vital vigor is imparted to the organism; thus, as the day advances, the energies naturally increase; but, on the theory I have advanced, the reverse of this should have been the case, and how, then, am I to explain this fact, or overcome the difficulty it presents?

The answer and the explanation is simply this: The fundamental error of mistaking our feelings for actual bodily conditions has again been made; we have mistaken our expenditure of energy for its greater, actual potential capacity. Now, we have seen elsewhere (pp. 261–2), that precisely the reverse of this is the truth; and I might, perhaps, answer this objection most effectually by asking a question. Thus: When thus feeling highly elated, at the close of an exciting evening, following a day of strenuous work, would you be willing to go back to the morning hours, and begin it all over again—the drudgery of work; the meals; the preparations; and the evening of excitement; do you think that you would be better enabled to reënact all this without a night's sleep than after indulging in one, merely because you *feel* better and more energetic—more stimulated and elated—at that time than in the early morning? If so, I can only say, try it! You will soon find out your mistake! The reaction will be doubly pitiful without the subsequent night of sleep; and yet, theoretically, we ought to be enabled to go through it again more easily since, (1) we feel better enabled to do so; and (2) because we now have more vital energy than in the early morning—having received such energy from the oxidation of food elements throughout the day. And we should be enabled to continue, in this way, *ad infinitum*, without ever sleeping at all! For what does sleep do for us, on such occasions, except to (apparently) weaken us?

It is the old fallacy of mistaking the body for a steam engine, instead of an electric motor; and it is only when we thus carry the argument to its logical and unavoidable conclusion that we perceive what a monstrous absurdity it is. I may add, in passing, that we feel better as the day progresses whether we eat anything or not, so that the increased vigor noted cannot be due to the oxidation of food eaten during the day.

And now, if we actually *do* not possess more energy in the evening than we do in the morning, why is it that we *appear* to do so? Why are we apparently stronger and more vigorous at that time than at a time when we are, actually, weaker?

Doctor Haig has, it seems to me, found the first link in the requisite chain of explanatory argument, in his theory of uric acid formation, and its stimulative effects upon the system, which he thus states, in his "Diet and Food in Relation to Strength and Power of Endurance," pp. 39–41:

"Stimulation is not strength, but force rendered a little more quickly available; and it is always followed (and must be so) by an exactly corresponding amount of depression, when the force used up is not available, and has to be replaced. . . . Quite an exaggerated and erroneous estimate has been formed of the power of meat to produce force, because its stimulating effect has been mistaken for power, and the depression which follows has either been overlooked, which is possible at first, or later has been counteracted by alcohol, tobacco and other more harmful stimulants. . . Another very common effect of meat eating, whether alcohol is added to it or not, is a certain amount of dullness, heaviness and disinclination for mental or bodily exertion in the morning hours, often associated with more or less irritability and mental depression. In fact, the meat-eater is never quite himself or to be seen at his best till the evening, when rising acidity clears his blood for a time from excesses of uric acid; and that is, I think, at least one of the factors that has caused our morning and evening hours to grow progressively later and later, as we have come to live more in towns and eat more meat."

I say, I think this is the "first step" in the explanation. Doctor Haig fails, however, like almost all physicians, to realize the true relations of living and dead matter; and to see that the drug is always that which is *acted upon*, never that which *acts* (pp. 32–3). And so Doctor Haig puts down the results observed to *chemical* instead of to *vital* action; to the effects of the acid upon the nervous system, rather than to the effects of the reaction of the nervous system against such uric acid poison. And, theoretically, there is all the difference in the world between these two statements of what actually occurs, for the one truly explains, and the other does not. Let us pursue this line of argument a little further. The presence of this uric acid in the system in increasing quantities, has aroused an increased vital resistance, or action, which is, as a matter of fact, the "stimulation" observed. That is, the vital powers of the body are, of sheer necessity, being expended and wasted uselessly, in this resistance of accumulating poison; the energies are becoming more and more diverted and changed from the potential form into the active channels of expenditure. This expenditure of energy continues to increase, as the day advances, but, as we have seen (p. 41), that we invariably notice energy in its expenditure, never in its accumulation, we apparently continue to get stronger and stronger, whereas we are, in reality, becoming weaker and weaker—our stock of vital energy lower and lower —more and more depleted.

There are many facts of daily life that seem to bear out this interpretation of the facts, and to show this position to be the correct one. For example: It has been frequently remarked that we can think more clearly and rapidly when our eyes are open than when they are closed—better in the light than in the dark—and the reason for this is obvious. A portion of the brain is kept constantly active, in the former case, by the stimulation of the sight centers, and the brain is enabled to expend more energy *pro tem.*, for the reason that it is working at a higher rate of speed, and under a greater degree of stimulation. The work it is enabled to temporarily perform is greater; but the potential energy must be less, since a part of our nervous energy is being constantly diverted into another channel; yet we *feel* that we have a greater amount to expend than formerly. Again, we see that energy is only noticed in its expenditure, never in its accumulation, and that just in proportion to the extent of our apparent gain in strength, we are, in reality, weaker; and *vice versa*. Says Dr. James M. Gully:[1]

"It is not the less true that the patient must be made apparently weaker in order to be made absolutely stronger. Nor should he (the doctor) be led away by the locomotive energy of the patient, for that is for the most part fictitious, and depends on the unnatural excitement of the brain and spinal cord, urged in their office by the unnatural irritations propagated toward them by the digestive nerves. Patients in this state have, in fact, *impulse*—not *sustained energy*. They talk, walk and eat rapidly, but each has the effect of thickening the spittle, drying the tongue, and rendering the pulse sharp, hard, and rapid." (p. 87.)

Says Dr. A. T. Schofield:[2]

" . . . Constant movement is in itself a sign of weakness in the higher centers. A baby is always in motion. As we grow older, we get quieter, and the man with the strong brain only moves for a definite purpose. Repose, not movement, is a sign of brain power."

The fact that we feel more energy as the day progresses is also due to the fact that the stored-up energy finds a greater and greater facility for expenditure as the day proceeds. It is a well-known fact, *e.g.*, that the passage of a second impulse down a definite nerve tract is accomplished more easily than is the first impulse; and each succeeding impulse is allowed to travel more and more freely. All the laws of *habit* are based upon this fact. It amounts to saying, in reality, that the same nervous impulse may, because of its repetition, be carried and find expression with less noticeable effort or fatigue. And I have

[1] "Water Cure in Chronic Diseases," p. 91.
[2] "Nerves in Disorder," p. 59.

only to bring this law into practical application in order to explain my meaning in the present connection. As the day progresses, *i.e.*, the stored-up energy finds a readier and easier (because of its more frequent) mode of expression, and the nervous impulses consequently seem more powerful—though they may be, in reality, of equal or even inferior strength. Their apparent increase of strength is due solely to their readier means of expression—to the greater facility with which the nervous impulse is rendered manifest to us.

To return, however, to the main theme under discussion. It will be remembered that we have only half settled the question why certain persons rise in the morning fatigued and exhausted, when they should be at their brightest and best? That point we must now consider at somewhat greater length. Undoubtedly Doctor Rabagliati's explanation is, in part at least, quite true when he says:

"We wake tired in the morning because too much material has been finding its way into the blood from the digestion, and because during the quiet of sleep the blood has taken the opportunity to drop in the connective tissue that excess of material which was oppressing it. As the connective tissue forms the coverings of the muscles, bones, joints, and nerves, the consequence is that the whole locomotor system is in such circumstances overloaded, so that whenever we begin to move we are tired."[1]

But I feel that there are other reasons for this feeling of depression upon arising in the morning. One of the chief of these is undoubtedly the sleeping for many hours at one time in the same atmosphere[2] and this is most enervating and unwholesome—even if the ventilation is fairly free, and, unfortunately, in the vast majority of cases, this is not so—the close, foul air of the bedroom being considered preferable to the fresh, pure air of "God's out-of-doors." (pp. 356–8.) Then, too, there is

[1] "Air, Food and Exercises," p. 312. Says Henrietta Russell ("Yawning," p. 168): "Fatigue is stagnation, unremoved débris, decay; and all decay, physiologically considered, is disgusting. . . . When a man is tired, he has, either by inactivity or over-activity, committed a chemical, physiological, and psychological violation of the laws of economy." (p. 61.) Says Dr. R. T. Trall ("Health Catechism," p. 21): "Laziness is an indication of disease."

[2] "Six hours of sleep, in a well-ventilated room is worth more than ten in an unventilated one." ("Fruit and Bread," p. 171.)

the possibility of sleeping under too many bed clothes (a very common error); and the depleting effects of this practice (in choking the pores of the skin, and preventing all access to it of the outside air) must be enormous. There are doubtless other important factors—especially the continued wasting, through the night, of what energy has been accumulated, in processes of digestion, etc., and none of these must be left out of account in considering this question of morning debility.[1]

But the greatest and most potent factor of all I consider to be yet unmentioned; and, as it is one that explains the seeming paradox—even supposing none of the above-mentioned factors be at work—I propose to state it here as briefly as possible.

The amount of vitality and strength we feel in the morning, upon first waking, and before the body has begun its activities, of thought or motion—before, in short, it has begun to be *stimulated*—is the amount of vitality and strength we *actually* possess—all else is false strength, stimulation; this is the true gauge of our vitality—and the degree of actual strength we possess at that particular time. The increasing strength we perceive as the day progresses is, in reality, due merely to the increased stimulation; *i.e.*, waste of vital force—being perceived by us, as force—only in this process of expenditure; we really becoming constantly weaker instead of stronger as the day progresses—which we apparently do. But our *real* strength—the amount we actually possess—is, in reality, just what we feel it to be in the morning upon awakening, whether it be much or little. If much, and we wake up feeling strong, active and alert physically; bright and clear mentally—then we are in good health, and have an abundance of vital power to expend during the day, without drawing upon our vital stock or capital. If, on the other hand, we awake feeling depressed, weak and sluggish, physically, and torpid mentally, we may be assured that that is our true physical condition—so far as our vital energy goes—and that all the strength we per-

[1] I cannot here go into this question of the hygiene of sleep and sleeping except in so far as it directly influences the theory under discussion. Should any reader, however, feel an active interest in the matter, he will find it very well discussed in "How to Sleep," by Marion M. George; "Sleep and How to Obtain It," by F. Davis; and in the chapter on "Sleep" in "You and Your Doctor," pp. 224–43.

ceive during the day, over and above this amount, is due merely to stimulation, and is the result of our drawing upon our vital capital—instead of merely spending the interest—as we should. And, instead of continuing to draw upon this capital, we should take such steps as will replenish it; instead of which—merely because we feel stronger as the day progresses—we believe that we are increasing our stock of vital force, while we are, in reality, wasting it more and more.

There are three sets of facts that would seem to bear out this interpretation of the case. (1) If we merelv *think* of some exciting event, we immediately feel this sensation of strength and power, and this, no matter how tired we may be at the time. The effects of the stimulation are here clearly manifest. (2) A cold bath will arouse the energies in a similar manner; and (3) as the day progresses, we feel this added strength, no matter whether we eat anything during the course of the day, or not. Evidently, the strength, in such cases, is the result of stimulation, and is not indicative of force added to the system.

And the difficulty experienced in awakening, and in getting the body into "working order" is thus readily explained. The human motor is being at such times *reversed*—so to speak—the process of accumulation ceases, and that of expenditure begins. And if the system is in a healthy and normal condition, this reversal is effected easily and naturally—without notable physical or mental disturbance; but if, on the contrary, the system is more or less diseased, choked with mal-assimilated food material, and obstructed throughout with effete matter, calling for elimination—then the reversal is most labored and difficult, and throws the system into a confused and weakened condition in the most forcible attempt to adjust these vital processes. And this I conceive to be the chief reason for this feeling of depletion in the morning.

It may be objected that this is mere assumption—that we do gain strength as the day progresses from our food. To this I reply that we feel this increase of strength as the day advances —whether we eat any food or not, which would seem to negative this supposition.

It may further be urged against my theory that sleep and rest do not invariably refresh, recuperate, and strengthen, for the reason that, when we occasionally stay in bed, because of sickness, or for some other reason, we become very weak—and can hardly walk about when we again try to do so. If my theory were correct, this would hardly be the case, and yet so it is. How is it to be explained?

First: I would point out that sickness is, in itself, a debilitating process, and that we should doubtless be somewhat weak at the end of three days (say) whether we stayed in bed or not. Still, I do not contend that this is the whole explanation of the above phenomenon. We are doubtless weaker than if we had not so stayed in bed. And to the further question—why should this be? I have the following theoretical explanation to offer. When we continue to stay in bed, we break down an almost imperceptibly small quantity of tissue—so small as to hardly need any replacement at all, in fact. The vital force is, on the other hand, very considerably reduced because of the state of illness existing. If, therefore, we are to continue to keep to our beds, we should, under these circumstances, eat practically no food at all—even granting that the system were in a proper state to assimilate it—which it is not. But, as a matter of fact, we do almost invariably eat nearly as much as though we were actively engaged in the hardest manual labor! And practically no reduction at all is made in the daily intake of food—certainly nothing like the proportionate reduction that should be made in order to balance the great reduction in the physiological wastes of the tissues—due to the lessened activity—or even to the amount we should by right ingest, even in healthful activity. And what is the result? Most certainly the vital powers are grievously taxed, in order to dispose of this mass of food material—uncalled for by the tissues, it must be remembered—without engendering more disease, by clogging the tissues and the circulation, and poisoning the general system by auto-infection from decomposing food products. And, even then, it is most doubtful if it succeeds, entirely. On the contrary, I am persuaded that many cases of chronic disease and death are due to this very cause. And so the weakness we experience, as the result of our stay in bed, may not be due to any other cause than this one—

and probably *is* not. I offer here this suggestion; that, instead of staying in bed and eating as usual, we *fast*, and then see whether the weakness generally experienced be present or not. I can state positively, from personal observation, that such would not be the case.

My idea is, indeed, that, when we are ill, we should practically divide our time between recharging the system with energy (sleeping); and using such energy as has been accumulated in cleansing the system, through increased functioning of the eliminating organs—these having been kept constantly active by bathing, enemas, etc. Instinct teaches us to do this; and, this being the case, why should we keep diverting all the energy we can accumulate into the processes of digestion—and *useless* elimination? Surely this should be against all reason, no less than instinct?

There is one other objection which must be considered, in this connection; and that is the fact that a lower temperature is frequently if not always observed in the morning than in the evening; while, if the energies are, as I claim, at their highest in the morning, this should not be the case. I have discussed this question (to me, for many months, one of the most baffling and insoluble of paradoxes connected with fasting and its phenomena) on pp. 457–9; and, as it would be impossible to discuss that problem here without going into the question of bodily temperature in considerable detail, and since I there do so, I must ask my reader to temporarily dismiss this objection from his mind, and be content to await until we can discuss it more fully in the light of the further *data* there obtained. For the present, I shall only say that this fact does not in reality, and when rightly understood, contradict or disprove my theory at all—but, again, if anything, confirms it.

I must add here a few words by way of *proof* of my theory, now I have answered the principal objections thereto; to showing how it synthesizes and explains satisfactorily a number of hitherto sporadic facts. Thus: One curious phenomenon in connection with fasting is the frequently observed lack of all desire for sleep and, apparently, the lack of necessity for it. In some cases, to be sure, this is not the case—Mr. J. A. Shaw, *e.g.*, writing:[1] "Sleep continues restful and unbroken, and every morning finds me ready for the day's duties, and with no weariness." This fact proves, to my mind, the extent of the nervous energy expended in "getting well"—in ridding the system of the mass of impurities it contains. But, in many cases—and these are the interesting studies of which I spoke—far less sleep is indulged in than is normally taken, or even none at all for considerable periods of time at a stretch; and the necessity for such sleep is at no time felt, nor do any noticeably bad effects follow. Thus, in several cases that I have observed, but very little sleep was called for or taken, nor did the patient miss the sleep to any appreciable degree. Perhaps one of the most remarkable cases of this kind is that given us by Mark Twain (seriously, for once!), who, in his "My Debut as a Literary Person"[2] has recorded one of the most intensely interesting cases of fasting imaginable; and, though the true philosophical deductions that could be drawn from the facts did not, probably, present themselves to their author—or rather recorder—they are, nevertheless, of monumental importance and significance, and could not possibly have been guessed correctly or foreseen by anyone who had not actually and faithfully recorded the facts in the case, as observed. But let Mr. Clemens speak for himself. He says (pp. 109–10):

"A little starvation can really do more for the average sick man than can the best of medicines and the best doctors. I do not mean a restricted diet; I mean *total abstention from food for one or two days.* I speak from experience; starvation has been my cold and fever doctor for fifteen years, and has accomplished a cure in all instances. The third mate told me in Honolulu that the 'Portyghee' had lain in his hammock for months, raising his family of abscesses and feeding like a cannibal. We have seen that in spite of dreadful weather, deprivation of sleep, scorching, drenching, and all manner of miseries, thirteen days of starvation 'wonderfully recovered' him. There were four sailors down sick when the ship was burned. Twenty-five days of pitiless starvation have followed, and now we have this curious record: 'all men are hearty and strong, even the ones that were down sick are

[1] "The Best Thing in the World," p. 56.
[2] "The Man That Corrupted Hadleyburg, and Other Stories."

well, except poor Peter.' When I wrote an article some months ago urging temporary abstention from food, as a remedy for an inactive appetite and for disease, I was accused of jesting, but I was in earnest. 'We are all wonderfully well and strong, comparatively speaking.' On this day the starvation regimen drew its belt a couple of buckle-holes tighter: the bread ration was reduced from the usual piece of cracker the size of a silver dollar to the half of that, and one meal was abolished from the daily three. This will weaken the men physically, but if there are any diseases of the ordinary sort left in them they will disappear. "

In this narrative, also, there is recorded the case of one man who went without sleep for the incredible time of twenty-one days at a stretch (p. 124), and noticed, during that period, no desire whatever for sleep, and no evil effects—either then or afterwards from this lack. No evil effects whatever from omitting twenty-one nights of sleep, *while fasting*, when the omission of even seven nights is practically fatal, when food is being regularly eaten! How ludicrous, in the light of such facts, is the contention that we derive our strength and our energy totally and exclusively from the food we eat! Do not such facts, in themselves, completely disprove the current theory that our energy is derived from the food we eat?

And the logical explanation of such facts should now be obvious enough. In the case of Mr. Horace Fletcher, so frequently referred to, we saw that far less sleep than usual was required or necessitated, for the simple reason that less energy was expended during the day in digestion, and consequently that there was less call for replacement. All the energy that was usually expended in the process of digestion was thus saved and conserved, and we can readily see that the less energy there is expended, the more will be thus conserved, and consequently the less the need for replacement—though I do not at all agree with Mr. K. S. Guthrie, in his view that sleep might be ultimately displaced and dispensed with altogether[1] for the reasons elsewhere mentioned.

[1] "Regeneration Applied," pp. 182-3. "How to Conserve Energy During Waking Hours," and "How to Conserve Vital Energy During Sleep." It *is* possible, however, that the greater amount of sleep called for and necessitated in winter is due to the increased amount of food ingested at that time—this calling for a greater outlay of digestive energy, calling, in turn, for replacement.

But, in fasting, when *no energy at all* is utilized in the processes of digestion, all that amount of energy is conserved and no need is present for its replacement. This, I think, is a logical and common sense explanation of the phenomena observed.

It must always be remembered, however, in this connection, that—inasmuch as the internal muscular functioning never ceases—there is always a *slight* expenditure of energy going on in consequence, even in the deepest sleep; *i.e.*, always a slight connection[1] or bond between the body and the external source of energy; and, so long as that bond lasts, life is present—forming a connecting link, so to speak, between the soul and the body, and tying the former to the latter, and rendering the connection inseparable so long as this continued slight connection exists—so long as the vital or life energy continues to flow into the body from its external source. Conversely, it might reasonably be urged that death is the result of the severance of this bond of connection, since the external Cosmic energy ceases, at that time, to have any connection with the body—its expenditure being no longer necessitated. It is only when this thread of communication is cut — the channel closed—that the soul is finally and irretrievably separated from the body, and "death" takes place.[2]

Of course, the actual *manner* of the connection of the external energy with the body will doubtless always remain a great and an unsolved mystery—as much so, indeed, as "the connection of mind and matter"—of which dispute there is no end! But, it might be conceived, I suggest, that the interaction of mind and matter, of the vital energy with the body, is rather that of a series of *point-connections*, so to speak, than a continuous,

[1] "There is the important fact that the vital functions, although they fall to a low ebb, are never altogether suspended. Thus, the breath comes and goes, and the heart continues beating. . ." ("Premature Burial," by David Walsh, M.D., p. 6.)

[2] As a striking coincidence between Eastern and Western thought, I quote the following passage from Swami Abhedananda's "Self Knowledge" (p. 81), which I had not read when I wrote the above passage. I regard the coincidence of thought and even language as striking. "In dreamless sleep . . . the life force is not entirely separated from the central part of the body, because the subconscious activity of the Prana is then manifested in the heart beat, in the circulation, digestion, and in the respiratory process. If that force which causes the motion of the heart and lungs stops, there is absolute separation of the Prana from the organs, then we do not wake. This is death."

whole, inter-communication; a series of touches or impulses given to the material body by the energy dominating and guiding it. Several facts of daily observation seem to verify this supposition. Every organ or tissue of the body; every muscle or gland, works and rests alternately; there is a period of rest and a period of work; as previously stated, *rhythm* seems to be the all-pervading law of the organism.[1] This, then, would seem to indicate that the periods of work are the direct results of the impulses of energy from the mind[2] while the periods of rest are respites, or intervals, between such impulses. The idea is, of course, purely speculative and somewhat crude, but may serve to indicate the position assumed.

[1] Says Dr. J. Butler Burke ("Origin of Life," pp. 150–2): ". . . rhythm, which prevails throughout the organic and inorganic worlds, which appeals in so inexplicable a fashion to the inmost depths of the very soul itself! It is by rhythmic disturbances that the flow of energy of the ultimate source or the vital unit would be affected; the connection between rhythm and the flow of vital energy in very many physiological phenomena being most remarkable. . . . Deeper than the rhythm of art is the rhythm of Nature, for the rhythm of Nature is the rhythm of life itself." For, says Dr. Wesley Mills ("Animal Intelligence," p. 107): "Rhythm seems to be at the basis of all things organic and inorganic. . . ."

[2] Unconscious mind: Myers' "subliminal consciousness."

CHAPTER III

DEATH

§ 1. *Theories of Death*

LET us now turn to a consideration of the problem of death—its physiological aspect—in the light of the theory of vitality above advanced, and see whether we cannot form some clearer conception of the problem than has heretofore been possible—because of the erroneous theory held of the nature and causation of the bodily energy. No consistent and logical explanation of the cause of death has as yet been forthcoming, and I do not think that any completely satisfactory explanation was ever possible before this theory of vitality and its relation to the organism was advanced. The *immediate* causes of sudden death were often obvious enough—a ruptured artery, a paralyzed nerve, a general poisoning—all such conditions as would produce sudden death are well known and have been carefully studied. But though M. Brouardel, in his excellent and most interesting book "Death and Sudden Death," devotes many scores of pages to the narration of such cases, and to the tracing of the deaths to their immediate causes, he rarely or never attempts to trace the origin of the condition that rendered this cause of death possible—the "cause of the cause," so to speak, and until this has been done, it certainly is little more than a farce to speak of an "explanation" of death, when it is, in fact, no such explanation at all. To the question: what is the cause of the paralyzed nerve or the ruptured artery?—science has had a reply in but the rarest of cases. This is a question into which I should like to enter in considerable detail, but my space does not permit.

Aside, then, from all such considerations of sudden—and consequently premature—death, the great question still remains: what is the real physiological cause of natural death? In cases of death from "old age," *e.g.*, what processes are involved that render death possible at all? what changes take place at that time? in short, what is the real *modus operandi* involved in such cases? To these questions science has as yet no definite answer, nor, since cases of "natural death" are so extremely rare—being, probably, just as rare as cases of "perfect" health—is this to be wondered at. Science has never had the opportunity of observing any number of such cases, and without such observations, nothing definite can be known. Physiologists can but advance theories, or "speculate" upon such conditions, and such speculations have been remarkably barren of result and displayed but little ingenuity. It is largely due to the scarcity of *data*. Says Metchnikoff:[1]

"Natural death in man is probably a possibility rather than an actual occurrence. Old age is not a true physiological process, but exhibits many morbid characters. That being the case, it is not surprising that it seldom ends in natural death. It is probable, however, that natural death occasionally occurs in very old men."

And on p. 241 this author writes:

"I think I am justified in asserting that senile decay is mainly due to the destruction of the higher elements of the organism by macrophags."

The germ theory again! Is it not more probable, I ask, that the causes which produced senile decay also rendered possible the growth of the macrophags?

Dr. E. Teichmann states[2] that death results "because they (the aged) are no longer occupied with life"—hardly an illuminating theory! Carl Snyder's seems to me to be even less plausible, when he says:[3] "When all the atoms of creation find their atom-grabbing proclivities satisfied, all chemical action, and consequently all life, will cease. Saturation is death." See also the suggestion in Dr. John D. Malcolm's "Physiology of Death," etc., p. 86. Now, while I cannot claim to have advanced any

[1] "The Nature of Man," by Elie Metchnikoff, Professor at the Pasteur Institute, p. 277.
[2] "Life and Death," p. 115.
[3] "New Conceptions in Science," p. 282.

theory that can be considered as in any sense a complete or a satisfactory one, I shall outline briefly, in the following pages, a theory which is at least consistent and explanatory—so far as it goes—and does not contradict any of the accepted principles of physiology and psychology—provided that my theory of vitality be true. The acceptance of that theory places us in a position to perceive the possibility of the theory of death to be immediately advanced.

§ 2. *Author's Theory of Death, and Facts Supporting That Theory*

Let us go back a little in our argument. Doctor Dewey conclusively showed that all disease is but the result of a gradual process of accumulation—of "evolution in reverse"—the climax of which was generally understood to be the "attack" of the disease, more or less acute and severe. We then saw how fasting would, simply because of its purifying, cleansing action, at once stop this process of "evolution in reverse," and set the body on the high-road to health again. (pp. 154–8.) That is, whenever the powers of *de*struction are more powerful, *pro tem*, than the powers of *con*struction, then the process of accumulating disease continues; that body "dies" faster than it becomes vitalized, in fact, and this may continue to the point of death. And, conversely, whenever the powers of construction are, *pro tem*, more powerful than those of destruction; when, in short, that body is becoming vitalized or recharged with life at a more rapid rate than it is dying, then we are getting well, or being cured of our diseased condition; or, if such does not actively exist, we are adding life and vitality to the system. It is simply a question of balance—in the vital scales. This theory is, I believe, so far intrinsically true. But if we accept the theory I have propounded—that, during a fast, such a rebuilding, revivifying process is always under way, and always acting more powerfully than the destructive forces (were it otherwise, we should not, of course, get well), then, we might argue, it would only be necessary to take a fast, whenever indisposed or ill, in order to successfully combat sickness and old age indefinitely, and, in fact, to live forever!

At first sight, such a conclusion appears to be the only logical outcome of my theory, and the position into which we are, in fact, forced, if we decide to accept that theory and all that it implies. And the defense of this position has not wanted its modern champions, who contend that such an idea is logical, and is also defensible, in spite of the fact that death is universal, so far as we can see. Notable among such champions is Mr. Harry Gaze, whose book, "How to Live Forever," is most daring and ingenious. Accepting the principle that death is always due to the predominance of the de- over the con-structive factors in our bodily organisms; and accepting, also, the conclusion that, if we could reverse this process, "immortality in the body" would ensue; and believing that old age and death are always due to such predominance, he takes the bold stand of asserting that perfect, ideally correct habits of life, and *ditto* the mental control conditions, would insure a man living forever, so long as such conditions were maintained. Mr. Gaze knows, apparently, little or nothing of the phenomena of fasting, which would put a far more potent weapon in his hands than he now has, *viz.*, ideally balanced diet, both as to quality and quantity; right conditions of exercising, rest, etc. But I leave his argument as it stands, *pro tem*, and for presentation. He says, in part:

"As natural activity does not wear away the body, but simply brings a change, so man is not made old by normal changes. . . . The centenarian and the little child are both continually building the body from equally new food and material. The mental conditions, however, are very different, and determine the great difference that is manifested. The centenarian thinks that his body is one hundred years old, while the child believes his body to be but a few years old. Neither is correct. The human body cannot exist for centuries or even for years. The body of the centenarian, which seems to be very old, in reality is new. . . . The fact that the body is incessantly changing demonstrates that old age is not caused by the passing of years, but by a lack of proper adjustment."

This theory is, it seems to me, most striking and ingenious, and the position is at first sight impregnable. Nor is it so intrinsically absurd as it appears, when first read. Many of our most brilliant and noted physiologists have frankly confessed that they are totally unable to explain why death should ever come upon a perfectly healthy body; and, so long as this ideally high standard of health is maintained, this remark may be said to apply. Thus, Dr. William A. Hammond once made the statement that "there is no physiological reason at the present day why men should die." Dr. W. R. C. Latson also said: "While his (Mr. Gaze's) conception of life and the possibility of physical immortality is unique, there is nothing in the accepted facts of physiological science, by which his position can be refuted." G. H. Lewes in "The Physiology of Common Life," also said: "If the repair were always identical with the waste, never varying in the slightest degree, life would then only be terminated by some accident, never by old age." Doctor Munro asserted that "the human body, as a machine, is perfect it is apparently intended to go on for ever." Doctor Gregory, in "Medical Conspectus," wrote: "Such a machine as the human frame, unless accidentally depraved, or injured by some external cause, would seem formed for perpetuity." These quotations are sufficient to show that there is no known reason why the human body should not go on living indefinitely, provided health be maintained, or why death from old age should ever result.

I have said above that this position of Mr. Gaze's is *at first sight* impregnable. There is a fallacy in it, however, which was perceived, or rather foreseen, and pointed out by Doctor Graham, with his customary marvelous foresight, as far back as 1843. He then said:[1]

"Were the constitutional principles upon which this renovating capability of the vital economy depends, in themselves inexhaustible, then were these bodies of ours, even in the present state of being, capable of immortality; and by strictly obeying the laws of life, we might live on forever, in the eternal ebb and flow of vital energy, and the unceasing incorporation and the elimination of matter. But this is not so. *The vital constitution itself wears out.* The ultimate powers of the living organs, on

[1] "Science of Human Life," p. 352

which their replenishing and renovating capabilities depend, are, under the most favorable circumstances, gradually expended and finally exhausted.

"Through the vital energies and the sensibilities, therefore, which we exhaust to-day, are replenished to-morrow, yet of necessity the process has taken something from the measured fund of life, and reduced our vital capital in proportion to the frugality or the profligacy of our expenditure. However proper the nature and condition of our ailment, however completely all the laws of external relation are fulfilled, however perfectly the functions of our organs are performed, and however salutary their results, yet every digestive process of the stomach, every respiratory action of the lungs, every contraction of the heart, draws something from the ultimate and unreplenishable resources of organic vitality; and consequently the more freely and prodigally we expend the vital properties of our organs, the more rapidly we wear out the constitutional powers of replenishment, and exhaust the limited stock of life. Nothing can, therefore, be more dangerously fallacious than the opinion which is too generally cherished and too frequently promulgated—that our daily trespasses upon the laws of life are as the dropping of water upon a rock—wearing, indeed, but so slowly and imperceptibly as scarcely to make a difference in the duration and comfort of our lives."

And so the fallacy lies just here. No one atom of our body is ever replaced by an *exactly* duplicate or similar atom, but *always by one vitally lower in the scale;* either vastly or infinitesimally lower—according to the degree of health or of disease of the body at the time. This is the true explanation, I think, of this otherwise inexplicable difficulty. But how are we to account for the facts if we refuse to take into our account the vital factor? As we have just seen, we cannot then account for the facts at all.

I have digressed to this extent because such digression was necessary in order to show that such an absurdity as "immortality in the body" is not, in reality, the logical outcome of my theory, and because I wished to forestall and answer this objection which, I felt sure, would be raised by some acute critic, and my whole theory held up to ridicule in consequence. Having now shown, however, that no such deductions are possible, or in any way warranted, I pass at once to a consideration of death from its purely physiologic aspect, and to an attempt to formulate my theory of its cause.

As before stated, science has to-day no true explanation or even theory of the cause of natural death. Is life, at death, transformable into one or other of the physical forces? It would be a daring scientist indeed, who would bluntly answer "yes" to the question thus bluntly put, and indeed, the evidence is all the other way. ("Life and Matter," p. 115.) Professor Hibbert has so well criticized this theory, and so completely disproved it[1] that it is hardly necessary for me to go over the same ground here, and I shall but refer the reader to those pages for an answer to this question. And if "yes" is not ventured, in answer, what then? Has science any rational—truly rational—theory of natural death—its causes and phenomena, to offer?[2]

Presuming that the answer to this question will be in the negative, I might, perhaps, advance my own view somewhat as follows:

We have seen (pp. 249–50), that, according to our theory, the individualized vital impulse, called life, is capable of manifesting to us and to others through the bodily organism—using that organism merely as the vehicle or means of its expression; as it is only in this manner that its existence can ever be made known to material beings, on the material plane. We have also seen (pp. 251–4), that the degree to which this life is capable of manifesting is, *ceteris paribus*, in direct proportion to the condition of the bodily organism—the purer and cleaner the body, the greater influx of vital power—of mental and physical life—is possible, and *vice versa*. When the body is in its best condition, an abundance of physical vigor and of mental force is present; when, on the other hand, such a body is diseased, then weakness and debility result, and mental sluggishness and moral perversion. And we have only to pursue this idea to its logical conclusion, I believe, in order to arrive at an understanding of what death may ultimately be. *It is that condition of the organism which renders no longer possible, the transmission or manifestation of vital force through it*—which condition is probably a

[1] "Life and Energy," chapter "Is Life Energy?"

[2] See H. M. Alden's "Study of Death," pp. 12, 326; "Conservation of Energy," pp. 200–1.

poisoned state of the nervous system, due, in turn, to the whole system becoming poisoned by toxic material absorbed from the blood. When such a poisoned[1] or obstructed[2] condition is present, then it is no longer possible for the vital energy—the life force—to manifest through it; the severance of the vital principle and the material body takes place; *i.e.*, death has resulted. The transmission of the life energy, *through* the body, its transmission into the world, so to speak, is no longer possible. Thus, I conceive, the body is really dying first, before the life principle and mentality leaves it; and that the latter vacates the organism only on this account—that its tenancy there is no longer possible. It is not the old notion of the "soul vacating the body," as Doctor Hartmann expressed it,[3] that is defended, be it observed, but the idea that the body acts as a sort of medium for transmission of the life energy, and that when such a medium becomes totally incapable of transmitting the life energy, death then ensues—for the reason that its manifestation *through* that organism is no longer possible. Such a theory explains all the facts in the case, and is in direct accord with my theory of vitality; while it does not contradict any known laws of physiology or psychology—and, has, further, many outlying facts which tell in its favor, and indirectly prove it to be correct.[4]

[1] Says Doctor Brouardel ("Death and Sudden Death," p. 292): "Death supervenes when poisons manufactured in the system, or unwholesome food that has been ingested, can no longer be adequately removed by the kidneys. . . . The individual is, therefore, poisoned either by his food or by poisons which are generated within his own body, *i.e.*, auto-intoxication."

[2] Says Doctor Kellogg ("Aristocracy of Health," p. 36): "The cause of old age is . . . the accumulation of waste matters in the body." Physiological degeneration, due to chemical changes, was the explanation offered by Haeckel ("The Wonders of Life," p. 106); while Doctor Trall favored the idea that death ensues when "the solids are so disproportioned to the fluids that the nutritive processes can no longer be carried on." ("Physiology," p. 203.) Doctor Rosenbach contends that: "Death, . . . is that condition of organized matter in which all processes of causation have come to such a state of rest that they can no longer be put in motion, since the grouping of the atoms in the molecule has become so firm that the liberation of fixing force would be associated with a destruction of the molecule." ("Physician *vs.* Bacteriologist," pp. 82–3.) Doctor Evans contends that: "Induration and ossification are the causes of 'old age' and 'natural death.'" ("How to Prolong Life," p. 29.) Dr. Benj. Ward Richardson assumed a position half way between that of Doctor Evans and Doctor Trall. (See his "Diseases of Modern Life," pp. 103–4.) It will be observed that *blockage* is the principal factor in all the above theories.

[3] "Buried Alive," p. 82.

[4] See, *e.g.*, "Common Disorders," by W. R. C. Latson, M.D., pp. 8–10; "Shall We Slay to Eat?" by J. H. Kellogg, M.D., pp. 43–4, etc.

CHAPTER IV

BODILY HEAT

§ 1. *Current Theories of the Causation of Bodily Heat by Food*

As I have previously stated, the position I occupy and shall endeavor to defend in this question is that, not only the bodily energies are independent of the food supply and not derivable from it, but that the heat of the body is also independent of this supply—a far more difficult thing to prove—and that the bodily heat, no less than the bodily energy, is not dependent upon food combustion for its maintenance — as is universally held. Let me state the current theory, in order to avoid misunderstanding, as I did in the case of the theory of the relations of food and bodily vitality. Kirke, in his "Physiology" (pp. 494, 496), thus expresses the current views:

"One of the most important results of the metabolism of the tissues is the production of the heat of the body. It is by this means that the bodily temperature is raised to such a point as to make life possible. . The heat which is produced in the body arises from the metabolic changes of the tissues, the chief part of which are of the nature of oxidation, since it may be supposed that the oxygen of the atmosphere taken into the system is ultimately combined with carbon and hydrogen, and discharged from the body as carbonic acid and water. . . . The more active the changes the greater is the heat produced and the greater is the amount of carbonic acid and water formed. But in order that the protoplasm may perform its function, the waste of its own tissue (destructive metabolism), must be repaired by the due supply of food material to be built up in some way into the protoplasmic molecule. For the production of heat, therefore, food is necessary. In the tissues, as we have several times remarked, two processes are continually going on: the building up of the protoplasm from the food (constructive metabolism) which is not accompanied by the evolution of heat, possibly even by its storing, and the oxidation of the protoplasmic materials resulting in the production of energy, by which heat is set free and carbonic acid and water are evolved."

Or as a more lucid and less "scientific" writer put it:

"In the human body and in the locomotive the fuel is burned by the aid of air, the oxygen of which unites with the combustible part of the fuel, and the potential energy it contains is trans formed into heat and power. The power of energy is used for muscular work; the heat is used to keep the body warm."[1]

This is the position I propose to attack; and I may as well come to the point at once and raise the issue between my own views and those of the scientific world, as a whole, by stating my position in the problem, and the ground I propose to defend.

§ 2. *Author's Theory of its Causation and Maintenance.*

My conception of the relations of food combustion and bodily heat, then, is somewhat as follows: the oxidation of food liberates, in the process of chemical combustion, a certain amount of heat, which is, of course, imparted to the organism *as heat* (not energy). Thus, it is true that our food supplies heat to the body, and this I do not deny. But my contention is that life is not *dependent* upon this heat for its maintenance, or preservation; I believe that, wherever life is present, and manifest, there the bodily temperature is maintained, food or no food, combustion or no combustion. So long as life lasts, this temperature is maintained. Now, when we die, the body cools to the temperature of the surrounding air—whatever that may be—and we consequently see that the bodily temperature is, in some mysterious manner, dependent upon the presence of *life*, or vitality, for its continuation and maintenance. The body is thus maintained at a uniform temperature of about 98.4° F., so long as life lasts[2] and, I submit, quite independent of the supply of food. To be sure, food, in its combustion, does impart heat to the

[1] "How to Keep Warm," by Albert Broadbent, F.S.S., p. 4.

[2] "Experience has satisfactorily shown that the heat of the blood in health is the same in all climates and in all conditions of atmospheric temperature." ("Food and Diet," by J. Pereira, M.D., F.R.S., etc., p. 8.)

organism; that I have admitted; but the heat is not necessary to support life, and it is again given off, from and by the body, as heat. Thus: heat is imparted to the organism; and this heat is again given off by it—losing nothing in its passage through the body. The heat imparted must again be given off, and the more heat is imparted, the more must be given off: and this forcible cooling process necessitates a very great and useless expenditure of vital energy.

But the question may be raised: if our bodily temperature is not dependent upon our daily food for its maintenance, upon what does it depend? *Some* force is at work, keeping the body maintained thirty or fifty or seventy-five or even a hundred or more degrees above the temperature of the surrounding atmosphere; and this force must, of necessity, be exceedingly powerful. What is it? I am not prepared to answer this question fully at present (might I ask if anyone else is able to do so?) but I think that a first crude attempt might be made at its solution. Let us consider the problem a little more closely.

The only thing definite that we know concerning the bodily temperature is that it is nearly uniform, and is present, *ceteris paribus*, in almost direct proportion to the degree of vitality—of life—present in the organism, at any one time. Life can function most perfectly when the temperature-conditions are most perfect; *i.e.*, when above or below the normal, the perfection of its manifestation is marred.[1] But it is upon *the presence of life* that the temperature is dependent; and, so far as we know, upon that only.

And what is life? That, of course, is unknown. But I venture to think that we shall not go far wrong should we conceive it—on its physical side—for of its essence we are quite ignorant—as a species of *vibration*.[2] Now, if we could extend our idea,

[1] "Temperature and Life," by Henry de Varigny, p. 407.

[2] Says Doctor Burke ("Origin of Life," p. 49): "Life might be described as a specialized mode of motion, the specialized mode of motion being, that of a complex system of molecules in a dynamically unstable state . . ." Similarly, Spencer defines life as: "The continuous adjustment of internal relations to external relations." ("Principles of Biology," Vol. I., p. 99.) It is amazing to me that such loose statements as these could be seriously considered definitions of life by any scientific man. Yet they are—Spencer's definition having been the one more universally accepted than any single definition of life that has ever been advanced. Yet is it not obvious that

and imagine that, in some way, corresponding to this vibration, is a certain, measurable quantity of *heat,* we might, I think, form some faint idea of the relation of life to the bodily heat, noticed by us. Life can manifest most perfectly at a certain rate of vibration (life cannot function in a cold body). We must assume, then, that this rate of vibration is in some way equivalent to the 98.4° F. of the thermometer. Above and below this rate, life is impeded in its manifestation; its powers are weakened. And this perfection of the rate of vibration depends, in turn, upon the degree of health and cleanliness of the physical organism. (pp. 251–4.)

We know that an electric current heats a wire along which it travels to do work, and I suggest that, by analogy, *the vital energy heats the body in flowing through it* (the nervous mechanism) to do the mental and physical work of the organism—the work of the world. At least I can see no vital objection to this hypothesis. And there are many facts which support the theory. First, let us take into account the heat that is generated by exercise. It has always been asserted that the heat noticed at this time is due to the added combustion of food material; more food material is being burned up in the body, and consequently more heat is imparted to it. This is the prevailing theory, and it is supported by the undoubted *fact* that, when we exercise, we do get warm; and when we remain stationary, we get cold. So far the prevailing theory would seem to hold good—though contradicting what has previously been written in its defense. (pp. 230–1.) But I venture to suggest that my theory can account for the observed and undoubted facts equally well—that the heat is not derived from the food at all, nor its combustion within the organism, but that the heat is due to the warming of the body by vital energy passing through it more or less rapidly, as it is enabled or permitted to do so by the physical condition of the organism, and the degree of its activity. And

this definition gives or states merely the *effects* of life—its phenomena—and does nothing to state what its real essence is at all? The movements, the "adjustments" *are* the phenomena—the *results* of life—what life *does;* and no more states what life *is* than we would define it when we say "I breathe" or "I hit" or "I perspire"—specific acts or adjustments. They are obviously the *effects* of life—not its cause or essence. In other words: Life is *that which adjusts*—not the adjustments themselves.

this would derive much support from the fact that all organs are warmer when they are active than when they are passive and reposing from active work.[1] Thus, the greater heat observed during exercise is due, not to the extra combustion of food material within the organism, but to the fact that more vital energy is being expended, and so more passes through the body, by way of the nervous system—warming it, in transit, just as the Cu. wire is warmed by the passage of the electric current. The nervous system is the medium through whose instrumentality the body is heated, and not by the oxidation of food material. The extra heat is due to the increased passage, through it, of vital energy; and, just as electric energy runs more easily through a warmed or heated wire than through a cold one (in fact, it warms it as it runs), so vital energy manifests more easily in a warm body—and this would explain why it is that athletes have to "warm up" by a few exercises before entering for the event in which they are engaged.

There are still other facts that would seem to indicate that this hypothesis is the true one. Thus; if true, we could account for the observed fact that the cerebrum is heated when thinking is intense,[2] by conceiving that this added heat be due to an extra nervous effort, rather than to the fact that any great amount of additional oxidation of food is taking place within the brain. It is much more easy to conceive my theory than the prevailing one, in cases of nervous action—more easily than in cases of muscular activity, where the combustion of food elements is certain, and consequently the greatly increased oxidation of food elements is certain. Then, too, we could understand the low temperature in certain patients. It is due to the fact that but little energy flows or can flow into the organism—which is not heated to such an extent, in consequence. The low temperature would thus correspond to the lack of vitality—which proves to be actually the case. (*v.* pp. 449–50.) It would also enable us to understand the low temperature in paralysis, *e.g.*, where but little energy can reach the affected part. (Kirke: "Physiology," p. 502.) On the other hand, we

[1] "Temperature and Life," p. 411.
[2] "Occult Japan," p. 312; Kirke "Physiology," p. 498.

can understand, to some extent, the *rationale* of fever. That condition might be, in part at least, the result of the forcible recharging of the body with energy—rushed into it—as it were —in order to assist in freeing the body from its dangerously diseased condition. We should thus have a clear conception of fever, which is certainly lacking to-day.[1]

From all the facts so far presented, then, I think I am justified in maintaining that life is innate, and its accompanying phenomena are but resultants; and that one of these resultants or phenomena is the manifestation and preservation of animal heat. No extra amount of food can perfect the process of the manifestation of life, nor do aught else but cramp and hinder it.

§ 3. *Facts Supporting This Theory*

It will thus be seen that the mere fact of supplying heat to the body means nothing; the more heat is imparted, the more is and must be given off. We derive no benefit therefrom—nothing, beyond the fact that more heat has passed *through* the system in the one case than in the other, and that the vital forces are consequently wasted more in the one case than in the other. The best way to maintain the bodily heat is to conserve the energies; to eat only those foods which will entail the least expenditure, the least waste, of energy, and these are, certainly, our natural foods.

Inasmuch, then, as the heat merely passes through the body, (which thereby acts merely as its transmitter); and, inasmuch as this process must involve a considerable outlay of nervous energy,[2] it is evident that our ideal food—that which will enable us to maintain the greatest amount of energy—the most vigorous and robust health—is that which imparts (and consequently needs the elimination of) the *least* amount of heat; and this, it will be noticed, is our natural food—fruits, etc.—which indirectly proves the accuracy of the contention that this is man's natural diet. Conversely, those foods that (apparently) furnish the greatest amount of heat are those which should be most carefully avoided—as likely to waste the vitality, and ultimately

[1] See, *e.g.*, "On Inflammatory Fevers" (Toner Lectures), p. 10

[2] Heat is always equivalent to energy *expended*. See Thurston's "Theory of Energy in the Living World," p. 540.

debilitate the organism, in all cases of acute or chronic disease.

The prevailing idea that heating, readily combustible foods are needed in cold climates is thus shown to be without foundation and false; for our capacity for resisting cold is in direct proportion to the degree of our vitality; and whatever will best enable us to keep this at the highest possible standard will also best preserve the bodily heat. (p. 342.)

If the food maintained the heat of the body, then we might surely suppose that those foods which would furnish the greatest amount of heat would be most essential to the organism, and those which would be, naturally, our staple foods; and, further, we might also suppose that such foods—because of the fact that they are so essential—would scarcely be *harmful* at any rate, and harmful, too, in almost direct ratio to the quantity eaten (as fats, sugar, etc., are, when eaten in any quantity). This would seem to indicate that they are harmful, although they are so essential; *i.e.*, the more perfectly they fulfill their duty (of heating the system)—the more heat they supply to the body—the more intrinsically unwholesome they are! Could anything be more contradictory, not to say absurd? To suppose that a food is unwholesome in exactly the same ratio that it performs its legitimate and normal function!

The theory that combustion took place in the lungs, which acted as a sort of stove, in fact, was held for many years by physiologists and strenuously defended by them. It is now practically given up, however, since physiology has shown us that a very small proportion of combustion takes place in the lungs, but usually in the body as a whole. It will help us to understand the real problem, however, if I briefly epitomize the theory, as then held, and point out the sources of error—inasmuch as many of the arguments may be utilized in refutation of the theory held to-day. The great champion of the older view was Liebig—whose theories ruled the scientific world for many years, and was considered to be so firmly grounded, and was defended by so many eminent men, that Doctor Graham wrote of it: "There never was an erroneous theory more ingeniously constructed or more plausibly supported." ("Lectures," p. 183.)

Upon the publication of Liebig's elaborate work on "Organic Chemistry," the idea at once became generally prevalent among the scientific circles, and, from them, it was promulgated among the non-scientific people—that the production of the animal heat is a mere chemical process; the lungs serving as a stove or fireplace, and the carbonaceous substances of the food serving as fuel "to be burned in the lungs." According to this theory, fatty substances, animal oils, and other matters containing a large proportion of carbon are not only useful but absolutely necessary to keep up the requisite degree of animal temperature. The position seems to me as almost self-evidently absurd, and it has certainly led many persons into the most egregious blunders practically, and at the expense, too, of their own common sense and common observation.

All the organic functions of the body—the vital processes—are in one sense chemical. They are not, however, such chemical decompositions and recombinations as are performed in a chemical laboratory. They are not such as the chemist can ever demonstrate or imitate. They not only change the relative proportion of elementary matters, but absolutely transmute elements into each other, reduce several of what we call elements to one, and separate one into several. All the chemico-vital processes—respiration, digestion, circulation, secretion, etc.—are attended by the elimination of heat; or, in other words, latent caloric becomes sensible by these changes of matter. But all the organs, by virtue of their own specially presiding centers of nervous influence, are, to some extent, self-regulating in their temperature, while the entire body possesses a general self-regulating power. The principal organ whose function serves as a universal regulator and equalizer of animal temperature, is the skin. When in vigorous and healthy condition, it throws off the surplus heat, or retains the deficit, according to the necessities of the organism. There is no need of a fire and boilers to warm up the blood, as the water is heated by the machinery of a steam engine; and for this simple reason I think Nature has not provided them.

The error lies here. Liebig and his followers have mistaken an excrementitious or cleansing process for a nutritive and supplying one. They have misconceived the function by which the body rids itself of waste matters, and called it a useful and indispensable condition of vitality! They have supposed the chemical process by which Nature throws off the effete carbon through the lungs to be a method of furnishing animal heat! This, I think, can easily be made manifest.

According to the theory of animal heat I am controverting, fat, suet, tallow, lard, marrow, grease, butter, blubber, and fixed oils, should constitute healthful food; and such is, indeed, the conclusion of Liebig's followers. But the common experience of all mankind is against it. Common observation says that these articles, though to some extent sufferable, are not strictly wholesome; and further, medical men generally disallow these articles to their patients when they are very much reduced with disease; at the time that the animal temperature is very low, and requires such food, if ever. Again, corpulent persons who are surcharged with carbon, do not bear cold better than lean persons, who have little; in fact they are, other circumstances being equal, more sensitive to it. Greasy matters, though composed mostly of waste, useless and excrementitious materials, which have accumulated in the cellular repository, because the process of alimentation was increased beyond that of elimination, are not strictly poisonous. They contain, doubtless, a very small quantity, yet very impure quality, of substances convertible into nutriment. But as food, they are to be regarded as next to venous blood in grossness and impurity.

They contain about eighty per cent. of carbon; hence, when freely taken into the system, the lungs, as the principal excretory organ for effete carbon, have an additional duty to perform in throwing it off. This increased labor is, as a matter of course, attended with an increased temperature of the body, simply because there is a greater amount of matter that is natural or necessary to be disposed of. But this, as in the case of alcohol, is an extraneous, useless, and exhausting labor, which wears out the machinery of life with inordinate rapidity. If the excessive quantity of carbon is constantly supplied in the diet, the organism must prematurely wear out, or break down with disordered action. If fatty matters are only occasionally eaten, the temporary increase in temperature will be followed by depression and debility precisely as with alcohol, though much less in degree. The lungs, however, do not "burn up"—oxidate—all the surplus carbon of grease, oils, gravies, etc., for we see in most persons addicted to their free use, pimples, blotches, eruptions, swellings, boils, and cancerous ulcerations, with evidences of bad blood, torpid brains, and glandular obstructions, clearly traceable to this habit, and curable by its discontinuance. The principal injurious effect, therefore, of animal oils and fats is not from their large quantity of carbon, but from their intrinsically impure character. In all pure, healthful, and natural alimentary substances, the system can appropriate what carbon it requires, and dispose of the remainder without injury, obstruction or excitement, be the quantity contained in the alimentary article more or less. All the grains, esculent roots, and fruits, as well as the flesh meat of animals, contain exactly the right proportions of carbon in their composition for perfect nutrition, respiration, and animal heat, however much their respective quantities of carbon may vary. They are also universally allowed to be "easily digestible," and innocuous to the stomach in all normal conditions of the digestive powers. Not so with greasy matters.

Pereira himself says, directly in the face of his argument in favor of the use of grease, for the benefit of the lungs:

> "Fixed oil or fat is more difficult of digestion, and more obnoxious to the stomach than any other alimentary principle."

Can any body tell why an alimentary article which is so necessary to the lungs should be so obnoxious to the stomach—unless nature has made a very great blunder? The whole theory of a respiratory alimentary principle seems to me preposterous in the extreme.

It is further urged, in favor of this wild conclusion from a false starting point, that people in the cold climates—the Esquimaux, for example—consume immense quantities of blubber oil, tallow candles when they can get them, fatty matters of all kinds that they are able to procure, as well as enormous quantities of flesh and fish, as they can catch it; and simply because they do these things, and live in a cold climate where they can get little else, the inference is drawn that it is necessary they should so eat to get carbon into the body, "to be burned in the lungs" to support the animal temperature! It is very true that a cold, vigorous climate enables the digestive organs to *bear* what would destroy life very soon in a warm climate. It is also true that these blubber oil eaters, and all the tribes of men whose dietetic habits are similar, are a very inferior race, and in them nothing is developed, scarcely, save the mere animal nature; hence their stomachs have all the nervous power, almost, of their whole constitutions. More than this, their animal nature is itself actually inferior, in muscular power, to that of those tribes and races of men whose general regimen is comparatively free from fats and animal oils.[1]

From all the arguments and facts I am able to gather the conclusion is unavoidable that this notion of pouring carbon into the stomach to support respiration and manufacture animal heat is just as absurd as the common fallacy of heating, peppering and stimulating the stomach with spices, pills and spirits, to "aid digestion." Moreover, the theory of the combustion of carbon in the lungs sufficiently to heat up the body is positively disproved by the fact that most of the carbonic acid expelled from the lungs is really formed in the tissues distant from the lungs.

There is no doubt that the oxygenation of the tissues throughout the system, and the combination of oxygen with the carbon, are sources of animal heat, in common with all the organic functions and chemical changes which take place in the body. All the conditions requisite to the due regulation of the animal temperature, are good digestion, free respiration, vigorous circulation, proper assimilation, and perfect depuration, in two words—*good health.*

The ordinary temperature of the body ranges from 98° to 100° F., varying but few degrees above or below, when the surrounding atmosphere is greatly elevated or depressed, or when the most violent fevers or extremes of debility and emaciation are present.

[1] See Smith, "Fruits and Farinacea," pp. 194–5; Pereira, "Food and Diet," pp. 10, 223, 269–70; "Physical Culture," Vol. IX., p. 13.

That cutaneous respiration is subservient to the maintenance of the equal temperature of the body, is evident from the fact that if the hair of animals be shaved off, and the bare skin covered with varnish, the temperature instantly *falls*.

Let me illustrate further:

Consequent upon the ingestion of food, there is, almost invariably, a rise in the bodily temperature, which is due, it is asserted, to the increase of the bodily heat—resultant, in turn, from the increased oxidation of food material. In every book on nutrition so far published, it has been asserted that foods produce a certain quantity of heat, when "burned up" in the system, and investigators claim to be able to calculate to the calorie the amount of heat that will be produced when this combustion of food takes place. Thus, we read, *e.g.*, that apples "supply" per pound, only 190 calories of heat; lima beans 540 calories; roast beef (rump) 1,090 calories, etc., etc.[1] And about the same may be found in any book on nutrition that has so far appeared.

Now, all this I conceive to be entirely erroneous for the reasons I have pointed, and shall point out, *viz.*, (1) that energy is always noticed in its expenditure, *i.e.*, waste, never in its accumulation—hence could not possibly be manifested, while being added to the system's store of energy; and (2) the fact that heat is not produced or maintained by the rapid combustion of food is completely refuted by the fact that the patient's temperature is as high and frequently higher at the end of a protracted fast than before entering upon the fast, and just after the ingestion of a substantial meal.[2] This point my observations and experiments have proved conclusively. Now, my claim is that the degree of heat noted in any organism, consequent upon the ingestion of food, is always manifested, in the vital economy, in direct proportion to the friction, or abnormal functioning, of more or less congested organs, or by a great excess of normal

[1] "Principles of Nutrition and Nutritive Value of Food," pp. 16–18.

[2] It has never been pointed out why hot *water* would not supply this heat, if that is all that is needed (and we have the statement of Doctor Kirke that death from starvation is, after all, little more than death from loss of heat!) As Doctor Keith said ("Facts of an Old Physician," p. 70): "It would take a considerable amount of carbon fuel, say in bread and butter, to produce the quantity of heat in a tumbler of hot water."

functioning by them—accompanied by the necessary expenditure of energy. All heat noticed at that time would thus represent a more or less congested, abnormal, or overtaxed condition of the digestive system. The degree of heat manifested would, therefore, represent the degree of the excessive functioning, and consequently of energy expenditure; and it may readily be seen that the more of this there is, the worse for the vital economy in the long run; and shows, indirectly, that any foods that will produce such abnormal conditions are not the best foods for the human being, nor those best suited for the conservation of (human) energy and the prolongation of life. The heat manifested is, in plain words, "the fever of *in*digestion," indicating vital expenditure, rather than the fact that heat has been supplied or added to the body. It detracts from, but does not and cannot add to the heat or vitality. This being the case, we should, of course, select those foods which cause or occasion the *least* manifestation of heat; *i.e.*, those foods which would digest with the least expenditure of energy, and these might justly be considered the most normal and most wholesome foods, whatever they may be.

Bearing these facts in mind, let us now turn to the various tables of food products, with their corresponding "fuel values" in calories, which have been repeatedly worked out and tabulated. I select for quotation one of Prof. W. O. Atwater's efforts in this direction[1] partly because of the eminence of the author, and partly for the reason that it has been officially stated by Mr. A. C. True, director of the U. S. Dept. of Agriculture, to be "a useful summary of available information on the subject." (p. 2.) It would, consequently, represent the latest views on the question, from the most "orthodox" point of view.

In the light of the above facts, then, we might expect, *à priori*, that the most natural foods would be digested with the minimum outlay of energy—and consequently the least manifestation of "heat and energy." Conversely the most gross, stimulating, and unnatural foods would necessitate the expenditure of more energy in their digestion; more "heat and energy" is manifested

[1] "Principles of Nutrition and Nutritive Value of Food." (U. S. *Department of Agriculture Bulletin, No.* 142.)

to the senses, consequently; and a close inspection of the table of food materials completely justifies this view.

Thus: while the fuel value of our natural foods (fruits) is extremely low—showing that they cause but little derangement of the digestive organs, during the process of their digestion—vegetables are far higher in the scale; breads, meats, and dried fruits still higher; while certain highly stimulating articles of diet are far and away the highest of all—furnishing more than twelve times the "heat and energy" of *e.g.*, a porterhouse steak! (pp. 16–18.) Apples, *e.g.*, "furnish" (supposedly) 190 calories per pound; raspberries 220 cal.; strawberries 150 cal.; muskmelons 80 cal.; and watermelons only 50 cal.; while parsnips "furnish" 230 cal.; sweet potatoes 440 cal.; lima beans 540 cal.; white bread 1,200 cal.; dried apricots 1,125 cal.; ribs of beef 1,135 cal.; mutton chops 1,415 cal.; fresh ham 1,320 cal.; bacon (smoked) 2,715 cal.; salt pork 3,555 cal.; and chocolate (a stimulant!) 5,625. I can conceive no better proof of my main contention than is afforded by a careful study of the above figures. Here we have a steady increase in the energy of digestion—*expended*—precisely as we should expect, *à priori*, were my hypothesis true, and progressing in exact ratio to the degree of unwholesomeness, or "unnaturalness" of the food; *i.e.*, the more the food diverges from the normal, or natural food of man, the greater the waste of energy necessitated in order to appropriate it for the organism, and consequently the more heat we notice, accompanying such waste or expenditure.

We clearly perceive that, as the food becomes richer, heavier, more unsuited for digestion—more indigestible, in fact (not more nutritious, be it observed), the greater the number of calories supposedly imparted to the organism; while, upon a plain, wholesome, non-stimulating diet, the number of calories is proportionately low. This is strikingly illustrated, *e.g.*, in the case of poultry. Here, while boiled chicken supposedly furnishes but 305 cal., and fowl 765 cal., the far richer, greasier, and obviously still more unwholesome flesh foods, turkey and goose, "furnish" respectively, 1,060 cal. and 1,475 cal. The above facts fully corroborate my contention, and sustain the theory advanced, most forcibly.

Throughout the above argument, I have been laboring to show that, if the accepted theories were carried to their logical conclusion, they become self-contradictory and absurd, and the presumption is certainly strong that we derive no heat whatever from the daily food—which presumption becomes almost a settled fact in view of the evidence to be presented in the remainder of this book, and especially in the chapter on "The Temperature." (pp. 448–59.) It now remains for me to indicate, briefly, a few additional facts tending to confirm my theory.

First, I ask, if our bodily heat comes from the food, how is it that the body always remains at a more or less *uniform* temperature—and that, regardless of the amount of food we daily consume? If the temperature be dependent upon food combustion, then, surely, the more food we eat, the higher the bodily temperature should be, and *vice versa*. And the fact that such is not the case is one of the standing wonders of physiology. And it appears to me that the current theory is practically disproved by the fact that the bodily temperature does not sink, but rises, during a fast—when no food whatever is ingested that can be oxidized. (pp. 452–3.) And if it be asserted, in answer to this, that it is possible that the bodily heat be maintained, under such circumstances, by the oxidation of our own tissues, then, I ask, why is it that the temperature is *higher*, after a fast of several days, than before such a fast was entered upon? It is readily conceivable that an equal—or slightly reduced—temperature might be maintained for some considerable time by oxidizing off our own tissues in this way; but, I ask, why is the temperature higher than before the fast? (For proof of this, *v.* pp. 452–3.) Can the current theories explain this undoubted fact? How easily it might be interpreted on my theory will be apparent immediately.

Now for a few confirmatory facts.

"It is a matter of common observation," says Dr. Wesley Mills,[1] "that when an individual exercises, the skin becomes flushed, and so with the increased production of heat, especially in the muscles, there is a provision of unusual escape of the surplus; at the same time sweat breaks out visibly, or if not, the

[1] "Animal Physiology," pp. 464–6.

insensible perspiration is generally increased; and this accounts for an additional increment of loss; while the lungs do extra work and exhale an increased quantity of aqueous vapor, so that in these various ways the body is cooled. Manifestly there is some sort of coördination between the processes of heat production and heat expenditure. Certainly, any theory that will imply that vital processes are more under the control of the nervous system than has hitherto been taught, will, we think, advance physiology. . . . The fact that the whole metabolism of a hibernating animal is lowered, that with this there is loss of consciousness much more profound than in ordinary sleep, of itself seems to indicate that the nervous system is at the bottom of the whole affair."

Here, certainly, it is acknowledged that the current theories are insufficient to account, in a satisfactory manner, for the phenomena observed; and the necessity for a new theory—one more in accordance with all the facts—is patent. As Doctor Broadbent remarked:

"When the body is clogged by over-eating, the production of heat is impeded. . . . I am often asked what food gives warmth and heat. No food does this. Food may stimulate and produce sensations of warmth, but the body only is the heat producer."[1]

Dr. John D. Malcolm, in his "Physiology of Death from Traumatic Fever," (pp. 1–2), brought forward evidence tending to show that the production of heat in the body depends entirely upon the nervous system and its activity. In part, he says:

"The development of heat in living structures depends on tissue changes, and it has been shown that the temperature of the body may be raised at will by the stimulation of a portion of the brain substance to the 'medial side of the Corpus Striatum near the Nodus Cursorius of Nothnagel.' . . . With the production of heat, a mechanism for its elimination is intimately associated; and there is reason for believing that the heat-eliminating function is also under the control of the thermal nervous system."

Another proof that the heat of the body is dependent upon the degree of activity of the nervous system, rather than upon

[1] "How to Keep Warm," p. 9.

the oxidation of food, is found in the fact that, in sexual excitement, when the nervous system is excited to an exceptional degree, (yet when there is little reason to suppose that the oxidation of food is going on at an equally rapid rate—proportionately rapid, so as to account for the facts) the body becomes excessively hot, and frequently perspires, within a very few seconds. This would be perfectly intelligible on the theory that the heat of the body is directly proportioned to the degree of its expenditure through the nervous mechanism (*see below*), but hardly explicable on the current theories.

Again, it has been stated that:

"When a man does no muscular work (save, of course, the internal work of respiration, circulation, etc.), all the energy leaves his hody as heat; but when he does muscular work, as in lifting weights or driving a bicycle, part of the energy appears in the external work thus done, and the rest is given off from the body as heat."[1]

Now, if this were the case, then those persons who take the least exercise should be the hottest—for the reason that, all or most of, the energy would be available for purposes of heating the body—when less is expended in the production of energy for exercise and other wasteful purposes. This would be a perfectly logical deduction from the premises; but of course, such is not the case. Again, on the current theories, the facts appear self-contradictory and absurd; but on the theory to be outlined immediately, it all appears rational and consistent enough.

Another confirmatory fact, which I quote from Doctor Rabagliati's "Functions of Food in the Body," p. 39, is this. In part, he says:

"I have known . . . the bodily temperature elevated by as much as 3 degrees F. from 96 to 99 degrees, and to remain up for an hour or two, by taking a cup of simple hot coffee. It is, of course, physically impossible that half a pint of coffee at 110 degrees F. could have raised 120 pounds of the bodily tissues of a man through two or three degrees, and have maintained it at

[1] "Principles of Nutrition and Nutritive Value of Food," by W. O. Atwater, Ph.D., etc., p. 11.

that level for some hours. As a question of thermal physics it is impossible. How then did the coffee act? It did not contain any nutrient material in the conventional sense. It is inconceivable that the nutrient material contained in the coffee, if there was any (there was neither sugar nor cream in it), could have directly, by its oxidation, raised the bodily temperature. What it did do, I suppose, was to stimulate the body to use up some of the materials already accumulated in it in excess; and, by freeing the body of them, to allow bio-dynamic or vital energy freer play to raise the temperature. I infer that nutritive material existed in the body in excess at the commencement of the experiment, because the temperature was sub-normal by two degrees of more—the bodily functions being choked or depressed by this cause. I have known a glass of hot water have the same effect in raising the bodily temperature, though not by 2 or 3 degrees. "

Proof that the bodily temperature is dependent upon the degree of vitality, and not upon the extent of the food combustion, is furnished by numerous observations of the phenomena of fasting. (pp. 452–3.) Here we shall see that the temperature is always directly proportional to the amount of the patient's vitality, and to nothing else.[1] We cannot, therefore, gauge the bodily temperature by any standard of food analysis—only by far subtler considerations. We know that we cannot *permanently* increase the bodily heat either by changing the quality,

[1] It is conceivable, of course, that food does supply a certain amount of heat to the body, under certain conditions; but my claim is that this is more of a pathological than a physiological process; and that it would never occur if normal bodily and climatic conditions existed. The vitality should never be so low—nor the temperature so cold—as to necessitate this; and if these conditions do exist, it would prove, merely, that they are unnatural conditions which the organism must counteract by adopting some extreme measures; and would not at all prove that these measures are normal ones. The fact that we eat more—and especially more fatty foods—in the colder weather might perhaps be accounted for in this manner—though I have on pp. 341–2 endeavored to show that the popular idea that we must "stuff" ourselves in the winter time is a gross mistake. Thus, we might conceive that some food is, under these circumstances, transformed into heat; but, as stated, it would not prove that this was a normal process—merely that living in such an extremely cold climate was distinctly unnatural to the organism. It would merely be an illustration of the way in which the organism should *not* function. I am convinced that this process is abnormal, and a waste of energy, and that any long-continued practice of the kind would ultimately tend to shorten the life of the individual—which seems to be borne out by the fact that all who live in the arctic regions are notoriously short-lived.

or adding to the quantity, of the food ingested,[1] since we know that while they occasionally increase the heat to an abnormal degree (fever), these methods frequently *lower* the temperature, by lowering the patient's vitality (by plugging up the connective tissue with an excess of food), when it becomes obvious that the reverse process is the correct one to follow, because the temperature of the body is frequently higher at the end of a protracted fast than it was at its commencement. A normal temperature indicates a normal condition, and the presence of sufficient vitality; and when the temperature is above or below this, abnormal conditions are present. In either case, our object should be to elevate or to reduce the temperature to normal, and this can only be effected by removing the causes that rendered it ab- or sub-normal; and this is done by removing the excess of effete material (food material) which is clogging the system, and rendering its fullest capacity for life and enjoyment impossible.

[1] "We cannot raise the temperature of animals above the normal standard by increasing the supply of hydrocarbons in the food, nor can we arrest the production of heat by depriving animals of the so-called calorific principles." ("The Source of Muscular Power," by Austin Flint, M.D., etc., p. 14.) Says Doctor Walter ("The Exact Science of Health," p. 173): "The fact is, the quantity of heat possessed appears to bear little relation to the food eaten, showing that there is some other source of heat in the human body than chemical affinity. Heat is the product of vital activity just as surely as of chemical action."

BOOK IV

HYGIENIC AUXILIARIES AVAILABLE DURING A FAST

BOOK IV

CHAPTER I

AIR AND BREATHING

IT MAY almost be said that the only point upon which modern hygienic and orthodox medical writers even tend to agree is the advocation of an unlimited supply of fresh, pure air. Even here, the agreement is but partial; it is by no means complete. For, whereas the hygienic physician advocates a plentiful supply of pure air at all times—from the moment he is born[1]—and in all places, the orthodox practitioner frequently denies his suffering patient this privilege, and for the same absurd reason that he administers poisons, *viz.*, that the same agencies are not good for the well and the sick alike; and what is freely acknowledged to be beneficial to the well man, is denied the sick patient, who stands in far greater need of every assistance which hygiene and Nature can offer.

Before I proceed, then, I wish my position to be distinctly understood; *viz.*, that out-of-door, pure air is not only admissable, but absolutely essential to the patient, at all times, under all circumstances, in all diseases.

It would be impossible for me to thoroughly justify my position in the limited space that I can devote to it, in a work of this character; but I cannot help making a few comments upon this greatest of all blunders—shutting off the outside air, under the impression that it causes "colds," or in other ways aggravates diseased conditions. Let us go back for a moment to

[1] Says J. P. Muller ("My System," p. 19–20): "My two little boys are bigger and healthier than any other children of the same age I have ever seen. The elder only slept with closed windows the first ten days of his life . . and the younger has never, either summer or winter, been in a room with closed windows since the night he was born"

some primary considerations. First, it must be understood that air is, in a sense, our most important *food.* "We can live for weeks without solid food, for days without water, but only for a few minutes without air." Deep, full breathing is of the very greatest importance at all times. One reason is that it thoroughly exercises the diaphragm and the muscular walls of the chest; and a thorough action of the diaphragm acts very beneficially in massaging the bowels, and in exercising the entire abdominal viscera. This would enable us to understand the beneficial effects of a "crying spell." Like laughter, this has exercised the diaphragm which, in turn, has stimulated the internal organs into greater activity. There is, therefore, a purely physiological reason for the good effects of both laughter and crying—the increased action of the diaphragm—and the results from such increased action must necessarily be beneficial —quite apart from all purely psychic influence.

It is true that the beneficial effects of a crying spell might be explained upon altogether different lines. Thus, Doctor Oswald, in his "Household Remedies" (p. 216), says:

"The Roman gladiators shouted and laughed aloud while their wounds were being dressed. A scalded child sobs and gasps for a therapeutical purpose: instinct teaches it the readiest way to benumb the feeling of pain. The physiological *rationale* of all this is that *rapid breathing is an anæsthetic.*"

Why this should be so long remained a puzzle, but the correct answer is probably that given by Doctor Kitchen, when he says:[1]

"With too rapid respiration the blood gets too much charged with oxygen, and the carbonic acid gas does not escape with its usual rapidity; and an excess of either or both of these gases in the blood acts as an anæsthetic upon the nerve centers."

On the other hand, we must remember that:

"A complete unconsciousness to pain is attended with an extremely feeble and sometimes almost imperceptible respiration."[2]

Feeble respiration in a lesser degree is, as we know, the cause of clogging of the lung tissue and of yawning.[3] This latter is

[1] "The Diaphragm," p. 52.
[2] Trall: "Popular Physiology," p. 151.
[3] "Yawning," by Henrietta Russell, p. 36.

a reflex action caused by bad air in the lungs, and it is the gymnastic chosen by Nature to awaken the respiratory organs into activity.

Upon respiration depends life, and we depend upon our lungs from moment to moment for the maintenance of our lives. As every plant and every living animal needs light and air for its healthful and perfect development, so man needs these agencies, and without them disease and death would soon result. As an example of the deadly effect of impure air upon the organism I need only cite one case. It is the following:

". . . It is stated, with much regret, that in a certain tunnel, notwithstanding every precaution being taken, all the men engaged in driving the drainage heading by means of a tunneling machine have died; and in the case of the first Vyrnwy tunnel crossing of the river Mersey—driven by Greathead shield under pressure—the mortality was great."[1]

For consider! With every breath inspired about thirty cubic inches of air are drawn into the lungs; and with every expiration nearly an equal amount of foul gases are expelled. And when we consider that a man breathes twenty times a minute, on the average, or 28,800 times every twenty-four hours[2] it becomes obvious what a tremendous task the lungs daily perform.

The blood, in passing through the lungs, has undergone certain chemical changes[3] becoming purified—being transformed from the foul, purple, venous blood, to the pure, scarlet, arterial blood—and giving up its impure matter in solution, which is expelled by means of the breath. The lungs are thus an important excretory or eliminating organ; and are commonly so regarded; but the extreme significance of this fact is hardly recognized by the majority of the medical fraternity. Let us take one case by way of illustration. A man is strangled—an operation which takes but a few moments, at the outside.

[1] "The Great Alpine Tunnels," by Francis Fox, M.I.C.E., p. 621.

[2] "Health, Strength and Power," by Dr. Dudley A. Sargent, p. 92.

[3] Not altogether chemical, as is commonly supposed. Says H. de Varigny ("Air and Life," p. 529): "Living tissues absorb oxygen indirectly and will not tolerate it when directly supplied." Although this fact would not actually prove that the process was *vital*, it very strongly suggests it, it seems to me—necessitating some sort of "digestion" in order to fit it for the organism's needs.

Here, death followed upon the exclusion of the atmosphere. Now, in this instance, death followed in an extremely short space of time; but for what reason? Is it because air, as such, was not admitted into the lungs, and they were not permitted to contract and expand, and to fill the air cells? By no means! Most people seem to imagine that they are constructed somewhat on the order of a pair of bellows, and that, when the forced draught is suspended, death results. But this is not the real cause of death. In such cases—as indeed in all cases of suspended breathing—death results from poisoning the system by toxic matter in the blood, which has failed to become aërated in its passage through the lungs. The blood of the strangled or suffocated man is nearly *black*—the deadly effects of allowing the blood to circulate even once or twice through the system without being purified. And this is sufficient to induce death! What a tremendous amount of toxic matter our systems must daily manufacture and eliminate for such a result to follow in so short a time! We can readily see how any disease may thus accumulate, consequent upon the inactivity or blockage of one of the eliminating organs; indeed, the only wonder is that the human race is as well as it is!

But to return to the influence of fresh air in diseased conditions. It is a well-known fact that about three thousand cubic feet of fresh air are needed each hour by each person,[1] and if this is not supplied by free circulation through open windows, evil results are bound to follow.[2]

There is a widespread delusion that fresh air—while it may be healthful and advantageous to those in a normal condition, or even in the majority of diseases, still, it is harmful, or even dangerous in others! Pneumonia is one of these. Surely, in no disease have so many antiquated notions been so long retained as in this. A patient suffering from this disease is carefully guarded from the slightest breath of cold, pure air. The clogged, diseased lungs are deprived of their chief hope and support, in their attempts to bring about a recovery. Only "stuffy," fetid

[1] "Hygiene," by Nodder and Firth, p. 30; "Hand-Book of Sanitary Information," by R. S. Tracy, p. 16.

[2] See, in this connection, Schofield: "Nerves in Order," p. 83; Gibbs: "Ambulance Lectures," p. 19; Page: "The Horse," p. 12; etc.

disease-soaked atmosphere is permitted the patient; every breath of cold air (that greatest of all arresters of decomposition, putrefaction, and diseased conditions) is carefully excluded—a course which, without doubt, is responsible for the fearful mortality in cases of pneumonia, and its almost universally fatal consequences. This superstition alone sends its thousands to the grave. Doctor Page's system of supplying the patient air that has been rendered extremely cold, artificially, by being passed through an ice-packed case, has been followed by him for years, with the result that the percentage of deaths from this disease, in his practice, is practically *nil.*[1] One would think that such an object lesson would have *some* influence over the prevailing treatment of this disease; yet it does not seem to have done so![2]

I have already spoken of this superstition of the evil effects of cold air in connection with "colds." The fear of "draughts" is one of the greatest and most harmful delusions of the age.[3] The mistaken idea that the cold is the disease itself, and not the process of cure; and the confusion of ideas existing between "caused" and "occasioned" is responsible for this widespread superstition—to the point, indeed, as Doctor Oswald so well said: "Of mistaking the cause for a cure, and the most effective cure for the cause of the disease." As this author says elsewhere:[4]

"The truth is, that cold air often reveals the existence of a disease. It initiates the reconstructive process, and thus apparently the disease itself, but there is a wide difference between a proximate and an original cause. . . . The vital energy of a person breathing the stagnant air of an unventilated stove-room is often inadequate to the task of undertaking a restorative process—through the respiratory organs, clogged with phlegm and all kinds of impurities, may be sadly in need of relief. But, during a sleigh ride, or a few hours sleep before a window left open

[1] "Natural Cure," p. 102.

[2] Since this was written, Dr. I. C. Fisher, superintendent of the Presbyterian Hospital, New York City, and other physicians have come forward as staunch advocates of the "open air treatment" of pneumonia. It is to be hoped their experiments and conclusions will shortly revolutionize medical practice along these lines.

[3] "Deep Breathing," by Sophia Marquise A. Ciccolina, p. 42.

[4] "Physical Education," pp. 249–50.

by accident, the bracing influence of the fresh air revives the drooping vitality, and Nature avails herself of the chance to begin repairs; the lungs reveal their diseased condition, *i.e.*, they proceed to rid themselves of the accumulated impurities. Persistent in-door life would have aggravated the evil by postponing the crisis, or by turning a temporary affection into a chronic disease. But in a plurality of cases Nature will seize upon even a transient improvement of the external circumstances: a cold night that disinfects the atmosphere of the bedroom in spite of closed windows, a draught of cold air from an adjoining room, or one of those accidental exposures to wind and weather which the veriest slave of the cold air superstition cannot always avoid."

Another subject I should like to mention in passing, whose importance is second to none. I refer to what some hygienic writers have so happily called the "night air superstition." The belief that "night air"—or, more usually, *damp* night air, is injurious, is so deeply rooted in the public mind that it will, in all probability, be many years before this silly superstition is fully eradicated. The belief that night air is detrimental to the patient can, of course, be most readily shown to be a preposterous delusion. As Doctor Densmore pointed out:[1]

"We cannot breathe any other air than night air during the night; all that can be done is to close the windows, and make the interior air impure by the exhalations from the lungs. It is just the same night air as that which is excluded by the closed windows; but while the latter is uncontaminated and invigorating, the latter is foul and debilitating; and whoever will make the experiment will find the same advantage in getting pure air at night as is found in getting it in the day time."

Indeed, it has been said on excellent authority that "of the twenty-four hours, the night air is by far the purest."[2] How can the oncoming of darkness affect the purity of the air? Its composition is certainly not changed; and this being so, the only possible objections that can be raised to night air are (1) that it is colder; and (2) that it is damper, than the air breathed in the day time. Let us examine these objections in turn.

[1] "How Nature Cures," pp. 80–1.
[2] "The Baby," by Marianna Wheeler, p. 16.

(1) Suppose that the night air is somewhat colder, what then? The fall in temperature is only that of a few degrees, as a rule, and, even were it considerably more than this, I ask, what then? Is not the temperature of the day air, in winter, far colder than night air in the spring or fall—to say nothing of the summer? And are we not accustomed to far greater, more severe and more sudden changes of temperature in the winter, when leaving a heated building, and emerging into the freezing atmosphere?[1]

No one thinks of such sudden changes because, forsooth, the sun happens to be shining at the time! It is not "night air" and consequently cannot be harmful! How ridiculous it is! What is the gradual and regular decline of a few degrees F. compared with this? Has not the position only to be stated in order to necessitate its own refutation?

(2) But the principal argument against night air is that it is *damp*. That such an objection ever gained public credence at all is due solely to the absurd doctrines universally prevalent. The air is dangerous because it is damp! Does not every medical man know that the mucous lining of the nose and throat *are purposely moistened by nature in order that every particle of air inhaled may be thoroughly dampened, before it reaches the lungs;* and that no air ever reaches the lungs, in health, that is not thus thoroughly dampened by nature, purposely? Says Dr. A. R. Baker:[2]

"Careful experiments have shown that no matter how dry the atmosphere inhaled, as soon as it has passed through the nostrils, it is completely saturated with moisture."

Further, when, for any reason, the passages become diseased or artificially opened—as, *e.g.*, in cases of "cut-throat," in which the wind pipe has been severed—the air must be rendered, not only warm, but *damp* in order to preserve, as nearly as possible, natural conditions! Thus, in detailing the treat-

[1] I myself have known this change to have occurred. While living in Minneapolis, Minn., I have suddenly emerged from an office building, heated to 80° F., on to the street, in which the temperature was 38° F. below zero an *instantaneous* drop of some 118° F.!

[2] "Coughs, Colds and Catarrh," p. 7.

ment for cut-throat (arresting the hemorrhage, etc.), Doctor Osborn goes on to say:[1]

"The patient must likewise be kept in a warm and moist atmosphere by means of a bronchitis-kettle placed on the fire in the room. Ordinarily the air passing through the mouth is freed from all foreign bodies, moistened by the saliva, and warmed by its passage across the mucous membrane of the mouth and throat, and the above directions are carried out to supply these several deficiencies."

All these facts are known to the medical man. Now, the question arises: knowing this (and he must) wherein lies the supposed danger of night air? In what possible manner can it prove harmful or dangerous? Our lungs merely receive air which has been partially moistened by atmospheric changes, instead of altogether moistened by the mucous membrane of our nose, throat and bronchial tubes. (We should never breathe through the mouth, under any circumstances.)[2] That this can be considered injurious and less healthful to invalids than the foul, disease-impregnated atmosphere of the closed-in room, will doubtless be looked upon as one of those singular delusions which dominated the human race for so long a time, when its clear-sightedness was, in almost every other direction, manifesting itself most markedly.[3]

Full, deep breathing, then, is one of Nature's sovereign remedies for diseased conditions of any character whatever; pure air, containing an abundance of oxygen, being the greatest of all germicides, of all disinfectants. On this question, Florence Nightingale doubtless went to the heart of the matter, when she said:[4]

"Let no one ever depend upon fumigations, 'disinfectants,' and the like, for purifying the air. The offensive thing, not its smell, must be removed. A celebrated medical lecturer began one day,

[1] "First Aid: Ambulance Lectures," p. 49.

[2] Doctor Densmore, in his "How Nature Cures," pp. 96–7, cites a long list of evils resultant from mouth breathing—diseased gums, teeth, and nasal passages, and deformed jaws being some of the most noticeable of these. See also Doctor Patchen "How Should We Breathe?" p. 16; Wagner "Habitual Mouth Breathing;" Yogi Ramacharaka: "The Hindu-Yogi Science of Breath," p. 25, etc.

[3] "Natural Hygiene," by H. Lahmann, M.D., p. 5.

[4] "Notes on Nursing," p. 23.

'Fumigations, gentlemen, are of essential importance. They make such an abominable smell that they compel you to open the window.'"[1]

Cool, pure air never hindered or aggravated any disease, nor retarded its progress; but the practice of excluding, of carefully guarding against fresh air, as though it were the greatest of poisons, is doubtless one of the most dangerous delusions of the age.

"The difference between fresh air in motion and stagnant indoor air is that between the pure water of a running fountain and the festering slime of a cesspool."

Or, as Doctor Oswald so well said:[2]

"The act of re-inspiring air, which has already been subjected to the process of pulmonary digestion, is thus precisely analogous to the act of a famished animal devouring its own fæces, and if performed habitually cannot fail to be attended with equally ruinous consequences."

See also Black: "Long Life and How to Reach It," p. 61–2. The question of cold air on the *surface* of the body (air bath), I shall consider on pp. 364, 375.

I shall close with two final reflections. (1) It has frequently been asserted that *conscious* breathing is essential if health is to be maintained. To this I would reply that no other animal but man breathes in this manner, yet all enjoy better health. If his food habits were managed differently, this breathing would not be necessary. (2) It has frequently been stated that no man need fear consumption who carries his chest well out. To this I would reply that apes and all monkeys are exceptionally flat and even hollow chested, in their native state, and yet never contract consumption until they enter captivity. This would certainly indicate that it is the foul air and the improper food that causes the consumption, rather than the position of the chest, in cases of this character. The chest may be almost as hollow as you like, provided the lungs are not called upon to oxidize off such an abundance of food material. I have discussed this question at some length, however, in *Appendix M.*

[1] It is interesting to note that the latest authorities tend to agree with this view; see Crandall: "How to Keep Well," p. 56.

[2] "Physical Education," p. 88.

CHAPTER II

BATHING

"Cleanliness is Next to Godliness"

THE skin is one of the most important depurating organs of the body; the amount of effete matter which is sometimes thrown off through this channel being almost incredible. As much as two pints of water—containing various noxious gases and other impurities in solution (and occasionally even much more than this)[1]—is daily eliminated from the body through this channel alone; and that its prompt removal is necessary, if health is to be maintained, goes without saying. The great importance of thorough and frequent bathing is becoming more and more recognized; yet most persons do not, I am persuaded, bathe half enough—even those persons who consider themselves models of cleanliness. For the average person, who does not consider him- or herself an invalid, and who follows anything like the usual dietetic habits of the majority, one Turkish (cabinet) bath weekly, and one or two baths daily, should be taken throughout the year; a cold bath in the morning, upon arising; and a warmer one in the evening, just before retiring—followed, invariably, by a cool sponge-off. At this latter bath, soap should be occasionally employed.[2]

[1] "The Skin in Health and Disease," by George Black, M.D., p. 31.

[2] I shall not attempt now to answer those hygienists who are opposed to the use of soap, on the ground that it "chokes the pores," "is unnecessary," etc. I am certain that, *under existing dietetic conditions*, much oily material is excreted which cannot be properly removed by water alone. In all cases of skin diseases, this is especially apparent, and a week's trial should convince the most skeptical that soap, containing some weak vegetable oil, is a highly important auxiliary to the bathing process. If the body were in a perfect state of health, and the diet simple, non-stimulating and abstemious, I quite agree that soap, as well as the quantity of bathing advocated, would be quite unnecessary. But these conditions are ideal—not real, at least so far as we find them in the vast majority of cases; and in all diseased conditions, the necessity is, of course, all the more urgent, since elimination is, at that time, proceeding with even more than usual rapidity.

The great fear of the average person is that "so much bathing is debilitating." Of course everything can be abused, no matter how good it may be, and bathing is no exception to this rule. Remaining for too long a period in water, at any temperature, is undoubtedly debilitating; but the bath should never be protracted to such extreme lengths. Cold baths should generally last but a few seconds, and never more than a few minutes, in duration; their tonic and stimulating effects upon the skin are all that are desired. If there is no reaction, you may be sure that harm, instead of good, results from the bath.[1] If swimming, the bath may, of course, be considerably lengthened, owing to the vigorous exercise taken. "Medicated baths" are of no greater value than plain water—the stimulating effects of the one being as easily duplicated by the plain water treatment, and I make this statement after reading the statements and theories advanced in, *e.g.*, "The Artificial Nauheim Bath" (New York). Warm baths, also, should last but a few minutes, the practice of lying and "soaking" in the bath being exceedingly reprehensible—rendering the skin flabby, anæmic and inactive. A quick scrub in hot water, followed by a cool shower, will produce only beneficial results; and, so long as this course is followed, the bath may be indulged in daily, throughout the year, without any fear whatever of its debilitating results.

These bathing processes should never by any chance be made too heroic. Kneipp himself warns us against this fallacy,[2] while Doctor Trall repeatedly urged that the treatment, both as to temperature and duration, be modified to suit the patient.[3]

Doctor Dewey, arguing against frequent bathing, contended that, since the material to be washed away is already on the surface of the body, it is unnecessary to bathe so frequently as we do—the effete matter, in other words, having been already eliminated when it reaches the skin. The sweat glands cannot absorb anything but the very smallest percentage of water, once eliminated in this manner—the sweat glands being eliminating, not absorbing organs—"little valves whose doors open in but one direction," so to speak. We must further remember

[1] "How to Take Baths," by Harriet M. Austin, M.D., p. 6.
[2] "My Water Cure," by Seb. Kneipp, p. 6.
[3] "The Bath," p. 12; "Water Cure for the Million," p. 20.

that these glands are spiral in shape,[1] and hence they cannot readily absorb any water or other liquid placed upon the surface of the skin—"rubbed into it"—the fallacy of "flesh foods," etc., thus becoming manifest.

Doctor Dewey contended then, that, for these reasons, the surface only need be kept clean, and the under-garments changed repeatedly in order to ensure perfect cleanliness and an active skin.[2]

This argument is open, I believe, to two objections. First, the fact is altogether overlooked that bathing *stimulates* the function of the skin, rendering the process of elimination more rapid and effectual than it would otherwise be. Second, granting that the valves open in but one direction, and that no matter once eliminated, can, consequently, flow back into the system—having once passed this valve (been eliminated)—it is obvious that we must, nevertheless, *keep the valve itself clean*, and prevent it from becoming choked and blocked with the effete material constantly passing through it. That this might happen, has, it seems, been altogether overlooked. I think it is also probably true that:

> "Water cure (Nature cure) provides, by provoking perspiration for the expulsion of diseased matter—excites the action of the skin and so enables it to fulfill its second function, the respiring of air."[3]

I am quite willing to admit, however, that were our dietetic and other hygienic habits perfect, bathing would be practically unnecessary. Even Doctor Trall, an ardent apostle of the water cure, acknowledged this when he wrote:[4]

> "If our habits were in all respects normal, the skin would perform its depurating function without bathing, as well as the mucous membrane, within, can do its duty without washing. But the improper ingesta and the foreign substances constantly taken into the system through the media of the digestive organs, lungs, and skin, necessitate more or less bathing, to enable the

[1] "The Skin in Health and Disease," by George Black, M.D., p. 14.
[2] "No-Breakfast Plan," p. 203.
[3] "Health and the Various Methods of Cure," p. 44.
[4] "Popular Physiology," pp. 210–11.

system to rid itself of some of them, through the cutaneous emunctory."

Constant bathing, in other words, is only rendered necessary because we keep filling the system with an excessive amount of impure and gross material calling for elimination; and it can readily be seen that by proper regulation of the diet, etc., we can dispense with such constant bathing; also to what extent *fasting* would act as a corrective measure, and hence never necessitate the water cure at all! And of the two processes of elimination, fasting is the safer, the more natural—in every way, the superior method. This is even acknowledged to be so, in certain cases, at least, by one of the greatest of American water-curists, Doctor Shew, when he wrote:[1]

"Now, in such cases, the water treatment, good as it is, comes in my estimation, far short of what may be accomplished by fasting alone. In these cases, and there are not a few of them, let the patient abstain resolutely from all food three or four days and he will be convinced of the advantages to be derived from the course."

The water cure, after all, treats only the *effects* of over-nutrition—and does not strike directly at the *cause*—as we do in the fasting cure.

Before entering into any details of the various bathing processes and their use as curative agents, in diseased conditions, it will be necessary for us briefly to consider the following facts: The skin of an average individual contains about two and one-half million perspiratory glands—the total length of which would, if added together, approximate two and a half miles.

"Each of its millions of sweat glands is actively and constantly engaged in separating from the blood impurities which would destroy life if retained. These foul products are poured out through a corresponding number of minute sewers, and deposited upon the surface of the body to the amount of several ounces each day, or several pounds, if the whole perspiration be included in the estimate, as is commonly done. The skin is also an organ of respiration; it absorbs oxygen, and exhales carbonic acid gas,

[1] "The Family Physician," by Joel Shew, M.D., p. 796.

with other poisonous gasses. The amount of respiratory labor performed by the skin is about one-sixtieth of that done by the lungs. In some of the lower animals, the whole work of respiration is performed by the skin. In the common frog, the respiratory action of the skin and of the lungs is about equal."[1]

It will readily be seen that these important changes and modifications should not be hindered in any way, but that, on the contrary, such organic efforts should be given free play. Clothing, when too heavy or too light, would very materially hinder all such variations (*v.* Chapter "The Clothing"), and insufficient bathing will also retard or materially check its healthful action. But the particular function to which I now call special attention is its power of *elimination.* The amount of effete material thrown off through this channel is sometimes extraordinary.[2] This material requires frequent removal or direful results will assuredly ensue.

The poisonous character of this excretion is perhaps brought home to us in those cases where, for some reason, the function of the skin has been altogether arrested—death invariably resulting, under such conditions, in a few hours. The cases of "tarred and feathered" atrocities are examples. In such cases death results from the poisoning of the system, due to defective elimination and undue retention of effete material generated within the body.

If, now, an active skin is so necessary for the restoration and preservation of health; and if the application of water is effective in bringing this activity and elimination into being, it is obvious that bathing, in its various forms, is of great value in thus assisting in the process of purification—and this fact is the basis of the much-scoffed-at "water cure." A more rational system of medication it would hardly be possible to conceive.

But if the baths are to afford the maximum degree of benefit with the least drain of the patient's vitality, they must be administered in a most judicious and careful manner. Simply "soaking" the patient in water will hardly have the beneficial

[1] "The Uses of Water," by J. H. Kellogg, M.D., pp. 18–19; see also "Muscle Beating," by C. Klemm, p. 14.

[2] "How to Bathe," by E. P. Miller, M.D., p. 42; Kellogg: "The Uses of Water," pp. 25–6.

results. The time required for the bath in each case; the character of the bath administered; the temperature of the water; the time of day, and a hundred other things, must be taken into consideration. This is no place to elaborate the various processes of the water cure, and the various methods of its application. For this I would refer the reader to Doctor Trall's "Water Cure for the Million," and the same author's "The Bath: Its History and Uses."

I must briefly indicate, however, a few of the more important and useful baths, treating only one method at length—the Turkish bath—for the reason that gross and often dangerous blunders can be, and often are, made in administering these baths. Much interesting material exists, and might be written, relating to all the bathing processes, but in a work of this character, such discussion would be out of place. For a description of the actual bathing processes, I cannot do better than to quote Doctor Trall, whose terse, lucid exposition might, indeed, be considered classical. He says ("Water Cure for the Million," pp. 13–19):

"*Bandages and Compresses.* These are wet cloths applied to any weal, sore, hot, painful, or diseased part, and renewed so often as they become dry or very warm. The best surgeons have, in all ages, employed 'water dressings' alone in local wounds, injuries, and inflammations. They may be warming or cooling to the part, as they are covered or not with dry cloths.

"*Fomentations.* These are employed for relaxing muscles, relieving spasms, griping, nervous headache, etc. Any cloths wet in hot water and applied so warm as can be borne generally answer the purpose; but flannel cloths, dipped in hot water, and wrung nearly dry in another cloth or handkerchief, so as to steam the part moderately, are the most efficient sedatives. They are usually employed from five to fifteen minutes. They are useful in such cases of severe constipation, colic, dysmenorrhea, hysteria, etc.

"*Hip or Sitz-Bath.* The water should just cover the hips and the lower part of the abdomen. Knead the abdomen with the hand or fingers during the bath."

As the Turkish (cabinet) bath takes the place of the wet-sheet pack, for all practical purposes, and as all the other baths are of comparative unimportance, I refrain from further quotation —merely adding one other method, known to but few persons. I might designate it the "salt-rub bath." Stand in the bath tub, which may, or may not, contain water. Take a handful of dry, coarse salt and moisten it slightly with water—just enough to dampen it, without rendering it slimy. Now rub the body vigorously and quickly with this salt, using the partially open hand as if rubbing the salt into the body. When this salt has been used up, take another handful and proceed as before. The entire body may thus be gone over in from two to three minutes, or it may extend to five minutes, if desired. Finish by sponging or spraying the entire surface with warm and then cool water; when a general invigoration or glow will be felt—rarely equalled in a lifetime, by those who have never taken such a bath. This may be followed, if desired, by an air bath, but that is not really necessary, since it practically constitutes one in itself.

The Turkish (Cabinet) Bath

The Turkish bath is also highly beneficial and an important remedial agent. The thorough flushing which the pores of the skin receive, during this bath, and the consequent elimination from the body of morbific material, render this method of treatment at once speedy and effective; and *physiologically* cleanses the cutaneous surface more thoroughly than any amount of washing could possibly accomplish,[1] since this latter method merely removes morbid material which has already been brought to the surface, without in any way assisting to bring it there, as does the former method.

The introduction of the cabinet (folding) bath is in one sense superior to all public Turkish baths, for the reason that, in the cabinet type, cool, pure air is available for the lungs throughout; and the head is also kept at a comfortable temperature. Two or three such baths may be taken weekly (if taken correctly) without the least fear of any debilitating effects. On the contrary, nothing but benefit will result from such a course. Baths

[1] Says Doctor Black ("Sea Air and Sea Bathing," pp. 10–11)· "Many a 'sweaty' laborer is actually cleaner than those who would call him dirty, and shrink from contact with him."

protracted for too great a length of time or improperly administered, may cause exhaustion and debility, but this will never happen if proper care be used. Profuse perspiration, such as the Turkish bath occasions, is frequently induced in violent or even moderate exercise in tropical climates, and this occasional flushing of the pores is in every way beneficial and of great assistance in exciting the over-torpid skin into action, and in assisting to rid the body of its overplus of impure material.

In taking this bath in the home, the following directions should be carefully followed—since the advice contained therein has been dearly bought, and is the result of repeated experiments and observations upon a large number of individuals.

Prior to entering the bath, copious draughts of water should be taken, and cool water should be drunk throughout the progress of the bath, whenever thirst or faintness seem to indicate its desirability. The object of this is to supply all the requisite fluid from which the system may draw while the excessive elimination of water (in the form of perspiration) is in progress.

Just before entering a bath, the head, the face and the neck should be sponged off in *warm* water, this having the effect (by reaction) of keeping the head cool when the bath commences. The result will be a cool head through the early stage of the bath.

No hesitation need be felt in wetting the scalp after the bath, the perspiration of the scalp rendering it moist, in any case. It has been repeatedly shown, moreover, that frequent washing and extreme cleanliness are as essential to the scalp as to any other part of the body—the effect of water upon the hair being beneficial and strengthening, however frequently applied, *provided the hair is thoroughly dried.*[1]

During the progress of the bath, signs of discomfiture may be allayed by the drinking of cool water and the application of cloths to the forehead which have been dipped in cold water and wrung out just sufficiently dry to prevent their dripping. If these transitory symptoms—faintness, etc.—are withstood, however, they will almost invariably disappear in a few seconds; and I believe that, in many cases, it is far better to allow the

[1] See Macfadden's "New Hair Culture," pp. 96–7; Mrs. Lee's "How to Care for the Hair at all Times," p. 37.

head and face to perspire freely than to check this action by continued cold applications. As in all other cases, this must, of course, be adapted to the idiosyncrasy of the patient.

The bath should be continued for from ten minutes to half an hour, according to the patient's condition and the effects of the bath upon him. Immediate and profuse perspiration will, of course, tend to terminate the bath far sooner than in those cases where perspiration is scant and laborious. This latter condition denotes a torpid, anæmic, inactive skin; indeed, it may almost be said that the extent of the patient's vitality and his bodily health can be gauged by the degree of responsiveness of his skin. Where the skin is vigorous and active, and the pores are open, and quick and effective response will ensue in every case.

The greatest care should be taken not to overdo this bath; that is, to make it last too long. Rather make it too short in duration than the reverse. Great harm may be done by prolonging the bath after the sensation of dizziness, faintness, lassitude, headache or nausea indicate that the bath has already continued too long, and that the body is being overheated to an uncalled for, or even a dangerous extent. This may even undo much of the benefit that has previously been obtained from the bath. Doctor Trall indeed, goes so far as to say:[1]

"The average time for its beneficial employment is from fifteen to thirty minutes. But if employed one minute too long, more injury may be received from it, the last minute, than benefit in the preceding twenty-nine minutes. So long as vigorous circulation is maintained, in the vessels of the skin, no harm can come of the vapor bath. But the moment the skin becomes so relaxed that congestion or engorgement takes place in the minute capillary vessels, and the millions of glands of the cutaneous surface, permanent injury is done. When these vessels are stretched to a certain degree beyond their normal diameter, depuration ceases; and if the heating process is persisted in, the system, instead of cleansing itself of waste and effete matters, pours out the serum of the blood to defend its surface against the excessive heat; and this overheating and oversweating become as exhausting to the vitality of the patient as drastic purging or copious bleeding."

[1] "The Bath: Its History and Uses," p. 28.

To one other matter I should like to call attention. Almost without exception, every book or pamphlet dealing with the Turkish bath has advocated the "sponging of the body with tepid water" after coming out of the bath. I am strongly opposed to this slack method of finishing an otherwise energetic treatment. From observation upon myself, and that of others whom I have persuaded to give the matter a trial, I have found that a thorough scrub in hot water is even more important at this time than at any other. The skin is intensely active. A very great quantity of effete material has been brought to the surface during the bath—some considerable quantity of which must be still upon the surface of the skin. Further, the pores, now working freely, are rapidly bringing to the surface this morbid matter for elimination, and, if these pores are suddenly closed—as by a cold water shower, *e.g.*—this elimination of effete material must be suddenly checked—the results of which cannot be other than detrimental. That a very large amount of "dirt" is present upon the surface of the body, even after a Turkish bath, with its consequent thorough flushing of the pores, is obvious to anyone taking a hot scrub bath as suggested. The color of the water will leave no room for doubt upon that point! It is inconceivable that anyone should again recommend a mere "sponging in tepid water" who has once tried the above experiment upon himself, or noted it in others.

CHAPTER III

CLOTHING

THE most important question that arises in considering this question of dress is that of practical utility. Of what *use* are clothes? What are their relations to the vital economy? For what reason do we wear them? The answers to all these questions will doubtless at once present themselves to my readers:

"To warm the body, of course; to keep the skin protected from the vicissitudes of the weather; to keep it warm and comfortable; to prevent the body from becoming burned or frozen—in a word, to protect the skin from the extremes of heat and cold, and to maintain the body in a state of perpetual natural warmth—these are the practical uses of clothes."

Though these statements are true in a general sense, they are not altogether true in the sense that most people imagine. Clothes do not add heat to the body under any circumstances whatever; clothes never *produce* heat; their sole purpose is to prevent loss of heat (by radiation and evaporation). No amount of clothing would warm a corpse, for the simple reason that there is no heat in the body to prevent escaping—clearly showing that clothes, *per se*, do not and cannot add one particle of heat to the body's natural warmth. Their sole and only use is to prevent undue loss of this bodily heat, and the clothes which will most effectually accomplish this are those which we should select *ceteris paribus*, for wearing purposes.[1]

Since man is the only animal who artificially clothes himself, and since lack of bodily warmth is the only reason—or the most

[1] I have been considering in the above only one side of the argument, *viz.*, that of keeping the body warm in cold weather, and have omitted all consideration of the other side, *viz.*, that of keeping the body cool in warm weather, for the reason that this is of so far less importance, for all practical purposes, that we can afford to ignore it. Throughout, in the text, I shall therefore, consider the other side of the argument only.

important reason—for his adopting and wearing clothes at all, it follows that only sufficient clothing should be worn to serve that purpose—any additional clothing merely tending to overheat the body and clog the pores of the skin by preventing their perfect and normal action. Whatever clothes are not actually needed, therefore, should be discarded, and it is only the prevailing prudishness and slavery to custom that prevents people from discarding practically *all* their clothes in the summer time. It is purely a question of habit. True hygienists everywhere look with contempt upon the vicious prudery which is rampant to-day; a fanatical desire to keep covered every possible portion of the human body; mere hypocrisy, under cover of which vices pervade all classes of society, and, I may add, always exist in direct (not inverse) ratio to this effectual bodily concealment.

If, now, the chief object of clothes is the purpose of keeping the body protected from extreme cold—they should be used for that purpose only; and should obviously be so constructed that they cover *evenly* every portion of the body, without undue superfluity of clothing in any one part, coupled with undue exposure in another. If any parts of the body are to be clothed more warmly than others, these should be the extremities—the arms and legs, the hands and feet, since these are the parts furthest removed from the vital centers, and consequently supplied with only a comparatively small quantity of blood and vitality, while the body proper, possessing by far the greater proportion of blood and vital force, should be kept comparatively cool, and clothed far more lightly than the extremities. In other words, since man is forced to live in what is, to him, an abnormal temperature, he must use artificial means to balance the circulation, and to keep it normal. It is hardly necessary, in this connection, to point out the fact that most persons follow the opposite course, wrapping up their bodies to an absurd and even dangerous extent—while recklessly exposing and neglecting their extremities. As Dr. Harriet N. Austin said:[1]

"   the arms being less thickly covered than the trunk, unequal distribution of blood is produced."

[1] "Health Dress," p. 2.

Unfortunately, this foolish and perverse custom is not only tolerated, but actually *advised* by the medical profession to-day.

If there is one part of the body that should be protected, it is the spinal cord, and if there is one part that can stand exposure with less harm than any other part of our vital economy, it is the chest. Yet doctors insist upon wrapping up the chest and protecting the least vulnerable portions, while paying little or no attention to the exceedingly delicate and sensitive spinal cord, with its intricate system of interweaving and outbranching nerves. "Whoever heard of anyone having a cold shiver down his chest?" humorously asked Mr. Warman. Who indeed!

And so, in recommending the use of "chest protectors," the medical profession once more proves the shallowness of its reasoning, and the absurdity of its methods of treatment—for the very obvious reason that every breath of air we draw into the lungs is (in cold weather) excessively cold, far below the temperature of the body, and must remain so, however great care be taken in breathing. This cannot be helped—it is a necessity, and obviously so. Here, then, we have the absurd practice recommended of protecting the lungs by wearing chest protectors of flannel, etc., though these same lungs are already protected by various thicknesses of clothes, by the ribs, and by the muscular and fatty tissue of the body, while, at the same time, we are, in breathing, taking cold air *right into the lung tissue itself*, and thereby bringing it into the closest possible vital contact with the nerves, tissues, and network of blood vessels throughout the inner surface of the lungs. Could anything be more absurd? Could any reasoning be more shallow, any treatment more ephemeral than this? And, the claim that all air breathed is warmed to the bodily temperature before it reaches the lung tissue is most certainly untrue. In mouth breathing, this is certainly not the case; and, even when nasal breathing is practiced, who has not noticed—when taking the first deep breath upon stepping out of doors, on an intensely cold day—that the cold air strikes the lungs most noticeably—giving rise to the instantaneous feeling of oppression, and even weight, upon the chest? Would this be true were the air rendered as warm as the lung tissue ere it encountered it? Certainly not.

The next question we must consider is this: all restrictive clothing should be abolished, as extremely injurious and detrimental. The use of garters, corsets, belts, tight collars, as well as too small gloves, shoes, etc., is altogether pernicious, and one of the greatest causes of disease, especially among women, that exists to-day. I cannot here dwell upon this point, merely referring the reader to the various books, magazines, etc., where the subject is treated sensibly, skillfully and at some length; but will note in passing that any article of clothing is too tight when it impedes the circulation of the blood in the slightest degree. Any article of clothing that is tight enough to be distinctly *felt* is too tight, and must ultimately lead to harmful and disastrous consequences—crushing the tissues, impeding the circulation, and rendering the muscles of that part of the body weak through inaction. It cannot fail to be decidedly injurious, and to render that part susceptible to disease, by lessening its blood supply, and consequently lowering its inherent vitality. "Every woman who has grown up in a corset, no matter how loosely worn, is deformed," says Doctor Kitchen.[1] "The pains and perils that attend birth are heightened, if not caused, by improper clothing," adds Dr. Mary Nichols,[2] while Doctor Peck asserted that "all cramping, binding, and confining of any part of the body weakens it."[3] These authors were arguing, of course, against the compression of our feet by leather shoes of improper fits and sizes, and in this connection I would call the reader's attention to the following argument against leather shoes which should call for the gravest consideration. It is:

"The foot should be as presentable as the hand, as healthy, sun-burned, and almost as pliable. It needs the purifying access of the air and the stimulating effects of the outdoor cold and heat. Instead of allowing it its freedom, we shut it up in a stiff, foul, unventilated prison, where its clammy pallor suggests vegetables that sprout in the dark cellar. We bind the toes together, and doom them to atrophy, until a foot is a thing to weep over."[4]

[1] "The Diaphragm," p. 87.
[2] "The Clothes Question," etc., p. 24.
[3] "The Dress and Care of the Feet," p. 99. See also Doctor Kahler's "Dress and Care of the Feet."
[4] "The Meat Fetish," by Ernest Crosby and Elisée Reclus, p. 18.

One can thus readily see why it is that "the nails of the feet are four times slower in their growth than those of the hands"[1] It may be interesting to note, in this connection—and it may strike my readers as a very novel view of the matter—that corns are caused, not so much by tight shoes, as by overfeeding! Says Doctor Rabagliati:[2]

"Corns are not due to pressure, but to pressure on toes nourished by a special sort of blood, *viz.*, by blood containing in it nutritive material in excess. The greater the excess of nutritive material, the greater the likelihood of the occurrence of corns. All blood must contain, or at least does contain, nutritive material in excess, and therefore may lay it down in the form of corns under the stimulus of pressure. But the blood can create nothing; it can convert many things, *e.g.*, nearly all sorts of food into all sorts of tissues. Corns are the indirect or reactionary effect of pressure, not the direct effect. The direct effect of pressure is to thin the skin, just as pressure thins or wears out the boot-sole. The indirect effect of pressure on living tissues is to thicken them."

I must now consider the subject of clothing from altogether another point of view. We have seen that clothes are useful only for the purpose of keeping the body warm; we know also that man is the only animal who artificially clothes himself. The question now arises: Why is it necessary for man to clothe himself in this manner—since no other animal does so? Inasmuch as man is not "naturally unnatural," why is it that he alone must provide himself and his progeny with clothes, when no other animal does so? Perhaps the answer might be given "Because man has no natural covering, such as fur, etc., which other animals have; his skin is more delicate and sensitive than theirs, rendered more so by generations of custom and habit." To this we may well ask, in reply: "How did man originally become thus sensitive and weak?" We can readily see that his thick covering of hair, which he shared at one time, undoubtedly, with his anthropoid brethren, may have become less thick and impermeable as clothes were adopted and worn, and its useful-

[1] "The Skin in Health and Disease," p. 29.
[2] "Aphorisms, Definitions, Reflections and Paradoxes," etc., pp. 184–5.

ness thus rendered unnecessary; but the question arises: "Why the necessity for clothes in the first place?" There must have been some period at which clothes were felt to be necessary for the first time, and, though this may have been partially due to the migration to and habitation of colder climates, by this prehistoric, semi-human race, it must have been partly due, I believe, to the lessened amount of vitality possessed by these tribes (due to—we cannot now tell what causes), and, when clothes were once adopted, a general weakening and degeneracy of the race would instantly commence—since, as I shall now attempt to show, the wearing of clothes invariably weakens and debilitates the organism of the wearer, lessening its vitality, and rendering it more or less diseased, or at least "predisposed" to disease.

"The skin exhales," says Doctor Reinhold,[1] "effete gaseous matter. Another portion is thrown off from the bowels in flatulence. The foul matter from both these sources is caught and condensed by the almost air-tight clothes, and a part of it reenters the skin, clogging the pores, and forming a layer of solid matter in and below the cuticle. This deposit depresses and stifles the action of the nerves, so that they desist from summoning the blood to the skin. Hence *the sensation of chilliness is only felt when the skin is inactive and anæmic.* The blood, having retreated from the surface, is congested within, and may lead to serious, even fatal results. Access of pure air to the skin stimulates its nerves, enabling all gaseous products to be removed as fast as they exude from the interior of the body. In this way the kidneys are relieved, and rheumatism, dropsy, etc., are avoided. . . . For health, the best underwear is none at all, and the worst, several layers of heavy woolens with extra protectors and pads of various kinds for special parts." (pp. 148–9.)

The main point is that the wearing of too many heavy clothes is undoubtedly a contributory cause of all diseases whatever, affecting most markedly and directly all skin affections, and greatly assisting in choking the body with impure material, by checking the healthy, normal action of the sweat glands and

[1] "Nature *vs.* Drugs," p. 145.

pores of the skin. Just enough clothes should be worn to prevent an undue and unpleasant sensation of cold; everything more than this is detrimental—whether the clothing be coats or underclothes in the day time, or night dresses and blankets at night.[1] We should accustom our bodies (by cold bathing, and by the exposure of the surface of the body to cold air), to withstand the changes of external temperature without discomfort—just as our hands and faces withstand it; and we should be enabled to expose our whole bodies with equal impunity—the results being altogether beneficial.

I have frequently spoken of the quantity of clothes as being too much. Suits, or, in the case of women, dresses, need not be altered to any appreciable degree—so long as they are not tight—or made of too heavy material. Overcoats may be of as heavy material as you like, provided the weather is really very cold, and, provided, also, that they are discarded immediately upon entering any warm apartment; and further, provided also that the underclothes are of the thinnest possible material consistent with cleanliness. Heavy woolen underclothing is not only unnecessary, no matter how severe the weather, but is decidedly prejudicial to health and in every way obnoxious and objectionable, for the following reasons.

I quote Doctor Densmore:[2]

"Recently . . . an agitation has been made in favor of linen underclothes instead of the woolen or Jaeger, which has heretofore been most popular. Woolen cloth, as long as it is dry, will protect the body against cold better than cloth made from any other material. However, wool, while slow to absorb moisture, is also slow to give it off, and after it has been worn for some hours, it has absorbed perspiration, and thereafter the body is clothed in damp garments. Linen is the best material for underwear; it absorbs moisture much more readily than wool, but it also more readily gives it off, and if the outside garments are in the least porous, the heat of the body soon expels all moisture from the linen, and the body is thus encased in dry,

[1] For an example of the actual danger of overdressing the body, see "The Training of Children," by James C. Jackson, M.D., pp. 38–9.

[2] "Consumption and Chronic Diseases," by Emmet Densmore, M.D., pp. 153, 165.

instead of damp, garments. Cotton is a compromise between wool and linen. It absorbs moisture much more readily than wool, and also is more readily dried bv the heat of the body. . . . The skin is thus enfeebled, has a poor blood circulation, and is poorly nourished; an exposure to a draught and a chill follow in due time, with the inevitable breakdown. Breathing vitiated air and wrapping our bodies in impervious garments have worked their fulll share of the havoc."

See also, in this connection, "The New Method in Health Culture," by W. E. Forest, M.D., pp. 320–3; and "Health In fluenced by Underwear," by Edward B. Warman, A.M., pp. 5, 6, 9, 10, etc. A discussion of the influence of the *color* of the the clothes on the health of the body is to be found in this book; in Doctor Babbitt's "Philosophy of Cure," and in Eaves' "The Color Cure."

CHAPTER IV

EXERCISE[1]

THE question of the amount of exercise desirable while fasting is a much disputed one; some hygienists claiming that, as fasting is, strictly speaking, a "rest cure"; and, as:

"Nature is able to restore the very sick to health without physical exertion, so she is able to keep the health duly maintained without special exercise."[2]

Others contend that exercise is as beneficial at this time as at any other—occupying the mind, and dispelling that languid feeling which so constantly attends the fasting cure. Writes Mr. Macfadden:[3]

"The first four days were the most uncomfortable. I did not seem especially hungry, but I was languid, except for a while after exercise, at which times I always felt strong and energetic."

The question, it will be seen, is therefore a vexed one, and requires careful consideration. Before proceeding to discuss the physiological effects of exercise on patients that are fasting, however, it will first be necessary for us to consider its effects in health, and its action on the normal body—meaning by this, the body which receives its daily allowance of food.

Exercise may be roughly defined as the use of the voluntary muscular system, by means of specific movements, more or less resistance being offered to the free play of the muscles involved in those movements. The alternate contraction and expansion

[1] Exercise, as we understand it, means muscular exercise, and voluntary exercise, at that. It is in this sense, accordingly, that I shall use the term.

[2] "No-Breakfast Plan," p. 98; "Experiences of the No-Breakfast Plan and the Fasting Cure," p. 38.

[3] "Fasting, Hydropathy and Exercise," p. 75; *Physical Culture*, Vol. III., p. 269.

of the muscle, and the extra amount of work involved thereby, breaks down an unusual number of cells in the muscular tissue thus exercised, and impure material begins at once to accumulate, as the result. This calls for an extra supply of blood to remove this effete material, which, in turn, necessitates a more rapid heart action. An extra amount of blood being thus forced through the lungs, these expand more fully, and perform their function more rapidly, in order to oxygenate the greater amount of blood forced through them; and thus we see that the effete material—the broken-down tissue—is removed as fast as created, and for this reason exercise is beneficial and not harmful to the organism. Further, it must be remembered, the blood, in circulating more swiftly and forcibly through the body, bathes and purifies every other organ or muscle, and every tissue and every cell in the body is indirectly benefited by the exercise of any one part, or set of muscles.

But this is but half the work which the blood performs—though a most important half. The blood, circulating through the tissues of the body in this full and rapid manner, carries with it the nutrient material for the up-building of the body; and it is from this material that the whole body is built; it is, in fact, entirely owing to this material that the increase in the size of the muscle is possible, and to which it is due; more food material is supplied, from which the tissues can draw nutriment, and they are consequently built up into the large, beautiful muscles observable in the body of the well-trained athlete. Add to all this the fact that the blood is more highly oxygenated during exercise (owing to the increased lung action) and we perceive, at once, why it is that exercise is so highly beneficial in all its aspects.

But a caution must here be emphasized. The muscular system should be exercised *symmetrically; i.e.*, every muscle should be exercised in turn, and evenly, throughout the body; and no one set exercised and the remainder neglected—leading to one-sided development, and eventually to very serious pathological conditions. For this reason, any one taking up a "course" of physical exercises should either make himself thoroughly familiar with the various muscles, their functions, and the different movements that will bring each one, in turn, into play; or (far better) place himself under the personal supervision of a thoroughly competent instructor—thereby obviating the risk of one-sided and unsymmetrical development; of becoming "muscle-bound," etc.

From what has been said, it should be obvious that suitable and vigorous exercise is one of the most beneficial of all Nature's reparative processes, and one of the speediest methods for the elimination of effete matter that could ever be devised. Active, systematic exercise is the great beautifier. It adds suppleness, grace, health, strength and shapeliness to the body;[1] fills out the "hollows" so much despised in the feminine figure; clears the skin of all pimples, etc., thus rendering the complexion clear, transparent and beautiful; it assists in removing superabundant fatty tissue (in the obese), or, on the other hand, adds healthy (muscular) tissue, in cases of extreme leanness and emaciation; it adds brightness to the eyes; poise to the head;[2] power to the brain;[3] alertness to the manner;[4] acuteness to the senses; power to the digestion; force to the character;[5] and largely assists in the formation of that all-powerful, indefinable something we term "Personal Magnetism."[6]

By increasing the peripheral circulation, in rate and amount, (thereby removing the effete matter clogging the circulation) we permanently relieve cold hands and feet—by removing their *cause;* while the diseased condition known as "that tired feeling" has no possible chance of long combating the beneficial effects of vigorous exercise. This last is purely an American disease—induced, no doubt, largely by worry and nervous tension; but also, beyond any question, by the habit of "bolting" large quantities of indigestible food, without proper mastication; and to too little bodily exercise. Most people take far too little. Walking is not enough—though a splendid exercise in itself.

[1] William Blaikie: "How to Get Strong," etc.; H. Irving Hancock: "Physical Training for Women by Japanese Methods," pp. 126–33.
[2] "Rational Physical Culture," by C. F. McGuire, p. 29.
[3] "Power and Health," etc., by George E. Flint, p. 210.
[4] "Jiu-Jitsu Combat Tricks," by H. Irving Hancock, *q. v.*
[5] "U. S. Setting-Up Exercises," p. 5.
[6] See "The Cultivation of Personal Magnetism," by LeRoy Berrier, pp. 66–89; Barnes: "Personal Magnetism," etc.

The arms, the chest, the back, above all, the muscles round the waist line should be thoroughly exercised daily—in fact, every muscle in the body. The more exercise we take, the more we can take; this is the peculiarity of the muscular system. Unlike anything else we know of, the muscular system does not wear out, through exertion and use; but, on the contrary, becomes bigger and stronger—though even if it did, it is better to "wear out," as Mr. Macfadden remarked, "than it is to rust out."

Works dealing with physical culture and exercise are now innumerable. Exercise, broadly speaking, may be divided into two classes, the active and the passive. Active exercises—those I have been discussing throughout—consist in the voluntary use by the patient of the muscles used; *i.e.*, he propels their movement himself by his own volition, and by the exercise of his own energy; while, in passive exercises, the muscles are "exercised for us" so to speak—by rubbing, kneading, slapping, etc.—this bringing the blood to the diseased part by manipulation. Such methods doubtless have their value, though I would point out, in this respect, that while such measures relieve congestion, etc., such congestion was brought about, in the first place, by the state of the blood—dependent, in turn, upon the quality and quantity of the food supply. Such measures, therefore, must always relieve the *effects*, and never remove the true *cause*—which can only be permanently effected by changing the diet.

Having now touched upon these primary questions relative to exercise, we must turn our attention more particularly to the question of its effects in cases of fasting, noting whether it is at such times beneficial or otherwise. We have seen in the opening paragraph of this chapter that the question is a vexed one; Doctor Dewey advancing strong and logical arguments for thinking that such would not be necessary, while Mr. Macfadden and others contend that exercise is as beneficial at this time as at any other—stimulating the circulation, and greatly assisting in the elimination of morbid material. Doctor Dewey's position I shall examine somewhat in detail presently, and will now offer one or two remarks of a general nature relative to exercise during a fast.

In the first place, it will be noticed that, since the prime object of the fast is elimination; and since exercise, by stimulating the various excretory organs, greatly assists in this useful work, it should be obvious that those who take the more exercise, while fasting, will succeed in totally eliminating the bodily impurities the more rapidly; and, since hunger invariably returns with, and only with, the complete cleansing of the system from morbid matter, and the restoration of healthful conditions, it follows that those who exercise the most will terminate their fast the soonest. Exercise, enemas, bathing—any hygienic device that will stimulate the depurating organs to greater activity, and help to cleanse the system, will assist in shortening the length of the fast; in causing it to terminate more quickly. I am convinced from my observations, that strict attention to these measures will shorten the length of time required for fasting from thirty-three to fifty per cent.; *i.e.*, the time required to terminate the fast, and induce natural hunger would be that much less if these cleansing measures were followed; and this will doubtless be most welcome news to the prospective and actual faster. Doctor Dewey, by neglecting these measures, needlessly prolongs his cases of fasting—from fifteen to twenty days to (*e.g.*) thirty days. Further, I greatly doubt whether, even then, the same clean and pure body would result as in the latter case, where these measures are adopted. (See Chapter on "The Enema.") Doctor Dewey's neglect of these auxiliary aids is, to my mind, a very great and extraordinary blunder for so keen an observer as he to have made.

The next point to which I would draw attention is this: That the body loses flesh, during a fast, at a far more rapid rate when much exercise is taken than in cases where but little is undertaken. This is only what we should expect, *à priori;* exercise wastes tissue, and but little new tissue is replaced during this period, since no new food material is taken into the system, from which tissue can be built, so that it must obviously decrease at a considerable rate. How great a loss of weight is sometimes experienced during strenuous exercise is well illustrated in the case of Prof. Gilman Low, who, during his marvelous record endurance lift (lifting a million pounds in thirty-four minutes, thirty-five seconds—a thousand consecutive lifts of 1,000 pounds each) lost five and three-fourths pounds during that brief period! Of course, such a case is most extreme; the rare exception. It serves to show, however, to what an extent the body *can* waste under the strain of great and prolonged muscular exertion. Consequently we find, during a fast, a far greater loss of weight and flesh in those cases where physical exercise is indulged in than where it is not. Thus, while the average loss of weight, during a fast, is about one pound a day (p. 468), Mr. Macfadden lost fifteen pounds during his seven-day fast—due, doubtless, to the great amount of exercise daily indulged in.

It will thus be seen that the daily loss of weight varies considerably, the extent of the variation being determined by many causes—such as the degree of grossness; the amount of fatty tissue accumulated by the organism; the type of the individual; but more especially by the amount of exercise daily indulged in.

The question now arises: How much exercise is beneficial during a fast? Granting that flesh and weight are thus lost, is it *desirable* that this should take place? or should we rather adopt Doctor Dewey's plan, and let the fast accomplish its task unaided? Should we expend our energies in this manner, during this trying period, or should we husband them the more closely?

Over this point there has been much dispute, as we have seen. But I think that this question may be decided by referring to first principles—bearing in mind the facts gained in our chapter on Vitality. We there saw that the *feeling* of strength does not by any means signify that more strength has been imparted to the organism, but rather the reverse; so that a feeling of lassitude signifies nothing. A right mental condition and active exercise will, on the contrary, invariably throw off such a condition; while, since we know the normal, physiological effects of exercise, and the benefits that arise therefrom; and since these effects must be very much the same during a fast, we come to the conclusion that a certain amount of active exercise[1] cannot fail to

[1] In cases of extreme weakness, passive exercises might be recommended instead.

benefit here, as elsewhere—the amount of the exercise being determined by the condition of the patient.[1]

To one further consideration I would call the reader's attention. That we should indulge in a certain amount of recreative exercise daily is unquestionably true; our muscles are provided for that express purpose, and all analogy would indicate this to be so. But why is it necessary for us to take more than that amount? Why is systematic exercise of the sort usually prescribed necessary at all?

It is for this reason. We must depend upon exercise or some similar active measure *to eliminate the excess of food material that would otherwise accumulate within the organism, and clog it sufficiently to produce disease.* In other words; it is a measure to rid the body of the excess of nutrition, forced into it! Since this is the case, it may readily be seen that precisely the same results would be attained by lessening the quantity of the food ingested—thus necessitating less active efforts on the part of the eliminating organs, and consequently a vast saving of vital force. This we should expect *à priori.* And in point of fact, such proves to be the case. Mr. Horace Fletcher, whose case I have quoted earlier in this book (pp. 113-14), is in perfect physical condition all the time, though taking no more exercise than is necessitated in daily walks about town. Says Mr. Fletcher:

"Did you ever try to reason out why it is necessary for athletes to go into training? Simply because, in order to get the best use of their strength, they are obliged to spend some number of weeks or months in overcoming false conditions which they have brought upon themselves. Any person who lives in accordance with the simple requirements of economic nutrition has nothing of this kind to overcome, but is in perfect condition all the time."[2]

[1] It is to be noticed that Mr. Macfadden modified his views on this question of exercise in his later writings. Thus: "As to exercises which should be taken during a fast of this nature, I would advise that one simply be guided by instinct, though it would be well to remember that not infrequently one feels very dizzy on rising and attempting to walk in the first few days of the fast. This, however, will usually disappear after continuing the endeavors for a short time. Walking is an especially valuable exercise when fasting, and of course toward the latter part of the fast it is about the only exercise that can be safely advised." ("Power and Beauty of Superb Womanhood," pp. 126-7.) In this he agrees with Mr. Purinton. ("Philosophy of Fasting," p. 112.)

[2] "A. B-Z. of Our Own Nutrition," p. 22.

It may be stated that this is the view held more or less indirectly by Rev. J. M. Buckley, Eustace H. Miles, Doctor Rabagliati, and Sir Benj. Ward Richardson.[1] See *Appendix M*.

Since our nutrition should be, *ceteris paribus*, directly proportioned to the amount of exercise taken, this should be a very much smaller amount than most of us are in the habit of taking, since our exercise is so limited. I quite agree with Doctor Page, when he said that:

"After all, excess in diet is, usually, only another term for lack of fresh air and exercise. "[2]

But I think the opposite statement is also true, as I have just shown. Or as Sir William Temple wrote long ago:

"In the course of common life, a man must either often exercise, or fast, or take physic, or be sick; and the choice seems left to everyone as he likes."[3]

As Mr. Purinton remarked:[4]

"A man can eat a lot if he exercises a lot. But what's the use? To eat less and also exercise less comes to the same end. With a saving of time, money, thought and vitality."

That this conclusion is both legitimate and true, our reason tells us (so do our bodies, occasionally!), and further, it has been proved to be correct by direct and actual experiment. It is a conclusion, however, which few of us are willing to accept, much less act upon; and, so long as this is the case, sickness and death will remain active and prevalent.

To one further consideration I would call the reader's attention.

"As a general rule," says Doctor Graham,[5] "the quantity of our food should, within certain limits, be proportionate to the amount of our active exercise; yet the athletic and active laboring man is, in our country, constantly in danger of taking too much

[1] See "Studies in Physical Culture," p. 18; "Muscle, Brain and Diet," pp. 30, 33; "Air, Food and Exercises," p. 458; "Diseases of Modern Life," p. 170.

[2] "Natural Cure," p. 83.

[3] "The Art of Living Long," p. 148.

[4] "Philosophy of Fasting," p. 38.

[5] "Science of Human Life," p. 581.

food. Indeed, it is unquestionably true that at least ninety-nine of the farmers and other laboring men of New England are prematurely worn out and broken down by over-eating, where one is thus affected by excessive labor or hard work." "Mental work, and even hard mental work is conducive to health and length of days," wrote Sir Benj. Ward Richardson.[1]

The truth is, it is not the overwork, but working in unwise ways, which does the mischief we so loudly deplore. It is not less labor that men want, but wiser methods of working—more varied occupation, better care, more frequent recuperation, and larger invoices of joy and mirth, with nobler incentives and hopes. As Doctor Trall so well said:[2]

"Much is said in these days of fast living, commercial energy, and the mad pursuit of immediate pleasures and sensuous indulgences, or overworked brains, as a course of dyspepsia. The true cause is *abused bodies.* The brain cannot be overworked, provided the vital conditions are properly attended to."

Dr. T. L. Nichols wrote, in a letter to Dr. M. L. Holbrook:

"Just now I am trying an experiment on the relations of work to diet, to test upon myself my theory that the trouble of overwork is chiefly, if not wholly, in the digestive apparatus. . . . I find my brain-weariness troubling me less and less, and my power for work increasing. I wrote yesterday a long article—a fair day's work, before breakfast—and I work twelve to fifteen hours a day with very little sense of fatigue. My stomach has such light work that all life flows freely to the brain, and I can work on, hour after hour I shall find the quantity that suits me best, which I expect will be from six to eight ounces a day."[3]

Of course this is not saying that one *cannot* overwork; far from it. The danger of excessive work, especially in the young, cannot be too strongly emphasized. (See Richardson: "Learning: and Health.") But, on the whole, its danger has been greatly overestimated. Were we to conserve our energies more, there

[1] "Diseases of Modern Life," p. 399.
[2] "Digestion and Dyspepsia," p. 137.
[3] "Hygiene of the Brain," pp. 168–70.

would be no such cry as to the evil effects of overwork. Says Carrica Le Favre:[1] "It is estimated that between seventy and eighty per cent. of the energy we generate, we also waste." I may add, of this amount, by far the greatest share is the waste necessitated in digesting and ridding the system of uncalled-for food.

[1] "Delsartean Physical Culture," p. 14.

CHAPTER V

WATER DRINKING

FEW persons realize probably that about three-fourths of their bodies are composed entirely of water!

"The blood and the brain are each about four-fifths water, while the fluid secretions and excretions contain more than nine-tenths of their weight of this limpid fluid."[1]

Water is constantly passing out of the body in the form of urine, perspiration, etc., while the fæces, and the breath also contain a large percentage of that liquid. It is evident, therefore, that a constant supply must be furnished the body in order to compensate for this loss, and this can only be supplied by food and drink—the amount absorbed by the skin or through the lungs being altogether insignificant when compared with the bodily needs. All foods contain more or less water, ranging from about two per cent. in the various nuts to upwards of ninety per cent. in such articles of food as asparagus, celery, cucumbers, lettuce, melons, rhubarb, tomatoes, etc., etc., while in many broths, soups, etc., the percentage is almost the whole amount. Fruits contain a very large percentage of water, and for this reason it has frequently been contended that persons living exclusively, or even largely, on a fruitarian diet, need little or no water in addition to that supplied by the food. But this question does not concern us now. The main point is that, in the usual "mixed" diet, consisting largely of so-called "dry" foods, a considerable amount of extra fluid is necessary, in the form of drink, in order to preserve the body in a state of health—the amount depending partly upon the nature of the diet[2] and

[1] "The Uses of Water," by J. H. Kellogg, M.D., p. 9.

[2] "The richer the food, the more liquid is craved." ("Rumford Kitchen Leaflets," p. 53.) Professor Chittenden also remarked that, with a diminished intake of proteid food, there was less thirst. ("Physiological Economy in Nutrition," p. 30.)

partly upon the bodily condition of the individual; and the amount must now engage our attention for a few moments.

It has been stated on good authority that we lose each day an average of two pounds or pints merely in perspiration[1]—not to speak of the losses through the urine, fæces, lungs, etc. It will readily be seen, then, that the food eaten does not in any way supply this loss, but that fluids must be taken in more or less large quantities to supply the deficiency here noted. There should also be, in addition to the amount actually required by the body, a certain surplus, even during health, for the purposes of dissolving impurities, facilitating function, and cleansing the system generally of its impurities—carrying them with it to the various excretory organs, there to be eliminated. In all cases of impeded functioning, and in feverish conditions (and in fact in all cases where a more or less morbid action is present) the amount of water drunk daily should be greatly increased—being, as a general rule, directly proportioned to the gravity of the disease. As a dilutant, as a solvent, as a diuretic, as a diaphoretic, as a quencher of thirst, as an equalizer of the circulation water has no equal.

If, then, water drinking is of such great importance, while the system is, comparatively speaking, "healthy," how much more important does it become in disease, and especially in acute disease—when all functioning is abnormally retarded, and the effete material is being conveyed to the eliminating organs faster than those organs can dispose of it! It will be seen that, under such circumstances, water drinking is of the very highest importance. In all acute diseases, the prompt administration of water, internally and externally, will undoubtedly save more lives than any other single and immediate measure that can be adopted.

The importance of drinking considerably more water than we at present do—which in acute diseases becomes a vital necessity—is becoming more and more recognized and accepted by all advanced physicians and students of hygiene. With hardly an exception modern writers upon these subjects are unanimous in contending that "less food and more water" would result in

[1] "The Skin in Health and Disease," by H. Black, M.D., p. 16.

benefiting mankind immensely. It is now known that one of the most universal and harmful ills from which humanity suffers, *viz.*, constipation, is very largely due to *insufficient water drinking.* An increase in the amount daily consumed, together with a properly reformed dietary, will relieve almost any case of this terrible disorder—the *bête noire* of modern society. See Doctor Parkyns' excellent remarks on this subject in his "Hypnotism," pp. 62–4.

Three important questions at once arise in connection with this subject of water drinking, which we must now consider: They are, *what kind* of water is best for us to drink? *how much,* and *when?* in other words the questions of *quality, quantity,* and *periodicity.*

(1) *Quality.* As to the first of these, its quality, the whole question may be summed up in four words—*the purer the better!* Absolutely pure water does not, for all practical purposes, exist in nature—the purest being rain water that has been collected in clean vessels—though even this is somewhat contaminated by its passage through the air, absorbing impurities, noxious gases, etc., in its descent. Filters are one hugh farce. They separate the *mechanical impurities* from the liquid, but the minute organisms—the "life"—in the water it absolutely fails to touch, as it does any elements or gases *dissolved* in the water. Boiling will generally have the effect of killing the micro-organisms (though even this is extremely doubtful), but does not remove the (now dead) organic matter in the water—which is consequently retained therein! The process has also other disadvantages. The only really pure water is *distilled* water; that is, water which has been evaporated into steam, leaving the solid ingredients behind, and reconverted into water in another, cooler vessel, into which the steam is made to pass. This process is without serious disadvantages (though even here it is contended that various gases, previously in solution, pass over with the steam); but at all events it is the best method known for obtaining water free from chemical, mechanical and organic impurities. It may be mentioned that the water found in fruits, vegetables and other organic compounds is almost absolutely pure.

Now the importance of *pure* water can hardly be overestimated As a dilutant, it is far more efficacious than water containing any mineral or other substances in solution. The drinking of large quantities of water containing various salts, gases, mineral substances, etc., in solution, as is done in Saratoga, Carlsbad, etc., *under medical advice*, cannot be too strongly deprecated. All such matter is highly injurious to the living organism, and cannot possibly fail to be otherwise. Says Doctor Trall:[1]

"Artificial mineral waters, and the saline, alkaline, ferruginous, sulphurous compounds of the 'medicinal springs,' are pernicious beverages for the sick or well. The drugs they contain are no better, and no different in effect, than the same drugs taken from the apothecary shop. Those water-cure physicians who *permit* their patients to use them may be justified in thus yielding to popular prejudice; but to *prescribe* them, argues strange ignorance of hygiene, or perhaps a worse motive." Again: "All the medicinal and mineral springs, from Saratoga to White Sulphur, and from Cheltenham to Vichy, are only modifications of the oceans, the great reservoirs of all the impurities that water can dissolve. No one thinks of drinking them when well, nor would any one be content to have his food soaked in them. But when sick, presto! the more earthy, saline, alkaline, and mineral ingredients they contain, the more they are in demand! Such is fashion."

As Dr. James C. Jackson so well remarked:[2]

"Every woman knows that she cannot wash clothes in hard water. It is scarcely less practicable to wash the blood in it."

In considering this question of the value of water containing mineral salts in solution, we have simply to ask ourselves this question: Are the mineral salts and gases contained in this water appropriable by the system? Either they must be utilized as food (in which case chemical changes must take place, altering the nature and composition of the salts contained in solution [and this we have shown to be theoretically impossible] they being inorganic substances); or, (2) the drug is not appropriable by the system, in which case it does and must pass

[1] "Hygienic Hand Book," p. xviii.
[2] "The Curse Lifted; or Maternity Made Easy," p. 16.

through it in its unchanged mineral condition, entailing considerable loss of energy in its expulsion, and clogging the system throughout with refuse matter—acting, in fact, in every way, as would a drug or mineral salt taken in any other form. Since they cannot possibly be beneficial, they must obviously be harmful; and the "cures" effected at the various resorts are undoubtedly brought about *in spite of* the injurious mineral waters drunk, and on account of the improved dietary and other hygienic rules adopted by the patients during this period of treatment. As Doctor Rausse said:[1]

"If, during a cure by mineral springs, a temporary recovery is affected, then it is not by virtue of the minerals in the water, but by virtue of the water in the mineral springs, by virtue of the out-of-doors exercise, of pure open air and of good living."

It is admitted that it is not known to what extent the drinking of mineral water *alone* would be of value,[2] while Doctor Arany admits that diet is a very important feature in the cure at Carlsbad. It would be highly amusing, were it not tragic, to learn that patients who visit the mineral springs, and get "cured" at them are considered in need of an "after cure"—a cure to cure the cure! On pp. 86–90 of the *British-American Guide to Carlsbad* are given a number of places that might be tried for the after cure!

If the same amount of *pure* water were drunk as there is mineral water now disposed of, infinitely better results would doubtless follow. And in support of this I might state that:

"It is worthy of remark that, at some places where 'miracles' are claimed to be wrought by the effect of the water—as, for example, at Malvern, the water used is remarkable merely for its great purity and almost absolute freedom from mineral ingredients."[3]

On the contrary, the direct and powerfully harmful effects of drinking water containing lime or other salts in solution is most forcibly shown in the following extract, which I quote at some length. It is as follows:

[1] "Health and the Various Methods of Cure," p. 65.
[2] "Hydrotherapy at Saratoga," by J. A. Irwin, M.D., p. 31.
[3] "Baths and Bathing"; *App. Health Primer*, p. 68.

"The solid earthy matter which, by gradual accumulation in the body, brings on ossification, rigidity, decrepitude, and death, is principally phosphate of lime, or bone matter; carbonate of lime, or common chalk, and sulphate of lime, or plaster of Paris, with occasionally magnesia and other earthy substances.

"We have seen that a process of consolidation begins at the earliest period of existence and continues without interruption until the body is changed from a comparatively fluid, elastic, and energetic state, to a solid, earthy, rigid, inactive condition, which terminates in death—that infancy, childhood, youth, manhood, old age and decrepitude, are but so many different conditions of the body or stages of the progress of consolidation or ossification—that the only difference in the body between old age and youth is the greater density, toughness and rigidity, and the greater proportion of calcareous earthy matter which enters into its composition. The question now arises; what is the *source* of the calcareous earthy matter which thus accumulates in the system? It seems to be regarded as an axiom that all the solids of the body are continually built up and renewed from the blood. If so, everything which these solids contained is derived from the blood. The solids contain phosphates and carbonate of lime, which are, therefore, derived from the blood, in which, as already shown, these earthy substances are invariably found to a greater or less extent. The blood is renewed from the chyle, which is always found upon analysis to contain the same earthy substances as the blood and the solids. The chyle is renewed from the chyme, and ultimately from the food and drink. The food and drink, then, which nourish the system must, at the same time, be the primary source of the calcareous earthy matter which enters into the composition of the chyme, the chyle and the blood, and which is ultimately deposited in all the tissues, membranes, vessels and solids of the body—producing old age, decrepitude and natural death.

"Common table salt which is used in the preparation of almost every kind of food, and along with many of our meals, contains a fearfully large amount of calcareous earthy matter, and is productive of very great mischief to the animal economy.[1]

[1] I cannot go into this question of salt eating here, but I cannot forbear offering one or two remarks on this terribly harmful practice. Salt is *never* necessary, under any conceivable circumstances, to the human organism; but, on the contrary, is decidedly harmful to it under any and all circumstances, and in proportion to the amount consumed. There have never been any reasons advanced by physiologists—showing that we need salt—that

"Spring water contains an amount of earthy ingredients which is fearful to contemplate. It certainly differs very much in different districts, and at various steps, but it has been calculated that water of an average quality contains so much carbonate and other compounds of lime that a person drinking an average quantity each day will, in forty years, have taken as much into the body as would form a pillar of solid chalk or marble as large as a good sized man! So great is the amount of lime in spring water that the quantity taken daily would alone be sufficient to choke up the system, so as to bring on decrepitude and death long before we arrived at twenty years of age, were it not for the kidneys and other secreting organs throwing it off in considerable quantities. These organs, however, only discharge a portion of this matter; for instance, supposing ten parts to be taken during a day, eight or nine may be thrown out, and one or two lost somewhere in the body. This process continuing, day after day, and year after year, the solid matter at length accumulates until the activity and flexibility of childhood become lost in the enfeebled rigidity of what is then called—though very erroneously—'old age.' A familiar instance of the decomposition and incrustation from water is observed in a common tea-kettle or steam-boiler. Every housewife knows that a vessel which is in constant use will soon

would stand the test of one moment's serious criticism, or which in any way proved that we need chloride of sodium or common salt, in the separate, inorganic form in which it is eaten, any more than we need lime, or potash or iron, or sulphur, or phosphorus, or any other mineral element—all of which, however, including common salt, are necessary for our welfare, and are supplied in organic, usable form in fruits and vegetables of all kinds. The one single fact that salt is a mineral substance, and, as such, is absolutely useless to and inappropriable by the organism, is proof positive that salt need not and cannot be utilized by the organism in that form. It can have no more effect upon the system than so much iron filings sprinkled over the food; but, like iron filings, it serves to clog the economy and ultimately shorten the life. It undergoes no chemical changes whatever in the body, and can have no possible use therein, as stated. This salt question will be found discussed at length in Trall's "Hydropathic Encyclopædia," Vol. I., pp. 336–9; in Dr. Susanna Dodd's "Diet Question," pp. 61–70; in Mrs. C. L. Hunt's "Salt;" in R. Y. Colburn's "Salt-Eating Habit," etc.; also in an excellent series of articles published in *Health Culture* Magazine, July–December, 1906. It is interesting to note that M. Dastre, in his "Salt and Its Physiological Uses" (P. 571), finally admits that salt plays no active part in the vital economy—though he is throughout arguing for its utility! His whole argument goes to show, merely, that "we should have salt"—to which all true hygienists would reply: Certainly, salt is very necessary; but all that we need is supplied in organic form in the vegetable kingdom. (*v.* "Saline Starvation and How to Avoid It.") Why, then go to the mineral kingdom for this substance, any more than for any other salt—since all are equally supplied in fruits and vegetables? It is interesting to note that salt is found in large quantities in eggs ("Eggs and Their Uses as Food," p. 13)—the very article of food that is usually salted the most heavily!

become 'furred-up' or plastered on the bottom and sides with a hard stony substance. Four or five pounds weight of this matter have been known to collect in twelve months. The reader must not mislead himself by thinking that because so much lime is found in a teakettle the water, after boiling, is, therefore, free from lime. It is true boiling water does cause a little carbonate of lime to precipitate, but the bulk of the sediment is left from *that portion of the water only which is driven off in steam, or boiled away.* This can easily be ascertained by testing the water both before and after boiling. It will be found to contain earthy particles however long the boiling may continue. Filtering it is also of no use, for this only removes what may be floating or mechanically mixed in the water, whereas the earthy matter which we have spoken of is held in *solution,* so that spring water, clear and transparent as it may appear, is nevertheless charged with a considerable amount of solid, choking-up matter, and is, therefore, in any form unfit, or at least is not the *best* suited, for internal use. The only means whereby it can be rendered perfectly pure and fit for unlimited consumption is distillation."[1]

(2) *Quantity.* The amount of water that should be daily consumed by the individual depends upon many and varied circumstances—such as the nature of the diet; the temperature of the atmosphere; the amount of its "dryness" or the reverse; the amount of exercise indulged in; the condition of the organism—whether healthy or diseased; etc., etc. If the diet is largely fruit or other substances containing a large percentage of water, it is obvious that less need be drunk than if food is of the dry kind, or if it be stimulating. In the hot weather we all drink considerably more than in the cooler, owing to the greater loss of water through perspiration; the same effect also resulting from vigorous exercise. Atmospheric dampness, or the reverse, would effect the thirst indirectly by its effect upon the bodily evaporation. But in all diseases, of whatever nature, water should be partaken of *ad libitum.* We should, in fact, encourage the desire for it in every possible way, and there is no disease whatever, in which pure water is other than decidedly beneficial in any reasonable quantities—provided that the diet be sufficiently restricted. The dread of water drinking is one of those

[1] "How Nature Cures," pp 251-5.

terrible superstitions which has doubtless sent thousands of unfortunate and deluded victims to a premature grave.

It is *possible*, doubtless, for anyone to drink too much water—especially if that water be of a low temperature. Water drinking should always be gauged by the degree of thirst, and a normal person will never crave more than is good for him. But I am assured that the real dangers of water drinking are entirely imaginary. Says Doctor Oswald:[1]

"The supposed peril of plunge-baths or draughts of cold water 'in the heat,' is one of the silliest bugbears of sanitary superstition. . . . Children, admonished not to touch cold water till they are cooled off, might as well be warned against falling asleep when they are tired."

It is hard, in reality, for any normal person to drink too much water at any one time—provided that the water be not too cold; and that a halt is called when the system cries "enough." I need hardly say that the idea of the injurious effects of drinking water and eating fruit at the same meal is pure superstition —containing no particle of truth—beyond that involved in the fact that drinking water and eating solids of any kind at the same meal is always unhygienic and harmful. Says Professor Schlickeysen:[2]

"I may mention in this connection an existing prejudice against eating fruit and drinking water at the same meal. This feeling has no justification in fact, and, indeed, one of the best tests of a sound condition of the digestive organs is the ability to receive uncooked fruit and cold water at the same time. Only a weak stomach will refuse them."

In all this it must be understood that I am not advocating the practice of drinking great quantities of water at any time during the day; of "drowning the stomach" as one author expressed it. Moderation and discretion must here be exercised, as at all other times. One mav have "too much of a good thing." All that is admitted. But I am persuaded, on the other hand, that, provided the water is pure and drunk only at proper times,

[1] "Fasting, Hydropathy and Exercise," pp. 97–8.
[2] "Fruit and Bread," p. 191.

it is practically impossible to drink enough water to seriously injure either the stomach, the kidneys, or any part of the digestive tract; while the effects of an occasional indulgence to the extent of two or three quarts may sometimes prove highly beneficial—thoroughly washing out and cleansing the stomach and intestines, which often cannot be directly reached in any other manner. This constitutes, in fact, a sort of second variety of enema.

But the quantity of water to be drunk is still an unsettled question; for, allowing for all the considerations at the commencement of this discussion, there must yet be some *approximate* amount which it is possible to determine. Upon this question opinions differ here as everywhere; but, without entering into the details, the *pros* and *cons* of the discussion, it may be stated that, on a rough estimate, and under ordinary normal conditions, from three pints to two quarts of water should be drunk daily,[1] in addition to any that may be contained in the food. It may safely be said that any great and long continued reduction from the *minimum* amount mentioned will sooner or later show itself in some form of acute or chronic disease.

(3) *Periodicity.* Coming now to the question as to the *time* when water should be drunk, we can lay down the definite and certain rule that it *should never be drunk at meals*, and preferably not for at least one hour after the meal has been eaten. The effect of drinking water while eating is, first, to artificially moisten the food, thus hindering the normal and healthful flow of saliva and the other digestive juices; secondly, to dilute the various juices to an abnormal extent; and thirdly, to wash the food elements through the stomach and into the intestines before they have had time to become thoroughly liquefied and digested. The effects of this upon the welfare of the whole organism can only be described as direful. At other times during the day or night, water may be drunk with comparative freedom, the quantity being dictated altogether by thirst.

It is advisable to drink a glass of water the last thing at night, just before retiring, and another in the morning, immediately

[1] That is, from six to eight glasses daily. A glass holds, as a rule, slightly less than half a pint.

upon arising, this tending to wash out the stomach by carrying the collected contents through, into the intestine. It is also advisable to take a few swallows of water shortly before a meal, for the same reason; but about ten minutes should be allowed to elapse, in such cases, before solid food is ingested.

During the fast, there are, of course, no meals to be taken into consideration, so that the water may be drunk at any time it is craved, the quantity being regulated, as always, by thirst. I shall return to this point (the quantity of water to be drunk during a fast) presently, but will, first, briefly discuss one other topic of interest and importance, namely, the *temperature* of the water drunk.

Water should be drunk either hot or cold—warm water being sickening, and for that reason is frequently used as an emetic. When hot, it should be as hot as can be *drunk* (not sipped) without undue discomfort; or capable of being held in the mouth under similar conditions. Cold water should be decidedly cool without being iced. This latter temperature is highly deleterious to the stomach, and ice water should always be mixed with water of a somewhat warmer temperature, before being drunk, in order to remove the extreme chill.

The question is: when shall hot water be drunk and when cold? Both systems have their staunch advocates, those of hot water drinking being especially and aggressively energetic in the defense of their pet hobby, and frequently deprecate the use of cold water entirely. Their opponents, on the other hand, almost invariably admit the *occasional* good effects of hot water drinking, but contend that cool water is the normal and healthful liquid for practically all occasions. My own view of the matter is that there is much truth in both these contentions; hot or cold water each being beneficial in certain conditions, and under certain circumstances—though I would contend that too frequent indulgence in hot drinks tends to render the stomach anæmic, just as too frequent warm baths render the skin anæmic. In certain, exceptional states, however, it would appear to me that the administration of either hot or cold water at these times would depend, (1) upon the temperature of the body, and (2) the degree of vitality present.

Let us consider these in turn.

(1) *The Temperature.* It is a well-known fact that warm foods and warm drinks, which we are discussing now, are craved when the body is unduly cold, and *vice versa.* The reason for this is, of course, that the drink imparts, or gives up to the body, the overplus of heat it contains (when more than the bodily temperature) thereby raising the latter; and conversely, cold water absorbs from the body, or the body gives up to it, a certain amount of heat—thereby raising the temperature of the water and lowering that of the body. The tremendous importance of cool water in plentiful supplies in all cases of *fever* is thus manifest. A glass of water, entering the body at, say, 40° F. and leaving it, as urine, perspiration, etc., some minutes later, at 98.5° F. has, in its passage through the body, deducted that quantity of heat from the body. A continued cooling process of this nature must obviously soon reduce the bodily temperature to normal, without the aid of any of the "antiphlogisties" of the medical profession.

(2) *The Vitality.* One other consideration must be mentioned relative to this question of hot *vs.* cold water drinking. I have already indicated that the degree of vitality present should assist in determining this point, as well as the bodily temperature, as indicated by the thermometer. The reason is this. Readers of the chapter on "Bathing" will remember that cold baths were always advocated as beneficial *so long as there was sufficient vitality to properly react from the shock.* Now the same rule holds good with regard to the stomach—where the temperature is always about the same. If the stomach can properly react, after drinking cold water, and no evil after-effects are noticed, I should then advocate the more hardy method of cold water drinking; but in case such reaction is lacking in promptness and completeness, or if discomfort be noticed, then hot water should be drunk temporarily; at the same time carefully attending to all the laws of health, in order to build up and maintain the highest degree of vital vigor.

Having now discussed the various points at issue relative to water drinking under ordinary circumstances (which discussion was nevertheless rendered necessary for a thorough understanding of the question), I now turn to a consideration of the question of water drinking *during a fast;* and, since water is the only substance of any kind that is allowed in the stomach at that time, a consideration of this question becomes of paramount importance.

First, let me answer a question which is sure to be raised by some acute critic. "Why allow water at all during the fast?" It may be asked: "If the contention is correct that anything entering the stomach draws the blood thereto, no matter how small the amount (p. 556), then would not water have this effect —thereby inducing hunger and virtually breaking the fast? In other words, does not the drinking of water involve a breaking of the fast, for all practical purposes?"

To this objection I would reply as follows: Only those articles of food need be considered which directly nourish the system by first undergoing the process of *digestion,* and it is this process of digestion which draws the blood to the stomach and involves the breaking of the fast. Now water requires no digestion in its passage through the alimentary canal. *It enters the system as water and it leaves it as water.* The differences noticeable, as a result of this passage, being due to the presence of certain salts and other matter in solution, which it has gathered up in its passage through the body. It has undergone no chemical or vital changes whatever in its passage through the body, and consequently no *digestion* is involved in the stomach and intestines, and consequently there is no breaking of the fast. This is the only substance, liquid or solid, of which this can be said— even air, strictly speaking, being "digested," and forming no exception to this rule.

Now, as water does not directly nourish the body and consequently cannot (if the accepted theories of the relations of food and bodily energy be true) in any way add to the bodily store of vitality, the fact that it *does so add* to the energy, is one of the most remarkable as it is one of the most easily demonstrable of facts. Doctor Tanner, *e.g.*, in speaking of his own fast said:[1]

"During my first fast my loss in weight was 1½ pounds per day, during the period when I abstained from water and food—14

[1] *Physical Culture,* Vol. V., pp. 209–210.

days; when partaking of water the remainder of the 42 days, my loss in weight was a little less than ½ pound per day. From my experience with and without water I hold aqueous fluids as among the most valuable of foods. It is not a tissue builder, but a great strength giver. When I left Clarendon Hall, in which my last fast was held, after fourteen days abstinence from water, I was very weak, scarcely able to walk down stairs without supporting myself with the hand rail. On that day I made my first visit to Central Park. There I found a spring of very cool and refreshing water, of which I partook freely. Returning to the hall, after an absence of one hour only, I climbed the stairs of Clarendon Hall two steps at a time with the nimbleness of a boy, I attribute that wondrous change to the water I drank and the pure air I breathed on that occasion.

"In my New York fast of forty days, I did not take as much outdoor exercise as during my Minneapolis fast, for the reason that my watchers objected; but still my strength kept up remarkably well. Returning from one of my many rides to Central Park and feeling greatly exhilarated by the water and pure air, I, on the seventeenth day, felt like loudly extolling the oxygen of the air and water as valuable foods. A medical student with more zeal than wisdom, took issue with me on the value of oxygen as a food, and flippantly remarked that however good oxygen might be, beef was far better. 'That is an assumption that demands proof,' I retorted. 'I challenge you to test your theory by taking laps around this hall until one or the other surrenders.'

"Round and round the hall we went, until the eighteenth lap, when the student fell out, blowing and puffing like a heavy old horse, leaving oxygen victor over beef."

Scores of similar cases could be cited; in fact every case of fasting would very readily demonstrate the truth of my contention. Without water it would be almost impossible to fast for any very considerable period without extreme discomfort, to say the least. The visible and tangible influx of energy, following upon the drinking of water, during the fast, is absolutely inexplicable upon the presently accepted theories of the relations of food and energy; while, since we know that water cools, soothes, allays inflammation, and rids the system of a large portion of its collected impurities, in its passage through it; in other words, that it *cleanses* it, we can readily see how, upon the theory advanced on pp. 249–54, this inrush of energy could be explained. Upon *that* theory it becomes perfectly intelligible to us; upon the other it is altogether inexplicable.

We now come to consider the question: How much water should be drunk by patients who are fasting?

Here again, we find considerable difference of opinion among the experts. Mr. Macfadden, and Doctor Page, *e.g.*, advocate a somewhat profuse drinking of water, whether indicated by thirst or not; their reason for this being that it assists in the process of elimination, and cleanses the entire organism—ultimately tending to shorten the fast, for these very reasons. Doctor Dewey, on the other hand, contends strongly against this practice. He believes in relying solely upon the indications of thirst, and insists that the drinking of too much water aggravates kidney troubles. Thus, in speaking of the case of Mr. Rathbun and his twenty-eight-day fast, he incidentally gives his views as follows:

"Again I had trouble with him on the water question, wishing him to drink only as thirst incited. He was differently advised by an eminent Boston physician, who, taking a great interest in the case, wrote him that he should have great care to drink certain definite amounts for the necessary fluidity of the blood. I had to respond that thirst would duly indicate this need; that in my cases of protracted fasts from acute sicknesses, not one had been advised to take even a teaspoonful of water for such reasons; that at the closing days before recovery of such cases there was only the least desire for water, and this with no indication of need from the blood. Mr. Rathbun did not escape some trouble from overworked kidneys, and he became convinced that my theory and practice were more in line with physiology."[1]

To this, in turn, it might be replied that *pure* water would not probably produce any such disturbances, while water that had not been distilled might. Further, I am convinced that no more work is required in passing (say) one quart of highly diluted urine, than is involved in passing (say) one pint of urine—more or less thickened with sediment. Indeed one might

[1] "No-Breakfast Plan," pp. 125–6.

suppose, *à priori*, that the task might be lighter. However, the point is somewhat obscure, and it is not safe to dogmatize in the present state of our knowledge, one way or the other.

Doctor Dewey's great point is that thirst will indicate the need of the tissues for liquid just as hunger indicates the need for solid nutriment. In this he merely advocates "turning to nature," and in that lies the great strength of his position. In this, I think, he is perfectly justified; but I should advocate the drinking of a greater amount of water than would be usuallv called for by thirst—were we merely to rely upon that indication. These statements, paradoxical as they may appear, may be reconciled as follows: Thirst, like hunger—and almost everything else in life—is more or less a question of *habit*. We can accustom ourselves to drink a very large or a very small amount of water daily, without noticing, for the time being, any especially good or especially evil effects from such a course. Now, if the appetite for water were more normal (it usually is highly abnormal), I am convinced that far more water would be drunk during the fast than is now the case; for the reason that there would be a greater thirst at that time. In other words, the patient would drink considerably more water than he drank before, but still only as much as thirst indicated; more being craved, however, owing to the more normal condition of the organism—the result of improved organic habits.

Surprisingly near to my own reasoning is that of Mr. Purinton, who, in his "Philosophy of Fasting," p. **111**, says:

"As to the amount of water taken internally, opinions differ. Instinct, here as always, may be assumed the only safe guide. In general we may say, however, that the one occasion when instinct might be forced is in the matter of water drinking, during a fast. Cultivate a desire for it. "

One or two remarks may now be offered regarding the drinking of water *during a fast*. I have already made some remarks on this subject, and will add one or two more, dealing more especially with this branch of the question.

First, then, I would suggest that water be drunk whenever a feeling of emptiness or "all-goneness" is experienced in the stomach. We shall see (pp. 549–52), that this is not true hunger, but a species of irritation due in turn to congestion, or other causes. Whatever the cause, however, the effects, the visible manifestations, may be speedily quieted and subdued by this process of drinking one or two glasses of water. This, and withdrawing the attention, by an effort, if need be, from that part of the body, will have the effect of speedily removing the cause, and relieving the unpleasant symptoms present.

After the fast has progressed some days, considerable difficulty may be experienced in drinking water of any kind, either hot or cold. Any impurities in the water will then be detected with the greatest ease, owing to the acutened sense of taste (pp. 505–7); an aversion to the water will invariably follow, which will continue so long as the water is unchanged, and other (preferably distilled) water be substituted. Even then the aversion may continue.[1] If cold water cannot be drunk, hot water will often be drunk with relish; but if even this is repugnant, *two or three drops* of orange or lemon juice in the water will have the effect, almost invariablv, of making it palatable, and of overcoming the flat, unpleasant taste of the water sufficiently to make it drinkable by the patient. These should be added to the hot water, not the cold, which should always be drunk plain and unadulterated. If the patient will merely *exhale*—instead of inhaling—before drinking, it will be found that nauseous liquids of any kind may be taken far more easily than is usually the case.

I have been careful to italicize, in the above, the words "two or three drops" of lemon, etc. The reason is this: were any *considerable amount* of lemon or orange juice added to the water, digestion would be called upon to deal with these substances —thus virtually breaking the fast (see p. 556). *Very small* quantities might be passed through the stomach, when thus

[1] Doctor Schrott's experience was somewhat different from my own in this respect. Thus: "There is experienced a strong, oppressive thirst soon after commencing. . . . Those who have been in the habit of drinking a good deal suffer most in this respect. As the cure progresses, or, in other words, as the body becomes more pure, the desire for fluid grows less." ("Family Physician," by Joel Shew, M.D., p. 789.) In Schrott's cases, however, it was a thirst cure no less than a hunger cure—so, perhaps, his cases are not so contradictory, after all.

thoroughly diluted, without any appreciable effect; while larger quantities would call for more effort on the part of the digestion, since it will be remembered that an almost infinitesimal amount of food will virtually break a fast as effectually as a full meal, since hunger will soon return in either case, as we shall see. Just enough should be used, therefore, to render the water drinkable, if decidedly unpleasant, without calling upon any energy for digestion—thus upsetting the process of the fast. For these reasons, also, I now advocate orange juice, instead of lemon juice, which I did formerly, for the reason that it is less irritating to the stomach. This was pointed out to me by Dr. J. M. Craig in a discussion upon this question, and I now beg to offer him my thanks for what I consider an exceedingly valuable suggestion.

CHAPTER VI

THE ENEMA

I NOW approach a branch of my subject which is by no means a pleasant one; *viz.*, a discussion of the bowel contents, and their influence upon the health of the individual. That constipation and its following train of ills is the cause of a very large percentage of the ills to which the flesh is heir has long been known to thoughtful physicians; and I cannot do better than to quote in this connection, the terse and forceful language of Dr. A. B. Jamison, a specialist of twenty-five years in diseases of the anus and rectum, and a man whose authority upon these subjects can scarcely be questioned. He says:[1]

"The putrid fecal mass of solid and liquid contents accumulated in the artificial reservoir at the end of the intestinal sewer, is one of the most common and serious pathogenic (disease-producing) and pyogenic (pus-producing) sources, which, by auto-infection, afflict man from infancy to old age. Here—in the dilated and obstructed sewer—the ptomain and leucomain class of poisons, and many of the poisonous germs, led by the king of morbid disturbers, the *bacillus coli communis,* find another and last chance to be taken up by the absorbing cells of the mucous membrane and returned to the blood; with which they are carried to all parts of the body, clogging the glands, choking up the pores and obstructing the circulation, thereby causing congestion and inflammation of the various organs. The action of cathartics, laxatives, etc., fills the ano-rectal cavity with a watery solution of foul substances; this solution is readily absorbed into the circulation, aggravating the auto-infection, (the established self-poisoned condition) already existing. Danger does not end with the absorption of bacterial poisons, as we have to reckon with the deleterious effects of the various intestinal gasses, resulting, with rapid augmentation of volume, from the putrefactive changes in

[1] "Intestinal Ills," pp. 25–6.

the imprisoned feculent matter. The system may absorb as high as three-fourths of this feculent substance in the colon; and this absorption is made possible by the obstructed or sluggish intestinal canal where disease germs are propagated and lodged; that these germs, along with a certain amount of excrement, invade the tissues by absorption; and that we thus have the system constantly saturated with poisonous germs and filth, re-excreted, re-absorbed and re-secreted—no one knows how many times—by the various organs of the body. (pp. 36-7.)

. It is not generally known among laymen, nor sufficiently appreciated among physicians, that the fecal matter normally evacuated from the bowels comes mainly from the blood; and that this mass is not, as it is usually supposed to be, the residue of the food that has been left unassimilated." (p. 99.)

Here then we have a picture which may verily cause us to sicken; one that may make us pause and realize—perhaps for the first time—the fact that there is within us at such times a veritable sewer—a tube "full of abomination" such as we dare not touch, nor smell, nor see—nor even think about! Yet this mass is actually within us! And the trouble does not cease here; it were fortunate, indeed, if it did. The bowels are not a closed, non-porous tube, but the very contrary. Yea, it is *from these very materials that our bodies are built!* That beautiful form; that God-like intellect; the very soul itself, is on any theory, dependent upon the material body for its manifestation, in this life; and *these* materials (and foul air), are the materials from which our bodies are built! Can it be wondered at, then, that sickness and premature death are ever present? and that bloated faces, blotchy skins, and foul breath are encountered on every hand—rather than the clean, sweet, healthy body that results from perfect nutrition, and a strict observance of hygienic laws?

And in stating this, I am drawing no fanciful picture. There is reason to believe—there is evidence to prove—that, were we to observe the laws of health; were we to eat only sufficient food for our bodily needs, and not to continually gorge and glut the bowels with such frightful surfeit; were we to eat just enough to furnish the bodily requirements, and no more; and food of the proper quality; there is every reason to believe, I say, that none of these foul conditions would exist—such as I have mentioned above. There is no *reason* why such conditions should exist; though we have so accustomed ourselves to them that few have ever thought of this fact. We have, in reality direct proof that such conditions need not and do not exist—provided that proper attention be given to the question of nutri tion, and that we sufficiently limit the food supply.

"Have you ever stopped to think," asks Mr. Horace Fletcher,[1] "why the excrements are foul and odorous? Simply because undigested food, which should have been so masticated as to give the body nourishment, is thrown off by the stomach into the intestines, there to decay and produce this unclean condition."

And again he says:[2]

"One of the most noticeable and significant results of economic nutrition, gained through careful attention to the mouth-treatment of food, or buccal-digestion is, not only the small quantity of waste obtained but its inoffensiveness. Under best test conditions the ashes of economic digestion have been reduced to one-tenth of the average given as normal in the best text-books on physiology. The economic digestion-ash forms in pillular shape, and, when released, these are massed together, having become so bunched by considerable retention in the rectum. There is no stench, no evidence of putrid bacterial decomposition, only the odor of warmth, like warm earth or 'hot biscuit.' Test samples of excreta, kept for more than five years, remain inoffensive, dry up, gradually disintegrate and are lost."

Here, then, is surely a revelation to the majority of persons who are accustomed to think of the bowel contents as *necessarily* offensive, and we are forced to the conclusion that, if proper attention were given to diet, and particularly to a sufficient *restriction* of it, there would be no need—either of the drastic purgatives of the "regular" school, or the more natural methods of cleansing the bowels described in this chapter; induced evacuations would be rendered quite unnecessary, owing to the fact that there would be no offensive or encumbering material present in the bowels, calling for removal.

[1] "A. B–Z. of Our Own Nutrition," p. 24.
[2] "New Glutton or Epicure," pp. 144–5.

It is true that I have been discussing so far an ideal condition; a condition which, in sick persons, *never* exists. In all cases of disease, things are very different! It will almost invariably be found that constipation, and subsequent auto-infection, is present; and that a foul condition of the digestive tract is present throughout. This may be inferred from the foul breath and coated tongue; but a far more tangible method is to cleanse the bowels, and notice the results. And in order to do this, it is not necessary to resort to that most harmful and in every way detrimental practice of taking "purgatives."

The objections to purgatives are manifold. I shall enumerate them briefly. (1) The "action" of the purgative being really, as we have seen (p. 32), the action of the bowel in expelling the drug poison thus introduced; it is obvious that this extreme and violent action must be followed by a period of abnormal reaction (p. 42), in order for the bowels to obtain their necessary rest. This constitutes constipation—an invariable consequent, as we know. Recourse must again be had to purgatives to remove *this* trouble (the result of the former "medication"), and so on *ad infinitum*—the patient's vitality, meanwhile, being sapped to the very core. (2) The purgative does not really accomplish its purpose. Thus, Doctor Jamison remarks:[1]

"After the system has absorbed 75 per cent. of the fecal mass, a 'remedy' is taken to excite the flow of watery excretions into the bowels, of which a portion will be retained in the colon, and especially the ballooned cavities, and reabsorbed; and every day the objectionable practice is repeated without any thought of the harm being done. . . . An abnormal amount of watery secretion is forced by the drug into the foul canal, to mix there with its contents, of which the major portion is retained and reabsorbed into the system. (p. 67.) . . . Drugs are prescribed to liquefy the hardened putrid remnant and absorption begins again; a fact very shocking to sensitive, even sensible, persons." (p. 70.)

Says Doctor Forest:

"What permanent good is a violent cathartic, which simply stirs up this mass for an hour, and then leaves it to accumulate again for days and weeks?"[2]

[1] "Intestinal Ills," p. 125.

[2] Forest "The New Method," p. 18.

(3) Who, with ordinary intelligence and an idea of cleanliness, would take or prescribe remedies to move the bowels, if it were possible to cleanse the foul cavities with water? We know that they can be cleansed in this manner, and that the only results are a great improvement in the condition of the diseased canals. (*loc. cit.* pp. 124–5.) (4) Constipation invariably results, as stated above. (5) The drug is in itself most harmful to the system—the water quite harmless. It is vulgarly supposed that the drug in some mysterious manner, passes directly through the stomach and passes at once and directly into the bowels upon which they "act." Apart from the fundamental error contained in this view, and pointed out in p. 32, it is, unfortunately the case that, before they can do so, they must pass through the *entire blood stream,* poisoning that, and inducing a general poisoned and abnormal condition of the system.[1] (6) The practice is founded upon an erroneous theory, which is liable to lead to further and graver errors. (7) The practice increases our belief in, and dependence upon, spurious medicines, and "cures," and away from hygiene and the true methods of cure. (8) Purgatives artificially and harmfully *force* an abnormal amount of watery secretion into the alimentary canal, in order to bring about an "action" (expulsion)—thus draining the system of much-needed fluids—while the enema, on the other hand, actually *supplies* the fluid—thereby removing one great *cause* of constipation—lack of sufficient fluid in the system—as well as the constipation itself. (9) An irritation of the bowel is set up which may result in local inflammation, and, if persisted in, far graver consequences—malignant growths, cancers, etc., having been traced, beyond peradventure, to this source. (10) The water indirectly benefits every portion of the system—especially stimulating the functions of all organs and nerve centers in contact with the colon—while poisonous drugs must invariably have the precisely opposite effect.

There is a far more physiological and healthful manner of cleaning out the bowels than this; a method that achieves far better results, both immediate and ultimate—without any of the

[1] See "Hygienic Treatment," by Dr. Archibald Hunter, p. 23; Dunlop: "Philosophy of the Bath," p. 242, etc.

drawbacks invariably accompanying the other method. This is the simple practice of *taking an enema*; of flushing, or washing out the bowels, that is, with water—just as one would flush out or cleanse, any pipe or sewer that had become clogged with an accumulation of foreign matter. Strange to say, there exists a prejudice against this method in many minds—some believing it harmful, *e.g.*—though they realize that man is made of more than three-fourths water, and that, in drinking, water passes into the bowels in just the same manner—only *per os* instead of *per rectum!* But this is not the place to defend the theory or practice of enema taking; such has already been done time and again, and all objections have been shown to consist in the greatest physiological absurdities.[1]

An enema is taken in the following manner. A large fountain syringe is filled with water—the temperature being suited to the case (pp. 412–13). The bag, being suspended at a height of several feet from the floor, the nozzle is inserted into the rectum, and the water is allowed to flow into the colon, thereby diluting and dissolving its contents. When the water is subsequently expelled, therefore (which is almost immediately after the injection is completed, as a rule), it carries with it all the effete material that had been retained in the bowels for hours, days—and some of it, by adhesion to the walls of the intestines, even for weeks, months or years previously! Can it not be seen what a potent, and at the same time, what a *simple* remedy this is? Here we have a mass of decaying and putrefying organic matter, lying within the intestine, constantly being absorbed into the system—thereby causing endless sickness and disease. What more rational method could be devised, then, of ridding the system of this accumulation of poisonous material, than flushing, or washing out, the intestine—just as we would cleanse any other vessel from its obnoxious contents, *viz.*, by thoroughly diluting and washing it out with an abundance of clean, pure water? The advantages and simplicity of the method are so obvious, and the objections so futile, that it seems unnecessary

[1] See, *e.g.*, "Intestinal Irrigation," by A. B. Jamison, M.D., pp. 108–119. Chapter "Objections to the Use of the Enema Answered," while practical illustrations of its utility are to be found in the same author's booklet "How to Become Strong."

to devote more space and time at present to what may be called a *defense* of the method.

I cannot now stop to consider the advantages and disadvantages of the various methods of taking the enema; the bodily positions advised by the various authorities upon the subject—for that would take a chapter of great length in itself. Thus:

"There are various positions that may be taken in flushing the colon; the simplest is to lie on the right side with the right arm behind and so turning the body somewhat. If this causes pain or the water is not retained, lie on the back with the hips elevated; or take the knee-chest position, resting the body on the knees and chest."[1]

"Where the bowels are loose and large and flabby, it is advisable to lie on the right side, with knees drawn up. This position relieves the descending colon and sigmoid flexure from the weight and pressure of the abdominal contents, and so favors the passage of the tube and the reception of water. Where people are thin, the Sims position is recommended—*i.e.*, lie forward upon the chest, with arms to either side, knees drawn upward toward the left, which slightly turns the hips, relaxes internal organs and gives freedom to both hands."[2]

Doctor Jamison, on the other hand, advises the "usual upright position" (seated) "for those physically able." I consider all these positions open to serious objection, but the matter is too complicated and extensive to discuss in any detail here.

I shall, on the contrary, confine myself to a statement of the method I personally would advise; giving my reasons for what I conceive to be the superiority of this method over all others, as we proceed. I would state, also, that the method of taking the enema here advised has been founded upon considerable personal and other experience, and by an analysis of the previous methods, and a discovery of their defects.

Take a four-quart fountain syringe and pour into it about half a pint of warm water, ranging in temperature from 100° to 105° F.[3] Hang this up about four feet above the couch upon

[1] "The New Internal Bath," p. 43.
[2] "The Internal Bath," by Laura M. Wright, M.D., pp. 10–11.
[3] This is a disputed point. Doctor Wright says: "The temperature of injecting fluid for flushings should be at all times as hot as can comfortably

which the enema is to be taken (the force of the water will depend upon the height at which the bag is suspended above the patient—the higher the bag the more forcible the stream of water, and *vice versa*). Allow the water to run through the tube for a second or two before using, in order to permit the escape of inclosed air. Oil and insert the nozzle[1] into the rectum.

Now lie upon the left side and gradually allow the water to flow into the bowel. Should pain or discomfort be experienced at any time, instantly check the flow of water until this has passed away. It is due to a sudden and forcible expansion of the intestine, which will cease instantly the water has made its way upward and has passed the dried and impacted fæces. The flow of water should then be allowed to continue—this process being repeated as often as may be necessary (frequently it is not necessary at all) until the half-pint is all injected. Having done this, withdraw the nozzle, and retain the water, if possible, two or three minutes, before expelling it—thus enabling it to dissolve and soften the contained fæces. Now rise and expel the water, and whatever fecal matter it may carry with it—the more the better. Next place into the bag about one quart of *tepid* water, and allow this to flow into the colon—as above directed—still lying on the *left* side. Should pain be experienced at any time, during the injection, temporarily stop the flow of water, as previously stated (five or six seconds will usually

be borne, *i.e.*, from 105 to 112° F. . . . ." ("New Internal Bath," p. 13.) For reasons that will presently appear, I cannot accept this advice as the best. Doctor Jamison recommends that the injected water be the temperature of the body—98.5° F. ("Intestinal Irrigation," p. 98.) Doctor Hunter ("Hygienic Treatment," p. 38), recommends that the temperature of the water be from 100° to 104° F., while Doctor Trall, in his writings, contended that tepid enemas were, as a rule, the best. Doubtless the temperature of the water has to be varied greatly to suit the patient and the disease.

[1] Doctor Wright is of the opinion that the short nozzle should be replaced, in colon flushings, by a long flexible rubber nozzle (from twelve to thirty inches in length), which, she insists, is far more effective than the "old" method. Her arguments seem to me to be very strong. Doctor Jamison's rejoinder to her arguments also seems to me very effective, and the choice must be left to each individual reader to decide. The subject cannot be discussed here—much as I should like to do so—but the arguments *pro* and *con* may be found in Doctor Wright's "New Internal Bath," pp. 8–10, and in Doctor Jamison's "Intestinal Irrigation," pp. 85–9, respectively—to which I would refer the reader for the full discussion. Meanwhile I suggest that, for all practical purposes, and especially in cases of fasting, the short, and usually procurable, nozzle will answer all requirements—*especially if the enema be taken as here suggested.*

suffice), then continue as before. Retain, and allow this to pass out. We now have the rectum, descending colon, and great sigmoid flexure fairly clear from impacted fecal matter, and we must now turn our attention to the cleansing of the transverse and ascending colon—which latter lies on the right side of the body—the transverse colon connecting the two. (In other words the direction of the colon is up the right side, across, and down the left side.) When undertaking to flush the colon, therefore, we must commence by cleansing the left, or descending colon, in order to effectually reach the right, or ascending colon, for the reason that, otherwise, the force of gravity would cause the first injection of water to flow across and into the right side—thereby infusing itself throughout the entire mass of fecal matter and "becoming lost," so to speak, amid so much material—defeating, thereby, its sole purpose of concentrated local action. The left side being cleaned of its contents, however, the passage is cleared for the direct flow of water to the right side, and a passage is left along which may flow the dislodged matter, unimpeded. It now becomes apparent why I recommended that the enema should be taken—first on the left, then on the right side—a most obvious measure, yet one which I have failed to find advocated in any book upon the subject that I have ever come across.

This third—and generally last[1]—injection should consist of the full four quarts of water, or as large a percentage of this as the bowels can hold without extreme discomfort. The amount varies, of course, in individual cases; some persons cannot take more than two or three quarts without experiencing a certain amount of tension and pain (relieved immediately the water is expelled) while others can retain two gallons or more without experiencing inconvenience.[2] It depends, of course, upon the individual; and should be administered accordingly.

The temperature of this third enema should be quite cool—in fact cold—provided that there is sufficient vitality to thoroughly react. In all feverish conditions, the enema should

[1] In all diseased conditions, the enemas should follow one another till the water comes away *clear*. These should be taken daily, at least; sometimes two or three times a day.

[2] *See* "Intestinal Lavage," p. 32.

invariably be quite cold—though never ice cold (except in very exceptional cases which cannot be discussed now). This cold acts as a helpful stimulant upon the jaded and relaxed vital centers, and does not leave them lax and flaccid, as a warm or hot enema would do. If a warm enema be taken, by all means end up with a small injection of cold water, which may be retained altogether if desired—being absorbed through the walls of the colon. This will serve to add tone to the bowels, and "draw up" the rectum —which might, otherwise, have a tendency to be inconveniently relaxed. If this is not done a cold sitz bath (p. 365), should be substituted instead, and will serve much the same purpose.

Many persons have a vague, superstitious fear of thus injecting cold water into the rectum; but, provided the system can properly react, this fear is altogether unfounded. Do we not pour glassful after glassful of ice water into our poor, abused stomachs without a thought of the consequences? And what is the stomach more than a mere bulging of one portion of the bowel? To be sure, ice water is not by any means good or healthful—even though it is so drunk by the vast majority of Americans (to the horror of their European neighbors), and is deprecated by most physicians. That is very true, and it will be noticed that I did not, and do not, recommend ice cold enemas; but stated, on the contrary, that they should be "cool." There is then no more danger in administering cool, pure water *per rectum* than there is in administering it *per os*. In each case heat is abstracted from the body, and for the same purpose; for it must be remembered that any water entering the body below blood-heat is raised to that standard before being expelled by the depurating organs (at bodily temperature) extracting, of course, this heat from the bodily tissues. In all cases of fever, etc., the extreme importance of cool enemas will thus become manifest—though it becomes more and more difficult to see wherein the supposed "danger" lies.

I have come across a few cases in which difficulty is experienced in expelling the water after the injection is complete. This very rarely happens, but it may do so. Should this difficulty occur, rise and walk up and down the room for a few minutes; or roll from side to side upon the couch, while keeping the arms stretched above the head. Kneading the bowels in the direction of the colon (up the right side; across the pit of the stomach and down the left) will almost invariably bring instantaneous results. Or a hot compress or hot sitz bath may be tried. In any case no alarm need be felt--since the water *per se* is perfectly harmless, and will be absorbed and eliminated by the system in exactly the same manner as water that is drunk, is eliminated. I have never heard of a case, however, in which this extreme retention is recorded, and much doubt if such could ever occur. The usual result is quite the contrary; and retention beyond even a few moments is impossible. I merely speak of it here as a condition that *might* occur—not as one that is *likely* to happen; as an extreme possibility, and to show that—even were so untoward a result to follow—no apprehension whatever need be felt on that account.

It occasionally happens, also, that slight sickness (of the stomach) may follow the injection—though, if the water is of the temperature advised—this very rarely follows. A glass or two of cool water will usually dispel this feeling; and the water should be checked and the nozzle withdrawn so long as it lasts. The enema should never be taken immediately before, or within two hours after, a meal; when provided reasonable care be taken, such unpleasant results need seldom or never follow.

It may, perhaps, be objected that this method of cleaning the bowels effects but one portion of them—the colon—leaving the stomach and the small intestine untouched. To a certain extent this may be true:

> "But there is no necessity," as has been pointed out,[1] "of reaching this directly if only the stomach and the colon are kept in order. The small intestine receives at its upper end the bile from the liver. Now, the bile is a decided anti-ferment, and if the stomach and liver can be made to do their work properly, the small intestine will protect itself against undue fermentation and poisonous absorption."

But, apart from such considerations, it has now been demonstrated that water injected in this manner *will* pass the ileocæcal

[1] "New Internal Bath," p. 38.

valve and enter the small intestine—even effecting its whole length. This has been definitely proved by Dr. W. B. Cannon's researches upon "The Movement of the Intestines Studied by Means of the Roentgen Rays."[1]

Here we read that:

"In every case antiperistaltic waves are set going by the injection, and the material is thereby carried to the cœcum, Small injections have never in my experience been forced even in part into the small intestine; but with the larger amounts, whether fluid or mushy, the radiographs show many coils of the small intestine containing the bismuth food. (p. 381.) . . . I have never seen food material pass back so far as the stomach, but once, about ten minutes after an injection of 100 c.c. of warm water, the cat reached and vomited a clear fluid resembling mixed water and mucus. In the fluid there were two intestinal worms still alive." (p. 382.)

From this we can no longer doubt that every part of the intestine may be thus cleansed by the injected water; and this cleansing process should always be assisted by copious water drinking.

The common sense—the philosophy—of this method of treatment is now, I trust, apparent. The whole secret is—*cleanliness;* a washing out of the intestine, as we would any other tube containing foul, obnoxious material. What possible harm can come from such a sane and healthful practice? In all diseased conditions this measure is of the utmost and very greatest importance; and even in health an occasional flushing of the colon is to be recommended. We know that absorption of this water takes place, as a considerable percentage of it is almost invariably passed off as urine, shortly after the enema is completed. For this reason also, "nutrient" or food enemas are frequently administered by the physician, after feeding *per os* has become impossible. Further, every particle of food which the body utilizes must, of necessity, be absorbed through the intestinal wall. Knowing these facts, then, is it not obvious that the foul, corrupt fecal matter must, to a very great extent be absorbed

[1] From the "Laboratory of Physiology," Harvard Medical School: Extracts from the *American Journal of Physiology*, 1902; reprinted in Horace Fletcher's "A. B–Z. of Our Nutrition," pp. 342–88.

also[1]—thereby leading to auto-infection, and a system infected throughout with filth, poison and disease? And does not the vast importance of a clean, sweet, alimentary canal become at once apparent?—its vital necessity proved, if health and purity of body are to exist? And does not the idea force itself more and more upon us, while considering this question, that a full, overcrowded and filthy alimentary canal is thus the basis and starting point of all diseases? "No need to journey to other localities for health," as Doctor Jamison has justly remarked,[2] "*so long as you carry so formidable a foe to health with you.*"

I shall make but one or two more remarks in this connection. It may be thought, by some, that an enema may be quite unnecessary in their case—for the reason that one—perhaps two—movements of the bowels occur daily, and with fair regularity. I must insist that this is no indication at all that constipation and other diseased conditions of the bowels do not exist.

> "The colon is loaded with waste and poisonous matter from one year's end to the other. There may be a discharge every day, even more than one, and yet the person may be badly constipated! Bear in mind that, accurately speaking, constipation means a loaded colon. Now, if from one end of this packed organ a small portion is discharged daily, the colon still remains full by the addition at the other end, and thus constipation is present and continuous even though there be a daily discharge. The discharge is from the lower end of the colon only."[3]

Further, we now have proof that fecal matter may cleave to the wall of the intestine, and there solidify and harden, permanently diseasing the bowel, preventing the nutriment taken from being properly absorbed, and poisoning the body;[4] yet, since the center of the passage is left open, and the bowel contents can, after a fashion, pass through it, and be finally discharged, constipation may never be suspected. It has been

[1] From two-thirds to three-fourths of the total amount, according to Doctor Jamison. ("Intestinal Irrigation," p. 60.)

[2] "Intestinal Ills," pp. 121–2.

[3] "New Internal Bath," p. 27.

[4] It is partly owing to this cause, I believe, that many persons are thin and anæmic; what food they eat "does them no good." Of course not—for they cannot appropriate or assimilate it, and we can now appreciate the full truth of Doctor Latson's remark—that an overfed man is "both starved and poisoned." ("Common Disorders," p. 120.)

shown that this process of accumulation and incrustation mav continue until almost complete stoppage of the bowel results—but a narrow bore being left along which fecal matter may pass—instead of a clean, sweet healthy bowel. Says Doctor Monroe:[1]

"Colons that are chronically impacted, lined with indurated fecal matter, are like an old stove when the ashes of many winters have formed clinkers in its sides that have to be chiseled off. These impacted colons present a small canal at the side or in the middle of the impaction, through which the fæces must pass, and such patients always have to liquefy their stools by drugs every time they obtain an action." Indeed, in some cases, we are assured that "diarrhœa may be present without removing the constipation, for the fecal matters are often so hardened and impacted that fluid dejections pass by them without solving or moving them."[2]

Doctor Depierris also says:[3]

"Constipation at times becomes so great that the intestines become covered with a crust of matter forming a solid and hollow tube, the thickness becoming greater, to the obliteration of the passage."

Are not such conditions obviously disease-breeding? And yet they exist, more or less, in almost all of us. Does it not behoove us, then, to keep this part of our bodies clean, healthy, and in such a condition that we are not *ashamed to acknowledge it as a part of ourselves?*

From the above, it will readily be seen that an enema, used in such cases, will have the effect of rapidly dissolving and carrying off this mass of effete material; and that the water may here have the effect of removing fecal matter which otherwise would never have been passed away from the system, but remained there until we died! Retention of this material within the bowel is one of the greatest causes of disease known to us—yet how common a disease it is! Constipation is all but universal. The amount of fæces that the colon may hold, without

[1] "Therapeutical Uses of Intestinal Lavage," pp. 19–20.
[2] "Digestion and Dyspepsia," by R. T. Trall, M.D., p. 52.
[3] "Aristocracy of Health," p. 248.

giving any notice of undue tension, is something prodigious. Thus, Dr. N. Chapman, in his "Clinical Lectures" (p. 304) says:

"The fæces sometimes accumulate in distinct indurated scybala or in enormous masses, solid and compact. Taunton, a surgeon of London, has a preparation of the colon and rectum of more than twenty inches in circumference containing three gallons of fæces, taken from a woman, whose abdomen was as much distended as in the maturity of pregnancy. By Lemazurier, another case is reported of a pregnant woman, who was constipated for two months, from whom, after death, thirteen and one-half pounds of solid fæces were taken away, though a short time before between two and three pounds had been scraped out of the rectum. Cases reported by Doctor Graves, of Dublin, which he saw in women, were from distensions in certain directions of the abdomen, the one was considered to be owing to a prodigious hypertrophy of the liver, and the other of the ovary; in the latter of which he removed a bucket full of fæces in two days. Mr. Wilmot, of London, has recently given a case where a gallon of matter was lodged in the cœcum, and the intestines perforated by ulceration."

I myself have known of cases reaching almost an equal amount, while M. Socquet has removed from the large intestine seventeen and one-half pounds of fecal matter.[1] This subject is not the pleasantest to discuss, but where disease and death are in the balance, we must discuss this question of nutrition in all its phases—looking on the fæces as so much "digestion-ash."

Now, one most interesting fact in connection with the fast is the almost uniformly complete lack of action of the bowels. After a fast has been entered upon, they seem hardly ever to move of their own accord, and unless coaxed or forced to do so by enemas, etc. Doctor Page informs us that:

"Tanner had no movement during his fast; Griscomb's experience was similar, and Connolly, the consumptive, who fasted forty-three days, had no movement for three weeks, and then the temporary looseness was occasioned by profuse water drink ing, which in his case proved curative."[2]

[1] "Death and Sudden Death," by P. Brouardel, M.D., p. 258.
[2] "Natural Cure," p. 112.

Now, from one point of view, this is only natural. Since no food is ingested, we should suppose, *à priori*, that none would be excreted; but this is a very superficial and, as we shall presently see below, a very erroneous view of the question. There frequently is much fecal matter present, but it is not voluntarily excreted—at least for many days. Mark Twain quotes a case, *e.g.*,[1] in which no action of the bowels was recorded for forty-four days! In this case, too, a very small amount of food was daily ingested. The system, of course, utilized practically every particle of this material, and there was none left to excrete. Again, Doctor Dewey mentions one case in which no action took place for twenty-four days.[2]

For the reason, then, that the bowels do cease to act, in this manner, I must insist that, while a patient is *fasting*, enemata should be constantly employed. Every organ of elimination works more rapidly and effectively while a fast is in progress, as we know (pp. 153–8); and the fecal matter in the bowels should be regularly removed to make way for the fresh material that is rapidly being deposited. It may be thought by some that—when once the food supply is cut off—no new material will be deposited, but this is a very great mistake. Says Doctor Page:[3]

"This movement, when natural, consists of waste matters secreted from the blood by the glands of the colon, and not, as is popularly supposed, of food substances, at least not to any considerable degree. When it does (and I am bound to say that this is the rule rather than the exception) it is because the person has eaten at least *that much more* than he ought."

And similarly Doctor Jamison says:[4]

"It is not generally known to laymen, nor sufficiently appreciated among physicians, that the mass of fecal matter normally evacuated from the bowels comes mainly from the blood; and that this mass is not, as it is usually supposed to be, the residue of the food that has been left unassimilated."

[1] "The Man That Corrupted Hadleyburg, and Other Stories," p. 124.
[2] "No-Breakfast Plan," p. 107.
[3] "Natural Cure," p. 111.
[4] "Intestinal Ills," p. 99.

Such being the case, we may readily see the necessity of constantly rinsing out the bowels—since the waste material continues to be deposited in them daily; and this, right up to the end of the fast—no matter how long, in duration, that may be. We thus have an explanation, also, of those facts that have puzzled so many observers of the phenomena of fasting, *viz.*, the extraordinary *length of time* that fecal matter may continue to remain within the bowel, even in spite of repeated and thorough flushings. I myself have known one case in which a very great amount of fæces were removed by an enema on the *thirty-eighth day* of a fast; and this in spite of the fact that thorough flushings had been taken almost daily! It proves to us how "far behind" was Nature in her accounts—requiring all this time merely to "catch up," so to speak, and how necessary in such cases must have been the fast!

We can now, I think, see the reason for these facts. In many cases, the fecal matter was *not* in the intestine at all, on the occasion of the previous flushing—but it was deposited there by the blood in the interval. Needless to say, this extraneous matter should be removed now, just as promptly as at any other time; and, since true health cannot return until the system is completely rid of *all* such material—and, as the fast will terminate naturally (as we shall see, p. 544), when such a condition of health is established, we can readily see that a frequent flushing of the bowels—say, once a day—will materially assist a return to health, and effectively shorten the fast.[1] It is a most important hygienic auxiliary to the main treatment; and, though so essential, Doctor Dewey hardly mentions the enema in any of his books; but its omission seems to me a very great fault, since we can see that its use will both shorten and lighten the period of fasting; and, for the fasting patient, these surely, are two highly important and much-longed-for measures; since I by no means contend that the fasting cure is either easy or pleasant. My contention is that it is a true and efficient *cure;* and this, I am convinced, is more than can be said of any other method now in vogue.

[1] Mr. Purinton's advice to "eat laxative foods only for several days preceding the fast" seems to me exceedingly sound. ("Philosophy of Fasting," p. 108–9).

It must be admitted, of course, that the enema is, after all, only a palliative treatment—removing the symptoms; and that, unless the diet is reformed (lessened in quantity and changed in quality) no permanent and effectual cure can result or be possible. The *cause* of the abnormal bowel conditions must be removed, if a true cure is to follow, and this can only be brought about by reforming the diet—the initial cause of the bowel trouble—which necessitated the enemas and even the fast.

CHAPTER VII

MENTAL INFLUENCES

The "influence of the mind upon the body" has become a hackneyed expression in medical literature, ever since Dr. Hack Tuke wrote his classical treatise upon the subject, bearing that title. "Suggestion"—hypnotic and other—is attracting the attention of the medical world to-day as it never did before. Keen interest is being manifested in the subject, and investigations have been conducted in this direction—a direction which will, I believe, ultimately prove far more fruitful and productive of results than any other that has so far been pursued. I am a firm believer in the great—the *very* great—influence of the mind in the causation and cure of disease, not only in mental and so-called "nervous" affections, but in the gravest of functional disturbances. As Dr. A. T. Schofield pointed out:[1]

"It is important to observe that a disease due to the imagination is not necessarily an imaginary disease, but may produce various functional and even organic disturbances."

That the mind exerts *some* influence over the body is too obvious to necessitate proof; the *extent* of that influence is the only point in dispute—the only matter to be decided. That this influence is vastly more real and potent than was formerly imagined is now conceded by all; and I shall briefly call attention to a few of the most well-known and obvious forms of this influence, in order to enable us, the more easily, to appreciate and understand the deeper set and more extraordinary phenomena, which we shall have occasion to mention later on in this chapter.

At no period of his existence is man severed from the active operations—the potent influences—of mind. Even before his birth this all-powerful factor is actively at work; prenatal

[1] "Nerves in Disorder," p. 6.

influences undoubtedly playing a large part in the formation of the mental and physical life of the unborn child.[1]

After birth, we begin to gain control of our bodies; to possess a personality; to feel the influence and the power of this inner "self." Thenceforward, the mind assumes a more and more important rôle. How great this control may be is not ever realized by the majority of mankind. The phenomena of blushing and of "turning pale" are two well-known instances of the effect of mental states over the circulation.[2] The influence of excitement upon the heart, the respiration, the excretory organs, etc., are also too well-known to require more than a passing mention. Fear frequently affects the kidneys; the bladder; and still more readily the skin—where a "cold perspiration" is experienced as the result of shock; excitement will stimulate the bowels to copious action; will increase the rate of respiration—thereby increasing the output of carbonic acid gas, etc.

Suggestion, hypnotic and other, has enabled us to produce most extraordinary effects. A quickening or slowing of the pulse has frequently been induced artificially. Krafft-Ebing's experiments (quoted more fully later on) are particularly surprising. "He succeeded in producing any temperature he pleased on his subject," wrote Dr. A. Moll.[3] Doctor Moll himself succeeded in "antidoting," as it were, the effects of purgatives by suggestion; or, on the contrary, inducing an action of the bowels by suggestions that such purgatives had been taken, when, in fact, none such had been administered at all. Thus we read (pp. 123–4):

"I have had several experiences of the facility with which the bowels of some hypnotics are affected by suggestion. I say to one of them, 'In half an hour after waking your bowels will act.'

[1] See "Foreordained," by An Observer; "Pre-Natal Culture," by A. E. Newton; "Human Personality," by F. W. H. Myers, Vol. I., pp. 455–8, etc.

[2] The circulation is, of course, regulated almost solely by the nervous system; and, by controlling the latter, we may, accordingly, regulate the circulation throughout the body. We thus see how valuable *suggestion* may be in some cases; for, by acting directly upon the mind, which controls the nervous system, which, in turn, controls the circulation, we may thereby equalize the latter—relieving congestion, and supplying one of the principal requisites for a true cure. (pp. 69–70.)

[3] "Hypnotism," p. 129.

The effect follows. 'To-morrow, between eight and nine, your bowels will act three times.' Exactly the same result, though the subject remembers nothing of the suggestion on awaking. It is interesting to note that the action of aperients can be checked by suggestion, though this does not often happen. A patient takes a dose of castor oil which is sufficient to produce copious action of the bowels. He is told in hypnosis that the medicine will only take effect in forty-eight hours. The suggestion is effectual, although with this person the dose habitually acts quickly and abundantly "

Dr. Hack Tuke gives the classical case in which the infant was poisoned, and died, as the result of the mother's milk becoming tainted—the result, in turn, of a fit of anger shortly before feeding.[1] We know that the secretions are often poisoned in this manner; the spittle of mad dogs well illustrating this point. Indeed, it has been demonstrated (if reports speak truly) by the experiments of Prof. Elmer Gates[2] and others, that certain mental states, such as anger, worry, fear, etc., actually create *poisons* within the system—poisonous precipitates being formed, and may be detected by the proper chemical tests. These precipitates are of various colors; the color depending, apparently, upon the character of the emotion or mental state invoked. Thus we see the physiological consequences of such mental conditions, and the delicate, yet potent, reciprocal action of mind and body. But this poison is and must be eliminated through the depurating organs, just as any other poison is, so that fasting and other appropriate hygienic agencies are as applicable in all cases of mental disturbance as in any other diseased condition whatever.

And in other ways is this influence exemplified. Cases of so-called "miraculous cures" may be found in the histories of all countries, but have always been scouted by the scientific men of the age as untrue, and as merely the results of mal-observation and ignorance. And it is only lately, when much these same results have been obtained artificially, by hypnotic suggestion, that they have become recognized as veritable truths, and as

[1] In certain foul conditions of the organism, the breasts become veritable eliminating organs! See Trall: "Sexual Physiology and Hygiene," p. 213.
[2] "The Mind and the Brain," p. 11.

worthy of serious consideration and study. Take, *e.g.*, the cases of stigmata recorded and generally attributed to "miracle." There are numerous cases on record where continued contemplation of and dwelling upon the scene of the crucifixion have resulted in the appearance of bleeding spots or patches in the skin, corresponding, in their location, to the wounds of Christ. This was first recorded in the case of Francis of Assisi; and there have been numerous other cases—one of the best known and most recent being that of Louise Lateau of Bois d'Haine, near Mons, France, which was much discussed in 1868.

"It appears," says Doctor Moll, in discussing this case, "from the literature concerning her, that the anatomical process was rather a complicated one in her case. Blisters first appeared, and after they burst, there was bleeding from the true skin (corium), without any visible injury. I will not enter into the question of simulation, which a Belgian doctor, Warlomont, decided was impossible, after personal investigation. Delboeuf and others believe that the phenomena were caused by auto-suggestion. Lateau directed her own attention continually to those parts of her body which, she knew, corresponded to the wounds of Christ, and the anatomical lesions resulted from this strain of attention, as in other cases from external suggestion. Virchow, as is known, thought that fraud or miracle were the only alternatives. In the well-known case of Catherine Emmerich, the bleedings are said to have appeared while she was looking at the crucifix."

Nor are these cases altogether exceptional. Many other similar results have been attained, sometimes as the result of direct experiment—by hypnotic and post-hypnotic suggestion, and by other means. Mr. Myers collected and published many interesting cases of this character in his chapter on "The Mechanism of Suggestion," published in the *Proceedings* of the Society for Psychical Research, Vol. VII., pp. 327–55.

But the most remarkable case of this character, undoubtedly, is that published by Krafft-Ebing, to which he devoted a whole book.[1] In this case the most remarkable phenomena were observed.

[1] "An Experimental Study in the Domain of Hypnotism," etc.

"Once at least," we are told, "she (the patient) was much injured and offended by the culpable act of a medical student, who laid a pair of scissors upon her chest, telling her that they were red-hot, and thus created a serious wound, which took two months to heal."

Krafft-Ebing made a humane variation of this risky experiment. Like Doctor Biggs, he ordered the production of red patches of definite shapes, which were to be formed without itching, pain, or inflammation.

"The history of the process thus set up is a curious one. The organism had to perform, so to say, a novel feat, which took a great deal longer than the rough and ready process of vesication. From February 24th to May 3d, 1888, a livid, red, hyperæmic surface, corresponding to the letter K was slowly and painlessly developing itself on a selected and protected area between the shoulder-blades."

I will cite one or two other cases equally extraordinary. Thus: Professor Beaunis and Doctor Krafft-Ebing have slowed the pulse by hypnotic suggestion; and these *savants*, as well as Professor Bernheim, M. Focachon and others, have produced redness and blisters by the same means. Doctors Mabille, Ramadier, Bourru, Burot, have produced localized hyperæmia, epistaxis, ecchymosis. Doctor Forel and others have restored arrested secretions at a precisely fixed hour. Doctor Krafft-Ebing has produced a rise of temperature at moments fixed by himself—a rise, for instance, from 37° to 38.5° C. Burot has lowered the temperature of a hand as much as 10° C. by suggestion. He supposes that the mechanism employed is the constriction of the brachial artery, beneath the biceps. "How can it be," he asks, "that when one merely says to the subject, 'your hand will become cold,' the vaso-motor nervous system answers by constricting the artery to the degree necessary to achieve the result desired? *C'est ce qui depasse nôtre imagination.*"[1]

Take again the following experiment, which was performed by Doctor Rybilkin, in the presence of his colleagues, at the hospital Marie, at St. Petersburg. Doctor Rybilikin had previ-

[1] "*Proceedings* of the Society for Psychical Research," Vol. VII., pp. 336–7.

ously experimented in the same way with this subject. The subject was Macar K., a house painter, aged 16, hysterical and almost wholly anæsthetic. He was hypnotized and it was suggested that:

"'When you awake, you will be cold; you will go and warm yourself at the stove, and you will burn your forearm on the line which I have traced out. This will hurt you; a redness will appear on your arm; it will swell; there will be blisters.' On being awakened, the patient obeyed the suggestion. He even uttered a cry of pain at the moment when he touched the door of the stove, which had not been lighted. Some minutes later a redness, without swelling, could be seen at the place indicated; and the patient complained of sharp pain on its being touched. A bandage was put on his arm, and he went to bed under our eyes. When the dressing was removed at ten next morning, we saw at the place of the burn two blisters, one the size of a nut, the other of a pea, and a number of small blisters. Around this tract the skin was red and sensitive." (*loc. cit.* p. 338.)

Thus we have been led by a gradual series of cases to perceive the potency and the extent of the influence of the mind over the body—that great influence which is now only just beginning to be realized, and put into practice by the medical profession. I cannot give any space to a detailed study of this subject, my object being to call attention to its importance rather than to attempt to establish any conclusion.

It may be thought by some that I have thus far given much too little attention to this branch of the subject, and far too much to the purely material or physiological side. I wish to say, in reply, that I do not wish to underestimate, in any way, that factor; but I have endeavored to make this a purely physiological work, dealing with the questions of health and disease from a purely material standpoint, and have purposely left out of consideration, *pro tem.*, the influences of the mind, as rendering the subject both more intricate and more detailed, without in any manner helping to elucidate the problem. I consider that the mental and the physiological are both most important factors in the causation and cure of disease, and that they travel along parallel lines, and must, consequently, be studied separately.[1] This book has undertaken the study of the material or physiological side only, and that is all that can be attempted in a volume such as the present.

I must confess, too, that I am much less favorably impressed with the evidence for mental cures than I was several years ago. The evidence is decidedly weaker than I once conceived it to be. Let me illustrate this and the reason for my decision. The Christian Science treatment, *e.g.*, is and must be erroneous in its principles because it aims at removing the symptoms rather than removing the causes—thus falling into the universal error of regarding disease (1) as an entity; and (2) as an evil to be overcome, rather than itself a beneficial curing process. And, further, when the symptoms have been relieved or removed, a "cure" is supposed to have been effected—this quite ignoring the fact that all symptoms may be removed, yet the true disease —the *cause*—still remain untouched. How fallacious this idea is, has been previously pointed out.

It may be objected that it is philosophically quite unwarrantable thus to divide up the mental and the physical in this manner, for separate study. "It is certain," it may be argued, "that there are not thus two distinct and separate factors, but that they are interblended and associated in the most intimate and inseparable manner." This connection and interdependence is one of the most certain and obvious of facts (albeit one of the most puzzling) with which philosophy has to deal. I fully realize the force and the implications of this objection. Indeed, I would go further, and acknowledge that, in reality, there may be no physical body at all, in the common acceptation of the term—it being but the symbol, counterpart, or external expression of the underlying, hidden reality—thought.

"If, at the present day," says Doctor Strong,[2] "there is a point on which philosophers show some sort of agreement, it is that

[1] "The force of suggestion is intended by Nature to be a powerful auxiliary, but no more." (Ebbard: "How to Restore Life Giving Energy to Sufferers from Sexual Neurasthenia," etc., p. 9.) Says Dr. T. J. Hudson ("Law of Psychic Phenomena," p. 164): "Theoretically, all the diseases which flesh is heir to are curable by mental processes. Practically, the range of their usefulness is comparatively limited." This is not in accordance with his later writings, it may be observed: see "The Law of Mental Medicine," etc.

[2] "Why the Mind Has a Body," p. 11.

matter *does not exist* in any such sense as the plain man supposes; that it has existence independently of mind."[1]

Thus the body—together with all other material objects in the world—may, indeed, be but the externality of thought—a modification of mind.

And that the whole visible universe is, for us, but a modification of mind can be proved, so to say, *ad oculos*. Thus: When I look at and apparently "see" a physical object, what really happens is something like this. Æther (light) waves, passing from the object to my eye, have caused the eye to vibrate, in turn, and this vibration, reaching the optic nerve, through the vibration of the vitreous humor of the eyeball, causes a nerve current to be set up, which travels along the optic nerve—reaching, ultimately, the center of sight, in the rear of the brain, where a certain brain change takes place (just *what* we are unable to say, but probably some sort of nerve vibration), and, corresponding to this nerve change, and coincidental with it, is the sensation of sight—of the object at which we happened to be looking at the time. But this brain change *is* not the object looked at, but merely its counterpart, or symbol; and, therefore, for every object we see, there is and must be this corresponding brain change, varying with and corresponding to the various objects seen. There is thus a series or succession of brain changes, corresponding point for point with the outer, external objects seen—of which they are the symbols, merely. But the mental state, the thought, does not, in any case, correspond with and to the external object, but with the brain change; with *this* it corresponds; with *this* it is intimately connected; and, if the mind can be said to "see" any physical thing in the world (so to speak), it is the brain change, and not the object. But the brain changes are, so far as we can see, as entirely dissimilar from the external object as possible; they are merely its counterparts, or symbols, as I have before stated. So that we do,

[1] Physics is now proving what philosophy so long held was the case—that matter does not exist in the sense that it is commonly supposed to exist. See Saleeby: "Evolution the Master Key," p. 346; Sir Oliver Lodge: "Modern Views on Matter"; Prof. J. J. Thomson: "Electricity and Matter"; Jones: "Electrical Nature of Matter"; Duncan: "The New Knowledge"; Hon. A. J. Balfour, M.P.: "Reflections Suggested by the New Theory of Matter," etc.

in reality, live altogether in a world of symbols—an inner, duplicate, mental world—which is thus the only world we do and ever can know. To take Doctor Strong's example:

"Suppose I am looking at a candle; the candle I am conscious of is a mental modification. How may I convince myself of the fact? By the simple process of closing my eyes. Something then ceases to exist. Is it the real candle? Certainly not. Then it must be the mental duplicate. By successively opening and closing my eyes I may create and annihilate the perceived candle. But the real candle continues unchanged. Then what I am immediately conscious of when my eyes are open must be the mental duplicate. If an original of that duplicate exists outside the mind, it must be other than the candle I perceive, and itself unperceived."[1]

But (and here is the rub) it does not follow that, because I believe all this to be *theoretically* true, I accept it as true for all practical purposes; for the pursuits and practical application of everyday life. That is the mistake the Christian Scientists have made, and I have no desire to follow in their footsteps. The fallacy has been so clearly pointed out and so beautifully illustrated by Sir Oliver Lodge that I cannot do better than to to quote his words, when he says:

"We cannot be permanently satisfied with dualism, but it is possible to be over-hasty, and also too precisely insistent. There are those who seem to think that a monistic view of existence precludes the legitimacy of speaking of soul and body, or of God and spiritual beings, or of guidance and management, at all; that is to say, they seem to think that because these things can be *ultimately* unified, therefore they are unified proximately and for practical purposes. We might as well urge that it is incorrect to speak of the chemical elements, or of the various materials with which, in daily life, we have to deal, or of the structures in which we live, or which we see and handle, as separate and real things, because in the last resort we believe that they may all be reduced to an aggregation of corpuscles, or to some other mode of unity. . . . The language of dualism or of multiplism is not

[1] "Why the Mind Has a Body," p. 186. See also Bradley: "Appearance and Reality"; James: "Psychology," Vol. I., pp. 219–20; Vol. II., pp. 617–89; Black: "Eyesight," p. 36, etc.

incorrect or inappropriable or superseded because we catch ideal glimpses of an ultimate unity; nor would it be any the less appropriable if the underlying unity could be more clearly or completely grasped. The material world may be an aspect of the spiritual world, or *vice versa*, perhaps; or both may be aspects of something else; but both are realities, just the same, and there need be no hesitation in speaking of them clearly and distinctly as, for practical purposes, separate entities."[1]

This so effectually disposes of the argument, I think, for our present purposes, that it is unnecessary for me to say more.

But, quite apart from all theories of a purely "spiritual" action, or of an extension of idealism sufficient to negate all disease—as a merely outward manifestation of morbid thought—one can quite see how, on the hypothesis that disease is a curing process, any mental stimulus would greatly assist in the cure—from a purely physiological standpoint. Granting that the mentality does (through the nervous system) affect the various tissues and organs of the body, the excretory organs must undoubtedly come in for their share of the stimulation, and hence tend to rid the body more quickly of the corrupt matter it contains. It must be remembered that all the excretory organs—together with all other organs of the body—are under the direct control of the nervous system, and limited in their functioning, not from lack of muscular power *per se* (if the expression be allowable), but from a lack of nervous, vital force lying behind such functioning, and regulating and controlling it. It must be remembered that the muscle contains no strength whatever in itself; the muscle of a dead person is absolutely useless, as muscle, and it only becomes capable of moving anything at all when still part of the living body, and influenced directly by the nerve currents of that body. Thus, the functioning power of any muscle or organ depends entirely upon the amount of nervous, vital energy supplied to that organ or muscle, and not in any special power inherent in the muscle or organ itself; and further, its power and activity are, *ceteris paribus*, directly proportioned to the amount of nervous force supplied. No matter how large and strong a muscle, or how perfect an organ, the

[1] *Hibbert Journal*, January, 1905, pp. 317–18.

nerves feeding these parts of the body once severed, paralysis instantly follows; no power, no strength, is there. On the other hand, stimulating the muscle or organ by increasing the nervous current to that part will have the effect of increasing the functioning power of that part, and stimulating it up to the requisite point for normal action. Thus, whenever there is increased nervous force or energy, there we invariably find increased functional ability and power for work.

Mr. Myers has pointed out, in this connection, that:

"The strong-willed, educated savant can sometimes compress the dynamometer more forcibly than the robust ploughman—not because his hands are stronger, but because he can at a given moment throw a greater proportion of his total energy into them."[1]

Thus we see that the degree of functional vigor of any part is due to the degree of life present in that part; and, by extending our view in this direction, we can surely conceive that a greater mental *grasp*, as it were, of the organism, may enable us to cling more doggedly to life—to turn the scale, it may be, in our favor, at the last, most critical moment, when life and death are in the balance; to live on by merely "willing" to do so.

Again, it is a well-known fact, that, whereas horses can outmarch men—the cavalry the infantry—in a single day's march, the reverse of this is true in cases of forced marches, especially when these are continued daily, for a considerable period. And we have Mr. Thompson-Seton's authority for stating that a man in perfect condition can invariably run down a deer, provided he follows it with sufficient perseverance for a number of days.

These facts suggest, of course, that the energy of endurance, (stamina), the real test of strength—is *directly proportioned to the degree of mentality which the animal possesses;* so that, given two individuals, equally conditioned as to heredity, physical condition, training, etc., the man with the greater mentality will invariably outlast and outstay the man with the less, in a contest of endurance. And experience tells us that such is the case.

The problem before us, then, in all such cases, is this: How can we best invoke this force, this added energy? We have

[1] "Human Personality," etc., Vol. II., p. 530.

already seen (pp. 249–50), that we cannot manufacture it; all we can do is to keep our bodies clear from poisonous matter, and to place ourselves in the most receptive condition possible—this alone favoring the greater vital influx. But can we assist in inducing this condition? I believe we can. And it is here that the great utility of *suggestion* comes into play. First, one can, by its aid, induce that quiet, restful condition which is, as we have seen, the prime requisite for the inrush of cosmic energy; and secondly, it is possible to utilize the energy thus gained, to direct it into the most helpful channels by "focusing" it, artificially, upon the affected part. The increased vital energy is centered upon the locality requiring stimulation, and kept there by constant suggestion. According to the susceptibility of the patient are these suggestions successful. If the patient co-operates with the suggestion, and allows them to take full effect, a vastly increased flow of nerve energy will necessarily gravitate to and center upon that part, stimulating the muscle or organ to greatly increased action—without necessitating any harmful relapse—as would any other form of stimulation. This is healthful, normal stimulation—inducing correspondingly healthful, normal action; and this is the only possible form of stimulation of which this can be said.

Now we have seen that, by suggestion, the blood is made to circulate more rapidly—thereby removing the effete matter and carrying it to the excretory organs for elimination. Thus, mental stimulation almost always has the effect of *cleansing* the system —by stimulating the eliminating organs—and rarely or never has the effect of *retarding* the expulsion of this matter. Now I ask, has anyone ever thought *why* mental stimulation should always act in the way it does? Has anyone ever penetrated below the observation of the mere facts, and seen the hidden philosophical meaning in all this? Few, if any, have grasped the true significance of such observations. The actual increase of function may, of course, be due to increased nervous action, greater blood supply, etc., but why should purely mental stimulation affect so largely and almost invariably the excretory organs —since the reaction might be supposed to affect the mind alone? Might we not suggest that, inasmuch as every mental act reacts on the body, and *vice versa*, Nature, in her wisdom, has foreseen this harmful reaction, and prepared for it by cleansing the system, so far as possible, of anything tending to hinder an easy and rapid recovery—when the reaction comes? And, in case this may prove too severe a strain upon the credulity of my reader, I might, perhaps, point to the closely parallel cases which may be observed daily. Thus, should any grief come upon an individual, the appetite is immediately withdrawn; hunger fails to appear—sometimes for days together; and this for no apparent reason save that the vital forces are wasted thereby, and they employ this method in order to restore the wasted energy. Does not this argue for a certain teleological action? Anger frequently has the same effect (*i.e.*, of removing the appetite), and this may be due, as Doctor Oswald suggests, to the fact that the "envenomed saliva has to be expurgated before the organism will trust it to assist the work of digestion."[1]

A short fit of anger is often enough not only to derange but to completely arrest the digestive process for a whole day. Close behind the stomach is a group of ganglia, the solar-plexus, which sends out a large number of nerve filaments that communicate with the brain, and thus suggest the physiological explanation of the curious phenomenon, though its final or teleological purpose is somewhat less apparent. Haller connected it with the fact that anger vitiates the saliva (*teste*, the virulent bite of enraged animals), and suggests that by a wise arrangement of Nature the suspension of the assimilative process may preserve the chyle from the contamination of malignant humors; and, in connection with the same subject, Camper mentions the circumstance that fear often acts as a sudden cathartic; perhaps for the purpose of easing the stomach, and thus preparing the body for emergencies—the necessity for flight, for instance. Speculations of that sort lead to a field of curious but rather recondite biological metaphysics.

There are many other instances of this effort on the part of Nature to right a wrong—which efforts we constantly pervert, because we do not understand them. Thus, Doctor Page pointed out that:

[1] *Vim*, March, 1904, p. 93.

"Scratching is, by a natural law, made agreeable, in order to insure such excitation of the skin as shall drive sufficient blood to the parts, to facilitate the absorption of noxious elements, that they may be ejected through some other channel. This is the true philosophy of all itching of the skin, and we here observe one of the manifold methods by which Nature essays to remedy our shortcomings."[1]

Again, we read·[2]

"If the person show signs of fainting, do but little to rally him, as fainting tends to stop bleeding."

For other examples of a somewhat different type, see Walter Kidd's "Use-Inheritance Illustrated by the Direction of the Hair on the Bodies of Animals."

Facts such as the above serve to indicate how marvelous are Nature's warning signals, which are displayed at every turn, did we but deign to notice them, and take the necessary pains to study them and interpret their meaning.[3]

And now, it may be asked, what is the object of this long preamble? Have I merely introduced this chapter to illustrate the influence of the mind upon the body? By no means! Is it to emphasize the extreme importance of the mind as a factor in the causation of disease, and of its efficacy as a means of cure? Again, no—though these subjects are both worthy of the deepest consideration. Doctor Dewey, *e.g.*, constantly reiterated the truth that "cheer is to digestion what the breeze is to the fire," and beautifully expressed himself upon the question thus:

"It may well be conceived that there are electric nerve-wires extending from the depths of the soul itself to each individual gland of the stomach, with the highest cheer, or ecstasy, to stimulate the highest functional activity, or the shock of bad news to

[1] "How to Feed the Baby," p. 136.

[2] "Accidents and Emergencies," p. 5.

[3] It has frequently been noticed that a desire is experienced, directly after a meal, to evacuate the bowels. This, I take it, is merely because the vital forces and the blood have been withdrawn from the bowels to the stomach, and consequently Nature, in her wisdom, endeavors to rid the system of that for which it has no further vital use. It is purely a question of the economy of the vital forces; Nature cannot attend to both processes, and consequently turns her attention to the more important, and neglects the less vitally necessary—the practically digested food elements in the colon.

paralyze. From cheer to despair; from the slightest sense of discomfort to the agony of lacerated nerves, digestive power goes down. Affected thus, digestive power wanes or increases, goes down or up, as mercury in a barometer, from weather conditions."[1]

But my consideration of this question is not for that reason, but for reasons much more practical, and dealing more directly with the daily life of each of us, and especially with the daily life while fasting. I have given especial prominence, in the foregoing discussion, to a consideration of the influence of the mind in controlling the circulation—and for a purpose. The chief and most important conclusion to be drawn from this chapter is the fact that we may, by constantly thinking of any one organ or spot in our bodies, thereby cause the blood to flow to that spot or organ in abnormal and excessive quantities—producing local irritation and congestion, or even more abnormal conditions. This being the case, it becomes obvious how necessary it is for us *to keep the mind occupied and away from the body generally, and especially from the stomach, while fasting.* For, by a morbid concentration of attention upon that organ; by the continual thinking of food, of eating, we unduly excite and irritate it, and may so influence it as to bring about a noticeably irritable state, which may be mistaken for hunger, and the fast broken long before true hunger has returned. There is a tendency to think about food almost continually—especially during the early days of a fast—and this is quite natural, seeing how great a break in the day a meal previously afforded. This, more than the actual omission of the meal, is what is most noticed during a fast. Many persons have, in fact, broken their fasts on this very account; it was not because they were hungry; it was not because they noticed any especial effects from the fast; it was merely because they became tired of the monotony of the day without the customary break, which the meals previously afforded! And so I must insist that, during a fast, the prime requisite—a consideration of the utmost importance—is, keeping the mind off the stomach, and away from the subject of food altogether, and busily occupied in some other question.

[1] "No-Breakfast Plan," p. 39.

"Keep *lifted up* in your mind," wrote Mr. Haskell. Doctor Oswald agreed as to the importance of the mental factor while fasting, and Mr. Macfadden wrote the very true words: "The benefits that result from fasting are unquestionably greatly lessened if the confidence in its efficiency is not sufficiently strong, and this graduated process of teaching its advantages can be recommended to those who are open to conviction, but who do not feel equal to a prolonged fast."[1]

At no time can purely intellectual and æsthetic pursuits be so successfully undertaken as at such times, and every possible method of distracting and holding the patient's attention should be brought into requisition and diligently employed. On the other hand, at no time is the lack of will power—from which humanity so sadly suffers—more manifest than during a fast—where, I admit, considerable determination is required, especially at first.

Indeed, as I have frequently stated, the greatest enemy we have to encounter during a fast is a more or less morbid mental condition—which results either from auto- or hetero-suggestion (suggestions given to ourselves, or those given us by others), generally given by our too solicitous friends and relatives, and which are, frequently, harder to bear than the fast itself "The trouble about fasting," wrote Mr. Purinton,[2] "is, there's no place in which to do it." Again (p. 106):

" every friend of a man on a fast becomes his direst foe. If they don't worry themselves into hysterics for fear you'll starve to death, they will at least comment on your looks, diagnose your symptoms, ask you to describe your feelings, in short, plague clean out of you the very life they are so solicitous to preserve."

We notice, in undergoing any such experience as this, which is a real call upon our powers, how extraordinarily small that will power is. A fast will make one realize the mental and moral weaknesses from which we suffer, no less than the physical ills; and to appreciate why it was that fasting was always regarded

[1] "Strength from Eating," p. 21.
[2] "Philosophy of Fasting," p. 129.

with so much favor as a means of penance. Fasting is not an easy and enjoyable experience—though Mr. Shaw told me repeatedly that he never felt so well as while fasting!—and I do not pretend that it is; but it is *really curing us*, and the process of cure is by no means pleasant or easy, on any system of medication whatever.

BOOK V

STUDIES OF PATIENTS DURING THEIR FASTS

BOOK V

CHAPTER I

THE TONGUE AND THE BREATH

IN THE present chapter, I propose to consider two symptoms of comparatively lesser importance, both of them being connected intimately with fasting in a manner peculiar to themselves, and both indicating that certain conditions are present, causing the symptoms to vary in a manner distinct from their variations in any other physiological or pathogogical state whatever. I refer to the condition of (1) the tongue and (2) the breath.

(1) A coated tongue has always been considered a sure indication of the presence of disease by the orthodox medical profession, while its cleanliness indicates, for them, a state of fair bodily health. The rule must be almost or quite universal, otherwise the examination of the tongue would be a farce—as indeed it is. In the light of the knowledge which we have gained, in studying cases of fasting, it may be definitely and truly stated that the reverse of this is frequently the case; that a coated tongue may denote a far *better* physical condition than is the case when the same is nearly or quite clear, and *per contra*, the tongue may be quite clean, and the system far more diseased and in a far fouler condition than when it was heavily coated.

The proof of this is to be found in the following fact. Immediately a fast is entered upon, the tongue—which may previously have been quite clean—*coats heavily*, and the thickness and the foulness of this coat may continue to increase as the fast progresses. Thus we see that, while the actual physical condition of the patient is far *better*, and his system cleaner, in the latter case (*i.e.*, after he has been fasting some days) than in the former, the tongue is far more heavily coated, and in a fouler condition in every way at the latter time; so that, were one to judge from this symptom, and follow the customary methods of diagnosis, the patient would be far worse instead of better! The tongue may, of course, have been coated more or less before commencing the fast; but in any case it will coat heavily as soon as this is begun, invariably; and continue to grow more heavily coated and fouler as it continues—up to a certain point, when it begins to spontaneously clean itself up. So long as the active elimination persists, just so long will the tongue remain coated; but when this elimination begins to decrease, the tongue will become clean, and stay so. A short while before the return of hunger, this cleansing process of the tongue commences, and continues until the tongue is perfectly clean, assuming a beautiful pink-red shade—rarely or never seen in the average man or woman; and the terminus of this cleansing process of the tongue is absolutely coincidental with the return of hunger and of health. By watching the tongue, one can thus gauge the condition of the patient, throughout the fast. A slight coating—heavy coating—very heavy coating—foul coating (continuing for a longer or shorter period according to the length of the fast necessary)—slightly cleared—rapid clearing—followed by a complete return to normal conditions, at precisely the period of the return of natural hunger: this is the almost invariable routine, and indicates, once again, how in accordance with natural, organic law this method of treatment is, and how clearly indicated are Nature's symptoms, were we but to heed them.[1]

This coating of the tongue may be temporarily removed by scraping the tongue with a wet tooth-brush, and rinsing out the mouth with a diluted mixture of hydrogen peroxide and water. This should never be done, however, before the daily examination, since it might lead the attending physician into forming erroneous conclusions—the tongue taking some little time to

[1] It is not generally enough recognized that this coated, foul condition of the tongue is indicative of the condition of the mucus membrane *throughout the whole alimentary canal*—since this membrane is most closely inter-related and connected; so that, when one portion is inflamed or coated with foul material, it indicates, to a great extent, the condition of the membrane throughout the rest of the alimentary canal. Says Doctor Harvey ("On Corpulence in Relation to Disease," etc., by William Harvey, F.R.C.S., p. 7): ". . . The state of the mucus membrane of the tongue indicates the condition of that of the stomach and intestinal canal."

become coated again. It might be suggested that a patient who was anxious to break the fast might thus artificially clean the tongue, prior to examination, and, a little later, claim the return of natural hunger. Such a ruse would not deceive the expert in fasting, however, owing to the presence of other symptoms, notably the breath, as we shall presently see.

Not alone the presence of the coated tongue but its *character* indicates the condition of the organism during a fast—thereby indicating indirectly the condition and degree of foulness of the patient's system, and allowing anyone, used to cases of this character, to predict, with approximate accuracy, the probable duration of the fast. A slight whitish-brown coating is, seemingly, the least important; while, as the color becomes more and more yellow, or of a deeper and deeper brown shade, a far graver condition is indicated. The *depth* of the coat must also be taken into consideration. A heavily coated tongue of a dark color, with dark red edges, indicates one of the worst conditions possible, and invariably indicates a putrid condition of the entire body, and the necessity for a careful, strict and protracted fast.

Schrott, in studying his fasting cases—in which, however water was denied—recorded almost precisely similar phenomena, and I quote his remarks in this relation, since they are of special confirmatory interest, inasmuch as they were written *circa* 1817 —though I had not read them at the time of writing the above. They are quoted by Doctor Shew, from whose work[1] I quote them:

"The tongue is dry and covered with a white coating for a time at first; but later in the cure, as the morbid matter of the body becomes more loosened or set free, it changes to a yellowish or brownish color, and is often covered with a thick slime. Not infrequently, too, this coating upon the tongue becomes quite black in appearance. The tongue loses the coating by degrees, beginning at its point, and as the purifying process goes on toward its termination, it takes on a beautiful and healthy reddish appearance. At first articles of food are insipid to the taste, and some nausea is experienced. Later, there may be a sour, bitter or metallic taste in the mouth; this last more particularly with

[1] "Family Physician," pp. 789–90.

those who have been much under the influence of mercury. Toward the last, the taste becomes saltish, which Schrott regards as a good omen. (This has not been my experience.—H. C.) The taste also improves in proportion as the inward purification goes on. During the course of the process, the teeth become whiter and the gums more firm and red, indicating an improvement in the digestive organs."

One other point deserves consideration. It has been stated that the tongue gradually coats, as the fast progresses, up to a certain period, when there is a more or less rapid cleansing up of that organ, accompanied by a return of natural hunger. This is the normal course of events. If, however, we were to artificially break the fast, at any time, for any reason, and with any kind of food whatsoever, that needs digestion (*i.e.*, anything else than water) the tongue would instantly become clear, and would not become coated again until another fast be entered upon. Water will not have this effect (p. 400) and may be drunk *ad libitum*, without disturbing the progress of the fast in any way; but this is the *only* substance that can enter into our stomachs of which this can be said. Any other liquid; any article of food whatsoever—needing digestion, however small in amount, will immediately check the progress of the fast, induce a return of hunger, and throw the whole machine "out of gear" so to speak—including the cleansing of the tongue, as formerly stated. An immense amount of damage can thus be done by an ingestion of a *single mouthful* of food. Nowhere do we see more clearly an illustration of the fact that all diseases, and all true cures, are both the results of long and tedious processes of evolution. Neither can result from any *sudden* cause—that preposterous theory advocated by the medical man of to-day—being tacitly admitted by him in the supposed cases of suddenly "caught" or contracted diseases, and positively affirmed in their present system of medicines that "act" instantaneously!

(2) A close scrutiny of the character and odor of the *breath* during a fast shows that it, too, in its own way, presents a set of phenomena paralleling the more tangible condition of the tongue. Here, also—though the breath may have been somewhat bad at the commencement of the fast, denoting, to the careful observer,

a more or less foul condition of the entire body—the breath is invariably sweet and healthful prior to a fast, in comparison with its extremely noxious odor immediately the fast is entered upon. In this case, the peculiar odor appears almost invariably, and continues throughout the fast—only finally disappearing and allowing the breath again to assume its normal, sweet condition when the fast is ready to be broken, and the system is once more restored to a normal, healthy state. Here again, we see Nature's dictates in the matter, and clearly perceive how unnatural and altogether uncalled-for is the prevailing system of breaking the fast before hunger indicates that it is ready to be broken; or that it has arrived at its natural, organic termination.

Throughout the fast, the parallel between the condition of the tongue and that of the breath is striking. Precisely coincidental with the heavy coating of the tongue—following immediately upon the commencement of the fast—is the greatly increased foulness of the breath, showing unmistakably that the lungs are assisting in the speedy elimination of all corrupt matter from the system with the greatest possible speed, and illustrating, in a beautiful manner, how Nature can and does utilize the energy thus economized in ridding the system of the foul material it contains.

Since every cubic inch of poisonous gas thus exhaled represents the freeing of the body from so much morbid material; and since our primary aim, throughout, is to purify the blood, it follows that pure air, both day and night, is most essential if health is to be restored speedily and effectually. If the breath is tainted by organic, decomposition products, and foul from absorbing such noxious matter as the gases generated in the intestinal tube (p. 409), it may readily be perceived that the health of others may be easily jeopardized by living in the same atmosphere as a patient undergoing a fast—unless the very fullest and best ventilation be allowed and maintained.[1]

[1] It is not true, as many persons believe, that bad breath comes from the stomach. "The passage to the stomach is always perfectly closed, except when something is going down, and even then it is open only where the mass is. A bad breath never comes directly from the stomach." ("In a Nutshell," by Dio Lewis, M.D., p. 120.) The sources of bad breath are (1) the nose; (2) the mouth; and (3) the lungs.

It has been previously stated that this increasingly foul condition of the breath is in direct proportion to the morbid coating of the tongue, and diminishes, also, in exact ratio. As the fast progresses, the breath frequently becomes more foul—emitting a peculiar and characteristic odor which cannot possibly be associated with any condition other than fasting—when once it has been noted and recognized, and associated with it. The odor is quite indescribable; but is easily recognized by anyone accustomed to such cases. Once noted, it cannot be forgotten! The breath is *sweet*, but not sweet with the fragrance of health; it possesses a peculiar saccharine element, wholly indescribable. It is more allied to the smell of chloroform than to anything else; always present and altogether repellent. Together with this, there is a (by no means faint) *odor* which can only be compared with carrion or decaying flesh, or decomposing animal tissue, and which is repulsive in the extreme! The combination may be imagined! The foulness of the fasting patient's breath is, at times, almost too great for words, and renders any close proximity to him unbearable. Doctor Dewey reported a case in which "the odor of the breath could be perceived some feet from the bed. This gradually declined, and was scarcely perceptible at the thirtieth day."[1] This condition gradually improves, however, as the fast progresses, until, when ready to be broken, a clean, sweet, pure breath is exhaled; absolutely untainted, and reminding one of the pure and healthful days of joyous childhood [2]

To the expert in fasting, therefore, the breath forms a unique and trustworthy guide to the condition of the patient, during a fast, being a kind of "organic barometer," and above all, supplies us with a positive test which may be applied in all cases of fasting where there is a doubt as to the genuineness of the patient's

[1] "True Science of Living," p. 85.

[2] Kirke ("Physiology," p. 508), noted that: "The exhalations both from the lungs and skin are fœtid, indicating the tendency to decomposition which belongs to badly nourished tissues . . ." Needless to say, this is entirely the wrong construction to place upon the facts, since it is not "badly nourished tissues" that give rise to the trouble, but tissues that have previously been surfeited with food material in excess, and the taint is the result of the efforts of the body to eliminate this morbid matter. This is easily proved by the fact that, if the fast be persisted in, this taint entirely disappears, whereas it ought to *increase*, on Doctor Kirke's theory.

honest coöperation—completely checking any such attempt at deception, by indicating at once that an absolute fast is not in progress. If it were, the breath would possess the peculiar and unmistakable odor spoken of above, and any attempt to break it, no matter how little is eaten, would instantly be recognized by the disappearance of this odor, together with the sudden and complete disappearance from the tongue of its coat, mentioned above. There are no two surer indications of fasting than these; and anyone accustomed to watching such cases cannot possibly be deceived by the patient in any way whatever. These symptoms furnish a complete "check," so to speak, upon the patient's physical condition throughout the fast; and, taken in conjunction with the more obvious and tangible phenomena (the loss of flesh and weight, etc.), form a chain of evidence which no patient has heretofore been sufficiently ingenious to break, and seem to form a perfect, conclusive and natural proof that the fast is being conducted strictly and uninterruptedly.

CHAPTER II

THE TEMPERATURE

For many years past, the regular practitioner has always acknowledged the value of noting and recording the patient's temperature, in all diseased conditions; and, whereas its importance has, without doubt, been greatly exaggerated, a thermometric reading is certainly helpful and suggestive, as indicating the general bodily condition of the patient at the time of making the observation.

The temperature of a patient—of any person, in fact—is "taken" by means of a thermometer, as any other temperature is measured. In this case, however, the observation is made by means of what is known as a clinical thermometer—which is simply an unattached glass tube, with the degrees marked on the glass itself. These thermometers vary somewhat in construction, but they range, as a rule, from about 94° to 110° F.—this being all the variation necessary, as a rule, in the regulation of bodily temperature—since the latter remains almost exactly constant, at about 98.4° F., and a variation of even 1° F., in either direction, above or below, denotes a distinctly pathologic condition.[1] The simplest and cleanest method of taking the temperature is that of inserting the bulb of the thermometer under the patient's tongue, and requesting him to gently close the lips—thereby excluding the air. Some physicians prefer taking the reading from the armpit or the rectum, but these are both unhandy, uncleanly, and, though the last named is probably a trifle more accurate, yet the reading from the tongue is certainly accurate

[1] In Asiatic cholera, the temperature may fall to 77° F. (Kirke: "Physiology," p. 495). 76° F. and 109° F. have been set as the "death limits," so to speak ("Baths and Bathing," p. 14). But, in Doctor Teale's case (reported in *The Lancet*, Vol. I., p. 340, and *Proceedings* of the Society for Psychical Research, Vol. IX., p. 206), the temperature, for seven consecutive weeks, never fell below 108° F., and for four consecutive days, had a temperature of 122° F.!

enough for all practical purposes. Such extreme nicety in diagnosis is quite unnecessary, and is altogether disproportionate to the subsequent empirical methods of treatment.[1] At the conclusion of the allotted time—from one to three minutes, generally—the thermometer is simply withdrawn, and the temperature noted. The normal temperature of the body, when in perfect health, is almost exactly 98.4° F. Variations above or below this point indicate that the body is not in a condition of perfect health; is more or less "sick" or diseased, in fact, and the severity of the disease is, *ceteris paribus*, in direct proportion to the variation of the bodily temperature; *i.e.*, the further the temperature is removed from the normal standard (either above or below) the greater is the degree of "sickness"—the graver is the condition of the patient.

Of course *slight* variations are always present; since no human being is, probably, in perfect health. (p. 63.) But, so long as the temperature keeps within the degree (98°-99°), it is comparatively unimportant. It is when the temperature rises or falls several degrees that concern need be felt, since this would indicate a decidedly pathologic process. Below 95° F. and above 100° F.—these begin to reach what may be called the "danger limits" of bodily temperature; and they cannot be maintained for any very great length of time without endangering the life of the patient.

Every fraction of a degree above or below the temperature indicated is of great importance, and should be carefully noted.

Fortunately Nature, in her bounty, would soon restore a fairly normal temperature, if left to herself, and the system not *kept* highly feverish—by administering food, drugs, etc.

Nearly everyone knows, I should imagine, that the bodily temperature is invariably raised whenever fever is present; according to the severity of the fever, so does the temperature increase. But comparatively few persons know the cause of a lowered temperature; know, *i.e.*, what is the reason for the

[1] "It should be always borne in mind that it is not the high temperature we are fighting, but the disease itself. The range of the temperature is simply a guide to the severity of the disease, just as the mercury in the thermometer indicates the temperature, but does not influence the temperature." (Forest "New Treatment for Fever," pp. 21-2.) It is not the high temperature, but the *cause* of the high temperature that we are fighting.

temperature sinking below the normal and remaining so, frequently, for weeks and months at a time. Nor, seemingly, have physicians sufficiently grasped the significance and importance of this phenomenon. This becomes apparent, however, when we realize that when the temperature is thus lowered, *it indicates depleted vitality;* and its gradual rise to normal shows a corresponding return to health.

But the average physician regards this low temperature as of comparatively little importance. He knows that such a patient can, and often does, live for months and years with his temperature continually below the normal (consequently it "does not matter" to any great extent, in his estimation); whereas in fevers, when the temperature is raised a few degrees, he knows death would soon result if a return to normal did not occur within a few days. And so he regards a rise in temperature as of far more consequence than a corresponding fall—of the same number of degrees.

I do not myself think that—looked at otherwise than superficially—this is by any means the case, and feel assured that, in the light of fuller knowledge, the order of cogency will be held to be precisely reversed. Paradoxical as this position may seem, I think it is substantiated by the following considerations.

Granting that high temperatures denote severe fever, and frequently need prompt treatment if the life of the patient is to be saved, still, all fevers, in the hands of skilled hygienic physicians, yield, within a few hours or days, leaving no evil after-effects whatever.[1] The temperature is speedily brought down to the normal (usually below the normal for a time), with comparatively little difficulty, and thenceforward the patient's health continues much as before. If there has been a sudden rise in the temperature (of several degrees, within a few hours) so also has

[1] No *observable* after-effects, that is. It cannot be doubted, however, that all disease, however successfully treated, leaves some evil traces, or "scars" in the organism, which ultimately help to decide the longevity of the patient. "It is not true . . . that a disorder from which we have recovered leaves us as before. No disturbance of the normal course of the functions can pass away and leave things as they were. In all cases a permanent damage is done—not immediately appreciable, it may be, but still there, and along with such items, which Nature in her strict account-keeping never drops, will tell against us to the end of our days." ("Vaccination a Crime," by Felix L. Oswald, M.D., p. 21.)

this high temperature been reduced to normal in a correspondingly short time, and without any permanent ill effects. Thus, while the high temperature cases demand prompt attention, their effects are but transitory and speedily rectified.

On the other hand, in low temperature cases, though there is no "crisis" to be surmounted, there is yet a long, tedious course of body-building to be gone through, before perfect health is to be attained. Depleted vitality is by no means restored in a few days, but frequently takes months of steady, persistent effort on the part of the patient, before "tone" is given to the system, and the temperature raised to the normal. Thus, whereas in the first case, the rapid rise of temperature is followed by an equally rapid fall; in the latter case, the gradual decrease of vitality—with accompanying loss of temperature—is regained only by a gradual process of restoration. And, while the former of these conditions (high temperature) is rapidly attained, and as rapidly dispelled, the latter (low temperature) is the result of weeks or months of cumulative evil, and is only dispelled by a correspondingly long system of treatment. The former of these conditions may, possibly, detract nine or ten days from the patient's life (*i.e.*, ultimately); the latter condition, as many or more years. Consequently I must insist that low temperature is vastly more important, ultimately, than a correspondingly high temperature; for, while the former's results are evanescent, the latter's are permanent and more or less indelible.

When, now, we realize that this depleted vitality is the result of choking or clogging the system with an excess of food material, and that the vitality is raised by its removal (pp. 253–4), we can readily perceive how it is that, by merely restricting the diet, or by fasting, we thereby elevate the patient's vitality and consequently his temperature. This will become more obvious as we proceed.

I now come to consider the question of bodily temperature *while fasting*. Thousands of observations have been made relative to the question of temperature in diseases of all kinds, but I have been quite unable to find any consecutive and systematic series of experiments conducted with a fasting patient—though I have consulted almost every work where such experiments would be recorded, including every book in print dealing directly or indirectly with the subject of fasting. Unfortunately, I myself have been unable to devote the necessary time and labor to this subject, in order to report any such results, but I now offer a few brief remarks upon this highly important subject, based upon my own observations and experience, believing that a comparative study of this question will be highly interesting, and will cast an entirely new light upon many long-cherished theories —completely revolutionizing our ideas as to the relations of food and bodily heat.

It will not, probably, be considered a very startling assertion when I say that, in all fever cases, when the temperature is above the normal, it falls as the fast progresses. That is what anyone would almost expect *à priori*. The fact that there is the ever-present striving on the part of Nature to return to the normal condition; the fact that the heat produced by the combustion of food (supposedly) is not added when the food is no longer supplied; the fact that the temperature would probably return to normal very shortly in any case; all these facts tend to make it obvious that the temperature should sink as the fast continues.

But while the foregoing may appear obvious, it will by no means seem so apparent when I state that the reverse of this is also the case; when I say, that is, that as the fast progresses, the temperature will slowly but surely *rise* until it reaches normal, when the fast is ready to be broken. Thus, supposing the patient's temperature be 93.8° F., at the commencement of the fast, it will gradually rise until about 98.4° F. be reached—though the fast may have extended over forty or more days! This statement will, I am sure, appear to the majority of my readers in the highest degree paradoxical. However paradoxical it may appear, however, it is a *fact,* and facts are stubborn things. It may be verified at any time, in any patient, who is undertaking a rigid and proper fast. Time after time, in case after case, I have watched this gradual rise in the bodily temperature of the patient; and in every case the temperature has not failed to rise as the fast progressed. At first, it is true, the temperature sometimes tends to fall, but let the fast be persisted in, and a return or rise to normal will occur in every case. In spite of the fact that absolutely no food is eaten by the patient during this time; in spite of the fact that the flesh continues to waste, and, to judge from the patient's own inner feelings, his vitality has greatly decreased; it is here obvious that, as the cause of the disease is expelled from the system, the patient's vitality—his life or vital force—actually *in*creases, until it reaches (almost) the normal standard.

Doctor Rabagliati discovered this fact that the bodily temperature rose with the fast, while observing some of his patients. To him, no less than to myself, when I first observed the fact, it was a great surprise. Thus, on p. 261 of his "Air, Food and Exercises," he writes:

"In point of fact, I raised the temperature of a man who was, besides, thin, emaciated, and attenuated by constant vomiting, lasting for seven years, from 96° F. to 98.4° F., by advising him to fast for thirty-five days."

See also pp. 45–6 of his "Aphorisms," etc. It will be observed that these are actual facts, derived from an actual study of cases, and flatly contradict the theoretical statements contained, *e.g.*, in Kirke's "Physiology," p. 507, and de Varigny's "Temperature and Life," p. 414. Experiments made on animals would invariably indicate the effects of *starvation*, not fasting—which distinction I hope will be clear in the reader's mind, before this book is completed. It is true that the temperature falls, also, when a person starves to death; but that is due (1) to the fact that starvation, and not fasting, has been undergone; and (2) since tissue is not replaced as it should normally be, the vital energy cannot manifest through it; hence the results noted. The theory of animal heat in its relation to the body is not disproved by such facts, because the two classes of phenomena are different.

Now this fact of the bodily temperature being raised and not lowered as a fast progresses, casts an entirely new light on the relations of food and bodily heat. For, although the medical world regards lowered temperature as (to a certain extent) lack of vitality, they consider that this is largely due to lack of nourishment—whereas its cause is really too much food—and so proceed to feed the patient; to "keep him up" on stimulants, food, etc., thereby keeping the patient's temperature *down*, or below normal.

Now, while I also regard the lowered temperature as a sign of depleted vitality, I must insist that this latter condition is the result of the disease (or causes of disease) present in the system; and that, as these causes of disease are expelled—by fasting or otherwise—the temperature rises accordingly. In other words: The lowered vitality (and consequently the lowered temperature) is due solely to disease; and the vitality (and consequently the temperature) is raised in exact proportion to the extent of the freeing of the body from the disease—or its causes.[1] As fasting is one of the surest and speediest methods of eliminating diseased conditions, by oxidizing off and otherwise eliminating the excess of food material previously ingested, and now choking the body —it follows that fasting must raise the temperature, since it increases the vitality—by ridding the system from the disease. Theoretically, this should be the case, and practically such proves to be so—the theory is in direct accordance with the observed facts.

There is another seeming paradox in this connection which needs some elucidation. Everyone who has fasted for any length of time (say three days) in winter, has probably noticed that he begins to feel the cold very keenly; it is difficult, in fact, for him to keep sufficiently warm; and, whereas he may have been content with a temperature of 70° F. at other times, he requires the house at least 10° F. hotter than that while fasting, in order to feel the same amount of warmth. As the fast progresses, this seeming inability to keep warm increases also; and consequently it would appear that the bodily temperature (and vitality) must be considerably lowered in order to affect the patient in this manner—thus apparently disproving my theory.

[1] Another proof that the bodily temperature is directly proportioned to the degree vitality present is found in the fact that the temperature falls as the result of the administration of drugs. (Mills "Animal Physiology," p. 467.) This becomes intelligible to us, when we remember that the action of drugs is merely the reaction of the system against the drug (p. 32), and consequently implies and necessitates waste of energy, and consequent lowering of vitality. This indirectly proves my point in a very striking manner. It is also strongly borne out by the fact that powerful emotions—fear, etc.—which, as we know tend to lower the vitality, also lower the temperature. ("Study of the Nature and Mechanism of Fever," by Horatio D. Wood, M.D., p. 20.)

This apparent coldness and sinking of vitality, however, does not, in reality, affect the bodily temperature in any way whatever. The latter does not sink as the feeling of increased cold creeps over the patient. It has nothing to do with the body's *actual* warmth. I have seen a patient complaining of "the cold," etc., whose actual temperature was 97.8° F. (or only .6° F. below normal), on the twenty-third day of his fast—this same man never having noticed the same temperature as being particularly "cold," while eating regularly—although his actual temperature was at that time nearly 2° F. lower! At first sight this may appear extremely paradoxical and extraordinary. If the vitality and bodily warmth *seem* less, why is it that the *actual* temperature is, by thermometric readings, shown to be higher than formerly? This is surely very extraordinary, but it is a fact nevertheless. I have never heard a satisfactory explanation given, in answer to this puzzling question. And indeed, what is the solution?

Personally, I am inclined to think that the feeling of cold, experienced in such instances, is due partly to a decreased peripheral circulation—a species of cutaneous anæmia—which, as we have seen, is always attended with the sense of chilliness.[1] It is probably also due, in part, to a keener perception of all variations of bodily temperature, since the senses are sharpened and rendered more acute in every single instance. Says Doctor Evans:[2]

"On one occasion, when living for five days entirely upon oranges, our temperature was lessened; still we felt a pleasant glow throughout the system; but to other individuals we felt cold; animal heat is, therefore, only *relative* . . . "

There are probably other causes for this feeling of cold, during a fast, also. It may be due, in part, to the lack of feverishness habitually present and necessitated in disposing of an excess of food material; to a lack of the excessive, injurious heat which frequently is present, almost constantly—a more or less perpetual fever, from which the patient suffers, and to which he is accustomed—noting its absence, of course, when not present, during the fast. In other words, it is quite possible, and in fact prob-

[1] Reinhold: "Consumption Curable," p. 280; Page: "Natural Cure," p. 166.
[2] "How to Prolong Life," etc., p. 80.

able, that what is now recognized to be the normal temperature is, in reality, a degree or so too high; which would seem to gain some support from the fact that persons living on a fruitarian (natural) diet are generally somewhat below the theoretically normal limit—though in perfect health, and always feeling perfectly warm.

Be the solution what it may, however, the fact remains that the feeling of cold experienced while fasting has nothing whatever to do with the body's actual temperature, which may be several degrees higher, by actual measurement, than before the fast was commenced. In writing on malaria, Dr. Susanna Dodds remarked that:

> "In this cold paroxysm there is a rise in temperature (which the fever thermometer will detect) some time before the chilling stage begins."[1]

As a further proof that the theory advanced in this chapter (that the bodily temperature tends, while fasting, to rise to normal when below it, and that food frequently retards or actually lowers the temperature, when it is not required, instead of causing it to rise, as has always been maintained), is correct, I must again refer the reader to Mrs. T. A.'s case, before referred to. In this instance the temperature was below 94° F. when the patient commenced her fast of thirty-four days, but had nearly reached the normal standard at the end of that period. When the patient began to eat again, the temperature immediately *dropped* more than a degree; and thence onward, whenever the patient had eaten bountifully, the previous evening, the following morning's examination revealed the fact that the temperature had invariably sunk from one to two degrees. A day's very light eating would bring it up again to normal. This did not happen occasionally, but invariably, from which facts the only conclusion to be drawn is that the bodily warmth does not by any means depend upon the combustion of food, as has always been contended, but is due to some other source.[2]

[1] "The Liver and Kidneys: With a Chapter on Malaria," p. 44.

[2] Doctor Keith observed a very similar case of his own, and wrote: "The great peculiarity in the case was chilliness coming on when he took anything like a meal." ("Fads of an Old Physician," by Geo. S. Keith, M.D., LL.D., etc., p. 168.)

Finally, it may be noted that the fact of the temperature falling to normal when above it; and rising to normal when below it; the fact of its reaching that point, in either case, just as the fast is completed and ready to be broken; these are but further proofs that fasting is a natural process, counseled by Nature, with its landmarks clearly defined, and but waiting to be recognized by man!

There is one point, however, which apparently contradicts my theory, and the force and the gravity of the objection I do not deny. I referred to it on p. 319. It is that, while the energy is potentially greater in the morning than at any other time; and while the degree of vitality is supposed to correspond to the temperature of the body, point for point, the fact remains that the temperature is frequently lower in the morning than later in the day,[1] which would seem to indicate a lesser degree of vitality —when precisely the reverse of this should be the case. This fact is, I admit, an exceedingly puzzling one, and it is one that has necessitated much thinking on my part in an attempt to solve it. At first sight, it presents one of the most formidable objections to my theory that has ever been advanced, because it apparently so completely contradicts it, by producing an undoubted *fact, viz.*—the lowness of the temperature. And that it does not, in reality, form any such objection at all is due, again, to the fact that, whereas the observation itself is indisputable, the inferences drawn from the observation are erroneous. Let me state my own view of the matter, and what I conceive to be a demonstration of its correctness, as follows:

It will doubtless be conceded that, if we were in the best of health—a perfectly normal condition—the temperature would also be quite normal in the morning, because there is no reason for its being otherwise; in fact, as the energies are, as we have seen, higher then than at any other period, the temperature should be correspondingly higher also. That is but logical. But the fact that the temperature is, in reality, lower at this time[2] proves, beyond all reasonable doubt, that this lower tem-

[1] "Temperature and Life," by Henry de Varigny, p. 416, etc.

[2] Of course I am speaking throughout of the actual temperature—not of the bodily feelings, which are deceiving. We doubtless feel cold in the evening and warm in the morning, because we have a greater stock of vitality at the

perature is due to some abnormal cause or condition, which renders it thus sub-normal. Now this, I take it, is actually the case; and is, indeed, the true cause for such abnormal temperature. The system is not normal; it is more or less diseased.

So far, all is clear enough. In order to make clear the remaining portion of my argument, I shall first quote the following passage from Doctor Gully's "Water Cure in Chronic Diseases," (pp. 330-1), which lays the foundation, I think, for our correct understanding of the facts in this case, and of the argument that follows. In part, he says:

"Fomentations, although directly lowering, are indirectly, a strengthening process. The inflamed stomach of a patient acts, by sympathy, as a spur to the function of the brain, which thereby exhibits a degree of impulsive energy that passes for power; the patient can walk or talk quickly, has incessant desire to move, etc., but all this is fictitious strength, just as the energy imparted by alcoholic liquors or tonic medicines is fictitious. Fomentations, by reducing the inflammation of the stomach, withdraw the spur from the brain; and the patient, feeling in consequence much loss of his locomotive propensity, says they are weakening him. But they are plainly only reducing his brain to its actual and genuine level of strength, by taking from it the morbid stimulant which gave it fictitious power. And, meantime, the digestive viscera, being strengthened by the reduction of their inflammation, will, as they improve, afford such natural stimulus to the brain as will give it a sustained energy. I dwell upon this, as patients often make complaint, in the first parts of the water treatment . . . whereas they are only weaker for a time in the animal nervous system, but are becoming permanently stronger in their nutritive nervous system "

And so here. When the vital energies are not being forcibly distracted from the internal, organic processes, into the external, active ones—where they would at once become more readily

latter than at the former time; and we feel cold in direct proportion to the degree of vitality present, and the more or less active or anæmic condition of the skin. (P. 375.) Even here our feelings frequently deceive us. Let any person strip himself entirely in a cold room; then walk into a warm room; still stripped. He will feel warm and comfortable in the cold room; but immediately he enters the warm room, shivering results, and the cold is noticed or "felt" for the first time. But I am discussing, in the text, the actual temperature; not what we feel it to be.

noticeable as energy; when the activities of the day, the stimulation of the senses and the organs are lacking; when the more or less feverish conditions accompanying digestion are not present —because their causes are absent; then the temperature should, I think, be normal, if the system is healthy and normal; and neither above nor below that point. But that it is very frequently sub-normal at this time proves, *not* that the bodily energies are lower than at any other period, but that *the low temperature represents the actual or existent bodily temperature—before it has been stimulated up to a certain higher point by the activities of the day;* and this sub-normal temperature is due to the fact that the vital powers are themselves low—which, in turn, is due to the presence of disease. Hence we see that the presence of disease, and not the lack of vital energies, is the cause of the lowered bodily temperature. And the proof of this theory would be found if, in removing the diseased condition, and consequently raising the whole vital energies up to normal, we thereby rendered the morning temperature normal also. And, in fact, this is actually the case. For, in the few cases of fasting in which such observations have been made, it has invariably been ascertained that this is precisely what occurs; and, as the fast nears its termination, the morning temperature—hitherto invariably sub-normal—now rises to normal, and is almost or quite exactly so at the conclusion of the fast. The morning temperature is no longer sub-normal, but normal! And the cause of this is obvious enough. So that the argument based upon this objection to my theory comes to nothing; and, so far from disproving it, does, when rightly understood, tend to confirm it in every detail.

CHAPTER III

THE PULSE

One of the first steps in diagnosing a case of almost any character is almost invariably to "feel the pulse." The pulse is merely the throb of any artery in the body, due to the heart pumping the blood through it in jets or spurts, as would any other pump. It is generally associated with the wrist, but this is only custom, since the pulse is necessarily present wherever there is an artery, and may be plainly felt in the neck, ankle, etc. The wrist is felt for the reason that it is the most convenient and plainly discerned. If, therefore, we count the number of beats per minute in the artery at the wrist, we thereby ascertain the rate at which the heart is beating.

The normal rate of the heart-beat varies greatly according to age, occupation, etc. In children it is considerably higher than in adults, and toward old age it is still further decreased,[1] and I suggest that, for this reason, the normal, middle-aged man or woman is probably more fitted for active work than at any other period of their lives—since they are thereby enabled to partake of abundant and vigorous exercise (without raising the pulsation to the danger point) and without noticing the effects of the sluggishness of the circulation present in old age.

Just here it may be noted that our rate of pulsation is, throughout life, in direct proportion to our natural vitality; greatest in youth; weakened, but still potentially powerful, in mature age; most feeble in old age—a fact which has, I believe, been universally overlooked, but which, of course, has a great practical bear ing on the question from our present standpoint. Its importance will become more apparent as we proceed.

The frequency of the pulse varies according to age, sex, the degree of health, etc., etc. In adults, it is usually about seventy

[1] "Animal Physiology," by Wesley Mills, M.D., p. 242.

to the minute.[1] Deviations from this, above or below, if long continued, show that the system is in a more or less abnormal condition. The causes for a more rapid pulse of temporary duration are manifold. Mental stimulus may greatly accelerate (or check) the heart's action; may "send the blood coursing through your veins," or may make your "heart stand still"—to use the popular expressions. Exercise invariably increases the heart's action; and, when the exertion is great, to an astonishing degree, in a remarkably short space of time. Diet has also a great effect upon the heart's action, though this, too, has been generally overlooked.[2]

If the pulse keeps generally above the normal theoretical limit, then we may take it for granted that some abnormal condition is present; some obstruction exists within the organism which the vital forces are thus (by increasing the rate and volume of the blood supply) endeavoring to absorb and carry to the excretory organs for elimination. This would seem to denote, therefore, the presence of a certain degree of fever, and I believe that this can invariably be shown to be present in such cases—if not noticeably on the periphery, then centered on some internal, vital organ. In this case, of course, the treatment consists, not in endeavoring to check the rapidity of the pulse —an indication, merely of the curing process going on—but by assisting in the elimination of effete material which was the *cause* of the rapid pulse, and, this once removed, the pulse will sink to normal of its own accord.

Thus far we have considered but half—and that the least important half—of the pulse variations; we have noticed the causes of an increased pulse, but have not yet inquired into the causes of a continually sub-normal rate of beat. Those of my readers who have carefully perused the chapter on "The Temperature" will find no difficulty in answering this much-neglected, yet highly important, question. *It is because the vitality is low*,

[1] "Anatomy, Physiology and Hygiene," by J. C. Cutter, M.D., p. 62.

[2] "It is a demonstrable fact that the heart of the habitual meat eater beats from seventy-two to eighty beats a minute, while that of the person living on a pure diet of fruits, nuts, etc., will be ten times less per minute. Fifteen hundred extra heart strokes every twenty-four hours makes a very appreciable strain upon the vital forces." ("Food Value of Meat," by W. R. C. Latson, M.D., p. 45.)

subnormal, depleted. Add to the patient's vitality, and you will raise the rate of pulsation to the normal in every instance. As with the temperature, so here. Above normal denotes feverishness; below, lack of vitality. In this respect, the two are largely inter-related, and the method of bringing them both up to the normal standard is also the same—namely, purifying the body, and causing it to return, thereby, to its normal condition of health and vital stamina. Here also the pulsation becomes either raised or lowered as the case may be, and finally reaches normal at the time the fast is ready to be broken. And the fact that this is the case clearly indicates that Nature and not man sets the time limits of a fast, indicating its duration by unmistakable symptoms.

This brings me to a timely warning. Theoretically, a fast, by cleansing the system, should bring both the temperature and the pulse up to normal together, and we should almost be able to gauge the one by the other—the thermometric examination revealing the approximate rate of the heart-beat, and *vice versa.*

"It is usual to have the temperature and the pulse rising and falling together, and it has been approximately estimated that, in fever, an increase of the temperature of 1° F. above 98° F., corresponds with an increase in the pulse of ten per minute."[1]

While this is very largely true, in a great number of cases, it is by no means universally the case—thus bringing us face to face with one of the most interesting of physiological problems. I have noticed that, where any tendency to heart trouble exists, *e.g.*, the temperature may be almost perfectly normal, yet the heart be beating at a most alarming rate of speed. In other cases, again, the pulse may be perfectly normal, but the temperature very low throughout the fast—as, *e.g.*, in Mrs. T. A.'s case, mentioned on pp. 195–7. While fasting, this tendency, is greatly increased—the pulse sometimes running up, under these conditions, to 110 or 120 or even more per minute, the temperature, meanwhile, remaining almost normal. Such was the case with Doctor B., whose pulse at one time rose almost to the latter

[1] "The Physiology of Death from Traumatic Fever," by John D. Malcolm, M.B., p. 9.

figure (120); and such also was the case with George Downie, who courageously undertook a fast, under my directions, while residing in Edinburgh Scotland — I being at that time in Minneapolis, Minn.—a distance of some five thousand miles separating adviser and patient. Surely, if cases can be brought to a successful termination under *these* exceptional circumstances, patients should have no fear of fasting, while under the daily observation of their physician![1]

While my own experience of fasting cases has most frequently resulted establishing the fact that the pulse was beating at an abnormally rapid rate, others seem to have met with very different results. Thus, Mr. Macfadden wrote:[2]

"I had one patient at the experimental health home whose pulse fell to twenty and was so faint that it could scarcely be felt, after a fast of three weeks. It quickly rose after the patient took some nourishment."

It is somewhat hard to account for such a case as this. The greatly enfeebled pulse may have been due to lack of physical exercise; or to a brooding mental condition; or to a peculiar anatomical abnormality, or to all these and other causes combined. Further, it must not be forgotten that food is a *stimulant*, pure and simple, at such a time as this. Every fiber of the body would be instantly revivified, owing to the artificially induced circulation. What toxic material the food contained (and no food is absolutely free from it) would also add to the stimulation, by greatly exciting the nervous system—and consequently the heart's action. Slight feverishness would result, and this, together with the mental stimulation and cheer at the prospect of renewed eating, would probably account for the increased pulse rate noted above.

But it must be remembered that all cases such as these are the exception—not the rule. The vast majority of patients will experience no personal inconvenience whatever during the fast,

[1] In this connection, I may be permitted to mention a somewhat humorous occurrence. At the time mentioned—though a young man and a layman I was instructing by mail no less than four regular physicians at one time, in different parts of the country, as to the course they should pursue in the treatment of fasting cases! They all later reported satisfactory results.

[2] "Natural Cure for Rupture," pp. 36–7.

either through greatly accelerated or greatly diminished heart action. In the vast majority of cases, the patient notices no peculiar effects whatever (slight differences of pulsation being rarely noticeable) and all quite insignificant when compared with the vast and beneficial changes that are taking place at that time within the organism.

When these abnormal symptoms are noted, however, they are generally accompanied by the feeling of extreme weakness, so that the patient can scarcely walk without great effort, and feels disinclined for any exertion whatever—and but little can be indulged in without producing great exhaustion. This exhaustion is, however, nervous, not physical. Quite apart from the theoretical argument—that exhaustion does not result from fasting, and is not a consequent of it—we have the best practical demonstration of this in the fact that, if the fast be persisted in, the weakness will gradually disappear. Were this weakness the result of physical exhaustion, such could hardly be the case, as the exhaustion would then simply increase as the fast progressed, instead of actually diminishing, and finally disappearing altogether, as is actually the case. In Doctor B.'s own person, we both noticed these symptoms very carefully, and watched for the results, whatever they might be.

It must be admitted, of course, that these symptoms are all very alarming, when they develop, during a fast—especially if the patient is not prepared for them, and half fears a collapse at any hour—owing to his imperfect understanding of the philosophy of fasting. I may here remark, however, that such extreme variations invariably denote some profound physiological change, taking place at that time—a crisis, in fact—and I shall accordingly speak of them under that heading (*v.* Chap. VII), and indicate the appropriate treatment. The fact that hitherto weak hearts are actually strengthened and cured by fasting proves conclusively that any such unusual symptoms, observed during this period, denote a beneficial reparative process, and not any harmful or dangerous decrease or acceleration, due to lack of perfect control by the cardiac nerve.

There is one other point of great importance that must be taken into consideration, when testing the rate of heart-beat, by means of the pulse. That is the *rhythm*. No matter how fast or how slowly the heart is beating, the rhythm should be perfect, *i.e.*, the time interval between each beat should be exactly uniform. If this is not the case, grave functional disturbances or organic defects are present—far more grave than any other variation whatever. The causes for this are again manifold, due sometimes to some organic defect in the heart, or to some obstruction of its proper functioning—in which cases fasting would prove of the utmost benefit.

Summing up, now, this chapter on the pulse, my readers may have come to the conclusion that these extremes are the usual accompaniments of a fast, and that one or other of them is almost always present—danger being present accordingly. If such an impression has been gained, I can only say that it is quite a mistaken idea, since the facts are altogether contrary. As I have before emphasized, and must here reëmphasize, abnormally high or low pulsation, during a fast, are quite the exception—*not* the rule. If I should have seemed to dwell somewhat at length upon the variations that may be observed at this time, it is because this highly suggestive, interesting, but, as yet, all but untouched field of physiological investigation has been neglected by hygienists no less than by regular medical practitioners; and it is with the hope of calling their attention to this most important subject, that I have undertaken these few brief remarks.

CHAPTER IV

THE LOSS AND GAIN IN WEIGHT

DOUBTLESS, the most marked result of the fast is the loss of flesh by the patient—a comparative and clinical study of which has never yet been undertaken—though the results of such an investigation would prove of the highest interest to all concerned. In the present chapter, therefore, I shall endeavor to lay before my readers the few somewhat crude observations I have been enabled to make—more with the hope that I may stimulate and direct the attention of those physicians who have a wide field of study and the opportunity for extensive experiments and research—than with the idea of making any permanent addition to our scientific knowledge, and indeed, with that very object in view have I written this book.

The popular idea that emaciation follows very rapidly upon the total withdrawal of all food is, of course, quite erroneous. We have seen, p. 124, that emaciation is almost invariably due to *disease*, and that it is physically impossible for a person to starve until the skeleton condition is reached; and we have also seen that this is a period of time covering at least four weeks, and which could, I firmly believe, be successfully extended over as many months, in certain exceptional cases. A study of the comparative loss of flesh in individuals at various stages of the fast, and its loss from the various parts of the body, together with the consideration of the causes of death occurring before the theoretical limit has been reached, forms the material for our study in this chapter.

Generally speaking, then, it may be stated that, as a general rule, patients possessing the greatest amount of fatty tissue lose the most weight during the early stage of every fast; while their more slender companions lose considerably less, and this is by no means so obvious a fact as might be supposed upon casually thinking over the matter. Fatty tissue does not, by any means, mean *heavy* tissue. On the other hand, fat of every kind is invariably known for its extreme *lightness*, and it is the same in the human body. Taking two men of equal height, but of otherwise different proportions, the stouter man may quite conceivably be the lighter of the two, the more solid and weighty bone and muscular tissue of the slenderer man more than compensating for the superiority in mere bulk of the other; and, this being the case, the stouter man might lose a far greater amount of flesh, as measured by the tape-line, but yet not so much as the other, when registered on the scales. Thus, it will be seen, my statement that the fatter man does lose, during the fast, a greater actual weight than the slenderer man, is by no meant so obvious a statement as might appear, but goes to show that the stouter man loses his fatty tissue at an *extremely* rapid rate, a considerable amount of which must be absorbed to cause any appreciable change in the balance.

Before proceeding to discuss the comparative loss of weight in different individuals, under various conditions, it will be necessary for us to see what is the average *proportionate* loss in the general run of fasting cases. Taking the first ten cases reported in Bk. II, Chap. VI, as representative of a wide variety of diseases and as great a dissimilarity of physique and temperament as it would be possible to meet, we arrive, by comparing the weights in the various cases, at the following results:

Name	Weight at Commencement	Weight at End	Days	Loss Weight
1. Geo. E. Davis			50	54
2. Mrs. I. Matthews			22	27
3. Rev. N. H. Löhre			10	13
4. Prof. F. W——			20	24
5. Mr. J. B——			23	11
6. Mrs. J. B——			8	8
7. Mr. G. W. Tuthill			41	36
8. Mrs. F. J. C——			28	33
9. Mrs. T. A——			31	25
10. Robert B——			17	17
	1531½	1286½	253	248[1]

[1] *i.e.*, 248 pounds of effete, diseased material eliminated!

It will be seen, from a study of the above ten cases, which may be taken as quite representative, in a period covering more than two-thirds of a year, that the total loss comes within five pounds of the actual number of days fasted—from which we are surely justified in making this important generalization. *The average loss of weight by fasting patients amounts, ceteris paribus, to one pound per diem.* It will be seen from the above table that this rule applied absolutely in cases 6 and 10, and almost exactly in cases 1, 2, 3, 4, 7 and 8—case 1 beautifully illustrating the point here made; the great length of time allowing a general "balancing of accounts," so to speak, within the physiological laboratory. In this case the loss was, for the first two weeks, far greater than one pound a day, but toward the end of the fast, fatty tissue becoming scarce—the loss was considerably *less* than that amount[1]—the average being found to be almost exactly one pound a day, at the conclusion of the fast, and so on throughout the list.

Interesting variations from this general standard may frequently be observed, both above and below, but the causes of these variations can almost always be easily discovered. Thus, in cases 5 and 9 (*v.* the above table), considerably less than one pound a day was lost—this being due to the fact that both these patients were previously somewhat emaciated from disease, and had but a small amount of fatty tissue left, comparatively speaking, to lose. On the other hand, in the case of Mrs. Jantz (St. Paul, Minn.), the almost incredible amount of seventy-five pounds was lost in twenty-one days—an average of almost three and one-half pounds a day throughout; the loss being, of course, far greater than this during the first few days! This result was due to the fact that the patient had a tremendous store of easily assimilable tissue—being "fat" in the accepted sense of the term. A similar loss was observed in the case of Mrs. A. E. R. (Minneapolis, Minn.), who lost forty pounds in three weeks, this while fasting only three days at a time, and eating one very light meal on the fourth day throughout. (pp. 209–10.)

Briefly, then, I believe that it will be observed, in every in-

[1] This is almost invariably the case. A patient loses approximately one and one-half pounds *per diem,* at the very beginning of every fast for every one-half pound which is lost toward its close.

stance, that those who lose on the average *more* weight than the theoretical pound are those who are encumbered with an excess of fat, while those who lose less than that amount are those who are already somewhat emaciated from disease.

The question now arises, how much should the *normal* man lose? *More* than a pound a day is obviously too much—denoting obesity; while *less* than half a pound is too little—denoting emaciation. To "split the difference" would be convenient—but guess work. Moreover the average losses throughout do not come to twelve ounces a day, but to one pound, or sixteen ounces, as we have seen. As this question is a highly important one, for reasons that will appear presently, I shall proceed to discuss it somewhat in detail.

The fact that one pound *per diem* is the all but uniform loss of weight during a fast, would perhaps cause us to accept that weight as the "ideal," or average, were it not for one considera tion. It is this. *All patients who find it necessary to fast absolutely are already in a grossly abnormal condition, and their loss of weight must consequently be considered abnormal also.* One pound per day must therefore represent the loss of weight of a *diseased* body, and is by no means a *normal* loss. The amount is too great. A more normal man would, of necessity, lose less. *How much less* is the problem.

There seems to be no conceivable manner for measuring this "ideal" loss, for the reason that this would be the day's loss, in weight, of a perfectly healthy man, and, as we have seen (p. 63), a perfectly healthy man is almost, if not quite, impossible to find. *Fairly* healthy men are the nearest approach to this condition that we at present know of—athletes in training, for example. The few cases of the kind that have been recorded (athletes as a rule being afraid to fast during their training) present very contradictory results. Thus Mr Macfadden, during his week's fast, lost fifteen pounds;[1] while Miss Louise Kops of New York, lost *nothing at all* during a four days' fast (in May, 1904); and in the case of Mr. J. Estapper, Jr., a week's fast resulted in an actual *gain* of three-fourths of a pound![2]

[1] "Fasting Hydropathy and Exercise," p. 73

[2] This weight was very accurately ascertained, and there was no possible source of error through which a mistake could have been made. The

From such figures as these it is, of course, quite impossible to reach any definite conclusion, or even guess the approximate weight lost—these being all exceptional cases. From the fact, however that the average loss, *per diem*, of any great number of cases, taken together, is, as nearly as possible, one pound; and since this loss is doubtless abnormally great; from this fact, and from the fact that so small a loss as one-half pound a day is rarely, if ever, averaged throughout; and from a study of the loss of weight of those few fairly normal cases it has been my fortune to encounter; as well as from a consideration of what cases I have been enabled to find reported, and of the discussion of them by the attending physicians, in such cases, I think we are fully justified in asserting that a daily loss of *twelve ounces* would be the average loss of weight for those in good health, were they to enter upon a fast for experimental reasons. The remaining four ounces *per diem* would thus represent the rapid elimination of fatty tissue and morbid matter—of which the system has no use, and of which it is much better rid.

Now from the above fact (if fact it be, and I can see no valid reason for doubting it, after reviewing all the evidence at my disposal), a highly important deduction may be drawn; an extremely significant conclusion reached, which, in fact affects the welfare of the whole human race. If such be the case, *we have*

"faster" was, in this case, one of the competitors in the seven day fasting-athletic-contest held in Madison Square Garden during the last week in December, 1903, in which the measurements and weights were taken with the greatest care, and the contestants were under the strictest surveillance throughout the whole period, and were frequently observed and examined by New York physicians, and others. Nevertheless, it was found that, in this case, the weight actually increased, as stated, instead of decreasing. "This increase in weight can be explained," says Mr. Macfadden, "only by the fact that pure distilled water, which Mr. Estapper took in large quantities, was absorbed and retained by his strengthened assimilative powers." (*Physical Culture*, Vol. IX., p. 261, Mar., 1904.)

I have since come across several cases in which weight was gained during a fast; Mrs. Martin, of Stapleton, S. I., being one of these. This patient fasted eight days, and gained four pounds during that period. Doctor Rabagliati mentions a case in which a patient gained one and one-half pounds in three weeks on a diet of less than eight ounces of food a day, about ninety per cent. of which was water. ("Air, Food and Exercises," p. 204.) The explanation is in all probability this: In all such cases great denseness of tissue is present—it is obstipated, as it is called—and when such a person fasts, he or she oxidizes off a part of this too solid tissue, and fills in the interstices with water, which the patient is at liberty to drink, during the fast. This is, at least, the explanation which I have been driven to adopt—none other seemingly covering the facts.

here, at last, a scientific basis for calculating what the average intake of food should be by those in health (and who wish to remain in health); for, since we have seen (p. 165), that the amount of "income" should be exactly proportioned to the "outgo," if we are to retain "that just balance we term health," then it follows, as a matter of course, that *twelve ounces of nutriment daily* (Cornaro's allowance), *is all that the body needs in order to preserve its weight and to replace whatever tissue has been lost as the result of the day's muscular exertions or tissue destruction.*[1]

I have been careful to use the word "nutriment" in relation to this question of weight, it will be observed, for the reason that "food" is by no means all nutriment (even its edible parts), and it might require fifteen or twenty or more ounces of actual food to supply this twelve ounces of nutriment—this depending on the percentage of nutriment each food contained. What the system actually requires is twelve ounces of material, every particle of which it can utilize. From this it becomes obvious that, *ceteris paribus*, that food which contains the most nutriment with the least waste is the best for the body—requiring, as it does, the minimum amount of energy expenditure and organic wear and tear.

The importance of this conclusion, should it prove to be correct, is obviously immense. Knowing the theoretical amount of nutriment required by the system, and the percentage of such nutriment, it would only be necessary, thenceforward, to calculate the amount of each food necessary in order to supply this amount of nutriment, and thus to ascertain the quantity of any food necessary to properly sustain life (the quality is another matter); and when the amount daily consumed is greater than the theoretical limit here set (and allowing, of course, for individual fluctuations) then the process of accumulation of diseased matter commences, and continues either until it is forcibly eliminated in some form of acute disease, or until the system has had the opportunity to "catch up" that amount, so to say,

[1] I consider it a very remarkable fact that I had written the above passage before I had read Doctor Rabagliati's work, "Air, Food and Exercises," where he arrives at precisely the same conclusion, from a somewhat different standpoint. (See pp. 121; 286–8.) That two workers, the one in England and the other in America, each unknown to the other, should have reached results so exactly similar, is, to my mind, most extraordinary, and strongly confirms the supposition that these calculations are at basis true.

by eating just that much less food on some succeeding day. Thus, suppose a certain person's organism can appropriate twelve ounces of nutrient matter during the course of one day; fifteen ounces are ingested on one occasion—this representing a considerable increase in the actual bulk of food eaten. This extra food must either be disposed of through the eliminative organs, at the expense of the bodily energy, or it would accumulate within the system as morbid matter or fatty tissue. The process of disease has begun, either toward nervous exhaustion or toward foul accumulations, which must be later expelled—this depending upon which of the above methods Nature follows in the elimination of the excess of food ingested. This extra three ounces of nutrient material, or rather the bulk of food which contains that amount, having been passed into the system, there should be, on some following day, a *corresponding diminution* of food, if perfect health is to be maintained. If the constant surplus is, however, continually forced into the system, disease is sure to result—and *this, I am contending, is the real cause of all disease.* If, on the other hand, "that just balance we term health" is to be maintained, only nine ounces of nutriment should be ingested on the ensuing day—thus allowing the system to eliminate the three ounces in excess previously ingested.

But, it may be argued, the former amount may already have been eliminated from the system, owing to increased vital activity having stimulated the eliminating organs to unwonted labors, with the result that the food material did not lodge within the system, but was successfully eliminated. In this case, also, the rule holds good, for the reason that the vital powers, which were abnormally expended in ridding the system of this excess, are now allowed to recuperate to just that extent, for the reason that the energy which would have been expended in digesting and eliminating that amount of food, is now conserved and used to "balance the accounts," so to speak, against the previous expenditure; and if this balance were justly and evenly preserved, there is no obvious reason why we should not live on practically indefinitely.[1] (*v.* pp. 327–8.)

[1] It will be seen that it would be possible (did we but know how much, in weight, this morbid accumulation amounted to, within the body, and the length of time it has taken to thus accumulate), to calculate the length of

To return now to the study of the comparative loss of weight of individuals while fasting. It may be stated that, as a general rule, women lose slightly more than do men at such times—this being due, in all probability, to the greater amount of fatty tissue which a woman generally possesses; partly as a result of her more sedentary habits; partly because of her greater indulgence in sweetened foods. It has been stated that the fatter the person, the greater the comparative loss of weight (p. 466), and this applies to men and women equally. Some persons who would apparently lose a very large amount in a short space of time lose a surprisingly small amount, and this is undoubtedly due to the fact that these persons possess less fatty and more muscular tissue than would appear upon a superficial examination. Some sparely built individuals, on the other hand, lose a surprisingly large amount—this result being due, undoubtedly, to the presence of the opposite condition. Exercise greatly increases the daily loss of weight (*v.* pp. 382–3), and it is only natural to suppose that stimulating any avenue of elimination would have the same effect—this tending, ultimately, to shorten the fast. By neglecting exercise, enemas, and other methods of elimination, Doctor Dewey undoubtedly, though unknowingly, protracted many of his cases of fasting, and added many days of useless self-denial to the patients, under his treatment (*v.* Chapter "Exercise," pp. 384–5).

Another interesting fact to be observed is this: The loss of weight is always greatest at first and becomes less and less, daily, as the fast progresses.[1] Now, this is only natural; since the fatty tissue, being in excess at first, is eliminated before nature undertakes any other task—such as the purification of the remaining tissue. That this "toning up" process is intended to be last in order, is manifest when we consider that, for several

time it would be necessary to fast, in order to bring about a complete restoration of health. It is hardly necessary to say that, in our present state of knowledge, such a calculation would be quite impossible.

[1] This agrees with other observers. Says Doctor Keith: "A healthy man when he takes no food loses in weight at first about a pound a day, which is gradually lessened to half a pound if the abstinence is prolonged." ("Plea for a Simple Life," p. 37.) My friend, Mr. Shaw, who closely watched himself throughout his forty-five-day fast, wrote: "The loss of flesh for many days has been less and less, as compared with the earlier days of the fast. . . . The loss of weight grows less and less daily." ("The Best Thing in the World," pp. 26; 30.)

practically *no loss of weight at all* is noticed—showing that there are other vital matters to be attended to even after the fatty tissue and morbid matter have all been oxidized off and eliminated. Since, as we have seen (pp. 126–33), that all fatty tissue is *diseased* tissue; also (p. 161), that it is "physiologically impossible" to starve to death until the skeleton condition is reached, and that any one of us may consequently fast, with perfect safety, until he is reduced to the weight of his skeleton and viscera (which weight can only be determined by a careful physical examination of the patient with this end in view);[1] it becomes obvious that many obese persons could reduce their weight, without danger, (and, indeed, with only added comfort and safety to themselves) to any extent desired; in many cases, doubtless, as much as from one to two hundred pounds! That there would be no *danger* attending such reduction I trust my readers will now appreciate; that it is *painless* may easily be verified by personal experience and observation; while the only remaining objection worth considering—that the skin would wrinkle or "sag" during and after such a fast—is completely negatived by the well-known fact that, in the cases of persons who have starved to death, and consequently have reduced their stock of flesh to the minimum—the skin is invariably drawn tight, stretched to its utmost, over the protruding bones of the ghastly corpse!

The objection is frequently made that, while fasting may thus be admittedly good for the extremely obese, it is, and must necessarily be, nevertheless, of doubtful advantage, if not obviously and necessarily dangerous and useless, to the emaciated, and to those already lacking in flesh and muscle. This reasoning is founded upon a gross misapprehension as to the nature of disease, as such, and of the causes of emaciation. *Abnormal or excessive emaciation is always due to disease*, and the degree of the emaciation exactly corresponds, *ceteris paribus*, to the severity of the diseased condition. Obviously, therefore, the most rapid and effectual way to check the emaciation is first to rid the system of the diseased condition present; and, since this can be done,

[1] Two-fifths of the total weight, according to Doctor Kirke. ("Physiology," p. 507.)

as we have seen, more rapidly and effectually by *fasting* than by any other method, it follows that this is the surest method of ultimately checking the emaciation! After the fast is broken, when normal functioning recommences; and the whole system, including the digestive apparatus, is restored to health—enabled to exercise its legitimate functions, the body will then be built up, owing to the fact that the digestive apparatus can *now* assimilate the food which previously it could not; and consequently, failed, for this reason, to nourish the system. Theoretically, therefore, fasting would be the best *cure* for emaciation, for the reason that it is the surest way to stop it, and to enable the system to ultimately increase in size and muscular development, which, in point of fact, is absolutely the case.[1]

As a proof of this I may quote two cases previously mentioned (pp. 189–94, and pp. 210–11). (1) G. W. Tuthill, though greatly emaciated, physically weak, and weighing, at the *commencement* of the fast, but 108½ pounds, yet *fasted forty-one days with marked benefit!* At the expiration of that time, though reduced to the skeleton condition (see Figs. 1, 2, 3, 4, pp. 192–3), and weighing but seventy-two and one-half pounds![2] was yet far freer from the paralysis than at the commencement of the fast—it being possible to observe the daily improvement in his condition—especially toward the end of the fast—to the very last day! In his case, then, there is obviously no possible escape from the admission of the fact that the fast benefited the patient up to the last minute, though protracted for nearly one thousand hours—the patient *commencing* only when already greatly weakened and reduced in flesh from the wasting of disease! Could proof be more positive? One other case! (2) Mrs. R. T. (*v.* pp. 210–11), in very much the same weak and highly emaciated condition at the

[1] Compare Doctor Dewey: "*Overweight* is always due to food in excess, and by fasting or limited daily food, it can be reduced in the easiest way to any desired figures; the cure of other ailings going on at the same time. *Underweight* is due to disease, for which fasting is the cure, and, with digestive power restored, the normal weight is regained with the luxury of eating" ("Experiences," p. 32). This would seem to remind us, on first reading, of the familiar "heads I win, and tails you lose"—but a little serious consideration will show us that the position here defended is fully justifiable and quite correct.

[2] A largely built, big-boned man could never, of course, reduce himself to this weight, by any amount of fasting—Mr. Tuthill's small bones enabling him to reach this really very extraordinary weight.

commencement of the fast, and weighing but ninety-eight pounds clothed,[1] yet fasted for eighteen days with marked benefit throughout, and with but little loss of weight as a result! Unfortunately an accurate weighing was not made at the completion of this fast, so the *exact* figures cannot be given—much to the detriment of science!

In these two cases, especially, were the results most striking and obvious; and, agreeing as these two cases do, with the theoretical point of view, and, in a lesser degree, with all other cases of a similar character noted by me, they explode, once and for all, the utter fallacy that only the obese can fast to advantage, and show us how ludicrous and absurd is the popular idea that the average well-fed person, weighing, let us say, 140 to 160 pounds, would run the risk of "death from starvation" as the result of omitting half a dozen meals!

The loss of flesh from the various parts of the body, and a comparison of the amount thus lost at different stages of the fast, and in various individuals, forms a most interesting study, but is a subject which cannot here be discussed at any length; partly because my observations have led to no definite conclusions (being too uncertain and contradictory to allow of any such being formed) and partly because of the comparative unimportance of the subject, from a practical standpoint. One or two brief remarks may not, however, be out of place. Those parts which are most rapidly and noticeably affected are the cheeks, the neck and the throat, while the arms and thighs come next—all of which parts are affected almost entirely by the absorption of fatty tissue, and the elimination of morbid matter from the localities indicated. The most noticeable reduction, however, is almost invariably observed over the abdomen, where, in addition to the above mentioned causes, the thorough emptying of the bowels (of their contents) must be taken into consideration. (*v.* pp. 420–3.) This obviously causes a very great and rapid reduction in this part of the body, and is one of the most noticeable and characteristic symptoms of fasting; furnishing a fairly reliable "cheek," and enabling the physician to tell

[1] Clothes average about ten pounds in winter, at which time this fast was undertaken.

whether the patient is really fasting conscientiously or no. (See also pp. 446–7.)

Reference has already been made to Louis Kuhne and his ingenious theory of "facial diagnosis." (See pp. 589–91.) Since these morbid deposits are present in the system, it is only natural to suppose that those parts most laden with this morbid matter would be the ones most affected while fasting; that is, the reduction of morbid tissue would be most noticeable in those parts. This fact is so obvious that it seems hardly necessary to say that, in practice, the facts are found to agree with this theory in every detail.

Gain in Weight

Thus far we have considered one side of the question only; that of the *loss* of flesh and weight, during the fast, and have taken no account of the *gain* in weight after the fast is broken. This must now claim our attention for a few moments, for the reason that it presents some very interesting paradoxes. Theoretically, of course, all increase in weight is derived totally and invariably from the food eaten (liquid or solid), the increase always commencing upon the breaking of the fast and the ingestion of the first meal. Generally speaking, this is, of course, the rule; the more or less rapid decrease in weight, during the fast, being counterbalanced by the correspondingly rapid or slow gain in weight after it has been broken—this continuing until nearly, or quite, or more than, the former weight has been reached. But to this general rule there are many exceptions. One patient may, during a fast, lose flesh and weight with extreme rapidity, but regain it extremely slowly; while, on the contrary, another patient may lose surprisingly little, and when the fast is broken, gain rapidly and shoot up far beyond his original weight. The former of these peculiarities is no doubt due to the fact that the patient's body was encumbered with a very large amount of easily eliminated foreign matter and fatty tissue, which, being once eliminated, did not again accumulate under the improved bodily conditions—elimination, not retention, taking place; while the latter condition is, no doubt, due to the fact that, in such cases, the patient's digestive system is improved by the fast to such an extent that it can afterwards digest and assimilate the food which it could not utilize previously. The small loss of weight is due to the fact that the body had but little tissue to lose; and the fast benefits such cases, not so much by ridding the system of foul material (though this is a highly important factor) as by enabling the vitality to recuperate sufficiently to properly assimilate and eliminate the food eaten. In such cases the benefits that thin persons may derive from a more or less protracted fast are obvious.

The variations in the gain of weight are most interesting to watch. Some patients will, as stated, shoot up, upon breaking the fast, far beyond their original weight—showing that this latter weight is the normal condition of such persons, and that their previous "leanness" was due to emaciation; to lack of nourishment; to "starvation from overfeeding." (See pp. 168–9.) Others, again, will never regain their original weight—showing that, normally, they would weigh considerably *less* than they did before entering upon the fast—the extra weight being due, in such cases, purely to the retention of morbid matter within the system, which had no place there, and was the cause of the diseased condition—rendering the fast necessary. The majority, however, will probably regain their previous weight, or nearly so, and continue at that weight indefinitely.

Weight is usually regained, upon breaking the fast, at an almost incredibly rapid rate, due, no doubt, to the fact that the digestive organs can assimilate, and the system utilize, every morsel of food ingested. Indeed, in some cases, more weight is apparently gained than there is food eaten! And this raises one of the most puzzling questions I have ever met with, relative to this question of fasting. It is one of those paradoxes to which I referred on p. 477, where I said: "Theoretically, of course, the increase in weight is derived totally and invariably from the food eaten (liquid or solid), the increase always commencing upon the breaking of the fast and the ingestion of the first meal." I have now some facts to bring forward which would seem to show that this is *not* invariably the case. Doctor B. both lost and gained weight with astonishing rapidity. In four days this patient lost eight and one-half pounds—more than two pounds a day. On breaking the fast and resuming a fairly abstemious diet, she, nevertheless, in the next two days, gained eight pounds on three meals and a plate of soup! In this case, I feel quite positive that the food eaten certainly did not amount to four pounds. Another extraordinary case was that of Mrs. C., above referred to (pp. 194–5), who broke her fast on November 16, 1902, weighing 103 pounds, and on November 22d—an interval of six days—weighed 113 pounds—an increase of ten pounds. The case is remarkable when we take into consideration the fact that for these six days, the patient had partaken of *no solid food whatever*, a liquid diet *only* being eaten throughout, consisting entirely of broths and fruit juices! (No milk whatever was drunk during this period.)[1]

Now, although the foods partaken of in the first two cases were not (unfortunately) weighed at the time, I feel morally certain that the *total bulk* of the nutriment taken into the system did not, in either case, amount to anything like the total weight gained by the patient during the period under consideration. Omitting whatever water may have been drunk during this period, which as we have seen (p. 400) does not theoretically supply lost weight, inasmuch as it supplies the tissues with no actual nutriment—the *total amount of food ingested* most certainly weighed far less than the actual weight gained; while, if we were to calculate the amount of "nutriment proper," and omit the "ashes" in these cases (which cannot add to the weight unless retained in the intestines, which they were not, in these two cases), we arrive at a figure very far below that which was actually reached. In other words, we find that the sum-total weight of the food eaten is far less than the total weight gained.

The question now arises: whence is this additional weight derived? Both air and water were partaken of in as liberal doses during the fast as after its completion and breaking; so these must, apparently, be left out of account; while, if the

[1] Doctor Nichols mentions a case in which a patient of his gained weight on less than three ounces of solid food *per diem*. See his "Diet Cure," p. 20. Dr. J. S. Cooley wrote me, on December 23, 1906, stating that he had observed a case in which a patient of his gained two and three-fourths pounds a day for ten days. I was not informed as to the nature of the diet.

increase in weight exceeds that of the food ingested, from what is this extra weight derived?

My idea is that both air and water *do*, to some extent, actually prevent loss of weight—not by supplying nutriment from which tissues can be built, but *by preventing waste of tissue from emaciation*. These two essentials, by keeping the body well supplied with the materials from which vitality draws, in order to effect a cure, prevents the harmful, ghastly emaciation that would follow, were we deprived of water or a plentiful supply of fresh air, during a fast. Were these conditions present, the loss would be exceedingly rapid—very far greater than the one pound a day previously estimated. Thus, had we any means of ascertaining what might be the "gross" or total loss of weight *per diem*, when deprived of water, air and food (were such a thing possible) and fix this as the "zero point," so to speak, we should find that, with both air and water allowed *ad libitum*, the "net" loss would be very much less than such a figure, varying in accordance with the condition of the patient. We thus see that the prevention of loss of tissue which the presence of these two elements occasion, represents, roughly speaking, just that amount of weight gained. There is thus a constant *gain* in weight throughout a fast, but this is nevertheless neutralized and altogether eclipsed by the far greater loss which deprivation of food occasions, and in fact necessitates.

The whole subject is a most puzzling and complex one. As Doctor Nichols pointed out:[1]

" . . . there are facts in physiology which physiologists have not satisfactorily accounted for; this, for instance:—Doctor Carpenter, in his "Animal Physiology," p. 177, gives a case of a young jockey who, being weighed before a race, was allowed to take a glass of wine shortly after. On being again put into the scales, the jockey was found to be some pounds heavier. Another rider, two hours after taking a cup of tea, was found to have gained ix pounds in weight. Mr. Hands, a surgeon, says:—'I once knew a woman (Mrs. Smith, East Street, Manchester Square) who, in the course of thirty days, discharged from the stomach, bladder, and bowels, fluids, etc., nearly equalling the weight of her whole

[1] "The Diet Cure," p. 20.

body, and this without eating, and almost without drinking.' He adds that 'Doctor Hooper relates similar cases.'"

Now, we have seen that the body can, under certain conditions, gain weight at an astonishing and altogether unaccountable rate. And there are cases on record, also, where a similar *loss* of weight has been noted; where, too, no exercise or other physical exertion has been taken, to render apparent the means by which such loss has been rendered possible. The *wasting of disease* is just such an illustrative case—emaciation sometimes rapidly ensuing, in the absence of all exercise, and while there is an abundance of easily assimilable food within the organism. Rear-Admiral George W. Melville, U. S. N., quotes a most interesting case,[1] in which a man allowed himself to be sealed into a glass-covered coffin for the period of one hour—his breathing space, for that period being but two cubic feet. The patient lived; and, though he did not take any physical exercise whatever, he nevertheless lost five pounds during that brief period. In a controversy I had with Dr. Duncan MacDougall, of Haverhill, Mass., over this case, he contended that such a result might have been brought about by profuse sweating on the part of the man shut in the coffin (*Journal* of the American Society for Psychical Research, May–June, 1907, pp. 276–83; 343–7), and it is possible that such might have been the case. But nothing is proved on either side, for lack of evidence. In short, there are so many varied and extraordinary cases on record, the explanations of which seem more or less obscure, that my own cases should find but little difficulty in receiving recognition and in gaining acceptance. While my own speculations in this field cannot be considered as of any permanent value, they will, I trust, help to divert the attention of the scientific world to a study of this most interesting and all but totally neglected problem; and if I succeed in doing that, I shall consider that my object has been accomplished.

[1] "The Submarine Boat," p. 723.

CHAPTER V

PHYSIOLOGICAL EFFECTS—I

The Stomach.—The stomach is, of course, the first organ in the body to feel the beneficial effects of a fast, for the reason that it is into the stomach all the food we eat enters. The first act of Nature, then, in the absence of food, is, undoubtedly, to thoroughly empty and cleanse the stomach; to rid that organ of the mass of corrupt, putrefying matter it contains, and to pass this material on through the bowels—there to be dealt with by the powerfully antiseptic intestinal juices. Occasionally, however, the stomach is unable to rid itself of the fermenting mass which it contains; in which case, the contents of the stomach is vomited—to the great relief of the patient. Physiologists have almost invariably contended that an ordinary meal is digested in from two to five hours; but I must emphatically dissent from this conclusion, as I have frequently found that (especially when a slight indisposition is present), food is retained for a very much longer period; the stomach being unable to rid itself of its contents. Says Doctor Rabagliati:[1]

> "Indeed, food is occasionally, or even not infrequently, still in the stomach twenty-four, thirty-six, and even forty-eight hours after it has been taken."

I have personally known of cases in which large quantities of food matter were thus ejected at the end of a three days' fast, and in spite of profuse water drinking! What state must the stomach of this man have been in to render such a result possible? What a foul condition must have prevailed, preventing the digestion of this food for seventy-two hours—it lying there meanwhile actually decomposing, rotting! And in what condition was this man's stomach to receive food? Would it not seem a common

[1] "Aphorisms," etc., p. 26.

sense procedure to wait until this mass of food rubbish was removed before again adding food, only to still aggravate the diseased organ, by adding to the bulk of its poisonous contents? And as the effete matter had, in this case, remained at least three days before Nature could rid the system of the decomposing material, a fast of *at least three days* was, therefore, necessary, in order to cleanse the stomach of this fermenting mass, preparatory to normal digestion. And yet this man was not fasting for stomach trouble at all, but for an altogether different malady, and his stomach had never troubled him in the least! How many of us may possess like stomachs if we but knew it![1]

Dr. W. E. Forest, in discussing this question, says:[2]

"In the first place, the stomach should be so treated as to require no treatment. There should be no trouble in the stomach and there would be none if only proper food were taken at proper intervals and in a proper manner. . . . If improper foods and purgatives are taken, or other conditions violated, there is trouble in the stomach. If too much food is taken, the stomach is distended, the muscular activity cannot take place, fermentation sets in, the acids which are generated by decomposition become irritants, and the stomach becomes diseased and cannot do its work. If the second meal is taken before the first has left the stomach, digestion of the first is suspended, and before the new supply is reduced to the same condition as the first, fermentation again sets in, and these partly digested products are retained instead of being passed on. This condition sometimes requires help; in the first place there should be fasting, giving Nature a chance to make matters right, and as an assistance the stomach should be cleansed."

These cleansing processes continue until the stomach is thoroughly empty, and is in a completely disinfected and, comparatively speaking, sweet condition. The walls of the stomach, meanwhile, have been coming into closer and closer proximity, as the emptying process continues; finally collapsing and coming into contact, remaining practically in that condition until the

[1] A case is given by Dr. E. P. Miller ("Dyspepsia," p. 53), in which "among the principal substances vomited, . . . were mucus, acid fermentations, bile, unchanged food, pus, blood, poisons of various kinds, fecal matter, and animal parasites." A pretty collection truly!

[2] "The New Method," pp. 23-4.

end of the fast—as pure water passes directly through the stomach, and into the intestines, without calling for stomach digestion, or distending it for any appreciable period. (p. 400.)

And I must here answer an oft-recurring objection to fasting that is made on this very ground. "The idea of allowing your stomach to get into this weakened and collapsed condition," I hear my reader say, "it's a wonder that you are ever able to digest anything again! Think of the weakened condition the stomach must be in to assume this condition, with every muscle slackened and inactive; it's a wonder you ever recover!" This objection is, of course, based upon an altogether erroneous idea of the functions of the stomach, and the relative amount of work it should perform. Many people believe (*why*, Heaven only knows) that a man should, in duty bound, keep his stomach at work every hour in the day and night, and that if he should happen to leave it empty for a few minutes, it would immediately commence to "weaken," until not sufficient strength is left therein to resume, properly, its functions, when eating is again resumed. Where such a curious hallucination could have originated, it is hard to see. That it has no foundation whatever in fact can easily be demonstrated by physiological argument; yet the vast majority of persons hold this view, I am convinced—and for the usual reason, in these matters, *viz.*, they have never thought or reasoned about the matter at all, but simply followed, like a flock of sheep, wherever popular prejudices and opinions lead them. Put aside prejudice and preconceived opinions, reader, and listen to the voice of reason—which is the voice of Nature! Is not the stomach a *muscle*, in that it is composed almost entirely of muscular fibers? Most assuredly it is. And why should we not rest *this* muscle just as we do any muscle in the body? When the muscles in your arm become tired from overwork, you rest them until they are thoroughly refreshed and recuperated, and ready for more work. Why should this not apply to the stomach also?—since the stomach is, most certainly, overworked all the time, in the majority of cases. As Dr. T. L. Nichols so well remarked:[1]

" . . . that much abused organ, the human stomach, needs

[1] "The Diet Cure," p. 17.

many hours of rest every day. It turns and churns; it pours out gastric juice; it absorbs liquids of all sorts that are poured into it; it shields its delicate surface from pepper, mustard, salt, vinegar, hot things and cold things, and the narcotisms of tea, coffee, alcohol, and tobacco, as well as it can; and its fellow organs salivary glands, liver, pancreas, and the myriad glands of the *prima via* (the whole nutritive system)—do their work as well as they are able; but they all need rest—they must be nourished as well as the rest of the organism. Blood vessels and nerves must build them up. And what rest can there be for a poor stomach with five meals a day, ending in a hearty supper, just before going to bed?"

What possible harm can result from resting this muscle any more than any other muscle in the body? Would not rest simply have the effect of strengthening and rejuvenating this organ, just as every other muscle is strengthened and rejuvenated through rest? If not, why not? Can a rational answer be found to this question? No; it cannot, since such an answer does not exist! It is in the understanding of the fact that the stomach is a *muscle,* performing certain complicated actions, and that in resting this muscle we naturally strengthen and invigorate it. that the whole secret and difficulty lies. No possible harm can come to this organ, any more than to any other organ in the body from its non-use for a short time—say, for a certain period every day. That nearly every organ receives its proper amount of rest is a fact of daily observation. Rest and work, work and rest—*periodicity*—is the law of the human organism. Every part or organ of the body is governed by this law, and the stomach is no exception to this rule. From this we must conclude, *à priori,* that the stomach should not be worked uninterruptedly, but should work and rest alternately. Consequently, the stomach should receive some hours of rest—some "sleep" —during every twenty-four; and, if worked uninterruptedly, is sure to break down sooner or later, as would any other organ that is forced to work without intermission. From this it is obvious that the stomach should, for some time every twenty-four hours, be empty and resting—giving it a chance to recuperate and gather strength for the next day's digestion.

Many of my readers will, no doubt, contend that some portion of every night is thus devoted to rest and recuperation; that the hours between midnight and breakfast are thus spent, and that this is all the rest that is required. In answer to this I must reply that this length of time is *not* enough; that under the usual régime, a heavy dinner eaten at night is by no means digested by midnight, but keeps the stomach at work the entire night at least, and often far into the next morning,[1] and I believe it can be positively demonstrated that food often remains in the stomach, undigested, for a period of three days, or even longer. Doctor Beaumont stated that:

"Food taken in this condition of the stomach remains undigested for twenty-four or forty-eight hours, or more, increasing the disarrangement of the whole alimentary canal, and aggravating the general symptoms of the disease."[2]

It must be remembered that all this was without pain or discomfort, and without the patient's knowledge that indigestion of any sort was present. And in support of my thesis I may cite the case previously referred to in this chapter, and repeat that this case is by no means so very exceptional, but might be frequently observed in cases of fasting, and indeed often has been observed by hygienists, who have watched such cases. Nor was this man an excessive eater. The fact that food frequently remains in the stomach of quite light eaters when they are indisposed, and "out of condition" is certain. Take my own case, for example. Several years ago, when taking a short fast, because feeling indisposed in this manner, and though eating at the time but two fairly light meals a day, and a simple vegetarian diet, I vomited up solid food after fasting more than thirty hours, and while drinking freely of water, throughout that period! In what condition, then, must be the stomach of those diseased individuals who perpetually overfeed themselves on gross,

[1] Says Dr. W. B. Cannon ("A. B.–Z. of Our Own Nutrition," pp. 385–6): "The statement is . . . made that at night, even without sleep, the intestines are almost entirely at rest; that this is their normal time for repose. I have seen both large and small intestines actively at work, however, from half-past nine until half-past ten o'clock at night." (They were observed by X-Rays.)

[2] Bellows: "Philosophy of Eating," p. 255.

stimulating foods, three times daily? And who would dare to question the assertion that such a stomach needed rest, not of hours, but of days? Surely no one who is in possession of the facts.[1]

Having now cleared the ground, so to speak, of the objections to fasting which are based on the absurd notion that it is harmful to rest the stomach, etc., we must turn to a consideration of another objection. It has been held, by those ignorant of the facts in the case, that, since the glands of the stomach secrete gastric juice, which normally acts upon the food eaten, promoting digestion, this gastric juice—being powerful and an acid—would injure the mucous coating of the stomach, were no food introduced for this juice to act upon; that it would, in short, eat away the lining of the stomach! This objection is completely refuted, however, by the now well-ascertained fact that, so long as food is withheld, and the stomach is empty, no gastric juice is secreted. The secretion ends with the evacuation of the last morsel of food from the stomach, and does not recommence until food is again ingested. It will thus be seen that this objection is also without foundation, and is made in ignorance of the recognized laws of physiology.

Thus far we have considered but one side of the problem, however, and have confined our remarks to one aspect of the case—to proving, namely, that the stomach cannot, by any possible line of argument, be shown to sustain any injury, or be weakened in any way, as the result of the fast. The opposite side of the question now demands consideration; *viz.*, does the stomach derive any benefit from its protracted non-use? That it does derive benefit, we might almost conclude *à priori*, for the simple reason that it received no injury; for nothing in the universe is stationary—evolution or devolution, progress or retrogression, is the invariable cosmic law, from which there is no escape, to which there is no exception. From this fact alone, therefore, we

[1] Prof. Anthony Barker, on p. 59 of his "Physical Culture Simplified," says: "In every case of which I have had personal knowledge, a fast of four days or over has been a decided and lasting injury." I question this statement. I challenge Professor Barker to produce his patients; and, if produced, to prove that it was the fasting that injured them. Were the subject rightly understood, such absurd statements could not possibly be made—or such as those on p. 283 of "The Great Psychological Crime."

might argue that the stomach, since it receives no injury, must receive benefit; and we should be quite justified in so arguing. But this line of argument is not necessary. Physiology shows us that the stomach, as a muscular organ, must, by analogy, recuperate and gather strength when rested, as any other muscle does; and this applies also to the glands. That these glands must gather strength and recuperate, because of their rest should be as obvious as anything can well be. At all times the fundamental truth cannot be too much insisted upon, *viz.*, that *the gastric juice is secreted not according to the amount of food swallowed, but according to the needs of the organism*, and since this is, in sickness, practically *nil*, this fact is, in itself, enough to forbid our eating during this period, or until the recovery of health, when hunger notifies us that the glands of the stomach are operating again and "ready for business."

It is for this reason that sick persons have no appetite. They are absolutely unable to digest food, normally, even when swallowed, owing to the lack of digestive fluids. Professor Pawlow proved that the mere *thought* of food—provided the system was ready to receive it—was sufficient to cause an extensive flow of the gastric juices.

"The passionate longing for food, and this alone, has called forth, under my eyes, a most intense activity of the gastric glands."[1]

And yet mechanical excitation—swallowing food, *e.g.*, when there is no appetite, has no effect upon them! (p. 233.) Further, strong emotions, such as fear, anger, etc., will have the effect of totally stopping all digestion. (pp. 338–9.) This fact also explains why it is that "the value of any food is partly determined by its flavor. No matter how nourishing a food may be, if it possesses little or no flavor, it is comparatively useless as a common article of diet."[2] It may be added, parenthetically, that the so-called predigested foods on the market, made so by artificial "peptonization," etc.,[3] are practically useless. They can save the digestion little or no energy, since the bulk of food

[1] "A. B.–Z. of Our Own Nutrition," p. 203.
[2] "Dietetic Value of Bread," p. 136.
[3] "Hand-Book of Digestive Ferments," etc., by Fairchild.

ingested has to be churned and handled by the stomach and intestines in any case.

Taking all the above facts into consideration, then, and remembering that the digestive juices are normally secreted, in times of sickness, in but very small quantities, should we "tempt the appetite" with delicacies, and *force* the secretion of this precious fluid, at the expense of the vital forces, when every drop of this fluid, thus forced, is obviously abnormal; or should we rest these organs, this delicate mechanism, until it returns rejuvenated, spontaneously and naturally, to the normal performance of its functions? Can there be any two answers to this question?

A final objection to this theory of rest is the following. It might be urged that every muscle should receive its proper amount of work, and that disuse of the muscle means, invariably, its atrophy and final degeneration. We neglect our muscles anywhere, and this degeneration is sure to follow. This is true, and the simile might stand, were it not for the following consideration. The analogy is not correct. The stomach is not, in this case, a *normally* worked muscle, but an *over*worked one. Its rest is not the rest of disuse, but the rest of recuperation from over-exertion. As has been shown, it frequently receives no rest, owing to our modern artificial methods of living; hence all rest received is clear gain. Again, how long does it take for our muscles to degenerate, and weaken from disease? Not days, nor weeks, nor months, but years! When the proof shall be forth coming that a stomach has rested absolutely for *that* length of time, it will be time for me to consider this objection—not before!

But a further and a practical proof that the stomach is strengthened, and not weakened, by fasting, is to be found in the fact that the stomach, though weak and dyspeptic, prior to the fast, is able to perform almost any amount of work when once more fairly started on the task of digestion, at its conclusion. Doctor Tanner (very foolishly) ate "sufficient food in the first twenty-four hours after breaking the fast to gain nine pounds, and thirty-six pounds in eight days, all that I had lost."[1] He

[1] "Physical Culture," Vol. V., p. 210.

suffered no apparent evil consequences from this rash proceeding. I cite this case in order to show what the human stomach *can* perform, when properly rested, and not to endorse Doctor Tanner's foolish experiment, it must be understood. Everyone, moreover, who has ever fasted for any length of time, has invariably noticed that almost an unlimited amount of food can be easily and thoroughly digested for many days after the breaking of such a protracted fast; and, indeed, until a surfeit of food has again rendered this organ unfit to perform its proper functions, by completely exhausting the stock of accumulated vital force which lies behind all muscular action. In other words, the stomach must be *re-abused* to a certain extent before it can again be "made sick"—before it can again become troublesome or dyspeptic.

A closer insight into the physiological action of fasting would make this clear. The moment the last morsel of food is digested, and the stomach emptied, a general reconstructive process begins; a new tissue formation, owing to the fact that the broken-down cells are being replaced by healthy ones—which is Nature's method of repairing any destroyed or injured part of the organism. This replacement of cells means gradual replacement of tissue; replacement of tissue means that a *new stomach* has been created—a stomach in every sense of the word *new*—as new in every anatomical sense as is the filling in wounds, or between the fractured ends of bones.

From this chain of reasoning follows a most important conclusion. It has frequently been stated, in works on physiology, that the body changes its composition once every seven years, owing to this very process of cell change; *i.e.*, at the end of that period the entire body will have undergone a complete reconstruction as to its tissues, and a new body will be the result. Now I ask, why seven years? Is there any mystic power attributed to this number which would, *à priori*, incline us to believe that the "magic seven" must complete our cycle, biologically; or is it not rather that calculation has shown us that, under the existing modes of living, the complete change is effected in about that time? Surely the latter! But does this necessarily prove that this is the right and normal length of time which should be occupied by the vital forces, in effecting the change? Most assuredly no. *Under the existing modes of living;* we must remember that. Now, since the present modes of living are monstrously abnormal; and since our bodies are, consequently, distinctly abnormal in composition and function throughout our lives, it follows that all such changes will be abnormal also, and that the length of time occupied in all such changes is, at the present day, and under existing conditions, entirely abnormal. Medical men have here, as elsewhere, taken our present diseased and unnatural condition as the standard of health, instead of realizing that our present condition is both artificial and abnormal *ab initio.* Hence their erroneous theories of health; hence, also, their lack of appreciation of the fact that the whole human race is diseased more or less all the time—even in apparent health, as we have previously seen. (pp. 61–4.)

And it is upon such foundations: deductions drawn from a study of more or less diseased organisms; that all such calculations as the above are based. If, however, the present mode and rate of tissue building is abnormal, it is only reasonable to suppose that "statistics" such as the above are calculated from erroneous premises, and consequently wrong. The question is this: Since the present rate of tissue building or replacement occupies an abnormal length of time for its completion, what, under normal conditions of living, would be the normal time? Every fact in this book goes to demonstrate that the length of time would be very greatly *reduced,* since the less the quantity of the food eaten, and the simpler it is in quality, the greater chance have the vital forces to repair damages by tissue replacement. Looking about, then, with these facts in mind, and considering all the *data* available, which are afforded by experiment and analogy, I became convinced (though I can offer no complete vindication of my belief) that, living on foods of proper quality, and partaking of them only in the proper quantity, man's body should be reconstructed throughout once a year, and this has grown to be a settled conviction with me.

Observations of the phenomena of fasting have thrown a flood of light upon this subject, and brought out a number of most suggestive facts which were quite unascertainable by and hidden from those who had never observed cases of protracted fasts either in themselves or in others. Hence the ignorance of the medical profession on this subject. They have never observed, nor availed themselves of the opportunities for observing, these phenomena; and consequently cannot be expected to draw the vastly important chain of philosophical deductions resulting therefrom. It is my contention that, were cell change not stunted and at times almost checked by the almost entire monopoly of the vital forces for the purposes of digestion and elimination, it could be definitely ascertained that the body changes with the seasons, as does the snake's skin, and I look for the not far distant day when science shall prove this to be a fact—by the observation of *normal* men and women, instead of diseased ones —the method now in vogue.

Now my point is this. Granting that the rate of tissue change may be thus reduced, in the body, from seven years to one, by adopting a simple and abstemious diet, might it not be possible to effect this complete change within two or three months, while on an absolute fast? From what we know of the extreme rapidity of elimination and purification and tissue change during that time, I think we should be quite justified in contending that practically the entire body (or at least every part of it which was in any way morbid or diseased) would have been replaced by healthy tissue in that length of time, under this strict régime. A new stomach may thus have been created, in the time mentioned; or any other organ, or any set of tissues whatever may thus have been easily and surely replaced.

There is one other point to be noticed in connection with the influence of fasting upon the stomach and its functions. After the fast has been broken, there immediately appears a ravenous appetite, which must be kept under control at all costs for the few days during which it lasts. If withstood for that period, however, care being taken to masticate all food eaten very thoroughly, this extreme and voracious appetite will disappear, in the course of a few days, and will not return. (pp. 558–9.)

This dangerous period once past, it will be noticed, invariably, that there is no desire for the great *bulk* of food which previously existed, and the stomach seems to rest content with only a fraction of the amount formerly eaten, in order to compose the meal. There is no desire to surfeit, to "stuff." In short, the appetite has become normal, for, as Doctor Oswald so well said:[1] "Only natural appetites have natural limits." Moreover, the appetite is more under control, and no craving is experienced for the hot, or spiced, or stimulating viands before indulged in. Of course this desire can be developed again; but it must be cultivated. Our normal taste must again be perverted in order for these desires to again arise; and every sane man, perceiving this, and noting the beneficial results to himself from discontinuing their use, and having a "start," so to speak, which he is unlikely to have again (for some time, at least) would surely seize the opportunity here presented, and discontinue their use entirely; together with the previous "stuffing"—which rendered his fast necessary. Henceforward, it would only be necessary for him to observe abstemiousness and obey the general laws of health in order to insure continued good health for the rest of his days—an absolute immunity from all disease, together with robust and vigorous health.

The reason for this (*i.e.*, that the stomach does not desire either the quality or the quantity of food craved before the fast was undertaken) seems to be, partly that the whole system is, by reason of the fast, toned up and rendered more normal; partly in the fact that the patient has learned to control his appetite; but most of all because of the fact that, of late, the stomach has not been so constantly overstretched and distended that it is not "comfortable" until it is in this abnormal condition. At the close of the fast, this organ, having shrunk to its natural proportions, refuses to be again distended and engorged to the previous unnatural and disgusting extent without protest; hence the inability to eat the amount of food formerly ingested. Says Dr. C. E. Page:[2]

"Accustomed to distention from the bulky character of the old diet, if only a physiological ration of the pure and more nutritous food be swallowed, the stomach misses the stimulus of distention: time will be required (in some cases) for the stomach to

[1] "Physical Education," p. 58.
[2] "The Natural Cure," p. 213

remodel itself as regards size—unless a large proportion of fruit is used in conjunction with the cereals."

And Dr. Russell H. Chittenden wrote that:[1]

"In the latter part of September, 1903, Doctor Underhill attempted to return to his original methods of living, but found difficulty in consuming the daily quantities of food he had formerly been in the habit of taking."

[1] "Physiological Economy in Nutrition," p. 78.

CHAPTER VI

PHYSIOLOGICAL EFFECTS—II

The Lungs.—Fasting seems to affect the lungs at once more speedily and more effectually than almost any other diseased organ—the exception, being, perhaps, the stomach. It must be remembered that the lungs are themselves the great purifiers of the blood; besides which, they are one of the most important eliminating organs we possess. Now since, as we have already seen (pp. 154–5), all the eliminating organs can and do perform a vastly greater amount of work, during a fast, than under normal conditions—owing to their being unimpeded by the constant deposit in them of unnecessary material, and the greater vitality at their disposal—it follows that the breath will be far more heavily loaded with organic impurities than it generally is—which, as we have seen, is the case. Elimination, by means of the lungs, is carried on with almost incredible rapidity; lung tissue seeming to possess the inherent power of healing itself in a far shorter time, and more effectually, than any other organ which may be diseased. I have repeatedly observed that, in all cases where a fast has been undertaken, in order to cure lung troubles of any description, such fasts have always terminated more speedily and satisfactority than in other cases; and such fasts are also undertaken far more easily, and the deprivation and lack of food noticed even less, in such cases, than in any other cases whatever.

All this enables us to perceive the extent to which we must have abused our lungs, in order for them to have reached their present diseased condition.

Consumptive cases, it is true, are apt, apparently, to collapse, more or less frequently, when a fast is entered upon; an extreme degree of debility being noticed. This, I think, may be due to a number of causes. (1) They have, in all probability, been "kept up" for some time past on stimulants, tonics, drugs, etc.; and the reaction from such stimulation must, of necessity, be severe. (2) Their food (milk, eggs, etc.) is also highly stimulating, and reaction would follow the withdrawal of that also. (3) The *real* condition of the patient *is* extreme weakness and debility—which condition the fasting but renders manifest, or brings to the surface. (pp. 520–3.) Owing to the disease, and to its treatment, extreme debility has resulted, and the fact that this debility is not apparent, is due entirely to the fact that the patient has been "kept up" on stimulants, food, etc.—the process of weakening and exhausting the vital powers continuing unchecked and unabated. Now, when this stimulation is withdrawn, "collapse" would invariably follow; but this is due to the fact that the fasting has merely brought to the surface or rendered apparent such a condition; and not that the fasting has itself caused or induced such a state. It was already there; and the fasting has but exposed it to our eyes—opening them to the true condition of the patient.

What has just been said, taken in conjunction with the theory of fasting, previously outlined, will enable us to perceive the true *rationale* of the cure. We can almost see and feel the lung tissue of the diseased patient (so easily can we understand what happens) eliminating the effete and foul material, with which it is more or less saturated. We can readily perceive how the process of purification continues; the gradual cleansing and purifying of the tissues—they being unhampered by the deposits of constant, fresh supplies of food, calling for and necessitating aëration. Once withdraw this additional supply, this overplus of food material, which necessitates constant labor on the part of the lungs, to properly aërate it; conserve the energy, by relieving the system of "its great, its principal strain—the digestion, assimilation, and elimination of food matter, in excess of bodily needs," and we have the rational basis for the cure of all pulmonary troubles laid bare before our eyes.

No accumulation of impurities could, under this treatment, long remain embedded in the lung tissue; no inflammation that could not be speedily reduced; no "tubercle bacillus," but that would be speedily starved out, for sheer lack of sufficient nutriment to render the perpetuation of its life possible.

The great sense of freedom which is experienced in the lungs, and the ability to talk and sing with greater clearness and facility, and with greater range and depth of tone than has been experienced, perhaps, in months and years, will amply testify that the lungs are far sounder and more normal than they have been perhaps ever!

Liver and Kidneys.—What has been said above, regarding the lungs, applies, in a sense, to these two great purifying organs. *Overeating* is the cause of their clogged and diseased condition—the excessive work imposed upon them in order to filter and eliminate the great amount of material forced into the circulation—thus causing this premature breakdown.[1] The *rationale* of the cure is the same and as obvious for all. A constant elimination of impurities, organic and inorganic, unimpeded by the addition of other material needing "filtering" (purification), together with the added stock of vital force from which these organs can now draw—all these causes working together must bring about a speedy restoration of health, and a freedom of those organs from their diseased condition. Examples of cures of these organs will be found on pp. 195-7 and on p. 222.

The Bowels.—We now come to consider the effects of fasting upon the remaining great eliminating organ—the bowels. But little need be said, in this relation, beyond referring the reader to what has been said in the chapter on "The Enema"; merely noting here some few important points that belong, more particularly, to this branch of the question—the influence of *fasting* upon the bowels.

We have seen (pp. 420-1), that, after the digestion of the last meal, prior to the fast, the bowels practically cease to function, and continue in that condition for days—often until the completion of a protracted fast.[2] As Doctor Oswald observed:

[1] "Liver and Kidneys," by Susanna Dodds, M.D., p. 16.
[2] Kirke: "Physiology," p. 508. This does not agree altogether with Doctor Schrott's experience, however; see "Family Physician," by Joel Shew, M.D., p. 792.

"The colon contracts, and the smaller intestines retain all but the most irritating ingesta."[1]

This remaining material must be removed by enemas.

The principal effect of fasting upon the bowels is, therefore, to force them to become more or less emptied, and remain so throughout the fast. The intestinal walls become cleansed; while the other great requisite for a successful cure is also supplied, *viz.*, rest. Once the bowels become empty—rid of their poisonous contents—the work of purification and revitalizing progresses rapidly, while the soothing effect of the water injected (in tepid enemas) will greatly assist in allaying any inflammation that may be present. No case of inflammation of the bowels; no case of ulceration; no case of the dreaded (and grossly maltreated) appendicitis[2] could fail to be cured by profuse water drinking, copious tepid enemas, proper massage and a protracted fast. (In cases where the wall is not actually ruptured.) There is no case of piles that could fail to be benefited or entirely cured by this treatment.[3] Doctor Shew wrote, on this subject:

"There is nothing in the world that will produce so great relief in piles as fasting. If the fit is severe, live a whole day (or even two, if necessary) upon pure, soft, cold water alone. Give, then, very lightly of vegetable food. Those who have suffered the agony of this affection, if they will but have patience to try this means, will find the truth of my remarks."[4]

I may add that I have observed some most striking examples of such cures myself.

Again, I do not know of any cure that is so potent in all cases of chronic constipation or enervating diarrhœa as this of fasting;

[1] "Fasting, Hydropathy and Exercise," p. 53.

[2] "Sir Frederick Treves contends that this distended state of the cœcum encourages catarrh of the appendix by dragging upon it and blocking its orifice, as well as by twisting it and thus interfering with its blood supply." ("A. B.-Z. of Our Own Nutrition," p. 141.) Gilbert Barling also traces the relationship between appendicitis and diet. "In a considerable number of cases," he writes, "the attack of appendicitis can be directly attributed to unsuitable food—pork, mackerel, over-ripe and under-ripe fruit, uncooked vegetables." (*Brit. Med. Jour.*, Vol. I., 1903, p. 61.) Doctor Rabagliati has contended very strongly against the present system of operations for cases of appendicitis; see his "Air, Food and Exercises," pp. 519–20.

[3] See "Piles and Their Treatment," by James C. Jackson, M.D.

[4] "Water Cure in Pregnancy and Childbirth," pp. 79–80.

and I know of no case that has failed to be entirely cured—to disappear utterly—when once their cause has been removed—the morbid condition of the colon, and whole alimentary canal.

I wish to say a few words, in this connection, suggested by the recent utterances of Professor Metchnikoff—representing, to my mind, the result of the extreme anti-vital doctrines at present in vogue, and leading to pure nonsense, when carried to their logical conclusion. Thus, realizing that the condition of the large intestine is a source of infection, auto-intoxication, and disease in many cases, he goes on:

"The fact that a human being was capable of carrying on an apparently normal life for thirty years in the absence of a large intestine is good proof that the organ in question is not necessary to man, though it has not yet become rudimentary."[1]

He consequently advocates cutting this organ out entirely! (pp. 74–5.) Could anything be more preposterous than this? One might as well contend that because some men have been enabled to live with a portion of their cerebrum missing, that, consequently, the brain is an unnecessary organ—and it assuredly would be, in such reasoning as the above! One would think that, instead of cutting out the organ in question, because it was in a more or less diseased condition, the more rational course would be to leave the offending intestine *in statu quo*—only to cleanse it, and render it sweet and clean by proper food habits. This is the position taken by Mr. Horace Fletcher, and by Doctor Higgins; see his "Humaniculture," pp. 85, 176, 239.

The ills arising from proctitis, and the auto-infection resulting from a foul and diseased colon are too numerous to be mentioned here; it can be stated, merely, that judicious fasting, continued until the return of natural hunger, cannot fail to completely cure every case of any such disease, where recovery is possible.

One objection must be answered before passing on. It has been urged that this complete emptying of the bowels is by no means a desirable condition—if not a highly dangerous one—

[1] "The Nature of Man," p. 71.

the bowels being normally somewhat distended, and their complete collapse might injure them and render them unfit for work, when again called upon to digest and eliminate food material.

What has been said in the chapter on "The Stomach" will also apply here. Most people have an idea that their bowels are constructed like telescopes, and that they will collapse as soon as the gases and fæces contained within them are withdrawn. How absurd such a contention is should be clearly perceived by anyone having even a rudimentary knowledge of physiology. From the practical standpoint, of course, all cases of fasting—as well as such cases as that of Mr. Horace Fletcher—absolutely disprove any such fantastic and erroneous notions. Doctors Woods and Merrill found that the fæces were of practically the same chemical composition throughout a two days' fast. See *Report of Investigations on The Digestibility and Nutritive Value of Bread*, pp. 39–40.

The Heart.—I need say little here beyond what has already been said in the chapter on "The Pulse." The greatly increased or lessened pulsation there noted was due, of course, to the increased or lessened action of the heart—Nature raising or lowering the rate of pulsation as best suits her needs for the occasion; and the reason, though we cannot always perceive and understand it, is, we may be sure, a good one. That the heart is invariably strengthened and invigorated by fasting is true beyond a doubt; and, in the nature of things, it must be so; first, because of the purer blood which the heart is called upon to pump through its chambers; the heart itself being nourished by this very blood; and secondly, because the amount of useless and fatty tissue, etc., which the heart is called upon to supply with blood has been greatly lessened and reduced—calling for a less powerful stream of blood to reach all the parts of the body, than formerly. Thirdly, because constant stimulation of the heart is now lacking. (*v.* p. 461.) For these reasons, then, and for others which I need not here enumerate, I take the stand that fasting is the greatest of all strengtheners of weak hearts—being, in fact, its only, rational, physiological cure.

The Muscles.—We need say nothing further regarding the effects of fasting upon the muscles than has been already said in the chapter on "Exercise," pp. 378-87.

Sexual Organs.—In all cases in which I have had the opportunity of personally questioning the patient undergoing a fast of any considerable duration, the answer has always been the same; *viz.*, that all sexual intercourse, during a fast, becomes a practical impossibility, after the first few days. While in progress, it renders the patient practically impotent, and seems to sap the vital center of life to its very roots. A temporary suspension of this function seems to exist; a complete lack of sexual energy being manifest,[1] and continuing until the fast is ready to be broken—when this function returns, in its full vigor and force, together with hunger, etc. For this reason, fasting patients must be allowed the greatest latitude; they should be "pampered," and allowed whatever they desire or crave. As Mr. Purinton so well remarked:[2]

" . . . A fourth common error lies in neglecting to provide against *the strain on the soul.* It is no light thing to controvert in the space of a few weeks all the habits of a lifetime and the thought-heritage of a race; you may have seen newspaper reports of people 'made insane through fasting'—through *faulty* fasting. There must first be an inner incentive, second an outer wisdom. Forced starving is more fatal than forced stuffing—since both soul and body protest. You must want to fast more than you want to eat, before you can fast with absolute safety."

I may add that in all diseased states that condition prevails. But to return. This lack of sexual energy seems to be almost invariably present during a fast of any duration; and is altogether independent of the general feeling of vigor, which may be practically unabated. This distinction must be kept carefully

[1] Doctor Hunter remarked that "in the case of strong sexual passions meat must be eaten in small quantities, and the starving process for a time will prove highly beneficial." ("Manhood Wrecked and Restored," p. 219.) "And," says Tolstoy ("The Morals of Diet," p. 31), "a man who overeats himself is not able to struggle with laziness—and a man who overeats himself and is idle will never be able to struggle with sexual lust. Therefore, according to all moral teachings, the aspiration after abstinence commences with the struggle with the lust of gluttony—and it begins by fasting."

[2] "Philosophy of Fasting," p. 101.

in mind. The energy apparently lost, during the fast, is sexual vigor *only*, and may or may not correspond to the *general* feeling of nervous laxity—this depending, apparently, upon other considerations.

My readers will, of course, urge that this complete loss of sexual energy—this feeling of lowered vitality—argues that such vitality has actually been lost, and refutes my position that no energy is, in reality, ever lost during these trying periods. At first sight, I admit, the evidence seems conclusive; there is no energy where formerly there was—more or less, according to circumstances. This much is admitted. But, if we examine the facts a little more closely, I think we shall find that no energy is, in reality lost, in this instance, any more than in any other case of apparently lessened or weakened functioning.

In the first place, I would draw attention to the fact that every form of artificial stimulation—both liquid and solid—has now been withdrawn; while the mental influences and environ ment without doubt greatly assist in keeping the patient's attention centered upon his body, from a purely scientific or medical point of view; and away from all other morbid cravings and outside suggestions and distractions, which would ordinarily have great influence over him. He is occupied in getting well. All these causes doubtless unite into an appreciable and weighty factor.

In the next place it must be remembered that the fasting patient is a *sick* patient; often highly diseased, and lacking in vitality at all times—such energy as is usually manifested being largely a matter of stimulation. When this is withdrawn, the patient naturally collapses, until sufficient vitality is again accumulated to become manifest.

Third, what energy there is present is diverted solely into the channel of cleansing and purifying the system; it is *withdrawn* from the sexual organs to be utilized elsewhere; and, such is Nature's economy, every useless expenditure or even maintenance of vitality (and there can be no maintenance without expenditure), is discontinued for organic, vital reasons; and this energy is used in ridding the system of the foul material which is the cause of the diseased condition—and of the fast. There is, therefore, no actual loss of energy, but *redistribution, and its utilization elsewhere.* And, as an example, I may quote the following fact, which tends strongly to support my theory as correct. It is that in certain cases (*e.g.*, that of Mr. Patterson, mentioned on pp. 213–15), the finger nails practically ceased growing, while, at the same time, the organism was evidencing great vital power—in that the patient was rapidly regaining his health. Thus, while there can be no questioning the fact that the vital powers were unabated, and even augmented, certain indications would seem to point to a contrary conclusion.

Fourth, that this theory is correct is demonstrated by actual practice. If the energy were actually expended or totally lost and gone from the body, it could only return with the resumption of eating; *i.e.*, *after* the first meal has begun to be assimilated. The fact is, however, that this sexual vigor returns (together with hunger) at the conclusion of the fast, and *before* the ingestion of the first meal. On the theory of complete expenditure or loss, this would be quite inexplicable; while, on the theory defended in this book, it affords a complete practical proof of the theory, and demonstrates, beyond all reasonable doubt, that withdrawal—not loss—has been the actual process involved.

Lastly, that my theory of the case is correct is conclusively proved by the fact that many persons—practically impotent at the beginning of the fast—regain their full sexual vigor as it progresses—it being completely restored at its close. The vigor and healthfulness of these parts have thus been regained, together with that of every part of the organism. If it were true, however, that we received our strength and energy only from food, how impossible such a result! And how completely this fact disproves that absurd notion, and indirectly proves the theory of vitality elaborated on pp. 225–303.

The Uterus and Female Generative Organs.—This subject has been well and fully discussed by other authors who have treated the question from the hygienic standpoint, and to these authors I refer the reader. See Dewey: "New Era for Women," pp. 170–353; Trall: "Uterine Diseases and Displacements;" Macfadden: "Power and Beauty of Superb Womanhood," etc.

The Secretions.—In discussing the effects of fasting upon the stomach (pp. 482–94), we saw that the secretion of the gastric juice was entirely suspended during all cases of fasting; and, in any cases where food is withheld, the secretion is withheld also—so long as food is not ingested. To a certain extent, this may be said to be true of all the other secretions also. The amount of these secretions is at most times very large. Says Dr. A. B. Jamison:

"The amount of gastric juice secreted in twenty-four hours is from six to fourteen pints; of pancreatic juice, one pint; of bile, there are two or three pints, and of saliva, one to three pints. It is estimated that the juices secreted during digestion in a man weighing 140 pounds, amount to twenty-three pounds in twenty-four hours. These fluids are poured back and forth in the process of transforming food into flesh and eliminating waste material."[1]

The intestinal juices certainly cease to be secreted to any great extent—save in some cases of deranged liver, where bile seems to be secreted in unusually large amounts, occasionally finding its way backwards to the stomach, where it is vomited—to the ultimate great relief of the patient. The bile in such cases is invariably evil-smelling and poisonous; the secretion being tainted, and indicative of the foul conditions present.

The saliva also ceases to be secreted in such large amounts as is usually the case; and, in this instance, we have the analogy of sleep to guide us, where, as we know, the secretion practically ceases altogether—another illustration of Nature's economy in vital matters; while in Kirke's "Physiology," we are informed that, during a fast, alkaline saliva gradually becomes neutral. (p. 301.) Sometimes, however, the saliva flows quite as freely as usual, and in some cases this secretion is tainted and extremely unpleasant in taste. In the case of Mr. Davis, *e.g.* (pp. 183–6), so unpleasant was it, indeed, as to almost excite vomiting on numerous occasions. This unpleasant symptom will gradually lessen, however, and disappear altogether before the fast is ready to be broken. The only measures we can adopt, in such cases, are those indicated in the chapter on "The Tongue and the Breath."

[1] "Intestinal Ills," pp. 5–6.

Doctor Schrott, on his study of fasting cases, noted that:

"Those patients whose digestive organs have suffered a long time, throw off an incredible amount of expectoration while undergoing the strong cure. This matter is first thick, tough, gelatinous, transparent, white, and slimy in character. Later it becomes gray, yellowish, or greenish, pus-like and offensive in quality. At times an increase of expectoration comes on, followed or attended by a febrile excitement of the system. At this time large lumps, as it were, of tough, slimy substances are thrown off, which almost choke the patient at the time. By degrees this expectoration grows less, and at length ceases during the cure."[1]

In such cases we clearly perceive how Nature adopts every possible avenue of elimination, to serve her purposes—the ridding of the system of the impurities it contains, the real cause of the disease.

The Senses.—In man, the senses are comparatively speaking dulled—this condition being due, no doubt, to his abnormal habits of living. In all other animals, and even in birds,[2] the senses are most acute, and are immensely superior to man's. But, in times of fasting, the senses are acutened, and that remarkably, in every case without exception that I have ever observed, or of which I have read. So distinctive a sign is this, indeed, that it has been looked upon, by those conversant with hygienic literature, as a more or less certain indication that the patient is fasting; the acuteness of perception being most marked in practically every case observed.

Now, this acuteness generally depends, I believe, almost entirely upon the degree of vitality present, both in the sense organ itself, in the sense centers of the brain, and in the organism as a whole. Nothing is more clearly established than the fact that poor health and depleted vitality go hand in hand,[3] and

[1] Shew: "Family Physician," p. 790.

[2] See X. Raspail: "The Sense of Smell in Birds."

[3] That lack of vitality is harmful, even dangerous, has always been known to the medical profession; but it has been deplored chiefly upon the grounds that it renders us unable to successfully "combat disease," or, more recently, that we could not "withstand the attacks of disease germs." But, since we now know that such beliefs are ill-founded, for the reason that the disease is the process of combating itself; and that germs are but friends, no apprehen-

correspondingly weaken and deaden the sense perceptions. This being the case, it follows as a matter of course that the acutening of the senses indicates an increased amount of vitality—thus indirectly proving, in the strongest manner possible, my contention that the ingestion and oxidation of food does not in any sense increase our vitality, but on the contrary, detracts from it.

Among the particularly noticeable symptoms are the following: The eyes become clear and bright (an invariable sign); the sense of touch and that of smell are also very greatly sharpened—this latter frequently resulting from a thorough physiological cleansing of the nasal passages from catarrhal matter, etc., which had not been effected, perhaps, for many years! That the sense of taste has been greatly acutened is evident to the patient directly the fast is broken (though there is, of course, no direct way of ascertaining this *during* the fast) by the fact that his taste will have become far more sensitive and discriminating than before, and to very marked degree. In all cases these four senses are rendered far more acute by fasting; and, as before stated, I never have known of a case, directly or indirectly, where they have failed to be benefited in this very noticeable manner.

But the greatest and most wonderful results of all are, perhaps, noticeable in cases of acutened *hearing*. The restoration and extension of this sense, during a fast, is little short of miraculous —sometimes restoring the sense to a better condition than it had been in for many years past, and enabling the patient to hear words, sounds, etc., which had previously been extremely faint or quite inaudible, and that for many years! Mr. Davis, *e.g.*, almost entirely restored his hearing (bringing it from an extremely defective condition to one of great acuteness, and

sion need be felt on these scores. But it is dangerous, and a cause of ill-health none the less, for the following reason. Lack of vitality—of the life force—enables but a small amount, an insufficient quantity, to reach the various bodily organs; above all, the organs of digestion and elimination, upon which always falls the bulk of the internal work. An insufficient amount of vital energy, therefore, being supplied to these organs, will cause them to function imperfectly; and the process of retention of effete material within the system (and consequent disease) will begin. Weakened and imperfect functioning of the organs is the greatest cause of disease that we know; and, invariably, this is due to the fact that the degree of vitality and the degree of functional activity of these organs is not equal to the amount of food material they are called upon to eliminate. The moment the balance is thus upset, the process of accumulation of disease begins. See, in this connection, "Dangers of Food" by A. Broadbent, p. 12.

extreme susceptibility), this being a case that had long been given up by the "specialists" as hopeless and beyond repair! The case of Robert B. (*v.* pp. 197–8), is another case in which hearing was restored in a most extraordinary and wonderful manner, as the details of the case plainly show.

The explanation of such cures is undoubtedly that involved in every case of a similar nature—the oxidation and elimination of the encumbering material present at the affected part, which was the cause of the trouble. Hence, its final elimination from the system necessitated final relief of the affected part. The trouble that is frequently caused by closure of the Eustachian tube—due to inflammation[1]—can, of course, be rectified by fasting, as can any other inflammation—thus rendering unnecessary the numerous operations that are now performed upon the ear.

The Blood.—Since the blood is the medium through which all changes within the organism are effected; the great channel through and by which is conveyed the effete and worn out material to the eliminating organs; the conveyor of nutrient elements from the digestive system to the tissues throughout the body; cleanser, purifier, we might almost say the life principal itself; it is only natural to suppose that the effects of fasting would be noticed at once and in a marked degree in this all-pervading medium. Such must be, and in fact *is*, the case.

Of the detailed chemical and microscopical changes that take place within the blood during a protracted fast I cannot speak, not, as yet, having had the opportunity to make such observations. Here, I suggest, is a wide field for investigation and research, and the importance of which cannot be too strongly insisted upon. Let us suppose, *e.g.*, that a small quantity of blood be drawn from a patient at the commencement of the fast, carefully analyzed and subjected to microscopic examination. The results are carefully noted. At the conclusion of the fast—at the return of hunger—the same quantity of blood is again drawn from the patient and subjected to the same detailed analysis. Now let the results be compared. The comparison would be most instructive. The complete change in the com-

[1] Black: "Hearing and How to Keep It," pp. 49–50.

position of the blood would at once and forever demonstrate the difference between this fluid in the diseased condition and in the normal state. Further, by collecting and analyzing a number of samples of such "normal" blood and comparing the results attained, a "standard" type of normal, healthful blood might be, theoretically, established—any deviation from which would show, beyond doubt, that the patient was in a more or less morbid and diseased condition. Still further, by a careful comparison of the results attained, in analyzing a number of cases of *one* disease, and by comparing such results with the normal, or "standard" blood, we should assuredly find, eventually, a uniformity of result, a constant deviation *in one direction* from the normal blood composition. This deviation being noted, and its microscopical and chemical composition being compared with that of numerous other cases of other diseases, we should thus, by comparison, obtain a detailed knowledge of the condition of the blood, in various diseased conditions; and, by comparing these results and noticing such differences and variations, we could thus, for the first time, have a new and infallible method of diagnosis—"diagnosis by the blood"—since we could invariably tell what disease existed, by merely analyzing the blood and noting its chemical composition and microscopical peculiarities in each case.

It may be asserted that this suggestion is by no means new, but that such analyses have often been made before, in diseased conditions, and diet and medicine, prescribed according to the results of the analysis. To this I reply that such analyses in the past have rarely had any practical significance (even in the *comparatively* few cases in which they have been attempted), for the reason that the medical fraternity has never had any "standard" of blood with which to compare the samples before them; all so-called "normal" blood being undoubtedly more or less diseased already, and by no means normal, since such "normal" blood only exists in the body of the patient who has just completed a fast, or who is living so extremely abstemiously and hygienically, and so in accordance with all the laws of Nature, that his blood is constantly normal and pure; and this does not happen probably as often as once in a hundred thousand cases.

The usual standards taken are those of "perfectly healthy men" (supposedly)—those who are enjoying apparent good health and have sufficient vitality to render them capable of undergoing a certain amount of fatigue, etc. Such men are usually more or less athletes. I have repeatedly pointed out that athletes are frequently far from healthy, in many respects, while their blood is undoubtedly more or less morbid in its chemical composition, since—eating meat, etc., as a majority of them do—it could not possibly fail to be otherwise.

Let me give a more definite example of my meaning. Suppose the blood is drawn from an athlete in apparently perfect health; this being taken as the "standard" or as near normal as it is possible to obtain. In the course of a few days this man develops a cold. The majority of persons will pay no attention to this fact! According to them the man *was* healthy at the time of having the blood drawn—the cold being "caught" in the interval. Such absurd and erroneous views as these will continue to block all real progress in medicine so long as they are held. They are based upon the present false theories held as to the nature of disease, and it is not realized that the system must be in a highly diseased or foul condition for days or even *weeks* before a cold becomes possible. The system must be clogged with effete material in order to render its expulsion necessary; hence, the blood of our "perfectly healthy man" is frequently by no means normal or healthy, but exceedingly gross and morbid throughout. Our "standard," therefore, is no standard at all; but, on the contrary, a sure indication of a diseased condition. The only objection that can be made to the above argument is that athletes in training do *not* develop colds in this way. This I unhesitatingly deny, and merely appeal, for confirmation, to any trainer, or to anyone at all who has had much to do with athletes in general.

Leaving the above detailed, and still problematical field, therefore, let us now consider, for a few moments, the effects of such changes, during a fast, as they become manifest to the observer. Since, at such a time, no effete material is taken *into* the system, and since that which is already in it is being speedily eliminated; while all this time the chemical composition of the blood is undoubtedly undergoing great modifications (being purified by the water drunk, the air breathed, etc.), the thickened fluid is, in this manner, gradually but steadily relieved of its overload of superfluous impurity, and becomes less gross and less thick in composition; in other words, *more fluid.*

Doctor Dewey, for some strange reason, takes the reverse view of the matter, contending that the blood becomes thinned during the progress of the accumulation of disease, and thickened as the fast progresses—this being due to improved nutrition.[1]

For many reasons I cannot agree with this view, and do not think that it is what we should expect, *à priori.* The point is too fine to be decided by anything but an appeal to actual analysis, as previously suggested, and this has not, as yet, ever been attempted. For the reason contained in the next paragraph, however, I do not think that this theory of the case is tenable; but on this point I leave my readers to form their own opinions.

The greater fluidity—which we must suppose the blood to have gained—enables it to penetrate the finer and more remote capillaries, the peripheral blood vessels, from which it had recently been partially excluded, owing to the blockage of these minute vessels by effete, encumbering material. A gradual absorption, removal and elimination of this matter would enable the blood to circulate with far greater freedom and more rapidity throughout these outlying structures, and finer tissues—the result being that a perfectly balanced and equalized circulation is present—reducing the labor of the heart to a minimum, and rendering the entire surface of the body smooth, and the skin a delicate pink color. A far greater percentage of blood is thus upon the surface than is generally the case—this being readily perceived by (1) the exquisite texture and color of the skin, and (2) the fact that the blood instantaneously and thoroughly responds to any pinch, scratch, etc., experimentally inflicted. This, the true "pink of condition," when observed (invariably toward the very end of the fast), indicates a perfectly healthy body, in very truth, a *mens sana in corpore sano.*

[1] "True Science of Living," pp. 190–91, 230, 230–2, 296; "New Era," pp. 172–3.

Further illustrating this position is the following passage, which I quote from Dr. Susanna Dodds' "Liver and Kidneys," pp. 28–9.

"An excess of hydrocarbons in the dietary thickens up the blood to such an extent often that it can scarcely circulate in the smaller vessels. The capillaries are half empty and the surface is cold. Patients of this class sometimes remark that their blood is too thin. They fancy that because the surface circulation is feeble, and the extremities cold, the blood needs 'enriching.' The doctor, too, has a similar idea, and he prescribes what he calls rich foods; usually there is an excess of oil in them. Just the reverse is what is needed. When the blood is so thick and tarry that it cannot make its way through the fine network of capillaries, the patient should use more fruits and fruit juices, especially of the acid varieties, and less solid materials in the dietary. We must never forget that three-fourths of the body is composed of fluids, or should be, at least."

Doctor Rabagliati has insisted upon a similar explanation of the observed facts,[1] and pointed out that fasting has the effect, generally, of increasing the number of the blood corpuscles. This fact is most significant, and causes us to modify our views on many points; see, *e.g.*, the facts discussed in C. S. Minot's "Morphology of the Blood Corpuscles."

The Brain and Nervous System.—While the substance of the nerve fibers and nerve cells is at once the most delicate, the most intricate, and the most sensitive of all that wondrous machine—the human body; it is yet a well-known fact that the nerve tissue is the last to be affected by, or show traces of, disease, in any of its acute or chronic forms. The vitality may be almost completely exhausted; the muscles too poisoned to move; even the very bones be rotting away or crumbling into chalk—yet the nervous system, especially the cerebrum, remains, oh! wonder of wonders! absolutely unimpaired—as an unaffected, and still remarkably brilliant mentality may show. The nervous system seems thus to be enabled to withstand the inroads of disease far better than the infinitely less delicate muscular tissue, or even the flint-like bone of the skeleton; and for this there must

[1] "Air, Food and Exercises," p. 290.

be a reason. The explanations that are commonly advanced for this phenomenon are altogether unsatisfactory.

Let us see, therefore, if an explanation of this fact cannot be found that is in accordance with the views and theories elaborated in this volume.

The table given on pp. 160–1 (taken from Yeo's "Physiology") and the reasons there advanced, prove beyond reasonable doubt, that the nervous system, in cases of starvation, loses no weight itself, but is capable of nourishing itself upon the bodily tissue until this latter is completely absorbed—maintaining, thereby, its own integrity. It is a *self-feeding machine;* (itself surviving and functioning perfectly); utilizing to that end the tissues of the body for self-nourishment and maintenance; and here, I suggest, is, at least in a great measure, a key to this seeming mystery.

That fasting should directly benefit nervous affections and effect a radical cure in the vast majority of cases may seem to some the height of absurdity—especially as practically all previous writers along these lines (even hygienists), have practically and uniformly recommended a "full" diet in all cases of nervousness (see, *e.g.*, "Hygiene of the Brain," by M. L. Holbrook, M.D., pp. 74–88). It is impossible for them to see how "purely nervous" affections can be in any way benefited by such purely *physical* treatment as that involved in the fasting cure. "Even granting," they say, "that the vast majority of functional disturbances may be readily cured by the method you advocate, still this is a *purely nervous* disease, and consequently cannot be treated on these lines!" In this objection we again notice the almost universal error which is unfortunately being propagated as truth by the medical profession—the error, namely, of thinking that any *one* portion of the system can be diseased without involving the entire organism. It is a failure to grasp the fact that the human body is one vast complex; a machine whose parts are so intimately connected in their workings and functionings that it is an utter impossibility for any one part to be affected without, in turn, involving the whole organism—either through the blood, or the nervous system, or (almost invariably) through both. The intricate inter-relation of all its parts must be fully grasped and accepted, as a working hypothesis, before any real progress can be made in the science of medicine.

In the next place I would point out, and insist upon the recognition of the following fact. The nervous system is not by any means so removed from the purely "physical" sphere as people imagine. Most persons seem to think that "the nerves" are in some mysterious manner inseparably connected with *thought*, and for that reason are (when it comes to their treatment), to be considered as, in some way, ethereal, mental, or spiritual in their character, and must be treated by some correspondingly delicate or non-physical method, rather than from a purely organic point of view. They do not seem to realize the fact that the nervous system, as such, is as purely physical as our muscles, bones, hair, or any other portion of our entire anatomy. The nerve fiber is as subject to cuts, bruises, lacerations, etc., as are our muscles. The blood supplies the nerve tissue and the nerve cells with the necessary nutriment, and without this nutriment, starvation and atrophy would invariably result.[1] The nervous system is, I must insist, as purely physical, and as subject to physiological treatment, as any other section of the organism, and, since the nerves are supplied and nourished, and their very life sustained by the blood—depending absolutely upon the blood supply for their existence—it is only natural to suppose—impossible not to believe—that their power, strength, vigor and functional ability, depend wholly upon the purity, composition and the quantity of the blood supplied to them.[2] Of course this is recognized by all regular practitioners—the old idea that eating fish is good for the brain (and mind) having originated in this idea. It was supposed that, by increasing the supply of phosphorus to the brain, improved mentality would result. This is, of course, the

[1] ". . . . The nervous tissue behaves in all respects like other tissues in its susceptibility to influences from within or from without, and to causes organic or inorganic. If other tissues become inflamed so may it; if they can be injured, so can the nervous system; if changing organic matter can poison the blood, it can also poison the nervous tissue . . . ." ("Some Remarks on the Classification and Nomenclature of Diseases," by A. Rabagliati, M.D., p. 58.)

[2] See, *e.g.*, Bain: "Mind and Body"; Ribot: "Diseases of Memory"; "Diseases of Personality," etc.

crudest materialism and the idea has long since been given up by advanced students. Says Dr. C. F. Langworthy:[1]

"There is a widespread notion that fish contains large proportions of phosphorus, and on that account is particularly valuable as brain food. The percentages of phosphorus in specimens thus far analyzed are not larger than are found in the flesh of other animals used for food. But, even if the flesh be richer in phosphorus, there is no experimental evidence to warrant the assumption that fish is more valuable than meats or other food-material for the nourishment of the brain."

Prof. William James considered this theory of the relation of brain activity and phosphorus, and found it to be pure superstition.[2] His position has been confirmed by recent researches. To my mind Mr. Purinton sums up the whole question very cleverly when he says:[3] "There is no such thing as 'brain food'—either fish or phosphorus. The less food, the clearer brain; the purer food, the stronger brain; that's all."

We are consequently forced into an acceptation of the doctrine that it is *through the blood* we must strike at the causes of nervous affections. We must adopt a physiological treatment, and upon the blood being purified, its chemical composition rendered normal, its being supplied in greater or lesser quantities to the nerve tissue, a true cure must and will follow, for the reason that we remove, in this manner, the real *cause* of the disease, and do not merely suppress the symptoms, by subduing the voices raised in protest against the highly abnormal conditions present and under which they have been compelled to function. (*v.*, my remarks on "Pain," pp. 25–9.)

It is now clear that the treatment of all nervous affections (as distinguished from the "purely" mental—granting such to exist), must hinge upon proper physiological treatment—upon the blood supply—and as we have abundantly shown that this medium is most radically and speedily reached and benefited by fasting, the mode of treatment advised becomes evident. I cannot, in this book, go into details regarding the effects of

[1] "Fish as Food," p. 22. (U. S. Dept. of Agriculture Bulletin.)
[2] See his "Principles of Psychology," Vol. I., pp. 101–3.
[3] "Philosophy of Fasting," p. 21.

fasting upon the cases of this character and will reserve such a discussion for a later work. But the theory is evident. Readers may consult pp. 21 and 55 of Dr. H. S. Drayton's "Nervousness: Its Nature, Causes, Symptoms and Treatment," for illustrative cases and examples of the effects of overnutrition of the nervous system. In all cases of nervous diseases the effects of fasting have only to be observed, to be appreciated. The extremely rapid and invariably successful results at once prove the correctness of the contention; while, if we take a rational view of the matter (regarding nerve fiber as so much organic tissue; the life or motive force, really lying in the brain), we cannot fail to see that fasting must benefit all cases of nervous diseases, just as it would benefit any other bodily affection whatever.[1]

As previously stated, it is almost invariably contended that one of the points considered to be of cardinal importance in the treatment of these diseases, is to "feed up" the patient, and to keep him "thoroughly nourished" throughout the course of treatment. The reason for this is that an increased nervous irritability is noticed immediately upon the discontinuance of the regular allowance of food—or even when lessening its quantity. For this reason it is considered advisable to continue feeding the patient—thereby checking all such manifestations of (supposedly) abnormal nervous action. My own view of the matter is that this method of treatment merely *smothers symptoms* whenever they arise, without making any attempt to remove their *causes*, and, at the same time, engenders diseases that must become manifest later on. I contend that the con-

[1] I quote, in this connection, the following most interesting passage from Doctor Rabagliati's "Air, Food and Exercises," pp. 159–60. "Whereas in the common carotid artery in the neck, before the internal carotid branches off for the supply of the brain, and whereas in the external carotid artery going to the face and *even to the brain membranes,* and in all the other arteries of the body, wherever they are distributed, the circulation is and remains synchronous with the pulsations of the heart, that is, heaving at the rate of, from sixty to ninety times a minute, the motion of the blood in the vessels of the brain itself is synchronous not with the heart's pulsations, but with the respiration, *i.e.*, it heaves and throbs only at the rate of from thirteen to seventeen or eighteen times a minute. The fact, so far as it goes, seems to have for its object, or, at least, for its effect, the limiting of blood supply to the brain. Now as blood is made from food, this seems to mean that persons who use their brain largely should not take much food lest they should make too much blood, which, finding its way in too great volume to the brain, might cloud and interfere with the finer and subtler working of that governing and controling and thinking and feeling organ."

tinued administration and enforcement of food, in such cases, merely checks the manifestation of nervous energy, by continually prostrating the vital powers (they being all utilized in the processes of digestion), to such an extent that no energy is left, at any time, to outwardly manifest (by symptoms) the inner, morbid conditions present. Take away all food, however, and relieve this tax upon the energies, and, while a nervous "storm" will doubtless be experienced for several days, this will gradually subside, with the restoration of normal conditions, and one thus cured is "cured to stay cured." The matter requires far fuller treatment, but that cannot be attempted here.

I cannot now stop to consider the effects of fasting upon the *mental life;* partly because of the very slight effects that are noticeable, calling for particular remark, and partly because I have considered this question at some length in Bk. IV., Chap. VII. on the "Mental Influences." I have elsewhere remarked upon the extraordinary extent to which the special senses are rendered acute (p. 505–7); and would here but draw attention to the fact that all purely mental operations are correspondingly improved. Attention, memory, association, the ability to reason with more than ordinary brilliancy[1]—all these are acutened and quickened to a remarkable degree. An added appreciation of the more spiritual forces of our nature, intuition, sympathy, love, etc.—all these expressions of our intellectual and emotional life are also quickened into being, and manifested to a remarkable and hitherto unknown degree. And it is obvious that such must be the case. Whatever view we take of our mental life, and its connection with the brain changes, the contention would hold good that any improvement in the texture of the brain substance and brain cells would benefit directly or indirectly the mental life; and the more perfect the condition of the brain substance, and the less gross and impure the blood that feeds it, the more perfect, the more spiritual, will the accompanying mental and spiritual life become. On the theory that the mental life is merely a product of the functioning of the organism, this must certainly be the case. And on the alternate

[1] "Fasting, Hydropathy and Exercise," p. 75.

theory, it must be equally true also. As Mrs. Annie Besant pointed out:[1]

"   The qualities of the soul working through the brain and the body take up something of the qualities of brain and body, and manifest their condition by the characteristics of that brain and that body alike" "Pessimism," says Max Nordau,[2] "has a physiological basis" "I believe," says Dr. Alexander Haig,[3] "that, as the result of a rational, natural and proper diet, producing the best circulation in the great power-house of the human body, we shall get not only freedom from gross disease, but we shall get, developing gradually, conditions of mind, thought, judgment and morality, which will, in the future, be as different from what they have been in the diseased and degraded past, as the light of heaven is different from the darkness of a dungeon; and that while there are to-day many things in human nature which all believers in the great and good and true can only most heartily deplore, I believe that in the future   . there will be more harmony, more strength, more beauty, more unselfishness, more love—in a word, a truer and greater and more complete sanity."

If anyone doubts the marvelous effects of fasting upon the mental, emotional, and spiritual life, let them but read Mr. Purinton's "Philosophy of Fasting."

From a purely physiological standpoint, we are forced to these conclusions—fasting demonstrating to us, in a remarkable manner, at once the independence and the inter-dependence of mind and body. And, with a cleansed body, purified blood, a clearer brain, and an unprejudiced and open mind, the patient can review his past life and clearly perceive how transgressed physiological law is the true and only cause of disease and suffering throughout the universe (a departure from which rendered the fast necessary), and how clear it is that Nature provides, in fasting, an unfailing, a sovereign remedy, always ready to hand, and that the mere following of Nature's dictates will and must render a return to health possible in every case where a cure is possible at all. See *Appendix N.*

[1] "Vegetarianism in the Light of Theosophy," p. 19.
[2] "Conventional Lies of Our Civilization," p. 17.
[3] "Life and Food," pp. 8–9.

CHAPTER VII

CRISES AND WHAT TO DO WHEN THEY OCCUR

IT HAS already been stated (p. 159), that judicious fasting is a great deal more than merely "going without food." If a fast of any considerable duration is to be undertaken—a protracted fast, as distinguished from the omission of a few meals, which is, of course, of little moment—if, I say, a protracted fast is to be undertaken, it is most desirable, if not actually necessary, to have some one constantly in attendance, who can explain and treat any outward symptoms that may appear—or rather the causes of such symptoms.

"An extreme fast," says Mr. Purinton,[1] "say from twenty to forty days, is just as apt to wreck a man as it is to rescue him. Unless, as I have mentioned before, it be properly conducted and completed."

A fast of this character is such an unusual experience for the patient; and his feelings and sensations, while undergoing it, are so entirely different from anything he has yet known; and his mental condition is usually (perhaps naturally) so perturbed, due to anxiety and uncertainty—all unfounded, yet present—that the appearance of any untoward symptoms (faintness, pain, vomiting, etc.), is apt to create something like a mental panic in the patient, and may even tempt him into wrong self-treatment, or, worse still, into breaking the fast. Such symptoms occurring at any stage of the fast will necessitate prompt and thorough treatment; but, when this is given, there need be no cause for alarm, since they indicate, merely, certain important crises that are being passed through; the momentary pause in the pendulum before it again swings free—in the reverse direction. The untoward symptoms do not necessarily indicate any dangerous

[1] "Philosophy of Fasting," p. 17.

condition—any "turn for the worse"—not by any means. They are merely the outward manifestations of certain internal, vital changes—changes which almost invariably denote a change for the better. But, the symptoms being taken for the actual disease, and their increase being looked upon as an indication that the patient is worse, instead of better, we can plainly see how the curative crisis might be mistaken for a turn for the worse—simply because the symptoms increase—and that the patient was in a highly dangerous condition, in consequence. Says Doctor Shew, in speaking of the first few days of fasting:[1]

"A feverish excitement of the system, together with a feeling of debility, faintness and depression is generally experienced. The patient becomes discouraged and melancholic, and is very excitable and sensitive to surrounding influences. He also experiences pains and soreness in the loins, feet, and sometimes in the joints. He becomes very tired of the sitting posture, and leans to one side or the other for support. But all these disagreeable symptoms, which are necessary in the process, grow by degrees less and less, as the morbid matter is eliminated from the vital economy. And when the body has at last grown pure, these unpleasant consequences disappear entirely, and the convalescent gains strength with inconceivable swiftness through the period of the after-cure."

Mental conditions here play a vastly important rôle; the smallest unpleasant and unlooked-for symptom being dwelt upon and magnified until the gravity of the resultant crisis is doubled, trebled, magnified a hundredfold—all due to the patient's morbidly active mental state. Here, as everywhere, the mind proves all-powerful—either for better or worse; consequently, the necessity for keeping and holding only the most cheerful, hopeful, optimistic thoughts. Nevertheless, since unlooked-for and misunderstood phenomena will sometimes occur, however cheerful the mind, or determined the will; and since the symptoms call for treatment, we shall now discuss, as briefly as possible, the various symptoms that may arise, together with the appropriate treatment in each case.

Before doing so, however, a few remarks must be made relative

[1] "Family Physician," p. 790.

to diseases already existent—their symptoms, and the effects of fasting upon these. If any diseased condition (of an eruptive nature, *e.g.*) be present, and the symptoms are active when a fast is entered upon, they will frequently—if not invariably—become more severe, or "worse" during the first few days of the fast.[1] And now, I insist, since most persons have only fasted for a few days at a time, if as long as that (*i.e.*, just long enough to bring to the surface these unpleasant symptoms), it may very readily be seen that fasting might, with them, gain the reputation of making all diseases "worse," and they consequently argue that this system of treatment is bad and should never be followed! This increase in the symptoms is, of course, accounted for, by them, as follows. The body is becoming weakened as the result of the withdrawal of food, and the disease is gaining headway in consequence—when, as a matter of fact, the symptoms indicate that precisely the *reverse* of this is the case, and indirectly disprove the theory that its advocates set out to prove and defend! The fallacy, of course, lies in the universal misunderstanding of the true nature of disease. Since, as we have seen, all disease is a curative process, and that its symptoms are signs of cure; and that the more active the symptoms, the more rapidly is the cure proceeding; knowing this, we can easily see that the increase of symptoms, noted at the commencement of a fast, is by no means an unfavorable sign, but the very reverse. It simply indicates that the stock of vitality is being increased; the depurating organs are working the faster; that the system is being purified the more rapidly; that the cause of the diseased condition is thus being expelled more forcibly; and consequently, that the cure is being more speedily effected. Instead, therefore, of checking the symptoms, they should be assisted; and they should be looked upon as one of the surest signs of speedy recovery.

Take an example: "Famine fever," *e.g.*, noticed, frequently, when entering upon a fast, indicates, merely, that the body is burning up and eliminating more rapidly than usual the surplus of mal-assimilated, oxidizable elements with which the system is clogged; it indicates a process of rapid elimination or purifica-

[1] Doctor Page noticed this, see his "Natural Cure," p. 169.

tion; and, as such, denotes, of course, merely a beneficial curative crisis—a process of cure. It is, as in the case of all other diseases, a curative crisis, and should be regarded as a favorable sign, in consequence. Instead, therefore, of seeing, in it, a proof of the evil effects of fasting (due to the system's weakened condition) we should see, in it, merely the indications of a beneficial, reparative process. As Doctor Rabagliati pointed out:[1]

"Fever and feverishness are due, not so much to the starvation, as to the fact that for a long time previously their bodies and blood had been loaded with waste and unassimilated materials derived from an excess of (even wholesome) food. The fever and feverishness are *occasioned* no doubt by fasting, but not *caused* by it. . . . If we cannot fast without fever, it is because we have been previously improperly fed."

Another point: Fasting will frequently bring to the surface (for elimination) conditions long latent, or diseases that have been suppressed—by drugs, etc. Thus, the patient may be on the verge of a cold, *e.g.*, when entering upon a fast. Under its invigorating and beneficial influences, the cure may begin at once; and with great rapidity, the cold will "develop" and the symptoms may become severe. In other words, the cure progresses rapidly, under the more favorable conditions, bringing to the surface, it will be observed, in this set of symptoms, a condition till then latent, and whose presence was unknown. In a similar manner, other symptoms may develop—all indicating that the process of cure has begun in earnest.

The anti-fasters have always argued somewhat as follows. That the cold was "caught" on the day after entering upon the fast, owing to the weakened condition of the system, resultant from the fast! How erroneous this idea is may readily be seen when we consider that "colds" have nothing to do with cold air (pp. 355–6); that they are not "caught," in any case, but developed (p. 11); that the system is never "weakened," but always invigorated, by fasting (pp. 225–30), and, finally, that the objection is based upon the currently false notions of the real nature of disease, and its cure. (pp. 1–13.) The cold is, moreover, *cured* by continued fasting! I need but state these reasons

[1] "Air, Food and Exercises," p. 122.

to demonstrate the futility of this objection; and to show that it is based upon anything rather than physiologic law.

As previously stated, one of the most interesting facts in connection with the fasting cure is that the symptoms of diseases long suppressed may be revived and become most troublesome, during a protracted fast. The reason for this is obvious. The *cause* of the disease was never really removed, but was suppressed, and remained latent within the organism. Partly owing to the persistent suppression of the efforts of Nature to bring about a cure (symptoms) and partly owing to the lack of vitality resultant therefrom, the system was unable to undertake the task of purification; but, under the purifying and invigorating effects of the fast, a cure—or at least an attempt at cure—became possible, and was accordingly undertaken. The process of purification begins; symptoms develop, depending upon the grossness or debility of the organism for their severity. Since the symptoms are not suppressed, but aided, in this instance, curative crises may develop swiftly and energetically—too energetically, sometimes, and they have to be regulated by the attendant physician. This may easily be done by artificially diverting the curative efforts from the organ of elimination most employed, *pro tem.*, to those less employed (as, *e.g.*, from the lungs to the skin, from the skin to the bowels and kidneys, etc.). Thus, the possibility must be constantly kept in mind that any disease once present, and suppressed by drugs, may become revived into activity during a fast; and the fast must never be blamed for the untoward symptoms that develop. Symptoms developing in this manner, and indicating any specific diseased condition, call for precisely the same treatment as though the disease was developed primarily. Water treatment, water drinking, enemas, exercise, deep breathing, etc., must be employed as usual, in such cases, while the fast should be persisted in, unremittingly. If the time is too limited to allow of a complete cure of the secondary or developed disease, prior to breaking the fast, this should be done, and followed by a very abstemious, non-stimulating diet—interspersed with frequent fast days. Persistently and conscientiously followed, this course cannot fail to produce a cure whenever such cure is possible.

A case in point is that of Mrs. Gertrude Y., referred to on pp. 202-5. In this case, it will be noticed, the disease for which the fast was undertaken (the paralysis) was completely cured before the fast was broken; but the long-suppressed syphilitic taint manifested itself, and proved that it had progressed so far as to render a cure impossible. In this case, of course, as in every other case, the patient died in spite of, and not on account of, the fast. Had the original disease been treated by fasting and other hygienic agencies upon its primary inception, it would have been eliminated, instead of suppressed—thus rendering the paralysis and the later treatment unnecessary. The real causes of the patient's death, it will be seen, were the drugs taken, and the vile medieval treatment received, rather than the consequent fasting, or other beneficial treatment administered or advised.

I now come to a discussion of the various specific symptoms that may arise during a fast, and their appropriate treatment. I shall first of all speak of:

Fainting.—Fainting spells, during a fast, whenever they may occur, should be treated precisely as are fainting spells under any ordinary circumstances—being due to precisely the same cause. The faintness is not due, as many think, to the weakness resulting from fasting, since no such actual weakness exists. (pp. 256-62.) Faintness is almost invariably caused by cerebral anæmia (*i.e.*, lack of blood in the brain), while the obvious antidote for this condition is the restoration of the cerebral circulation—to bringing more blood to the head—which can best be effected by placing the patient's head low and his feet high.[1]

The common practice of propping the patient up in chairs, etc., is dangerous in the extreme. The proper treatment in all such cases is to place the patient flat on his back, with the head low, and the feet slightly elevated; to loosen all tight and restrictive clothes; to allow a plentiful supply of fresh air—and leave the rest to Nature. The customary practice of dashing cold water over the patient's face, applying smelling salts, burnt

[1] Again we see Nature's wonderful provision, in such cases. When any person is seized with faintness, and consciousness is lost, the patient immediately falls prone—the very best position possible for equalizing the circulation.

feathers, etc., to the nose, and so on, are in my opinion decidedly harmful and deleterious. Such sudden shocks are unnatural, and a severe strain upon the nervous system; moreover, quiet and rest (not shocks) are obviously the conditions required by the organism. A simple chafing of the hands, fanning, and, perhaps, a *little* cold water applied to the forehead (if the insensibility lasts an unusually long time), is all the treatment indicated, and all that should be permitted.

Precisely the same treatment holds good in fainting "fits" occurring while the patient is fasting. The cause is the same, and the condition calls for the same treatment, precisely. The great point is, never to elevate the patient's head, but always to keep it as low as possible; this is the invariable rule in all cases of fainting.

Dizziness is very frequently due to the same cause as fainting, and may be treated in precisely the same manner. Since the condition is not so grave, the treatment advised for the latter cases would fully cover all such cases, also. It will readily be seen, I trust, how unjustifiable breaking the fast would be on account of any of these weaknesses, since they are mere outward indications of internal, vital adjustments.

Cramps in the bowels are most unpleasant, but seldom or never met with, in cases of fasting, since they are almost invariably due to an excess of fermenting food in the alimentary canal; and, during a fast, this is not present. Still, the *process of removing* this might, perhaps, cause cramp; and I mention it accordingly.

If present, administer a warm enema, followed by a small, cold injection; and insist upon the patient drinking a considerable quantity of hot water. In any case, hot fomentations are necessary, and should be administered promptly—applied as elsewhere directed in this book. (p. 365.) They should be changed as often as they become at all cool. Gentle kneading of the parts may also prove beneficial; and the application of the bare, open hand has frequently a wonderfully soothing and pain-allaying effect.

Retention of the Urine.—In one case I have known of a prolonged retention of the urine, occurring toward the end of a protracted fast. Whenever there has been no action of the bladder for (say) twelve hours, and provided that plenty of water has been drunk, we may safely diagnose "retention." In such a case, cold sitz baths should be administered; or alternate hot and cold sprays directed against the lower part of the abdominal wall. Gentle pressure and kneading might also be tried—following such treatment by dashes of cold water. Suggestion might also be employed; and the patient ordered to thoroughly relax all the muscles of the abdomen. These measures should be continued for some time; but should they fail (which is exceedingly unlikely) recourse must be had to the catheter.

Diarrhœa.—I have never known or heard of a case in which diarrhœa was present, after the first two or three days of a fast, and I doubt whether such a condition would not be a physiological impossibility. Costiveness is almost invariably present; the difficulty being to get the bowels to act at all. Nevertheless, if such a condition should arise, the treatment would be profuse water drinking, rest, and tepid enemas as soon as the bowels permit their use. Sitz baths should also be employed. Otherwise, the strictly "let alone" plan is all that is required.

Headaches.—I have elsewhere spoken of headaches; their causes and cure. (p. 28.) Since they are, again, but symptoms—troublesome at the time, but mere indications of a deeper cause—and since this cause is, most certainly, being removed by the fast, we can see that the simplest and shortest way to cure a headache is to let the symptoms alone, and to continue the fast—the speediest manner of removing the cause. Nevertheless, it may, perhaps, be somewhat justifiable, in such cases, to check the symptoms by various applications—thereby relieving the patient of the pain—since, to the psychic life of the patient, the pain is very real. I indicate some few of the leading hygienic measures that may be adopted to allay such pain in the speediest and most effective manner possible—without, however, breaking the fast. (1) Encourage profuse water drinking. (2) Administer a tepid enema. (3) Apply hot, warm, or cold cloths to the head—at the temperature most agreeable to the patient. Change as often as indicated. (4) A full, warm bath will often relieve this condition. (5) Suggestion might be tried—also soothing passes over the forehead. (6) Active friction or manipulation will often be all that is desired. (7) Sleep is the sovereign and generally unfailing remedy.

"*A bad taste in the mouth*" is due to various causes—all of which must be attended to, in order to effectually remove this unpleasant condition. The teeth must be kept thoroughly clean, and the throat gargled frequently. The tongue may be "scraped" with the toothbrush (See pp. 442–3), being careful not to do this, however, until it has been examined for its condition, etc. For a mouth wash, I know of nothing to equal diluted hydrogen-peroxide; but extreme care must be taken not to swallow any of the solution during this operation. Water may be freely drunk, also. This is about all that can be done until Nature has removed the cause—the foul material—when this unpleasant symptom will cease once and for all.

Insomnia.—It must be constantly borne in mind that the fasting patient requires, *ceteris paribus*, far less sleep than the average man or woman, living according to the general rule—the time for sleep being cut down to one-half, or even less, on occasion, with impunity. (pp. 320–2.) Consequently, insomnia need worry the patient but little, if it means but a few hours of sleep daily—and provided that this sleep is natural and untroubled by nightmare or other morbid dreams. The mere inability to go to bed and to sleep at the usual time is only to be expected, and is not at all an abnormal, or even (it will be seen) an unexpected sign. It is precisely what we should expect, if our theory of fasting be sound; and the fact that it *is* so forms a very important link in the chain of argument. It proves conclusively that all food eaten involves expenditure and loss of energy—which sleep is called upon to replace. Since, in fasting, this energy is not lost, its replacement is unnecessary.

But to return. Since less sleep is required, less should be sought; and the additional time thus saved may be spent in any way most pleasurable to the patient. Passively lying in bed, while the brain is active, is greatly to be deprecated; the nervous condition resulting therefrom often being a strong, predisposing cause to subsequent, genuine insomnia. All rest should be *earned* (like hunger!), and if the necessity for sleep is not felt, one night, by all means wait until the next, when unmistakable physical and mental fatigue will indicate rest; sleep being welcomed by the patient, under such circumstances, as the ideal goal to be reached. The loss of a night's sleep, while fasting, will be no greater hardship than the loss of three or four hours sleep under ordinary conditions, it must be remembered. It is only the blind acceptance, by the public, of that great bugaboo "regularity" which deters patients from attempting any such experiments upon themselves—rational as they might appear to their reason.

Granting, however, that a certain amount of sleep is required each night, in order to insure the best possible results, the question arises: How may we best assist Nature in wooing slumber, granting that a certain amount of insomnia be present—which, I may add, is very rarely the case? After attending to all the conditions requisite for inducing sound, healthful sleep—and if no particular symptoms are present, demanding treatment—the body and mind must be composed, relaxed, and utterly given up to the spell of sleep. A copious draught of hot water just before retiring will frequently induce sleep. Immersing the feet in hot and cold water alternately will also have this effect. Hot-water bottles should invariably be applied to the feet, if they show the least signs of being at all cold. A few minutes exercise will have the effect of inducing sleep in many cases; so also will a warm bath—followed by a cold spray and rapid drying, immediately before retiring. Suggestion is also a very valuable auxiliary indeed, in such cases—sleep suggestions being more potent than any others.

The object, in all the above methods of treatment, is the same; *viz.*, to withdraw the blood from the head, and to produce semi-artificial cerebral anæmia—which is, as we know, one of the prime requisites for sleep. Any measure which would tend to do this, without injuring the patient's health, may be legitimately employed—though it must be constantly borne in mind that I have been discussing, throughout, *possible* contingencies, not *usual* ones. So far as my own experience goes, I have never encountered an obstinate ease of insomnia during a fast (so the latter cannot be the cause of that condition as will be claimed, doubtless). The above remarks will all apply, however, to patients not fasting with equal propriety.

Pain in the Heart—Palpitation, etc.—This condition is almost invariably due to gases in the stomach, and other digestive disturbances, and so will not appear during a fast, except as a curative crisis. Says Doctor Schofield:[1]

"To understand what is the matter we must picture the heart sitting on the end of the stomach something like—to use a striking illustration—a donkey-boy sits on the hinder end of his ass; so that when the donkey kicks, the boy begins to palpitate on his back. In like manner, when the stomach kicks or is distended in any way by food, it often sets the heart off palpitating; and in this way the heart gets the blame while the stomach is the culprit."

Abnormally Slow Pulse.—This symptom is occasionally present—due, frequently, to extreme debility. For weeks, months, or years past the patient has been living under constant stimulation from both food and drink, which has the ultimate effect, in consequence, of sapping his vitality to the very dregs. When this stimulation is wholly withdrawn, therefore, as in a fast, abnormal symptoms at once develop. The long-deferred crisis is at hand. Either the patient will recover the expended powers, and live; or, if wasted to such an extent that recovery is impossible, will die, during the fast. This is the most frequent, if not the *only* cause of death that occurs during cases of protracted fasts, where death occurs before the return of natural hunger. Such cases never die from starvation; it is a physiological impossibility for them to die during a fast before the return of natural hunger—unless the vital powers have previously been so wasted as to render their recuperation impossible—death being due to this failure; and it will thus be seen that the real cause of death is, again, previous mal-treatment—death

[1] "Nerves in Order," pp. 63–4.

occurring in spite of, and not on account of, the fast. Had a fast been instigated, in such cases, at an earlier period, the vital powers might have been sufficiently strong to have withstood the shock—recuperation, instead of failure would have resulted; *i.e.*, life instead of death. This question is more fully discussed, however, on pp. 537–9.

To return, however, to the pulse. Apart from what has al ready been said in the chapter on "The Pulse," there remains the special study of the exceptionally rapid and the exceptionally slow pulse. The latter of these we are now considering. The only lasting and true cure in such cases is, of course, to remove the *cause* of the abnormal functioning; and this the fast is doing as rapidly as possible. There may arise occasions, however, when the pulsation reaches a dangerously low point, and this condition calls for prompt and vigorous (yet careful) treatment. Mild exercises are, perhaps, the best to prescribe, since exercise invariably quickens the heart's action. Deep-breathing exercises are also to be highly recommended. Extreme measures—such as throwing cold water against the patient's chest, etc.—I do not by any means endorse; the experiment is dangerous in the extreme. A hot bath, however, might be allowable. Says Doctor Kellogg:[1]

"The hot bath is a most efficient stimulant, in the true sense of the word. It will so excite the circulation as to increase the pulse from 70 to 150 in fifteen minutes."

Suggestion might legitimately be employed in such cases—especially when extreme weakness is present. Friction, massage, warm baths, may all be employed with great advantage. Under no circumstances, however, are stimulants or drugs permissible—the subsequent reaction leaving the patient in a lower and more dangerous condition than in the first instance, and without benefiting him in the least degree. (pp. 20–33.)

An abnormally rapid pulse may be due to various causes—all more or less normal. Thus, exercise, excitement, nervous shock, etc., will all have the effect of increasing the heart's action to a tremendous degree. In such cases, a return to the

[1] "Uses of Water," p. 60.

normal rate of pulsation will invariably return in a short time, without any assistance, and is of comparatively little importance. When, on the other hand, the pulsation is extremely rapid from what may be considered distinctly abnormal causes, it calls for prompt attention, and may be more or less dangerous, according to the rate of pulsation and the condition of the patient. The causes of the rapid pulse in such cases are, sometimes debility; inhibition by the cardiac nerve—due to disease or other causes; long-suppressed emotions; blood poisoning, organic defect, etc. An undue retention of urine, *e.g.*, seems to have an appreciable effect upon the pulse. These causes, supplemented by those mentioned above, will occasionally induce a rapidity of pulsation (*i.e.*, of the heart's action), which is truly alarming; and will, in fact, in some cases, unless treated promptly, be followed by a speedy and painful death. Provided that the *rhythm* is perfect (and if this is not the case, a very grave functional or organic condition indeed is present, which little can be done to regulate or assist, but which, of course, fasting has in no way *induced*)—if this rhythm is perfect, the rate may run up to 110 or more beats a minute without causing serious alarm; but when the pulse runs up to 120 or 130 or even a greater number—as is sometimes the case—every effort must be made to reduce the rate, by every means possible, and with the greatest rapidity—consistent with a steady, not an instantaneous decline. The following would be my advice, in cases of this character.

Upon finding that the patient's pulse is mounting up to an alarming extent, he should be placed in a bath of water at 100° F. —*not hotter or colder;*[1] and this must be regulated by a bath thermometer. Gentle friction may be applied to the skin, and the bath may be continued for about five minutes. As the water is *very slightly* above the blood heat, this will have the effect of *gradually* withdrawing the blood from the internal organs (including the heart) to the periphery, without either sudden shock, or harmful reaction. The patient should then be dried rapidly, put to bed, and covered up warm, with hot water

[1] Doctor Kellogg advises a cold or cool bath, at such times. He says ("Uses of Water," p. 60): "By the cool or cold bath, the pulse may often be reduced twenty to forty beats in a few minutes."

bottles to his feet; absolute repose, both of mind and body, is necessary, and great care must be observed to supply an abundance of fresh air, which the patient must breathe deeply, in *slow*, regular inspirations. A relaxed muscular system and a reposeful state of mind are to be insisted upon.

If the pulse is *already* beating at an extremely rapid rate, however, it may be impossible, or at least inexpedient, to follow these directions—though, in such cases, we must be guided by circumstances. In cases in which the pulse has already run up to a dangerously rapid pace, soothing treatment of every kind is the best, if not the only treatment possible. Placing the open hands over the spine, and gentle manipulation may be useful. Quieting suggestions may also be employed with great advantage, on occasion; their trial should never be omitted. Someone having a thorough knowledge of psychology and suggestive treatment can frequently do far more good, in these extreme cases, than can all the doctors in the world. The vital forces can be rallied, seemingly, and brought under the direct control of the will—turning the scale in the patient's favor. If the faintest traces of mentality remain, they should be thus appealed to; and even if not, the suggestions might still be given, with great advantage—they falling, in that case, directly upon the subconscious mind of the patient.

The pulse must be carefully watched, and all efforts directed toward preventing such a rapid pulsation as that mentioned above. This can nearly always be done if prompt action be taken at the commencement of the upward tendency. The practice of controling the heart's action by hypodermic injections, etc., will invariably result in the patient's death—since they simply "control" the heart's action by destroying the vitality upon which it depends; and, when once the effects of the poison have worn off, (if indeed, the patient does not die under its influence), the previous attack will return with even greater severity; and this is "reduced" with more poison—this process continuing *ad infinitum;* or rather, until the patient succumbs under the great prostration—resultant upon the poison administered. That the patient does not die in *every* case I admit; but this simply shows how wonderful are Nature's forces

—how strong the tendency toward recuperation—which can thus sustain life in spite of such barbarous treatment.

Vomiting.—This symptom will sometimes manifest itself during the first twenty-four or forty-eight hours of a fast. In such cases, the treatment resolves itself into the strictly let-alone plan—with the exception, perhaps, of copious water drinking, and hot fomentations to the pit of the stomach. The vomiting is merely ridding the stomach of a load of putrescent material, which low vitality and a superabundance of food have hitherto rendered impossible. It denotes but a transitory spasm, which will pass away, if left to Nature—just as will any other "fit of sickness" (curative crisis)

But there are exceptional cases on record where severe, even fatal, spells of sickness have occurred; and even toward the close of a protracted fast, which has progressed in every other way most satisfactorily, until this seizure—all the bodily infirmities for which the fast was undertaken having been removed. At the end of a thirty or forty days' fast, *e.g.*, such vomiting spells have been known to occur (though they are of extreme rarity), and have, as before stated, even terminated fatally. If there is any alarming symptom that can possibly develop, it is, most assuredly, this one. If anything might tempt the breaking of a fast, it is just such a crisis as this. After fasting for a considerable time, and noting nothing but improvement, nothing but continued gain in health, it is certainly quite excusable for any patient to become alarmed, should a severe vomiting spell suddenly develop, and continue for several days, with unabated vigor.[1]

While acknowledging that this condition is an exceedingly grave and critical one; still, fear and other morbid mental conditions can but tend to make matters worse, both *per se*, and by inducing the patient to attempt harmful self-treatment. Little

[1] While *attempts* at vomiting—"reaching"—must be understood by the word used, *actual* vomiting may occur, even after fasting a number of days—pus, mucous, large quantities of evil smelling bile, etc., being ejected, as well as whatever water may be in the stomach at the time. These substances often seem to initiate the vomiting spell, which afterwards generates, apparently, into a continued reflex spasm—as, long after the solids are all ejected, the attempts at vomiting continue.

can be done—but that little must be done promptly. The following is what I should advise in such a case:

Immediately upon the appearance of a vomiting spell, the patient should be given all the hot water he can possibly drink —two quarts, or more if necessary—the object being to facilitate the eructation, and to cleanse the stomach of the offending, irritating material—the probable cause of the sickness. All restrictive dress should be loosened. The patient should be removed at once to the outer air—of which he should breathe deeply and regularly. Rest, physical and mental, are important requisites. If the above instructions are followed promptly and energetically, they will be found to bring immediate relief in almost every instance. In case vomiting is not thus freely induced, however, the patient should, if able, continue to drink the hot water, even to the point of considerable discomfiture.

Free vomiting being thus induced, nothing should be attempted until the foree of the spasm or spell has ceased, and temporary relief follows. The obnoxious material being removed, the vomiting will undoubtedly cease, *pro tem*, and the patient recuperate.

If, however (as *might* happen—it probably *would* not happen once in a million cases), vomiting continues more or less steadily for three or four days, in spite of the treatment above recommended, still more decided measures must be taken. Hot and cold baths may be administered—the temperature being determined by experimentation. A little glycerin added to a glass of hot water and swallowed by the patient has been known to produce a remarkably soothing effect. Spinal manipulations, and the placing of the open hands over the region of the stomach for a considerable period; hot fomentations or cold compresses, or both alternately, over the pit of the stomach;[1] suggestion—all these may be tried—preferably in conjunction. Should all these measures fail, and it is noticed that the patient is becoming manifestly weaker, it might be permissible to break the fast, since the resultant evil consequences from such an action would be more than counterbalanced by the conservation of the patient's vitality (through stopping the vomiting)—the reaction

[1] Doctor Oswald recommends this. ("Household Remedies," p. 220.)

coming at a time when it could be comparatively well borne. It is, most certainly, a choice of evils. If the vomiting continues, despite all the above measures, which I hardly think possible, even theoretically, the patient may die from exhaustion. If, on the other hand, food is administered, the patient may die in any case—the food being ejected, and this action perhaps even hastening the patient's end. There is the possibility that the ingestion of food may, under such circumstances, break the spasm; in which case a recovery is highly possible. There is considerable risk attached to the experiment, of course, but no greater risk than the introduction of deadly poisons into a patient's organism, which are daily and hourly administered in regular medical practice—while such cases as the above occur, as stated, but once in a million times. In the only two such cases that I have ever heard of, in which death resulted, apparently from this cause (that of Mrs. G. Y., above referred to, pp. 202–5; and Mrs. Meyer, referred to by Doctor Dewey, "No-Breakfast Plan," etc., pp. 190–98), no thorough trial had been given the above-suggested methods of arresting such vomiting, and I am morally certain that if they had, death would not have resulted in either case. As against them, I might mention the case, spoken of by Doctor Dewey, ("No-Breakfast Plan," pp. 199–200), where nausea and vomiting commenced after more than fifty days of successful fasting, and where the food administered was promptly ejected without the slightest relief to the patient. There was nothing to do but to wait on Nature; with the glorious result that:

"In one day after the last vomiting spell there was a natural call for food—and this on the *sixtieth* day of the fast." (p. 200.) "Had this man died," continued Doctor Dewey, "such was his prominence—I should have been paraded as a criminal of the stupid kind in the entire press of America, except in the papers of my own city."

I may here mention, incidentally, that Doctor Dewey was exceedingly opposed to the idea of breaking the fast in such cases, under any conceivable circumstances. In a letter to me, written March 26, 1903, he wrote (in reply to a question from me, as to its advisability):

"Only God could break a fast where there is a sick stomach and there is no time to let Nature perform the task. Taking food into such a stomach is death-dealing. There is nothing to do but make the body and mind as comfortable as possible and Nature will cure, if the seal of Death is not set."

Besides the above-mentioned instances of acute crises, calling for treatment, I have known of one or two exceptional cases in which most interesting—though somewhat alarming—symptoms developed, either during a fast, or immediately following its breaking. These phenomena were merely transitory, however, and required no special treatment, beyond that supplied by good nursing; and I mention them here simply as curiosities worth noting, rather than as pathological phenomena likely to occur. Indeed, it is doubtful if precisely the same effects will ever again be observed in fasting patients—being due, in every case, to a peculiar combination of causes, all but impossible to duplicate again. It is for this reason that I am tempted to to record them here.

In one case, then, the patient became practically *insane* from the second to the fifth day of the fast (pp. 195–7)—normal conditions being restored on the fifth day! When once the crisis was passed, no indication of such a condition ever recurred; the mentality became, on the other hand, far clearer than in years—indicating that the condition was transitory and merely a curative crisis; one aspect of the vital upheaval, affecting, by chance, the mentality. In this case, the condition was undoubtedly brought about by the excessive, morbid action of the liver, which was greatly deranged, causing an excessive flow of bile; and to a disordered circulation. This was undoubtedly the cause, since the patient, also, turned almost *green* during these few days—her complexion becoming normal, as the fast progressed. In another case, again, a practical suspense of all consciousness resulted upon the ingestion of the first meal, after the breaking of the fast, and lasted some hours. In a third case, the patient stated she "saw double" for a time—just prior to breaking the fast—two visual images being perceived, instead of one. I have no theory to account for this fact, which is most singular, and worthy of being ranked, it seems to me, with the interesting cases collected by Dr. S. Bidwell—in his "Some Curiosities of Vision."

I must now point out and insist upon the fact that such crises need not occasion concern or consternation, and certainly afford no argument for breaking the fast. With careful nursing, the rest may be safely left to Nature; she will cure in every case, where recovery is possible.

The reader who has followed me through the above "chapter of accidents" may have come to the conclusion that, if a fast invites so many grave crises and perils, it is a thing to be left severely alone, and is far too dangerous to be attempted by the average individual, without a competent and experienced adviser at hand. If I have conveyed that impression, it is certainly not the one I wished to convey. While I strongly advise any prospective faster to procure the services of some doctor or hygienist who thoroughly understands and is in sympathy with the treatment here advocated; still, such is by no means necessary, provided that the patient himself thoroughly understands the *rationale* of the fasting cure, and has absolute faith in it, and in Nature; that he preserves a calm, unruffled mental condition, and knows what to do whenever emergencies such as these occur. It is with the intention of helping the student, or prospective patient in this last point that the present chapter has been written; to show him that, while peculiar phenomena and abnormal symptoms will sometimes show themselves and develop, they should not, as a rule, be regarded as serious, or even as extraordinary—being merely the outward signs or indications of internal, vital adjustments. Properly treated, the symptoms will, in practically every case, disappear shortly, without necessitating any special treatment; and need not occasion worry, breaking the fast, or the administration of drugs and stimulants.

That I have dwelt at some length upon the various symptoms that may arise, is not due to the fact that I regard them as serious, as a rule (for I do not), nor that all or any of these or other symptoms will manifest in the majority of cases which are treated by this method (for they will not). Such abnormal symptoms will not become manifest once in a hundred times; and fear of them need certainly not deter any patient from entering upon a fast with the full confidence that he will be restored to health in the speediest manner possible, and without the development of any of the untoward symptoms mentioned. This chapter is written with the object of assisting patients to treat themselves in a rational manner *if* such symptoms should appear, and not with any anticipation or belief that they *will* appear. They crop up so rarely as to be hardly worthy of serious consideration. I have given the rational treatment for whatever crises *might possibly* occur, and not for those which *will undoubtedly* occur—since they but rarely do so. In short, I do not intend to alarm my reader, and should feel sorry indeed if I have done so. The comparative risk from death from such causes as those spoken of in this chapter may be considered as something less, perhaps, than that involved in walking beneath a building in the course of construction—it is infinitesimal. On the other hand, the alternative (of not fasting at all) if followed, would often mean slow, but sure, death—painful and lingering.

Let me illustrate more fully my conception of the cause of death—resultant, apparently, from fasting. *Emaciation and disease have so far taxed the vital energies and wasted the flesh that, when the fast is undertaken, there is not enough tissue present to feed the brain a sufficiently long time for a complete elimination of this morbid material* (and consequently for the return of hunger) *to take place.* We see, then, that, in such cases, it is practically a *race* between the successful elimination of the diseased material, and the amount of flesh upon the body. If the vital powers are sufficiently strong; if there is sufficient tissue upon the body to last the brain, as food, until this complete purification and cure has resulted, then the organism recovers; health is regained. If, on the other hand, the bodily tissue is already almost totally lost (through emaciation due to disease) the brain system may not have enough food left to last or nourish it a sufficiently long time to enable the body to eliminate the impurities present.

In this manner, death may possibly result before hunger returns; but it will be seen that death is, in such cases, inevitable;

the body was so far diseased, so emaciated, that recovery was impossible in any case—whether the fast was undertaken or not. Death would soon have resulted under any circumstances. The body could not possibly hold out long enough—feed the brain for a sufficient length of time—to enable it to completely eliminate the excrementous material, and to allow hunger to return. It is purely a question of balance, of time; and the time was not sufficient. But, in any case, death would soon have resulted, since it was inevitable, and the only thing that can be charged against the fasting, consequently, is that it somewhat *hastened* the end. But there is always the possibility—nay, the certainty, almost—that the fast will not terminate in this manner at all; but, on the contrary, that it will restore the organism to complete health. For all but the very last stages of the most severe and dangerous diseases this is absolutely certain. In the few remaining cases, we may feel that we are, so to say, "taking the bull by the horns," or our life in our hands, in entering upon the fast. The patient might die, in such instances—die somewhat sooner than if he had not so fasted; but the fasting is, at any rate, his only hope—since death, at some near period of time, is inevitable; and he has the alternative, on the other hand, of a chance to completely restore his health and to recover entirely—which would certainly be quite impossible were the fast not entered upon, or undertaken. You balance a possible premature death against a strong and extremely probable presumption of recovery. The decision each patient must make for himself—bearing in mind that, in such extreme cases (and only in extreme cases does this apply at all) the hope for recovery afforded by the fast is the only hope he can possibly entertain.

The objection may be raised that death would not have resulted, had not the fast been undertaken—which must, therefore, be considered more or less the direct *cause* of such deaths. This is incorrect; the patient would not, perhaps, have died quite so *soon*, had not the fast been entered upon; but it would have inevitably and more surely have resulted a little later. The longer the period of time allowed to elapse before the fast was undertaken, the more doubtful the recovery. Were such cases taken in the early stages, but a very few days fast would have been necessary in order to bring about complete recovery; but the longer the time that is allowed to elapse before the cure is undertaken, the greater the danger that it will not be ultimately successful. Those cases which die under the fasting treatment are, indeed, merely examples of the complete neglect to undertake a fast at an earlier date, when a cure would have been effected certainly and quickly. As Doctor Dewey so well remarked:[1]

"In five fatal cases under my care in which there was no possibility of feeding, there was such agitation over the question of starvation as would have subjected me to violence had my city been nearer the equator. In all these cases I was compelled to have a post-mortem to silence heathen raging. . . . The physiology of fasting in time of sickness is so entirely new to the medical world that every death that occurs with those who practise it is certain to be attributed to starving. Fasting, because it is Nature's plan, will win the victory in all cases in which victory is possible; and yet, wherever it is adopted, to become known about, there will be the same confusion of tongues as would be were violent hands laid upon gods of wood and stone in heathen temples. 'Starved to death,' is the verdict."

In the last stages of many diseases, I do not doubt that a cure is quite impossible to effect, even by fasting—aided by all other hygienic auxiliaries.[2] But the case should not have been left thus long before treatment was begun. The cause of the patient's death is, therefore, not the fasting—from which the body derives extreme benefit in every case; but the previous, lengthy and neglected disease, which rendered the system incapable of being cured by any means; in fact, rendered the case absolutely hopeless. That so very few deaths result from fasting, then, shows the almost unlimited potency of this method of treatment; and shows, also, that death, in such cases, always results in spite of, not on account of, the fast having been ultimately undertaken.

[1] "No-Breakfast Plan," pp. 189–90.

[2] The very great importance of such hygienic auxiliaries—such as enemas, exercise, water drinking, baths, etc., will here become manifest—inasmuch as they all materially tend to shorten the fast (p. 382), perhaps enabling a cure to be effected, which, otherwise, would have been impossible.

CHAPTER VIII

HOW AND WHEN TO BREAK THE FAST

"In a very languid way it is admitted that we eat too much," says Doctor Dewey;[1] and that that fact is coming to be more and more recognized as time progresses, I am certain. Overeating is coming to be frankly recognized as one of the great besetting sins of the American and English peoples, and as largely responsible for the sickness and the prevalent diseased condition of those peoples. At the same time no particular effort has been made even by those who realize more or less the truth of these remarks, toward a betterment of the existing conditions—in their own persons! "Yes, I do think most people eat too much, undoubtedly," I have heard repeatedly· but the speaker never thinks of including himself as one of "the people!" It is always the *others* who eat too much! For ourselves, we are paragons of dietetic continence!

Unfortunately, Nature does not seem to think so, and will not enter into, nor cater to, our egotistical views. That we overeat she reminds us most forcibly, when the next sickness or pain intervenes. That most all of us do overeat, and that grossly, is, I think, sufficiently proved by the case of Mr. Horace Fletcher—before referred to (pp. 113–14); and by other cases mentioned in this book. And, as the results of this surfeit, come the evil consequences; the law is absolute, irrevocable, irreconcilable. "As ye sow, so shall ye reap!"

Reasoning closely akin to the above would convince the average person, probably, that a fast of a certain length of time would be beneficial, were it not persisted in for so *long* a time. A *little* fasting is good; that almost everyone will admit who has attended, or even seen much of, the sick for any lengthy period.

[1] "Experiences of the No-Breakfast Plan," etc., p. 40.

Many persons would believe in a fast of one or two meals, or perhaps a day, or even two or three days; but not in a protracted fast! "Moderation" is their cry. The same slackness that is observable in the previous reasoning, with regard to overeating; the same half-heartedness and lack of complete assurance in the system, if followed, is conspicuous here—indicating a failure to grasp the real *philosophy* of the treatment—necessitating, as it does, the complete reversal of all our preconceived ideas. The real or philosophic basis of the plan of treatment once thoroughly grasped, backsliding or uncertainty becomes a mental impossibility, and we no longer shrink from accepting the legitimate conclusions, deduced from our series of facts.

A word in explanation before I consider, in detail, the real subject matter of this chapter; a word both of explanation and defense. I do not pretend to deny—in fact, I have always contended—that, if we eat only our natural food, at proper times, and in the proper amount, these long fasts would be quite unnecessary. That I freely grant. If the system contains but little corrupt matter from which it must rid itself, but a very brief period will be required in which to accomplish that result. The ideally balanced diet and bodily condition is that in which no change in bulk of food is ever called for,[1] (the amount eaten

[1] No *proportionate* change is here meant. Living a uniform life the bulk of food craved and eaten should be, theoretically, exactly the same each day. This is the true basis of *regularity* at meals, and not the thoroughly erroneous, and very harmful idea held by the majority of people at the present day—and insisted on by doctors. The popular idea is that regularity consists in administering food at certain definite and set times by the clock; at noon, or six, or whatever hour is decided upon; and food is forced upon the patient, willy-nilly, at that time—quite independent of whether appetite is present, or food is craved. Food is administered and eaten because "it is time," and because "regularity is highly important," in feeding the sick, in keeping the human machine in running order, and in "keeping up the strength!" The stoking of the engine must be "regular;" thus reasons the medical man; thus, consequently, reasons the layman; and thus are a vast number of unfortunates hurried to their graves prematurely!

In advocating "regularity" at meals then, I do not mean the prevalent idea of a "meal time," at which food must be taken; and yet I am arguing for regularity! The paradox is easily explained. The medical profession has the cart before the horse. They have failed to delve deep enough into the question; and ask: What is the *origin* of the present belief in the regularity of meals, and its efficacy? On what is it founded? The answer is not far to seek. It is—*not* that a certain definite hour, a time of day, has arrived, at which food must be taken; but that if the food supply had been absolutely normal—as to its quality and quantity—natural hunger would appear, in the normal individual, at regular intervals—signifying that the last meal had been digested and absorbed, and that the bodily tissues were crying aloud

satisfying the system exactly, with no surplus and no deficit), and in which regularity is the predominant feature, the appetite—the call for food—being as regular as clock work; and deviations from this should represent, invariably, deviations in the bodily habits, or extraneous causes affecting the system—atmospheric purity, temperature, etc. Thus, a greater amount of bodily exercise than is customary will call for a greater bulk of food than is usually eaten, to replace the extra tissue destroyed, etc. But, in these cases, my contention is that the *proportionate* bulk of food is not altered; the *ratio* between the food and the bodily waste remaining precisely the same, as ever.

Doctor Graham seems to me to sum up the whole question in an excellent manner, writing:[1]

"If . . . an individual in civic life, with a perfectly undepraved system, regularly eats at stated periods his three meals a day, of pure simple vegetable food, and uniformly takes about the same amount of exercise, and at each meal eats just about that quantity of food which the alimentary wants of the vital economy really demand, the physiological condition of the stomach indicated by the sense of hunger will become a fixed habitude, and hunger will recur at its regular periods of eating with utmost exactness and precision. But, if at any time he takes considerably more nourishment into the stomach than the real alimentary wants of the vital economy require, or omits his customary exercise, or labor, hunger will not recur precisely at his next stated period of eating; and if he eats at that time, he will oppress and irritate the stomach, and trespass upon the gen-

for nutritive material, in the language of hunger. In other words; in the perfectly balanced diet, hunger would invariably appear at precise and stated intervals, owing to the fact that the previous meal had been digested and utilized in *exactly that length of time*, and for no other reason. Thus we see the appetite regulates the meal time, and not the meal time the appetite. Regularity is still the ideal; but the regulator is hunger, and the demand of the bodily tissues; not the wisdom of the doctor, or the hour hand of the mantelpiece clock. As Mr. George M. Bailey pointed out ("Nature's Law of Hunger," pp. 12–13): "Do we look at the clock when we are thirsty, to see if it is time for all of the members of our family to take a drink of water? Nature is kind, and *appears* to adjust us to this machine-plan of living, but she punishes this violation of her laws, just the same." And there is no more reason why we should eat by the clock than there is why we should drink by it. Yet meal times could be as regular in each case, the prime difference being that, whereas one system is artificial and death dealing, the other is natural and an indication of the highest degree of normal bodily health.

[1] "Science of Human Life," pp. 557–8.

eral physiological interests of his body; and, by continuing such transgressions, he will inevitably so effect the condition of his stomach as to bring on a preternatural appetite, which will eagerly receive food as often as his meal-time comes, and perhaps, even more frequently, whether his system really requires alimentation or not, and which will never be satisfied with such a quantity of food as the vital economy of his system can dispose of without embarrassment and oppression. Such an appetite, therefore, is something very different from that natural and healthy hunger which is a physiological manifestation of the real alimentary wants of the body; and it is of the utmost importance that this distinction should ever be kept in view when we are reasoning on the dietetic habits of man; for such an appetite is no safer guide for us in regard to eating—as to time, quantity or quality—than the drunkard's thirst is in regard to drinking."

To revert now to the main theme of my chapter. I must contend, and that strenuously, that the breaking of the fast prematurely is one of the most foolish and dangerous experiments that can possibly be made. The prevalent idea is that a fast should be undertaken, and persisted in, for a certain, definite period, which can be fixed upon before the fast is begun; and that the fast can be broken, and even broken to advantage, at the expiration of that period. How long a period that would be would vary with the belief of the individual. Some might contend that skipping one or two meals would be beneficial; but that (say) three days would be far too long a period. Others that two or three days might be advantageous in certain cases, but that a week would certainly be detrimental; and still others might be willing to admit that, in acute cases, five or six days, or even a week, might do "no harm," or might even benefit the patient, whereas a fast of four or five weeks would be (if not fatal), at least an extremely harmful and dangerous experiment, and of no permanent advantage. And who is there to decide? Were it thus possible to determine, *à priori*, the length of time the fast might be protracted, without harm resulting, or with benefit to the patient fasting, this system of treatment would be as blindly experimental, and as empirical, as the orthodox medical treatment of to-day—whereas it is nothing of the kind. Nature would institute no such senseless codes, no "law in which there is no law," and this I shall now endeavor to prove.

I wish to impress the following statement upon the minds of my readers, since it is one of the most important facts contained in this entire book; and the failure to appreciate it is, I believe, the cause of almost all the misunderstandings concerning the fasting cure—showing the complete ignorance of the philosophy of this method of treatment.

The statment is this: *Nature will always indicate when the fast should be broken*—and there can never be any mistake made by those who are accustomed to watching fasting cases, as to *when* to terminate the fast. Nature will always indicate when the fast should be broken by a series of symptoms which can never be misunderstood, and which she here displays most obviously —to all those whose judgment is not perverted by preconceived ideas, and who possess a sound knowledge of the phenomena and philosophy of fasting. These symptoms are, *inter alia*, the following:

The tongue, which has been previously heavily coated, now clears and assumes its normal, healthful appearance. (pp. 441–4.) The breath which, up to now, has been most offensive, and of a peculiar sweet odor, assumes its previous, normal state. (pp. 444–7.) A sudden and complete rejuvenation; a feeling of lightness, buoyancy, and good health steals over the patient in an irresistible wave; bringing contentment and a general feeling of well-being, and of the possession of a superabundance of animal spirits. Another important indication is found in the condition of the blood supply, and the degree of the reaction noted on the periphery. Thus, if the flesh, under the finger nails is pale in color (when the fingers are held out straight), then the circulation is poor and the patient is more or less anæmic. The capillaries are blocked and choked with an excess of nutritive material, and the blood cannot circulate freely to those parts. Fasting, by removing this obstruction, will enable the flesh to resume its normal, pink color; and the return of this condition invariably indicates a return to health. At the end of a fast, I have frequently observed this pink, healthful condition of the fingers—under the finger nails.

Another indication is afforded by the rate of the blood reaction on the surface of the body. Dr. Alexander Haig pointed out this fact, and, in his "Life and Food," p. 4, says:

"Let any one who eats meat and has eaten it for years, be touched, say, on the back of the hand with the point of the finger. A white mark is made, and the rate at which that white mark is obliterated by returning color gives the rate of the circulation in the skin of the person so touched. Now, if two men are com pared, one of whom lives on the natural food of the frugivorous animal, and the other lives on the unnatural of the carnivorous animal, it will be found by this test that the skin circulation of the carnivorous man is about twice as slow as that of the natural living frugivorous man, and it, of course, follows that the man with the slow circulation has a slow circulation not merely in his skin, which is seen, but in all the organs of his body which are not seen, including the great power-house of his mechanism, the frontal lobes of the brain. . . . "

I may say that all these remarks apply with equal or greater force to the man fasting; as in such cases the reaction is remarkably rapid and forcible.

But more than all these symptoms, and the surest symptom of all (that the fast is now complete and ready to be broken), is the fact that *hunger*, which till now had been altogether absent, returns and notifies the patient that the system is ready to utilize to the best advantage whatever food may be taken as nourishment.

That these statements are true can be proved by observing any case of a protracted fast; and they are well-known to those hygienists who have written on this subject—though no writer has, so far as I know, collected and presented in cumulative form these arguments for allowing the fast to assign its own limit—by the return of natural hunger. Nature will always indicate, by unmistakable symptoms, when the fast should be terminated, *and it should never be broken prior to these indications and to the return of natural hunger!* No matter how long a fast may be necessary, the same rule holds good in every case. Nature, in her wisdom, adopts this course and the rule is infallible. If a fast of only two days is necessary, in order to clear up the system and recover health, then hunger will return at the end of the second day. If, on the contrary, two weeks or two months are necessary—then natural hunger will not return until the expiration of *that* lengthy period. And thus we see that natural hunger will always return when, and only when, the cause of the disease is completely expelled from the system, and the body is once more restored to perfect health. Again Nature's wise provision for our safety is manifested; and again the complete demonstration of how in accord with Nature is the method of cure here advocated.

A two or a one month's fast, *e.g.*, is necessitated simply because it requires the system that length of time to "catch up," in the process of elimination, with the overplus of ingested food material. This process may—probably has—continued for years before the fast was entered upon; and is, in reality, a marvelously short time in which to rectify the condition present, and to recuperate. A week's fast, again, has been necessitated by a less extensive and gross abuse of the organism than in the former cases; a three or a four days' fast by still less abuse, and so on; a one day's necessitated fast indicating but a slight divergence from the normal. But my contention is that such long fasts as those recounted (and necessary) are only rendered necessary by a long continued evolutionary process—one in which overeating has been practiced for years before such a fast was necessary—or even possible. The first step in this evolutionary process is that of eating the first meal one minute too soon! And this rendered it possible, and in fact probable, that the next would be five minutes too soon; the next ten; the next fifteen; and so on—the system always running a little more and more behind in her "accounts," until finally a whole day's fast became necessary, in order to preserve the balance; then two days; then three; then a week; and so on, till these lengthy and extraordinary fasts became necessary. This process of evolution is, of course, very gradual, but that it is the process involved, I feel quite certain. It explains all the facts in the case, and has the additional advantages of being logical and consistent.

Another word of explanation is perhaps necessary. However long the fast may continue, no danger whatever from starvation need be feared, since *hunger will always return before the danger point is reached.* Thus, so long as hunger is absent, it is a plain indication that no food is required; but the instant the body is released from the impure matter, and its accompanying complications, causing the disease; the instant health is restored, in other words, the vital powers are released from their task; nervous equilibrium is restored, and the tissues then call for nourishment to replenish the waste; and this constitutes what is manifest to us as *hunger.*

I cannot too strongly impress this point upon my readers—that natural hunger, *and that alone* should indicate the terminus of the fast: when the fast is ready to be broken. That this signal is invariably given at the proper time, and in the proper way, and that absolutely no danger from starvation need be apprehended until this signal *has* been given, is absolutely true; and that these statements are true can be verified by anyone who cares to repeat my observations bearing on these points, or who is sufficiently unprejudiced and strong-willed to experiment on him or herself.

The artificial breaking of the fast; the taking of food in the absence of real hunger, for the reason that the ignorant attendant thinks the patient has "fasted long enough," is an abomination, and an outrage upon the system which cannot be too strongly deprecated. Perhaps I can best illustrate this point by a crude analogy. Suppose a watch had, in the course of years, become clogged with dust and other foreign matter; and suppose this watch possessed the power of *cleaning itself* by removing this matter (as our bodies do); then would it not be obvious that, so long as this cleansing process continued, it should not be checked or interrupted—but that, on the contrary, every moment that the watch was left alone, in its process of "cure," just so much improvement was certain. Would anyone think, under these circumstances, of voluntarily stopping the watch—in part at least—by introducing *more* foreign matter to be eliminated, on the ground that this would help to clean the watch, and eventually rid it of the impure matter the *sooner*, which is precisely what is done when we administer poisonous drugs? Ridiculous notion! Is it not obvious that *adding* to the material to be eliminated must eventually lengthen, not shorten, the process of repair?

And thus it is with the human machine—the human body. The sudden and artificial check to, or stoppage of, the process of cure (the fasting), would act just as detrimentally on the vital mechanism, as would the introduction of some foreign, unsought element—such as a pin—into the machinery of the watch. In both cases the result is the same, *viz.*, the stoppage of the vital mechanism, and the consequent check to the rapidly progressing process of cure.

An objection might here be raised to my analogy on the ground that food is not foreign matter to the body, in the same sense that the pin would be to the watch—inasmuch as food is generally capable of being appropriated and used by the system, in the process of repairing the tissues, whereas the pin must necessarily, and always, be damaging to the watch in and of itself. I may reply to this objection by pointing out the fact that, when the organs of digestion and assimilation are incapable of utilizing the food ingested (as is the case when a fast is badly needed), the one is just as harmful and as foreign to the organism as the other; both the food and the pin, at such times, representing a substance introduced into the organism which cannot be utilized to advantage; and which must be expelled before the process of cure can be continued. Besides, that is not my point. The food may be never so healthy and nutritious, and the digestive organs may also be capable of assimilating the food thus ingested, but the point is that the moment such digestion begins, the process of cure is necessarily retarded, or altogether checked in other parts of the body, and cannot be resumed until that meal is completely digested and the vital forces once more free to "turn their attention," so to speak, to the work of the purification of the system.

Human vitality may thus be conceived as an army defending an extensive line of fortifications. The more numerous the points of attack, the weaker the defense must necessarily be at each point; while, with the temporary complete withdrawal of the most constant and dangerous attacking force (the digestion), the army is thus left free to attack and demolish in detail the other harassing forces (the causes of the diseased condition); and, these once disposed of, be enabled again to concentrate its entire strength and energy upon the main attacking force (the digestion)—when again resumed—utilizing only a *portion* of the force available, and while keeping a considerable reserve on hand for any emergency (reserve force). The analogy is, of course, crude, but it will serve the purpose and is, I believe, at basis, true.

I have, throughout this chapter, been urging an abstinence from food until the return of "natural hunger." Now, it will be asked, what *is* this "natural hunger," and why do I thus carefully distinguish it from the hunger we experience every meal time, and which we are accustomed to associate with that name, and regard as true hunger?

The reason is this: That not one person in a thousand ever experiences natural hunger after reaching the age of maturity, and perhaps not even in youth or infancy; they have *never* experienced it! What they mistake for hunger is not real hunger at all, but a morbid craving, induced by an abnormal condition of the body—by stimulation, congestion, irritation, etc.

Let me make the distinction clear. *Normal hunger is never manifested in the stomach, but, like thirst, always in the glands of the throat and mouth.* Just as normal thirst is not experienced in the stomach, but in the system generally, and in the throat and mouth particularly—just so should normal hunger be manifested, and *is* so manifested, when normal.

"I have asked many thousands of persons, including many physicians, if they could describe to me the sensation of natural hunger," says Mr. Haskell,[1] 'Not one has been able to do it, unless he had obtained the knowledge through the "True Science of Living." They would always describe some sensation in the stomach, such as faintness, emptiness, or all-goneness; craving, gnawing, yearning, etc. These are the sensations of *appetite* and not of hunger, and are the results of wrong habits of eating. Like natural thirst, natural hunger is located in the mouth and throat, and is a sensation that food would taste deliciously. Natural hunger will come in the mouth and throat."

[1] "Perfect Health," pp. 45–7.

Horace Fletcher, in his "New Glutton or Epicure" (p. 107), thus distinguishes them:

"Its mark of distinction, to differentiate it from false appetite, is 'watering of the mouth' *for some particular thing.* False appetite is an indefinite craving for something, *anything,* to smother the disagreeable sensations, and frequently is expressed by the symptom of 'faintness' or 'all-goneness.'"

And, as Doctor Dodds insisted:[1]

"The sense of all-goneness in these cases is not from a lack of nutrient material, but owing to the absence of the habitual stimulus."

Natural hunger is never in a hurry, as Doctor Dewey reminded us; or, as another writer put it:

"False hunger is not likely to attack a man who lives simply and naturally upon unstimulating foods and drinks."

That this contention is founded upon correct observations and indubitable facts can be easily demonstrated. A close observation of many animals, and the more direct evidence of the few really normal adults and children who have been questioned upon the subject, have invariably led to the same conclusion; *viz.*, that true hunger and true thirst are both manifested in the glands of the throat, and never, under any circumstances, experienced in the stomach.

And it is here that true hunger is invariably manifested at the conclusion of the fast, when, if ever, we should expect to find genuine "normal hunger" present. The fact that it *is* so proves conclusively, to my mind, that normal hunger is manifest here, and here only; and inversely forms a complete and satisfactory "test" as to whether the sensations observed during the period of fasting signify real and natural hunger, or are merely symptoms of some morbid congestion, stimulation or irritation which would, if left alone, sooner or later pass away, allowing the fast to be continued, and thus conducted to its legitimate end. This last sentence furnishes the key whereby we may explain the unpleasant symptoms observable during the first two or three

[1] "The Diet Question," p. 87.

days of the fast—the empty, gnawing sensations nearly always mistaken for true hunger.

"No person," says Doctor Page,[1] "feels faint upon passing a meal, or has a gnawing stomach, except it be occasioned by an irritated or unduly congested state of that organ. It is a sure proof of dyspepsia, (using this term in its popular sense, as implying the condition of that organ). Strictly speaking, the term is a synonym of indigestion."

It may be objected that hunger is always felt in the stomach, and consequently must be normal—unless I am prepared to argue that normal hunger has never been experienced since infancy. I do not shrink from this conclusion; I *do* so consider it! Most persons have *never* experienced normal hunger in all their lives! Their appetites and tastes are perverted by overfeeding in infancy, and have never had a chance to become normal during the whole course of their lives—owing to the overfeeding being continued ever since. Says Doctor Dewey:[2]

"The first step in every disease is the very first moment when digestive balance is lost. With each one of you that evil work began *with your very first meal.* This meal was taken, forced upon you by the nurse, before Nature made any demand; in due time trouble began, every outcry was interpreted as a signal of hunger, and the oftener you were fed, the oftener the solemn stillness of all the air was broken by your nerve-lacerating music. Your meals, all through the first year of your life, were regulated by the tunes of crying."

That this gnawing sensation — usually mistaken for real hunger—is not *real* hunger is disproved, both theoretically and practically. Theoretically because true hunger comes, as we have seen, in the throat and mouth; and practically because these sensations will invariably subside, and altogether pass away, after these two or three initial days, when the habit of eating at certain fixed times is completely broken, and the new order of things is thoroughly planted in the mind (and body) of the patient. This gnawing sensation (supposed hunger) is

[1] "Horses; Their Feed and Their Feet," p. 28.
[2] "The True Science of Living," p. 200.

always greatest at, or about, meal time—if, indeed, it is not present at these hours of the day only. More strikingly than anywhere else is it here illustrated and demonstrated that hunger is purely and simply habit from beginning to end.

It must always be distinctly remembered, then, that neither this all-gone, faint feeling, nor the sensation of gnawing in the stomach are signs of true, normal hunger; but of a morbid, diseased appetite—either reaction from stimulation or indications of a diseased and congested stomach. And that this is the case is directly proved, it seems to me, by the fact that, in all cases of gastritis, *e.g.*, when food is invariably prohibited—even by the most "orthodox" physicians—and is known to be most harmful to the stomach at such a time—this feeling of gnawing and faintness and all-gonness is the very worst—proving beyond question that this sensation is merely a morbid craving.

This abnormal craving of the stomach may be carried to almost any extent. Doctor Miller mentions a case in which the patient "ate five full meals before dinner time and then, because food was denied him, he went to a barrel of offal and ate therefrom."[1]

The amount of food ingested (and allowed!) in some cases is almost incredible. Doctor Shew quotes a number of such cases in his "Family Physician." Thus, in one case, the patient ate four meals a day:

"Each meal sufficient for a stout laborer. Besides these four meals of meat and vegetables, he daily ate many pounds of dry bread, biscuit, and fruit. He had no sooner eaten a meal, than he denied that he had eaten anything, so that the more he ate, the more he desired. If he was not fed the moment he requested it, he sucked the bedclothes and bit his fingers like a child." (p. 93).

Again (pp. 283–4):

" . . . The quantity of food devoured in some cases of morbid appetite is almost incredible. Doctor Mortimer relates the case of a boy of only twelve years old, who from a feeling of inanition, had so strong a craving that he would gnaw his own flesh when not supplied with food; when awake, he was constantly

[1] "Vital Force," p. 39.

eating; the food given him consisted of bread, meat, beer, milk, water, butter, cheese, sugar, treacle, puddings, pies, fruits, broths, potatoes; and of these he swallowed, in six successive days, three-hundred and eighty-four pounds, eight ounces, avoirdupois, being sixty-four pounds a day on the average! The disease continued for a year; and that the hunger did not depend upon an extraordinary secretion of gastric juice, producing a rapid digestion, was evident from the fact that the food was usually rejected soon after it had been swallowed; but whether it passed into the duodenum could not be ascertained. . . "

Cases are also on record in which all kinds of abnormal things are craved—bullets, glass, stone, earth, pins, etc., being eaten with avidity. There are recorded cases of this disease in which there has been an inclination for devouring dirt, cinders, ordure, fire, spiders, lice, toads, serpents, leeches, bits of wood, hair, candles, and, as one author observes, "more literature in the form of printed books than is devoured by the first scholars of Christendom." Dirt eating is very common in some parts of Africa and South America.

Why such morbid appetites should be indulged, either by the physician or the family of the patient is an insoluble mystery.

But to return. The initial difficulty, in entering upon a fast, then, is due to the periodic recurrence of certain abnormal stomachic sensations, which are technically known as "habit hunger"; and must be successfully mastered and resisted at this time. Once this time is passed, the "danger period" as it is called, and all such abnormal and unpleasant sensations will completely disappear, and will not recur throughout a fast, however long it may be protracted, but will, instead, be terminated in Nature's own good time, by natural-hunger, as previously stated.

This habit-hunger (the "hunger of disease," as Doctor Dewey called it; "poison-hunger," in the language of Doctor Oswald) is absolutely abnormal in every single case, and is due to the confusion into which the stomach and digestive system is thrown, as a reaction from the incessant irritation and stimulation to which it has been subjected for a longer or shorter period of time. Just as a rum-tippler's system cries aloud for its customary stimulant, just so, here, does the abnormally excited digestive system call for its regular excitement, and if this is suddenly withdrawn, distressing symptoms are sure to follow. But these symptoms are processes of cure, and indicative of ultimate benefit, in both cases; and they should be so regarded. Eating food at such a time, and under such conditions, would be precisely the same, and as great a blunder as, "taking a drink," when the alcoholic reaction is at its height. Relapse, evil and disastrous, would be sure to follow in both cases.

In thus speaking of habit-hunger, however, I do not wish it understood that eating food at such times will not frequently relieve the sensation in that organ, *pro tem*, for it will. But that indicates nothing more than the fact that the patient has merely smothered the symptoms for the time being. As Doctor Page so well remarked:[1]

> "The fact that the meal affords immediate relief argues nothing against this position; it is the seventy-five or eighty per cent. of water contained in and taken with the meal that relieves the digestion. It forms a *poultice*, so to say, for the congested mucous membrane of the stomach; but unfortunately it can not, as when applied externally upon a throbbing, sore thumb, for example, be removed when it becomes dry."

Most people—who have never had the opportunity of watching the varied phenomena to be observed in cases of fasting—are under the impression that the undertaking of a fast is an extremely severe and trying ordeal. Popular fancy paints the unfortunate faster as suffering the most intense agonies from starvation—these increasing as the fast progresses, until the victim finally expires in the most excruciating agony! How false this picture is may readily be perceived by even a casual observation of a fasting patient, when viewed from a proper standpoint. In a fever case, *e.g.*, an absolute *aversion* to food of every kind is always present, and it would be far more cruel, in such cases, to force the food upon the patient, than to withhold it (as Nature indicates), since the wasting of the flesh continues with precisely the same rapidity in both cases—if anything, the patient who is fed loses flesh the faster of the two. If

[1] "The Natural Cure," p. 202.

food is withheld in such cases, the recovery is easy, rapid, and certain, and the patient at no period of the treatment misses his food in the slightest degree—in fact he feels, and is, infinitely safer and better without it. I have chosen fever to illustrate my point, for the reason that it is now all but universally acknowledged that the temporary withholding of food, in such cases, is beneficial and not detrimental to the patient, and the same remarks are applicable in every case of chronic or acute disease. And it is not even necessary for me to revert to such extremely and obviously pathological cases as these to prove the point here made. Anyone going into an experimental fast, or "physiological fast," as Doctor Dewey called it, can demonstrate this point for himself. Natural hunger is invariably absent throughout a strict fast, no matter how long this may last, and does not return until the fast is ready to be broken—this indicating that the system is rid of the cause of the disease. Schrott noted this, more than ninety years ago, and wrote:

"In the beginning of the process the appetite is almost wholly lost, so that two or three of the small dry biscuits are often sufficient for the whole day, the patient eating according to the inclination of appetite."

In his cure, he allowed a *very small* quantity of food to be eaten each day—mistakenly, I think.

This abnormal craving sensation in the stomach, occasionally experienced during the early days of the fast—may almost invariably be directly allayed by taking copious draughts of water; seeing that the abdominal muscles are thoroughly relaxed (they will often be found very contracted) and by diverting the attention from these organs into some outside channel. (See chapter on "Mental Influences.")

The "habit-hunger" spoken of above, generally lasts for two or three days before finally and completely disappearing, though the time naturally varies in each individual case. When once this period has passed, *no hunger will, in any case, be experienced until the fast is completed—is ready to be broken—and natural hunger then announces that the system is free from its previously diseased condition.* Though I have watched a great number of cases of fasting patients during the past few years, and have had, perhaps, exceptional opportunities for studying them, I have yet to meet with my first case in which (when plenty of water is drunk, and the mental influences are normal), these symptoms have persisted longer than three days. In several cases, to be sure, these distressing sensations have continued throughout a period of *almost* complete fasting; but in the "almost" lies the whole difficulty. Eating even a *mouthful* of solid or liquid food will have the immediate effect of unsettling the entire organism; stimulating the digestive organs into activity; exciting an intense hunger, and completely disorganizing and disturbing the whole progress of the fast—of "throwing the whole vital mechanism off the track"—as a friend once naïvely but forcibly expressed it.

Professor Parlow (when fasting for experimental purposes, and being afraid he would collapse!), wrote:

"Fearing that I should collapse, I resolved on the second or third day, to endeavor to create an appetite by swallowing a mouthful of wine. I felt it quite distinctly pass along the œsophagus into the stomach, and literally at that moment perceived the onset of a very strong appetite."[1]

The practice of eating "a little" daily, or irregularly during the fast, therefore, must be heartily deprecated for two reasons. First, because it prevents the complete and thorough cleansing process to progress satisfactorily and unimpeded. Secondly, because, by constantly drawing both the blood and the vital forces to the stomach when they should be engaged elsewhere, *it keeps the patient hungry.*

We have now seen that it is impossible to tell *à priori,* when to break the fast. No arbitrary time limit can be set; no definite date fixed upon beforehand and asserted that it would be the most advantageous for the patient were the fast broken on *that* day. Nature will always dictate when the fast is ready to be broken, if we but interpret her aright. The return of natural hunger is the great point to note, and the most important indication that the fast is ended, and the system is able and willing to digest and assimilate nutriment, in the form of either solid or

[1] "A. B.-Z. of Our Own Nutrition," pp. 243–4.

liquid food. The spontaneous and precisely coincidental cleaning of the tongue (pp. 441–4), of the breath (pp. 444–7), and the other and lesser phenomena which may be observed toward the termination of a "finish fast," all indicate that Nature, and Nature alone, is the authority to be consulted as to when the fast should be broken; and inversely proves conclusively that fasting is Nature's cure; counseled by her as the true remedial agent; and, when conducted under her care and according to her dictates, shows us that no danger can possibly result at any time during the fast's progress, and, indeed, that nothing can follow but beneficial results.

Proof of the correctness of this contention exists independently of the proofs cited above. In cases of paralysis, *e.g.*, or in diseases where the *daily* improvement can be distinctly and easily noted, we can clearly see and follow the process of cure; the rapid and successful elimination from the system of the morbid matter which forms, and is the real root and basis of, the disease. So long as the fast progresses, we can see this steady, daily improvement, and can clearly perceive the rapid and successful restoration of the patient to the normal, healthful condition. So long as the fast is allowed to progress undisturbed, this process of cure will continue undiminished. *But the moment the fast is broken this process of cure ceases; the improvement abruptly terminates and the patient is not cured completely, but is benefited just to the extent which corresponds (organically) to the actual time fasted.*

To illustrate: If, for example, a fast of thirty days is actually required in order to cure a given case of paralysis; and if the patient were to break his fast at the expiration of (say) ten days, under the impression that he had fasted "long enough"—and ignorant of the fact that normal hunger and vigorous health would ultimately arrive together, of their own accord, if only permitted to do so—this patient would then be, roughly speaking, only *one third cured;* that is, he would experience the benefit of the ten days he had fasted, but *that benefit only.* He would not derive a *complete* cure from the fast, which would have been the case had he "fasted to a finish." And this explains why so many patients are not cured completely, as they should have been, by the fasting cure; the fast has been broken prematurely. In many cases of protracted fasts, this is most clearly perceivable —every hour, almost every minute, restoring health and vigor to the system, and allowing us to almost *see* the effects of the elimination of the diseased material from the organism, and the consequent rapid return to normal conditions.

The question now remains: *How* shall the patient break his fast? Granting that he has followed it to its normal termination, and awaited the return of natural hunger (which may have arrived at the end of the third, the thirtieth, or the ninetieth day, as the case may be) of what food shall the first meal or meals consist? This is a highly important question, for it may easily be seen that however invigorated and capable the digestive organs are of performing their normal work; still, after such an unusual rest as they have had, we must begin cautiously, and only gradually increase the amount and the variety of food eaten, as time progresses. After any machine has been thoroughly oiled and repaired and put into perfect working order, it is never started at full speed *immediately*, but always allowed to increase in speed and gather momentum as the activity increases.

We have already noted the ill effects of the premature breaking of the fast; and attention must now be called to the evil consequences ensuing upon the *improper* breaking of the fast—even when done at the right time — the return of natural hunger. First, then, great care must be exercised not to eat *too much*. An extraordinarily vigorous appetite, and the apparent, and no doubt real, ability of the digestive system to successfully cope with, and assimilate, an almost unlimited supply of food material, may very readily induce us at first to indulge most gluttonously in food of all kinds; but this course must necessarily result in disastrous consequences, if persisted in. The organism will again become surfeited; the process of accumulating malassimilated food material and diseased tissue commence again —ultimately leading to a recurrence of the same disease (to cure which the fast was undertaken) or to a disease of another, and perhaps one of a worse and more dangerous character. This improper breaking of the fast is the real and the *only* danger connected with this system of treatment—since we have seen that the fast itself is not, and cannot be, anything but beneficial throughout.

When we come to consider the question: What foods are the best upon which to break a fast, we are met with a very puzzling question, and one concerning which there is no little controversy. Doctor Dewey has persistently maintained that appetite should guide the choice at that time absolutely; that normal conditions now being established, the appetite will only crave those foods that are beneficial to the organism, and that—thorough mastication being insisted upon—"there need be very little of restraint as to the bill of fare."[1] This view has received a most important reënforcement from the experiments and researches of Mr. Horace Fletcher, whose work has been previously quoted. It is most conclusively shown, in his writings, that, *when completely normal*, the appetite will crave *only* those foods which the system requires, and that this appetite can be safely and implicitly followed.

Doctor Dewey's position, as stated in his own words, is as follows:

"It may be said that the waste is so very trifling, especially with brain workers, that one may be a vegetarian, fruitarian, or even an eater of pork, without positive violence to practical physiology. There is this further very practical consideration, that when Nature is so fairly dealt with that she can speak in Natural tones, she will only call for those foods easily available along geographical lines."[2]

I am strongly opposed to this view of the matter, for many reasons—more particularly, perhaps, because of the following considerations: If the quality of food were suited to the climate man lived in, it would only be necessary for him to remove from one climate to another, in order to render "natural"—even "the best" for him—such complete change of diet as this change of climate would necessitate. To me this seems an inherent absurdity. Let us take a man, living in the tropics, *e.g.*, and living, let us say, on such fruits as the tropics afford. Let us now remove this man to the north temperate or frigid zone. It

[1] "New Era for Women," p. 115.
[2] "No-Breakfast Plan," p 108.

is contended that, simply because of this change, his nutrition should be completely changed, as though his physiological needs had undergone a complete change also—and within a few days! Would such mere change of external temperature alter, in any appreciable degree, his real digestive capacity and physiological requirements? Certainly not! As Doctor Schlickeysen re-remarked:[1] "Climate and surroundings cannot change the nature of man with regard to food." Again, we should not forget that man is naturally a tropical animal, since those were doubtless the regions from which he originally sprang. And it must also be remembered that fruit seems to be the natural food of certain classes of animals, throughout the tropics, and of man, almost exclusively. (pp. 81–9.) And the fact that this is man's natural food far outweighs the other fact that man *can live* (after a fashion) on other foods of all kinds—since that merely proves what a wonderful ability the body actually possesses of sustaining itself under the most adverse circumstances. No: man has a certain fixed, definite *type* of diet, just as every other animal has, and any prolonged and gross perversion of Nature's laws, in this respect, will ultimately and inevitably be followed by the penalties of such transgression.

Nevertheless I am persuaded that the appetite will frequently call for foods which are distinctly "unnatural," if not absolutely detrimental, at the period of breaking the fast. Thus Doctor Dewey (allowing his patients to eat at this time whatever their appetites craved), speaks of one case in which "soft toast, well buttered," was demanded,[2] and of another where the call was—"not for chemically prepared food, but for beefsteak."[3] Other cases are mentioned here and there among the writings of those who have observed fasting patients, of similar appetites and cravings—cravings which I must believe to be distinctly and demonstratively abnormal. (See Book II., Chapter I.)

Mr. Purinton's remark, in this connection, seems to me extremely pointed. He says:[4]

"People shrink from the fast because of the follies that usually accompany it. Milton Rathbun, for instance—Doctor Dewey's

[1] "Fruit and Bread," p. 207.
[2] "New Era," p. 145.
[3] "True Science of Living," p. 313.
[4] "Philosophy of Fasting," p. 17.

star case—fasted thirty-five days, then made his first meal of oysters, soda crackers, beef broth and oolong tea! All of which iniquities a really hungry man cannot crave. If the pupil of so famous a teacher didn't clarify his instinct any better than that, what could you expect from common folk, uninstructed and uninspired?"

Why such food should be craved, at this time, when the appetite should, theoretically, be perfect, presents an apparently hopeless paradox—yet one which can, I believe, be shown to be no paradox at all.

Our appetites and tastes undoubtedly depend largely, if not absolutely, upon our mental conditions; upon heredity and race impressions, above all upon the present and existing environment. Whatever food has been customarily supplied to meet the demands of the stomach—that food will be the one most naturally craved upon the return of hunger and the ability to eat. In other words, the food craved upon the return of hunger will be food which we were accustomed to eat before entering upon the fast—this being in turn dependent upon the environment of the patient. Thus, the native of India—whose staple food is rice—would crave rice upon the return of natural hunger. Similarly, the Esquimaux would crave for blubber; while the average American or Englishman would, in all probability, crave for roast beef and boiled potatoes! It is all a matter of habit and custom; environment and previous habits of life mold the appetite as surely as they have molded our characters; and our tastes and desires are entirely dependent, at such times, upon our previous habits of eating. Thus it is that the food craved, at the conclusion of the fast, may be—not the food which would be most beneficial to the patient, or that the system most requires, but the food to which the patient had been formerly accustomed, and to which his thoughts would naturally recur when hunger again made it possible for him to eat. It is thus all due to existing mental conditions—these governing the appetite to the extent that we actually crave those foods which we think we require—rather than those actually called for! On any diet whatsoever this is the case. The food craved will be that which we expect to crave. That vegetarians or fruitarians, who have thus fasted, crave their own particular class of foods, and none other, upon the resumption of eating, I can testify from personal experience. Mr. Purinton asserts that this was so in his own case also.[1] Sir E. Bulwer-Lytton observed this fact likewise. See "The Philosophy of Water Cure," by John Balbirnie, M.D., p. 138.

In another place,[2] Doctor Dewey refers to this very point, and (to my mind wrongly) remarks:

"At the close of long fasts for acute sickness, Nature never objects to the odors of the frying pan or the oven; she never calls for fruits, nuts, or any of those raw foods whose palatability and digestibility are increased by cooking."

Again I say, my own observations disprove this statement; though I do not deny the effect of the frying odors! But it must be remembered in this connection that the smell of frying will cause the flow of saliva and arouse the appetite as soon as we are awake, hence this is no argument against breaking the fast —unless Doctor Dewey should be prepared to admit that his whole theory of the no-breakfast plan is wrong—which is certainly not the ease.

Having now disposed of the theory that any food that is craved may be allowed, we again return to our question, which is still unanswered; *viz.*, what foods are the best upon which to break the fast? The food must obviously be light, for the reason given above (pp. 555–6), while the fact that it should be "natural" food goes without saying. For this reason, many prescribe fruit for a first meal—Mr. Macfadden having compiled, for that purpose, a carefully selected list of some forty-eight fruits, etc., especially suitable for eating at this time.[3] This is undoubtedly far nearer the truth than Doctor Dewey's method —which must be deprecated in any case; but I do not believe that, in spite of the numerous suggestions offered, the right diet has as yet been suggested.

Thus, Miss N. M. Pratt advocates: "Grape-nuts, a shredded wheat biscuit, or a dish of Force or Malta Vita."[4] Doctor Han-

[1] "PhilosophV of Fasting," p. 20.
[2] "The Art of Living," p. 20.
[3] "Natural Cure for Rupture," pp. 99–100.
[4] "The Body Beautiful," p. 61

ish, again, who is supposed to know something of the laws of fasting, advocates popcorn![1]

My own experience, and the experience of those with whom I have been associated in practice, or of fasters whom I have known personally, all seem to indicate this fact; that, at this time, and in the vast majority of cases, *liquid food only* should be taken—preferably in the form of fruit juices, freed from the pulp; and that this diet should be followed to the exclusion of all other food, liquid or solid, for the first day, and sometimes for the initial two or three days, after breaking the fast, when solid food may gradually be added. The great danger consists in overeating, and this desire must be repressed at all costs for these few days. No definite rule can, of course, be set, one that can be strictly followed in every case. Here, as everywhere, allowances must be made for personal idiosyncrasies. Nevertheless, I have never met a case in which the juice of an orange or a glass of grape juice (unfermented) was other than grateful and productive of beneficial results. They may be safely given, in practically every case, and, if "Fletcherized" carefully, will form a meal both satisfying and sustaining. Another such "meal" may be allowed about six hours after the first; and late the next morning, if hunger is experienced, and a desire for a more substantial meal be manifested, a light luncheon may be allowed, followed by an equally light supper. The next day a little more indulgence may be allowed in the patient's diet, and so on, guided always by the patient's hunger, and the kind and amount of food craved. If properly and thoroughly masticated, it is astonishing how *small* an amount of food will be called for, once this "danger period" has passed. Indeed this holds good at any period of our lives whatever—be it after a fast or no.

One other point may here be noted. The *distinction between fasting and starving* should now be clear to us. Throughout this book I have been advocating the theory of fasting; I cannot too strongly condemn the practice of starving! For they are not by any means interchangeable or synonomous terms, as many think. *Fasting* is a scientific method for ridding the system of diseased tissue and morbid matter, and is invariably accompanied

[1] "How to Fast," p. 11.

by beneficial results. *Starving* is the deprivation of the tissues from the nutriment which they require, and is as invariably followed by disastrous consequences. The whole secret is this. *Fasting commences with the omission of the first meal and ends with the return of natural hunger; while starvation only begins with the return of natural hunger and terminates in death. Where the one ends, the other begins.* Whereas the latter process wastes the healthy tissues, emaciates the body, and depletes the vitality; the former process merely expels corrupt matter and useless fatty tissue—thereby elevating the vitality, increasing the energy, and eventually restoring to the organism "that just balance we term health." As Doctor Dewey so truly and so pithily said:[1] "*Take away food from a sick man's stomach, and you have begun—not to starve the sick man, but the disease.*" There is the whole science and philosophy of fasting in a nutshell.

The Reaction After Fasting

The reaction after fasting, when once the fast has been broken, is typical, certain and speedy. The tongue, breath, pulse, etc., being—at the time of breaking the fast—practically *normal,* no improvement can be noted by the study of any of these otherwise very reliable indicators of the bodily condition; nor can the special senses be rendered more acute; but there is a general exhilaration consequent upon the ingestion of the first meal which is quite indescribable unless experienced. This will, I know, be looked upon as the "strength" which the food has imparted to the organism, but since, as I have endeavored to show (pp. 225-303), we never derive either strength or vitality from the food we eat, we must look for the explanation in some other direction, and, thus looked for, it is not hard to find.

The sudden apparent inrush of energy, consequent upon the ingestion, of the first meal, cannot be due to the "strength" which this meal has furnished, since food, on any theory whatever, *must first be assimilated* before its potential energy can be realized by the system; whereas the energy resultant upon the ingestion of this meal is manifested almost *immediately*—certainly far too soon for the system to have appropriated any of

[1] "True Science of Living," p. 5.

its nutrient elements, which would be necessary if the currently accepted theories were true. No, the food must react in an entirely different manner, and this I believe to be somewhat as follows:

At the conclusion of a fast, the circulation and vital forces of the body are almost evenly distributed throughout—the internal organs and periphery receiving as nearly as possible the proper proportionate amount, without an undue concentration of the blood and energies at any one point. Consequent upon the ingestion of the first meal, however, this entire equilibrium is disturbed. The blood and vital forces of the body are brought suddenly, and centered continuously, upon the stomach and digestive system—this being necessitated by the processes of digestion. The bodily energy at once begins to be expended in this digestion. The vital forces, so long latent, are aroused and forcibly concentrated upon one point. Now, since, as we have seen (p. 41), energy is always felt, appreciated or perceived in its *expenditure*, never in its *accumulation*, this energy, so long latent, is now aroused into sudden activity: the process of its expenditure begins—being then perceived by us, for the first time, for the reason that it is now being forcibly *expended*. In other words, the sudden arousal of the vital energies and their concentration at one point constitutes a species of *stimulation* which is, in reality, the "strength" which the food is supposed to have furnished.

It will thus be seen that, from a physical point of view, I regard *stimulation* as the true and sufficient cause for all the elation of spirits observed; an indirect proof being that, the more stimulating the food, the greater will this stimulation, or reaction be. Hot food will stimulate more than cold, for example. But there is also a highly important consideration which we must by no means omit to notice. This is the question of *mental influence*. So ingrained is the belief that food furnishes strength and vitality to the organism that it is next to impossible to rid the mind of the patient of that belief; and even though he may fully understand and appreciate the *rationale* of the fasting cure, there is, I believe, always present a kind of sub-conscious belief that an increase of strength and energy will result upon the breaking of the fast, which, of course, is found to be the case, but for the reasons mentioned above.

This constant auto-suggestion is bound to bring about, to some extent, its own realization. Add to this the fact that a certain peace of mind is present as a result of knowing that the crisis is past and that the cure has been effected—and the mental elation over the prospect of health, strength and consequent happiness in the future—and we have found, I think, the explanation (in a great measure at least) of the exhilaration which follows upon the breaking of a protracted fast.

There are still other reasons, however, which tell in favor of my theory (that stimulation is the cause of the renewed strength) and away from that generally held—that the food during the process of digestion, actually imparted energy to the system. One such consideration is the fact that an almost *infinitesimal amount* of food will seem to impart s amuch "strength" as will a far more elaborate repast. Now, if the accepted theories were true, this ought not to be the case, since, on that hypothesis, the amount of the strength imparted ought to precisely correspond to the amount of food eaten, when, as a matter of fact, it does not; a very small meal, or even a mouthful or two, generally producing practically the same results as a far larger meal, indeed, an even moderately heavy meal, at this time, will soon bring on a feeling of lassitude and physical depression; all of which is perfectly intelligible on the theory proposed on pp. 225–303, but absolutely incomprehensible so long as the present-day theories are clung to; these latter facts being especially significant when we take into consideration that the digestive organs, together with the rest of the physical organism, are, at the moment of breaking the fast, at the point of their highest attainable vital vigor.

Just here let me answer an objection which I can forsee will be raised by the critical reader, and which I did not perhaps elaborate at sufficient length on pp. 555–6. It may be contended that if the organism is, at the moment of breaking the fast, enjoying the greatest freedom from diseased conditions, the vital powers having reached their climax, digestion at this time should be *more*, not *less* easily accomplished than at any other subsequent period, and for precisely the reasons that I have given. A little reflection will, I think, convince any candid person that this is not necessarily the case. Let us see. For many weeks past the stomach and bowels have not been called upon to perform any work whatever (comparatively speaking), and the saliva, the gastric juice and the other digestive juices have practically ceased to be secreted. (See pp. 504–5.) The brain system has been called upon for no long continued taxation in this direction. The circulation has been "equalized away," if I may so express it, from the stomach and digestive system generally; in other words, this section of the bodily machine has, for all practical purposes, *ceased to operate.* Now the question I propose is this: should we, under such circumstances, start off the machine again immediately *under the highest possible pressure?* Should we not rather start the machine *gradually*, working it up to its greatest speed and pressure as the time passes? Every analogy points to this as the correct method. The printing press, or the steam engine, is not at once started at its greatest rate of speed (if it were, there might, and probably would be a break down), but is *gradually* worked up to that point—to its maxi mum speed, and I contend that it is only natural to suppose that the vital machinery should be treated in precisely the same manner. Did the printing press and the steam engine *gather energy* during their periods of rest, as does the body, the parallel would be almost perfect. But the simile is close enough for all practical purposes. The potential energy may be far greater at the moment of breaking the fast than at a later period, but the *facilities for expending it* are not so perfect, and they must be gradually "exercised back" into working order, before the machine can again be run at full speed; but when once this has been attained, it will be found that almost an unlimited amount of food can be eaten and utilized by the system before the vital powers are again lowered and the retention of effete matter recommences—before the body once more becomes diseased. Needless to say, this condition should never be reached, only sufficient food being taken to keep the body healthy and well supplied with nourishment.

Thus, while a certain amount of indulgence may be allowed

in the matter of food after the second or third day from the time of breaking the fast, considerable care must be exercised not to let the patient constantly overfeed. To do this would be to offset the beneficial effects of the fast, and to re-invite a diseased condition. While the body is perfectly normal, at the time of breaking the fast, it must be remembered that its *improper breaking* constitutes its chief, if not its only, danger; and there can be no guarantee to the patient that his former condition will not return if he abuses himself in this manner again. *Anyone can make himself ill very easily!* At the first sign of returning ill health, should such appear, a supplementary fast should always be undertaken—the omission of a few meals usually sufficing, in such cases, to completely restore the organism to vigorous health.

Long and Short Fasts

Any meal that is ever omitted, so long as natural hunger—the keenest of appetites—is not present, is clearly that much gain; and yet many persons worry because, *e.g.*, a member of the family omits a meal, through indisposition or aversion! There need be no worry, no trepidation whatever! All that it is necessary for the patient to do, in order to regain his healthy, normal appetite, is to omit that meal and wait for the next; and if he is not truly hungry then, await the next, and so on until a natural hunger *does* return. And why not follow out this exceedingly rational and simple system? What harm can possibly come to the organism from this omission of food? What is there to fear? Is it not obvious that the opposition is purely prejudice? Let us see what is lost and what is gained by this omission of a meal. *All that is lost is the amount of tissue which the food ingested would build up* (were it utilized completely and properly by the system, which, in diseased conditions, it is not). That, and nothing more! And what is gained? *The amount of energy or vital force that would otherwise have been expended in digesting and eliminating that amount of food matter, and in cleansing the encumbered system of the added effete material which imperfect digestion must of necessity produce.* Clear gain, no loss! It is entirely owing to the present false theories as to the relations of food and energy that renders it possible for beliefs to be held which are so completely at variance with philosophy and observed facts.

The same remarks apply to all cases of fasting of however long duration. Until the return of natural hunger, every minute during which the fast is protracted is that much gain, and cannot possibly be otherwise. Nevertheless there are individuals who would never undertake a strict fast of any great duration—but who might be prevailed upon to take several fasts of shorter duration; these fasts to be interspersed with periods of light eating. Thus, a two or three days' fast might be taken, followed by one day's eating; then another two or three days' fast, followed by another day of eating; and so on until a considerable time has elapsed (it may be several months), when a return of the normal condition is established and the days of fasting become no longer necessary

That this method will appeal to many of my readers as in many ways preferable, I do not doubt. It is a less severe strain upon the patient's will power, and eventually accomplishes very much the same result. We will, therefore, compare the above two methods of treatment; and I shall endeavor to point out that the latter is, in reality, an infinitely less satisfactory way of bringing about the desired result, both from a mental and from a physical point of view.

We have, in any diseased condition, a certain amount of foul material to be eliminated from the system, and the length of time required to complete this elimination—the duration of the fast—depends upon its nature, its amount, and the innate vitality of the patient.

Before health is restored *all* this foul material must be eliminated, and it is only natural to suppose that effecting this result in the shortest time possible would ultimately be the best method for the patient, and exhaust his vitality the least, since every day this material is retained must weaken the patient (ultimately) to just that extent. The best and most effective method of treatment, therefore, would be the one which would effect the elimination in the shortest time possible; and this can be done in no other manner so speedily and so effectively as by the absolute unbroken or "finish" fast.

For, when the vital machinery has once set upon its work of purification, all the digression or diversion of this energy must constitute a more or less effective "check" (see p. 556), and I believe that this "check" is in almost direct proportion to the amount of the food swallowed.

Since we know that we can go without nutriment of any kind with safety and benefit, and that for a period of time not less than several weeks (*v.* pp. 160–1); and since, in all diseased conditions, Nature will clearly indicate when food is needed, by sending up an urgent call for it; why not continue the fast to its legitimate conclusion, when it is once entered upon? since it will effect, by this means, in a few weeks, what would require double or treble that time on the other system. The unpleasant "dose" is taken all at once and effectually disposed of for all time, while the patient may have the satisfaction of knowing that this method is shorter, better and more effective than the other, which is the more unscientific method. No person would voluntarily undertake anything but a finish fast who thoroughly appreciated the physiology and philosophy of fasting; who understood the fact that no energy is lost during a fast; and that natural hunger will invariably indicate when the fast is ready to be broken—such hunger always appearing before death from starvation is possible.

But there are two other objections to this system of short fasts which I will mention here, though briefly.

First, it has been my experience that the system of alternate fasting and feeding is much *harder on the patient* (though he does not know it) for the reason that *it tends to keep him constantly hungry*. I have elsewhere pointed out (p. 556–7), that the first few days of the fast are the trying ones, in which "habit hunger" is noted, and the lack of stimulation felt, more than at any other period of the fast. Now, on the plan of alternate eating and fasting, practically *all* the time is converted into "first days," inasmuch as the patient is always just commencing a fast, when it is again broken off, to be again resumed at the expiration of the day of feeding. The result is that the patient is in a constant state of alternate stimulation and depression, which is really far harder to endure than the more simple and more effective method of omitting food altogether. The cure is no sooner commenced than it is again retarded. The old adage "Abstinence is easier than Temperance" applies here with even more than its ordinary force.

The *second* reason for my so strongly advocating a "finish" fast—as opposed to the series of shorter fasts—is this: In the latter method, the bowels never have a chance to become thoroughly emptied and cleansed—as they do in the former. Reference to the chapter on "The Enema" will show that the bowels often retain their fecal contents for weeks after no food whatever is permitted to enter them—and this, after repeated bowel washings. A complete emptying and purification can only follow a thorough and complete abstinence from all solid food; and I am convinced, from my experience and observations, that this is never satisfactorily accomplished upon the (otherwise unsatisfactory) method of a series of short fasts—broken into by alternate days of eating.

REFLECTIONS AND CONCLUSIONS

The task I set myself, in writing this volume, is now practically complete—so far, at least, as my limited knowledge enables me to complete it at all; and it but remains for me to summarize the results attained, and to add one or two further reflections that are suggested by the theories and the facts brought forward, which will, I hope, at least stimulate others to original research in these lines, even though the conclusions arrived at in this book be not accepted. As I have several times pointed out, the present book is intended to be merely a pioneer work in a hitherto neglected field of inquiry, and consequently cannot pretend to do more than indicate certain lines of research which might profitably be followed out in detail by others more competent to do so than I; also to offer a protest against the present materialistic scheme of physiology, and the theory that we derive our vitality and bodily heat from the food we eat—both of which doctrines seem to me to be palpably and demonstrably untrue. Other, more general, speculations will, it is hoped, not be without interest; and may possibly suggest lines for further inquiry and research.

In Book I. we saw that all disease is in reality a curing process—the various diseases, so-called, being but the various methods of elimination, from the system, of effete material—unduly retained therein, which should have been eliminated. This shows that all "disease" is, at basis, fundamentally *one;* and has a common cause—which is equally the cause of all disease. This cause is the material floating at large in the body, and this material must have been directly or indirectly derived from the food eaten, since the material must have got into the body and circulation in some manner, and we saw that the only normal way it can get into the circulation is through the stomach—through an excess of food and drink; consequently, that the source or cause of all disease must be the same at basis; *viz.*, some defect in the food supply—the various diseases, so-called, being but the various methods of ridding the system from the excess of this material ingested.

We saw that it was impossible, on this account, to "cure" disease by drugs, many reasons being advanced which show clearly that drugs can be of no possible benefit to the man diseased; but that, on the contrary, they may be of inestimable harm; all tonics and stimulants also being harmful, for the reason that the apparent strength resulting from their administration is merely fictitious strength, and ultimately tends to weaken and ruin the body. Passing, then, to the germ theory, we saw that the real cause of the various "germ diseases" was, not the germ itself, but that condition of the body which rendered possible the presence, within it, of the germ in question; and hence that the real disease, here, as elsewhere, is the bodily condition—this condition being, the presence of the same effete material, which is the cause of all disease. Consequently these diseases, no less than others, are shown to be due to the same primary cause—more or less direct over-nutrition.

Finally we saw that, the cause of all disease being the same—the retention, within the system, of effete material—the means of cure must be the same also—the removal of that material; and this once removed, the cause of all disease would be removed, in consequence; and, the cause once removed, the effects must cease; and the disease be cured. And the only way in which this can be accomplished is to eliminate this morbid material from the system—by oxidizing it off, and by eliminating it through the various depurating organs.

In Book II. we saw that the human race does overeat monstrously—enabling us to perceive that it is quite possible for the body to become choked and blocked with food material, after the manner described in the previous book. Thus we can see that fasting, or abstaining from food, must of necessity be the great, ultimate means of cure, for the reason that it enables the system to throw off this overload of impurities; increasing the vitality and enabling the eliminating organs to dispose of the mass of mal-assimilated material within the system, which is the cause of the disease; also it is clearly apparent that, if we did not ingest so much food in the first place, fasting and even disease would be wholly unnecessary and even impossible, for the reason that the causes of disease would be no longer in the body—not being supplied—and consequently could not possibly be eliminated from it.

The remaining three books cannot and need not be summarized here; since, the theory once established and understood, the detailed exposition of the theory is not necessitated. Many pet theories will doubtless be shattered, but that cannot be helped; if our ultimate goal be Truth, it cannot be helped if the means by which it is reached be over smooth ground or over stony. The truth will ultimately prevail, in any case, and it is immaterial to me whether it be reached through myself or through another. I certainly have no personal interest in any of the theories advanced, and if they can be shown to be false and untrue, no one will delight in the ultimate triumph of truth more than myself. It is simply in the hope of arriving at the truth that this book is written.

Turning now, to the physiological side of the question for a few moments:

It may be objected that I have exalted fasting to the dignity of—that bugbear of science—a panacea. That a panacea is an impossibility I deny. The panacea which has been the object of such continuous search for so many ages, and at the possibility of which modern science, so-called, scoffs, is to me an assured scientific fact. I pay no attention to the scoffs. Science has proved herself both wrong and arrogant too many times for the impartial searcher after truth to be turned aside from his researches, from what he considers the truth, by her taunts. I cannot accept the prevailing ideas on this question, of the possibility, or rather impossibility, of a panacea. It does not appeal to my sense of right, of the ultimate justice of things. I cannot conceive that a law of Nature can be broken without retribution following as its inevitable consequent—the retribution exactly corresponding, in extent, to the extent of the transgression. Try as we may, to get away from this truth, it is there nevertheless, fixed, unalterable. It pervades the moral, the mental and the physical worlds alike. Every analogy and the experience of our daily lives prove this to be the case. And the reverse of all this is, I must insist, as obviously and as necessarily true. Were we to follow Nature's teachings and live according to her rules, sickness and premature death would be utterly absent from our universe—quite impossible, necessarily absent, in the nature of things. I cannot conceive it otherwise. The universe would be altogether irrational were this not so—which, as we know, is not the case. There is no more absurdity in this statement than is implied in the former one. Both are merely opposite aspects of one great truth. The simplicity of it all is the greatest drawback to its acceptance. Will not the Universe prove simple when rightly understood?

Those who accept the above statement as fact (and I can see no reason for any rational doubt) and who accept the theory propounded on pp. 14–19 of the "Unity and Oneness of All Disease," and the consequent necessity of a uniform and single method of cure, can surely find no difficulty in accepting the possibility of a panacea—which is nothing more than this same method in operation. Why hesitate to accept it? Is it not rational and simple? Does it not cover and explain all the facts in the case? Why its inherent absurdity and the difficulty experienced in conceiving its verity and existence? To be sure it is decried by the medical profession, but, to the majority of the medical profession, the theory of the unity and oneness of all disease is as a sealed book. Once its pages are cut, why refuse to read? For my part, I cannot conceive that a panacea is not possible, or in fact anything but a most obvious certainty.[1]

In saying that fasting is a panacea I, of course, admit that even this most potent method has, and must have, its limitations. As I have before pointed out, and here reaffirm, while there is no such thing as an incurable *disease*, there may be incurable *cases*. It is possible that the patient's vitality is at so low an ebb that recovery is impossible, no matter what measures may be taken for his relief. The scale has already turned—and against him. In such cases, of course, nothing can be done but

[1] Doctor Rabagliati, in his "Air, Food and Exercises," p. 519, says: "Are there any diseases to which the same principles [of fasting] are not applicable? I do not know of any."

to make his last moments on earth as comfortable as possible. Again, if sickness be due to psychical defect or anatomical lesion (purely mental disease or mechanical obstruction or interference) fasting may, of course, be unsuccessful here also; but I should advise it in such cases even then, and for two reasons—or perhaps three. (1) We cannot ever tell whether a mental malady be "purely" such, or dependent upon an abnormal functioning of the brain, until the experiment be tried. If the latter, it would, as I conceive, effect a cure in every (curable) case. (2) The "suggestion" that fasting will benefit should be of the very greatest help—even in all cases of "purely" mental disease—if such exist; and (3) fasting will improve the general tone of the body, enabling it to successfully withstand and recuperate from any operation, etc., that might be necessary in cases of anatomical defect, due to accident, injury, etc. In such cases, fasting would prove of the very greatest benefit.

Again, it may be objected that this proposed method of curing all diseases, from the crown of the head to the sole of the foot, by fasting, by "striking only through the stomach," and depriving it of food, is absurd, inasmuch as it does not in any way treat the affected part directly. To this I reply that it is by no means so absurd as the habit of taking drugs into the stomach, for the cure of every imaginable ill—the alleviation of an ache or pain in any part of the body whatever—yet this is the all but universal practice! Secondly, fasting does not appear at all absurd, as a cure for all bodily complaints, when we realize the fact that the blood reaches every part of the body, and every part of the body depends upon the quality of the blood for its tone and general character, whether healthy or morbid, and can be diseased or rendered healthy by no other medium, through no other channel. And as the blood is, in turn, altogether dependent for its composition upon the character of the food supply, we can readily see how, by influencing the former, beneficially or otherwise, we thereby influence the latter, and thus effect a cure, no matter of what part—all parts being equally dependent upon the blood for their nutrition, their composition and character.

And it must always be borne in mind, in considering this question of a panacea, that, in all diseased conditions, no matter what, and in all stages of such diseases, practically the same conditions prevail; *i.e.*, insufficient vitality is present, and either an excess or a deficit of more or less morbid material with which to build the required tissue or structure. Thus the fundamental requirements for the cure of any disease whatsoever becomes at once manifest. Increase the amount of vitality available for the purposes of repairing the bodily structure; if too much, lessen, and if too little, increase, the amount of nutriment supplied to the tissues; and improve the tone or quality of the material thus supplied. These essentials must lie at the root of all methods of cure whatsoever; and, no matter what the disease, they must be the prime objects sought, and without them there can be no true cure in any case. Our only need our sole object—then, is to find them; and having found the method that will supply or fulfill all these requirements, then the panacea will have been discovered—for if not, why not?

Now, we have seen (pp. 225–303) that fasting does increase the bodily vitality—rendering available for the purposes of cure a vastly greater amount than is generally the case; and we have also seen (pp. 121–2) that fasting has the effect of either lessening or increasing the amount of nutriment supplied the tissues—decreasing the quantity, if necessary, in cases of surfeit, and increasing the quantity in cases of local anæmia—where such has resulted from the excess of material in the blood, blocking or choking the smaller blood vessels, and so effectually preventing the free passage of nutrient material to these parts where it is needed and which are starving because of the lack of it. And finally we saw (pp. 154–8) how fasting, because of its great cleansing and purifying action, freed the system from all morbid material, rendering a return to health possible because of this very action. And so we have, combined in this process, the three essentials for a successful cure, each in a very perfect degree. And, this being the case, I ask, what possible objection can there be to this method of cure, and in fact how can we escape accepting it as a true panacea—a method of treatment applicable alike to every case of disease equally, and to every state or stage of such disease? To me, this position seems the one into which we are driven and from which there is no escape. Philosophically, as well as practically, the panacea is a most obvious and positive reality.

One great objection will always be raised to this theory of fasting—an objection that will be raised equally against the use of enemas, against food reform, in fact against all hygienic agencies whatever. It is this: That, if people would only *think* correctly, everything else would be of secondary or subsidiary importance; that is, the "mental factor" is raised to the highest possible level—the position being that, if the mental conditions were adjusted properly, health might be preserved in spite of the most disadvantageous surroundings or unphysiological life; that the mind can, in short, overcome and rise above the harmful results that would otherwise ensue, and enable the body to completely offset and "antidote," as it were, the ills that would otherwise afflict the body because of the insanitary surroundings or unhygienic habits.

This is the position stated, I think, fairly—or perhaps I had better let one of the advocates of this school speak for himself. Says Charles Brodie Patterson:[1]

"So it is with everything in life. It all depends upon the way we do a thing, the way we *think* about it. If we could only see it, the tonic does not come from the physical exercise alone, and even the extraction of certain properties from the food we eat depends upon the condition of mind. Many will eat the most nourishing food and fail to derive any benefit from it. You may pay all the attention you like to your food, but you will never build up your bodies till your minds are thoroughly poised. . . . For a long period I had devoted myself to the subject of food and derived no good from it. Just so soon, however, as I put my faith in other things and forgot the body (in the sense of centering my care upon it), it became well and strong and has remained so ever since."

This is the position of a very large number of persons, and to them I am, of course, paying far too little attention to the mental factor and far too much to the physiological factors in the case. I have tried to show in my chapter on "Mental Influences," that I consider this factor as one of the very greatest

[1] "The Will to be Well," pp. 177, 178.

consequence, but it is not *all*-important, as its votaries would insist. I admit that a proper mental attitude is on every impor tant avenue toward the regaining and maintenance of health, but it is not the only factor. I agree with Mr. Salt, where he says:[1]

"There is a tendency among certain 'psychical' authorities of the present day to eschew the vegetarian doctrine as itself 'materialistic,' and as attributing too much importance to the mere bodily functions of eating and digesting. . . . Though it is true in a sense that spirit can sanctify diet, it is not true that a general sanction is thereby given to any diet whatsoever, no matter what cruelties may be caused by it, or who it be that causes them. . . . If food is one of the 'indifferent' things, why do you hold fast to your flesh diet, like a snarling dog to his bone?"

The position I would assume, then, is that the mental and the physical factors work side by side, in this question of health, and that one cannot be studied and practiced and the other altogether neglected—the practice alike of the Christian Scientists and the materialistic physicians. We must take into consideration *both* factors, and we cannot possibly neglect one of them.

But the point I wish to make just now is this: That, in taking the attitude they do (that the mind can, by certain concentrated effort, overcome the evil effects of an unphysiological life, and restore health to the organism), and even admitting that all this is possible, I would point out this fact which, to my mind, conclusively proves their position to be wrong. It is that these mental scientists are forced to admit the fact that *there are certain bad, unphysiological conditions to be overcome; i.e.*, that the body has become more or less abnormal and diseased, because of its unnatural modes of life, and it is this abnormal condition which the mind is called upon to cure. Now the point I make is this: Why should we cause or induce such abnormal conditions in the first place? Why should we allow the body to become diseased at all — thus necessitating its cure—by mental or any other means whatever? Would it not be much simpler to *prevent* the diseased condition from coming about by proper, physiological living, and not to necessitate its "cure" by mental effort

[1] "Logic of Vegetarianism," pp. 72–73.

or by any other means? It seems to me that, by thus allowing the body to become diseased, and then "curing" it by mental control (even granting that this is the case), we burn the candle at both ends, for the reason that we devitalize the body by allowing it to become diseased, and then waste more energy in the mental effort to get well again! I ask, is it not more simple as well as more philosophical so to regulate the life that such diseased states and such "cures" are not necessary—thus saving alike the vitality we should expend in becoming diseased and in becoming cured—in more profitable occupations and pursuits?

So, once more and finally, we are driven to believe that proper balancing and limitation of the food supply is the one all-important factor—compared with which every other is comparatively unimportant and even insignificant. The question of food supply—its quality and quantity—is the greatest question before the world to-day; and I think the sooner this is realized the better it will be for the community at large. The evil effects of overfeeding cannot, to my mind, be overestimated, and the solution of this food question will solve many other—social, economic and industrial—no less than physiological and scientific problems. The fact that we do not derive our strength and energy from food alone should revolutionize medical practice; and more than that, enable us to see that a purely materialistic scheme of this universe is probably insufficient to explain all the facts it presents for our consideration; and that, in fact, these very facts, once established, disprove it. For that reason, I consider that the theory has tremendous philosophic, no less than medical, importance—enabling us to see that surrounding this Universe, and pervading it, is a conscious, vital energy which is, in all probability, the energizing force of the Universe, and which, for want of a better name, we might call God. Whether or not future generations will verify this supposition remains to be seen; I have done all that I can by calling attention to those facts and arguments which seem to render that hypothesis at least a thinkable one. If the Universe is at basis spiritual and not material, that, at least, will be a consolation; and, it may be said, this position is one which has the support, both of philosophy and of the latest discoveries of Modern Science.

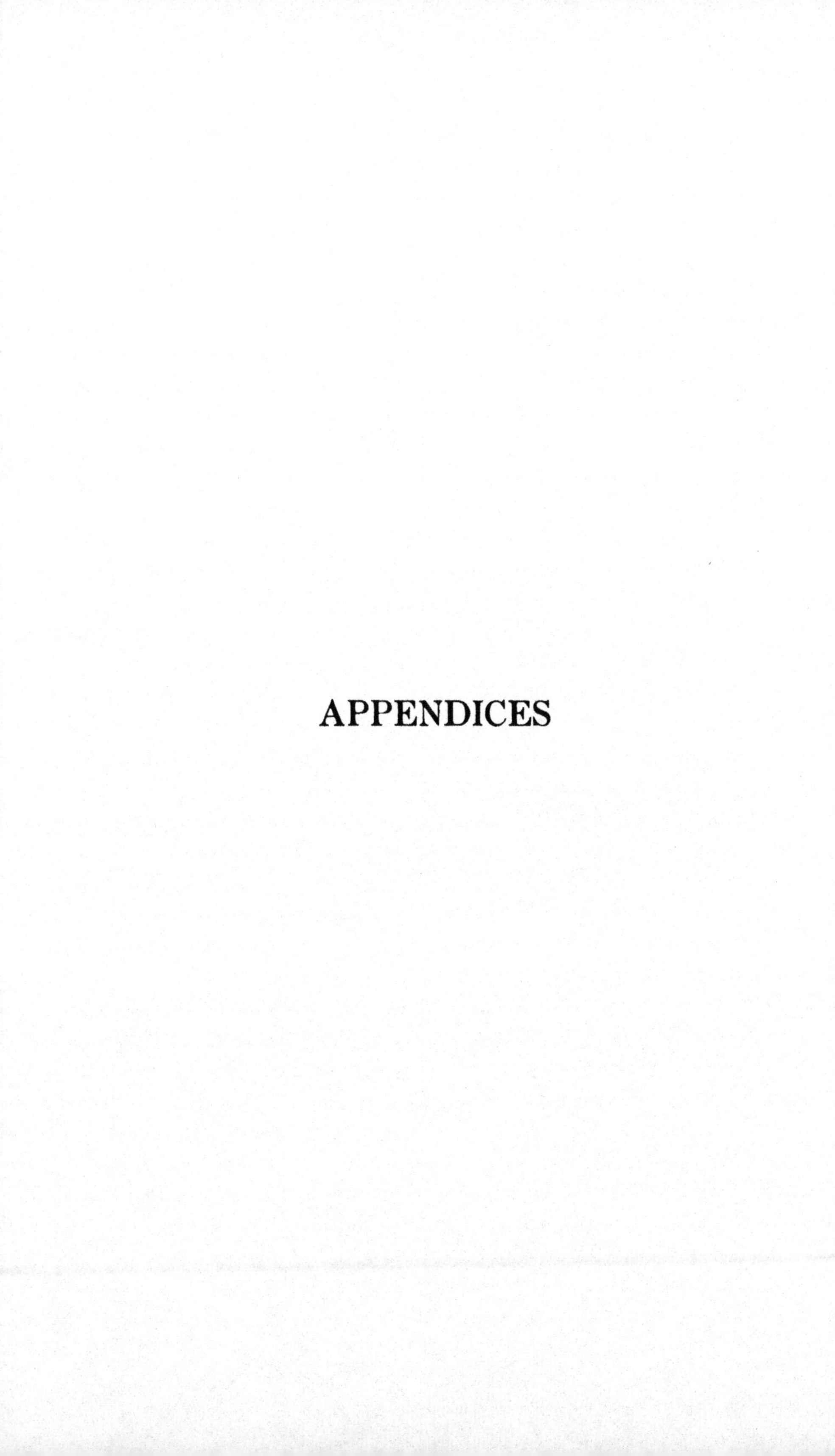

APPENDICES

APPENDIX A

I WISH it to be distinctly understood that I do not add this appendix with any intention of casting any slur upon the medical profession—as a profession—far less upon any individual, since I have the very greatest respect for them, in certain directions: my quarrel is entirely with their *system* and the present-day methods of curing disease, and not with the men following that system. I consider that the medical world is entirely wrong, in its treatment of disease, in its philosophy of medication; but it is against the philosophy and not the men supporting it, that my attack is leveled. That must be understood distinctly. My object in supplying this appendix is to show that the statements made in the text are not so radical and novel and revolutionary as might be supposed by many of my readers, but that many of the most learned medical men have always been discontented with the present system of medication, and leaned more or less to the theories outlined in this book. In order to strengthen my position in this respect, therefore, and to show that the present system of medication is anything but a "science" in its present state, I append a number of opinions and statements which emphatically condemn drug-medication and the systems at present in vogue. Such statements could be multiplied a hundredfold; but those which follow will probably be sufficient for my purpose. They express clearly and emphatically what I have stated to be the case in less forcible language in the text. Thus:

Bichat, the great French pathologist, in his "General Anatomy," Vol. I., p. 17, says:

"Medicine is an incoherent assemblage of incoherent ideas, and is perhaps, of all the physiological sciences, that which best shows the caprice of the human mind. What did I say? It is not a science for a methodical mind. It is a shapeless assemblage of inaccurate ideas, of observations often puerile, and of formulæ as fantastically conceived as they are tediously arranged."

Doctor Stille ("Therapeutics," Vol. I., p. 31) says:

"Nearly every medicine has become a popular remedy before being adopted or even tried by physicians; and by far the greater number of medicines were first employed in countries which were and are now in a state of scientific ignorance."

Sir John Forbes, F.R.C.P., and Physician to the Queen's Household, said:

"No systematic or theoretical classification of diseases or therapeutic agents ever yet promulgated is true or anything like the truth, and none can be adopted as a safe guidance in practice." ("Nature and Art in the Cure of Disease," p. 256.)

Sir Thomas Watson ("Practical Physic," Vol. I., p. 247) says:

" I remember the time when a surgeon, seeing a man in a fit, if he did not at once open a vein would be abused by the bystanders. To do so nowadays would be to incur the charge of murder."

Prof. Alonzo Clark, of the New York College of Physicians and Surgeons, says:

"In their zeal to do good, physicians have done much harm. They have hurried thousands to the grave who would have recovered if left to Nature."

Doctor Ramage, F.R.C.S., London, says:

"It cannot be denied that the present system of medicine is a burning reproach to its profession—if, indeed, a series of vague and uncertain incongruities deserves to be called by that name. How rarely do our medicines do good! How often do they make our patients really worse! I fearlessly assert that in most cases the sufferer would be safer without a physician than with one. I have seen enough of the malpractice of my professional brethren to warrant the strong language I employ."

Again, Sir John Forbes says:

"Some patients get well with the aid of our medicines, some without, and still more in spite of them."

And again, writing in the *Medical Journal*, he says:

"What a difference of opinion! What an array of alleged facts directly at variance with each other! What contradictions! What opposite results of a like experience! What ups and downs! What glorification and degradation of the same remedy!"

Professor Barker, New York Medical College, says:

"The drugs which are administered for scarlet fever kill far more patients than that disease does."

John Mason Good, M.D., F.R.S., says:

"The effects of medicine on the human system are in the highest degree uncertain, except indeed, that they have destroyed more lives than war, pestilence, and famine combined."

James Johnson, M.D., F.R.S., editor of *The Medico-Chirurgical Review,* wrote:

"I declare, as my conscientious conviction, founded on long experience and reflection, that if there was not a single physician, surgeon, man-midwife, chemist, apothecary, druggist, nor drug on the face of the earth, there would be less sickness and less mortality than now prevails."

Dr. A. O'Leary, Jefferson Medical College, Phila., Pa., says:

"The best things in the healing art have been done by those who never had a diploma—the first Cæsarian section, lithotomy, the use of cinchona, of ether as an anæsthetic, the treatment of the air passages by inhalation, the water-cure, the medicated baths, electricity as a healing agent, and magnetism, faith cure, mind cure, etc. Pasteur has no diploma, but has done more good than all the M.D.'s in France."

Doctor Quain, editor of the *Dictionary of Medicine,* said in an address to the British Medical Association in 1873:

"Diseases are curable, but we can not cure them."

Dr. Samuel Wilks, F.R.C.S., lecturer on medicine at Guy's Hospital, said:

"All our best treatment is empirical . . . I believe that we know next to nothing of the action of medicines and other therapeutic agents."

The celebrated Majendie, lecturing to his class, said:

"Gentlemen, medicine is a great humbug. I know it is called science. Science indeed! It is nothing like science. Doctors are merely empirics when they are not charlatans. We are as ignorant as men can be. Who knows anything in the world about medicine?"

A. E. Wright, M.D., late professor of Pathology, Army Medical School, Netley, wrote:

"That scientific knowledge which alone can avail in the conflict with disease is—practically all of it—still to seek."

Thomas A. Edison is reported to have recently said:

"Medicine is played out. Every new discovery of bacteria shows us all the more convincingly that we have been wrong, and that the millions of tons of stuff we have taken were all useless. The doctor of the future will give no medicine, but will instruct his patient in the care of the human frame; in diet and the cause and prevention of disease. Surgery, diet, antiseptics—these three are the vital things of the future in the preservation of the health of humanity. There were never so many able, active minds at work on the problem of disease as now; and all their discoveries are ending in the simple truth—that you can't improve on Nature."

Professor Gregory, of Edinburgh, author of a work on *The Theory and Practice of Physic,* said:

> "Ninety-nine out of every hundred medical truths are medical lies; and medical doctrines, are for the most part, stark, staring nonsense."

Doctor Evans, F.R.C.P., said:

> "The medical practice of our day is, at the best, a most uncertain and unsatisfactory system; it has neither philosophy nor common sense to commend it to confidence."

Quotations such as the above could be multiplied; but I forbear. Medical literature is so full of statements of this kind that nothing is to be gained by repetition. The above will at least surely tend to show that the so-called "science of medicine" is anything but that; and that the field is certainly open for any new system that can vindicate itself with a sufficient number of facts and arguments—which, I venture to think, is the case with the hygienic system.

APPENDIX B

THIS question of *colds* is a highly interesting and important one; and it is essential that this question should be thoroughly understood by the public—since more misapprehension exists on this question than on any other that is related to the public health. Like all diseases, a cold is, of course, a friendly effort on the part of Nature to rid the system of impurities; and as such should be looked upon as a friend rather than as a foe. It is an effort to rid the system of impurities. Says Dr. W. E. Forest:

"The main element in 'a cold,' accompanied with fever, is a disturbed condition of some part of the digestive organs. It is very doubtful if almost any amount of exposure to cold or chilling the surface will bring any other than temporary discomfort, provided the system is in its normal condition. If, however, the blood is charged with waste material, absorbed from the alimentary canal, if the liver is sluggish and the kidneys inactive, then a sudden interference with the action of the skin, due to cold, will cause a congestion of the internal organs that may result in a violent attack of fever."

Dr. C. E. Page proved this to be the case in his own person. He writes:[2]

"In order, however, to see if I could, by exposure, cause the well-known symptoms of cold, I have made many experiments, some of which I will name: I have walked in snow and slop with low shoes until both soles and socks were soaked through, and have thus sat for an hour or more; after wearing all-wool flannels during moderate weather, I have, upon the approach of *colder* weather, removed my undergarments, and have then attended to my outdoor affairs, minus the overcoat habitually worn; I have slept in winter in a current blowing directly about my head and shoulders; upon going to bed, I have sat in a strong current, entirely nude, for a quarter of an hour, on a very cold, damp night in the fall of the year; I have worn a flannel gown, and slept under heavy-weight bedclothes one night, and in cotton nightshirt, and light-weight bedclothes the next. These and similar experiments I have made repeatedly, and have never been able to 'catch cold.' I have become cold, sometimes quite cold, and become warm again—that is all. On the other hand, changing the form of my experiments, returning to my old way, the present style of living—a 'generous diet' and a full meal every five or six hours through the day— I have found no difficulty in *accu-*

[1] "The New Treatment for Fever," pp. 23–4.
[2] "Natural Cure," pp. 40–1.

mulating a cold, and within reasonable length of time could count upon it, although now a part of the programme consisted in taking the most extreme care to avoid what is commonly reckoned as exposures—keeping my feet very warm and dry, paying strict attention to wraps, etc." Benjamin Franklin once wrote "I shall not attempt to explain why 'damp clothes' occasion colds rather than wet ones, because I doubt the fact. I imagine that neither the one nor the other contributes to this effect, and that the causes of colds are totally independent of wet and even of cold."

One more word. It is in connection with the old adage—"Stuff a cold, and starve a fever." Since this is universally known, and so often quoted to those who believe in fasting by their anti-fasting friends; and as it was the cause—more or less—of considerable annoyance, Doctor Dewey went to the trouble of having the origin of this saying looked up by a friend of his, who was a classical scholar, and it was found that the sentence had got into the English language in a perverted form. The real meaning of the sentence is this: that "If you stuff a cold, you *thereby* have to starve a fever." I think this disposes of the difficulty, without further trouble.

[1] "Essays," p. 216. See also Dr. Alexander Haig's "Etiology of a Common Cold."

APPENDIX C

Louis Kuhne's Facial Diagnosis is based upon the fundamental principle outlined in Chapters I and II, *viz.*, that disease is itself a curing process; that all disease is necessarily one at basis; that the various "diseases"—so-called, are but the varying modes, faces, or methods of elimination of the principal cause of all disease—which cause is the retained, effete material which should have been eliminated. Accepting these theories as established, Kuhne went on to conjecture that this material would undoubtedly vary in composition, in the various diseases; and the various states or stages of each disease—according to the constitution and general make-up of the individual concerned, and, further, that such material would accumulate in certain portions of the body more readily and more certainly than in others—this, perhaps, corresponding to the particular form of disease present. Thus, he thought it might be possible to establish a definite connection between the size, character and location of the encumbering material, and the disease present—or even threatened—in any particular case. That this could be worked out in detail, and more or less definitely proved, he showed in his ingenious book on "Facial Diagnosis." Of his conclusions I can, unfortunately, give only the very briefest summary.[1]

Kuhne begins by drawing for us the theoretically ideal man—whose proportions he had calculated partly from ancient Grecian sculpture, and partly from modern athletes, who have received recognition as ideally developed men—and from these figures he arrived at a mean average, which may fairly be taken as "ideal." This, then, is the type of the truly normal man, and any great departure from such figures in any one direction, Kuhne justly felt to be due to a diseased condition of that locality; to a morbid accumulation at that point, of matter calling for elimination. This hypothesis was more or less decisively proved when—by pursuing the nature-cure methods, and thus regaining normal health—the patient thereby and invariably lost this accumula-

[1] Miss Florence Nightingale remarked that "there is undoubtedly a *physiognomy of disease.*" "Notes on Nursing," p. 117.

tion of morbid material in the part noted, and the part assumed its normal or "ideal" outline. This practically proved the contention made. Kuhne now set about studying the relations of the various accumulations to the diseases that followed; as well as the diagnostic value of the former. Into this I can go but very briefly. The case may be stated somewhat as follows:

All "encumbrances"—*i.e.*, deposits of fatty or effete material—are either front, back or side encumbrance. The front encumbrance is the least important, and most easily curable of all—material always having a tendency to settle there *first.* The forehead may be unduly padded with fatty-cushions; the face become bloated; the mouth and lips unduly protrude; and, most characteristic of all, and in fact a sure test of health in any organism—the jaw line (*i.e.*, the line which sharply defines the face from the neck) should be *clean cut.* If this is not so; if this space is filled up with fatty-tissue, or cushions of morbid material, *that person is diseased,* and this is a most infallible and invariably true sign. The neck is also subject to encumbrance—lumps forming on the sides, under the chin, and the head cannot readily be turned or thrown back. It is hardly necessary to say that the abdomen is readily disposed to be rendered abnormal in size—because of undue internal and external accumulations—and every such case indicates, most assuredly, the presence of disease.

Side encumbrance is present on the neck, or on one side of the body, (*i.e.*, more than upon the other side), the encumbered side then appearing uneven and larger than the other. Kuhne suggests that this is frequently caused by the habit of sleeping on one side—the morbid material in the body having a tendency to follow the law of gravity.

Back encumbrance is considered the most serious of all, as indicating a diseased condition more deep-seated and of longer standing than any other form of encumbrance. The back of the head and especially the nape line of the neck is particularly liable to this form of encumbrance; this latter being almost as ready a method of diagnosis of diseased conditions as the jaw-line, above mentioned. Whenever a person's neck, then, instead of curving in, from the back of the head, and then out again to the body, descends more or less straight, (this part being filled out with gross, puffy-looking flesh), you may depend upon it that person is diseased—and that gravely. I myself have noted these two tests repeatedly, and invariably found them to be correct.

Besides these modes of encumbrance, there is also the mixed or universal encumbrance, in which the body is throughout, more or less, evenly encumbered with effete material. This is, of course, the most serious of all. Such persons are "apt to die suddenly, though, on account of their appearance of stoutness (owing to the presence of so much foreign matter) they are usually thought to be in excellent health." (p. 59.) Finally, it must not be forgotten that the internal organs are also subject to this manner of encumbrance—and indeed, such diseases as fatty-degeneration of the heart conclusively prove that they are.

Other considerations must also be taken into account, in this connection. The *size* of the accumulation is, of course, of cardinal importance; the greater the encumbrance, *ceteris paribus*, the graver the disease. The *texture* is also of very great importance. So long as the encumbrance is soft, it is easily and certainly cured or removed, but "when the tissues begin to shrink and harden, recovery becomes more doubtful." (p. 59.) I might be permitted to remark, in this connection, that the difficulty experienced by all extremely thin or emaciated persons in gaining weight and recovering a normal condition, is because of the shrinkage and hardening of the originally soft tissue—rendering the case an extremely difficult one to cure—both because of the length of time it has necessarily progressed, and because of the refusal of the patient to acquiesce in any rational treatment—owing to the erroneous notion prevalent that he must be constantly "fed-up" and stimulated, in order to "support his strength."

APPENDIX D

It is an utter impossibility for human beings to deviate from the laws of Nature one iota without suffering in consequence. We acknowledge this to be true in all plant life, but we do not admit this applies to ourselves, because we can apparently withstand so much and yet live. And yet the law must apply to us also. Fixed laws must apply to the health of man no less than to every other living thing: the law of Health is as fixed a law as is any other law in the universe.[1] This being the case, we see clearly that so long as people persist in living in the perverse manner they do, there will be sickness and death in the world, and nothing can save them—no power, no medicine on earth can prevent them from becoming ill. It would be quite irrational to think there is. "Men do not die: they kill themselves," says the French adage.[2] "When the health is bad, Nature has been disobeyed." Miss Florence Nightingale insisted upon this point.[3]

One great trouble is that doctors have a habit of accepting our diseased humanity as representing the normal man and woman—and gauge their physiology and practice by this standard.[4] How far astray their conceptions may lead them is illustrated in the following passage, taken from Dr. Louis L. Seaman's "Real Triumph of Japan," (p. 100):

> " It may be said that in war it is the rule that four times as many are wounded as are killed; that from three to ten times as many soldiers are victims of disease as are wounded, and that four times as many die from disease as from casualties of war."

And this is called normal! Why should there be *any* sickness in camps any more than in any other locality? Were the principles of Fletcherism taught the rank and file of the army, there would be no reason whatever to think that sickness might not be reduced to almost *nothing.*

[1] Graham: "Science of Human Life," pp. 14–15.
[2] "Science in the Daily Meal," by Albert Broadbent, p. 5.
[3] "Notes on Nursing," p. 25.
[4] "Nature *vs.* Drugs," p. 32.

Again I must insist that the whole human race is ill. Also, every person dies before his or her appointed time—meaning by this, the length of time they should live, if the laws of life were normally and closely followed. Says Dr. E. Teichmann:[1]

" every man may die a natural, normal death. To be sure, it is freely granted that he never does it: he always dies before that time comes. "

Says Dr. James C. Jackson:[2]

"The great majority of the American people are either ill in health or ailing in health, or sick."

Says Mrs. Mary Foote Henderson:[3]

"'I am well,' says the man with his palsied palate, his want of relish for simple food, his defective eyesight, his fatigues, his depressions, his pessimism, his indigestion, his colds, his avoirdupois, his sensitiveness to weather, his need of a drug—alcohol, tobacco, tea, coffee, or pepper."

While we probably live longer now than ever, on the average, (Professor Dolbear affirms that the average length of human life was thirty, in 1800, and is forty, in 1901. See "Faith as Related to Health," p. 64), that is undoubtedly because of the improve ment in sanitary and hygienic conditions, health reforms, etc., and is not due to any change in the dietetic habits of the people, which are as bad, if not worse, than they ever were.

It is certain that the human race should live many times as long as it does; or, rather, the normal span of life should be much greater than it is. Says Dr. A. T. Schofield:[4]

"It is computed that, apart from disease, the ordinary span of life is five times that of growth; and fixing this latter at 21 years in the human race, men should die between 100 and 105 years. When we remember that the average duration of life here, with every advantage of sanitation, is still but 43 years (men 42, women 44), that within my memory it was only 36, that in the eighteenth century it was but 20, we see that a mighty work still remains to be accomplished in perfecting the science of hygiene, or prevention, as distinguished from that of medicine or cure. "

Says Professor Metchnikoff:[5]

"Natural death is probably a possibility rather than an actual occurrence. Attempts have been made to estimate the natural limits of human life. Flourens based a calculation on the duration of the period of growth. If the latter be taken as one-fifth the natural life, then human life ought to last a century. . . . In most cases it ought to be more than a hundred years, and only in rare cases ought it to be less than that term."[6]

[1] "Life and Death," p. 148.
[2] "How to Get Well," p. 3.
[3] "Aristocracy of Health," p. 3.
[4] "Nerves in Order," p. 16.
[5] "Nature of Man," pp. 277–78.
[6] See also Dr. E. Teichmann: "Life and Death," p. 158.

It will be observed that from 100 to 105 years is given as that of the *natural* termination of life; *i.e.*, without that person being considered as especially old. And all the faculties and functions should be preserved in such a person, also; since these should not begin to weaken and decay till very old age has been reached—if then. A hundred years of youthful activity! What might not be accomplished in that time! And the fact that the average length of life is something less than forty-three years; and that even during that brief period, it is full of diseases and weaknesses and fatigues and what-not, clearly shows that *something* is wrong with the human family, somewhere! And in what is it so wrong and perverted as in its food-habits—both as regards to quality and quantity? Surely further proof is scarcely needed that the whole human race is diseased, miserable, and prematurely short-lived?

Strong support of this view is afforded by those cases of old men who have lived simple lives, and who have lived to a great old age, in health and contentment. A number of such cases are collected together in Dr. DeLacy Evans' book, "How to Prolong Life, (pp. 100–35). The reason that more persons are not longer-lived is easy to see. "Few people," says Tracy, "Have enough self-control to become centenarians."

It is all very well for men to laugh at this question of diet—quality and quantity—and to say that "too much fuss is made about food," etc. It is the most vitally important question before the world to-day, not only because of its own innate importance, but because many other vices hinge upon and are the result of the food habits. (pp. 110–11.) Mr. Weinburgh well said:[1]

> "People exercise great care in selecting material from which to construct their house and much more in furnishing it, and in nearly all things they want the best; but when it comes to selecting the material out of which heart, brain, blood, bone, flesh, cartilage and muscle are made when it comes to selecting the material that shapes to such a large degree their sympathies, emotions and morals—all that is of real value in human beings, they exercise absolutely no choice—manifest no interest. All this is left to an ignorant chef, a negro or Chinese cook—it is of no importance."

Or, as Doctor Page humorously put it:[2]

> "'Nothing hurts me—I eat everything.' (Next year.) 'Nothing agrees with me—I can't eat anything.' Thus the dyspeptics' ranks are kept full with recruits who 'don't want any advice about diet.'"

[1] "Perfect Health," p. 315. [2] "Natural Cure," p. 157.

APPENDIX E

I MYSELF have followed this diet for many years, and a number of personal friends of mine are living in the same manner. I do not think anvthing could possibly persuade any of us to return to the ordinary cooked diet, (I mean vegetarian diet, of course, meat is out of the question). The difference between the two diets is simply beyond words! It is hardly necessary to remind the reader that whole colonies in California live in this manner and on this food. It is most amusing to remark that we, who live on the "low" and "innutritious" diet, never eat but twice a day, and many of us but once; and even less at that meal than the majority of persons in one of their three—yet, I need hardly remark, are far better, healthier and better nourished than they. Mr. Salt remarked this in his excellent little book, "The Logic of Vegetarianism," (p. 63), when he said:

> "If the chemist were a man of action, and not merely a man of study, the practical aspects of this question might at the outset give him pause. Had he known vegetarians, lived among vegetarians, and talked with vegetarians, instead of regarding them theoretically, he would be aware that the average vegetarian eats decidedly less in bulk than the average flesh eater . . . "

This is not the place, of course, to argue for vegetarianism, raw food, or any other kind of diet, but merely mention the diet in passing by way of strongly recommending it to my readers for a thorough trial. Should they care to look into the question seriously, they will find it discussed in all its aspects in the following books, *inter multa alia:*

How Nature Cures, by Emmet Densmore, M.D.
Health in the Household, by Susanna W. Dodds, M.D.
Food in Health and Disease, by I. Burney Yeo, M.D., F.R.C.P
The Philosophy of Eating, by Albert J. Bellows, M.D.
Our Digestion, by Dio Lewis, M.D.
Food and Feeding, by Sir Henry Thompson, M.D., F.R.C.S.
Diet in Relation to Age and Activity, by Sir Henry Thompson, M.D., etc.

Diet and Food, by Alexander Haig, M.D., F.R.C P.
What Shall we Eat? by Alfred Andrews.
Rumford Kitchen Leaflets, by Ellen H. Richards etc.
Foods for the Fat, by N. E. York-Davies, L.R.C.P.
Food and Work, by M. L. Holbrook, M.D.
The Diet Cure, by T. L. Nichols, M.D.
Natural Hygiene, by H. Lahmann, M.D.
The Key to Health, by A. G. Hinkley, M.D.
First Lessons in Food and Diet, by Ellen Richards.
Strength From Eating, by Bernarr Macfadden.
Uncooked Foods, by Mr. and Mrs. Eugene Christian.
The Perfect Way in Diet, by Anna Kingsford, M.D.
Every Living Creature, by Ralph Waldo Trine.
The Food of the Future, by C. W. Forward.
The Foundation of all Reform, by Otto Carqué.
The Dietetic Value of Bread, by John Goodfellow, M.D.
Muscle, Brain and Diet, by Eustice H. Miles, M.A.
Fruits and Farinacea, by John Smith, M.D.
Fruit and Bread, by Professor Schlickeysen.
How to Prolong Life, by DeLacy Evans, M.D., M.R.C.S.
Eating and Drinking, by Albert H. Hoy, M.D.
The Logic of Vegetarianism, by Henry Salt.
The Folly of Meat Eating, by Otto Carqué.
Dietetic Advice to the Young and Old, by Mrs. C. L. H. Wallace.
Salt, by Mrs. C. L. H. Wallace.
Vegetarianism, by Harriet P. Fowler.
Saline Starvation, by Chas. D. Hunter.
The Salt-eating Habit, by Richard Colburn.
The Whole and the Hulled Wheat, by James C. Jackson, M.D.
Flesh as Food for Man, by James C. Jackson, M.D.
Why a Hindu is a Vegetarian, by Swami Abhedananda.
Vegetarianism in the Light of Theosophy, by Annie Besant.
The Diet Cure of Cancer, by C. P. Newcomb.
The Morals of Diet, by Leo Tolstoy.
Food Value of Meat, by W. R. C. Latson, M.D.
The Meat Fetish, by Ernest Crosby and Elisée Reclus.
Vindication of a Natural Diet, by Percy B. Shelley.
Food of the Orient, by Alice B. Stockham, M.D.
The Diet Question, by Susanna Dodds, M.D.
Shall We Slay to Eat? by J. H. Kellogg, M.D.
Simpler Food and Athletics, by Eustice Miles.

Cancer and Uric Acid, by Alex. Haig, M.D., F.R.C.P.
Life and Food, by Alex. Haig, M.D., F.R.C.P.
Etiology of a Common Cold, by Alex. Haig, M.D., F.R.C.P.
The Drink Problem, by H. B. A.
Science in the Daily Meal, by Albert Broadbent.
Forty Vegetarian Dinners, by Albert Broadbent.
Hygienic Cook Book, by R. T. Trall, M.D.
Hygiene Home Cook Book, by R. T. Trall, M.D.
Testimony of Science in Favor of a Vegetarian Diet.
Death in the Milk Can.
Epitome of Vegetarianism.
Hydropathic Encyclopædia, Vol. I., by R. T. Trall, M.D.
Return to Nature, by B. Lust.
Nature *vs.* Drugs, by Aug. Reinhold, M.D.
Science of Human Life, by Sylvester Graham, M.D.

APPENDIX F

VARIOUS measures have been devised to check the habit of over-eating with the least unpleasantness to the patient.

(1) Dr. Dio Lewis advocated the following method:

"On sitting down at the table take upon your plate all that you are to eat, and when that is finished, stop."[1]

This is doubtless excellent advice so far as it goes, but its practice requires a certain amount of will-power—more, perhaps, than the average person possesses.

(2) *Standing up at meals* I most strongly advocate—at least until the new habits have been formed. (Have we not frequently noticed that the feeling of unpleasant "fullness" and distension after a hearty meal, is scarcely ever noticed until we stand up?) Standing up to the meal would obviate this difficulty, and materially assist in lessening the amount of food called for; and I am not sure but that this is the most wholesome and hygienic way to eat the meal, in any case. Doctor Schlickeysen advocated this method also, saying:[2]

"When one is not too weary, it is much better to take the food while standing or walking. This may at first thought seem unnatural, but in truth man is the only animal, or certainly the only one of the higher vertebrates, who habitually sits or reclines while eating, and there is no good reason why he should constitute an exception here more than in various other respects. . . . The usual position at table somewhat obstructs the circulation in the chest and abdomen, and this hinders digestion when it should be most active. It also admits of the stomach being overloaded much more readily and imperceptibly, the first sense of fullness being often experienced only upon arising."

I myself have practiced the habit of walking about at meals, (when alone!) and can say that these theoretical statements are certainly borne out by the facts.

(3) *Eating only one kind of food at any one meal* will also materially assist in reducing the bulk of food required or craved. The reason for this is the following. It is acknowledged that each

[1] "Our Digestion," p. 146.

[2] "Fruit and Bread," p. 184.

nerve responds to a certain stimulus, and to none other. Thus, Dr. George Black says:[1]

"As each kind of nerve responds to a special sensation, and has no concern with any other, the optic nerve can convey no other impression than that of light, and can no more conduct a sensation of pain than a nerve of ordinary sensation can see; hence, when irritated, as by galvanism, it responds by a flash of light." See also E. Hering: "On Memory, and the Specific Energies of the Nervous System."

For each tone and each color we have distinct nerve-fibers. Exercising our nerves causes pleasure, up to a certain degree; then rest must follow, or pain will ensue. Hence the ear enjoys a variety of sounds, the eye of colors, and the tongue of flavors. In partaking of any one dish, we arrive at a point when the stomach has received enough; then we ought to stop eating. But by presenting food of a different taste, new nerve-fibers are aroused, more food is taken, the stomach is loaded beyond its capacity, and in that way digestion is impaired, and the foundation is laid for many forms of disease.

(4) *Ceasing the moment that genuine hunger has been satisfied* is, of course, a rule of fundamental importance. But it is frequently hard to say just when this has been accomplished—perverted as our tastes are. Says Doctor Oswald·[2]

"It is an excellent rule to prolong the pauses between the several dishes of a full meal in order to give the stomach time to indicate the real wants of the system."

(5) *Never drink at meals.* If food is properly masticated, liquid will never be required, and should never be drunk—as it dilutes, unduly, all the digestive juices, and tends to wash the food through the stomach, into the intestine, before it has been properly digested. If eating were discontinued as soon as a call for liquid be felt, there would probably be very little over-eating and this, I think, is an important and far-reaching hint for health reformers.

(6) *Do not eat spiced or stimulating foods.* Says Doctor Oswald:[3]

"Wholesome food rarely tempts us to indulge to excess. We do not often hear of milk topers or baked-apple gluttons."

And again:[4]

[1] "Eyesight, and How to Care for It," p. 19.
[2] "Household Remedies," p. 68.
[3] "Fasting, Hydropathy and Exercise," p. 39.
[4] "Household Remedies," p. 66.

"Not the naturally palatable, but the unnaturally stimulating qualities of a dish tempt the dyspeptic to eat to excess."

Dishes of this character have a tendency to cause a forced or abnormal appetite—and to call for more food than is really required. Miss Ellen H. Richards remarked:[1]

"Condiments too often result in over-stimulation of the secretions, and thus cause the eating of more food than the body needs."

Dr. Burney Yeo has stated that "cooking increases the desire to take food."[2] Many writers have remarked that we can live upon far less food when uncooked than after it has passed through the culinary process. Thus, Mr. Christian remarked,[3] "we know that, as compared with cooked foods, it only takes about half the quantity of uncooked food to sustain life." From personal experience I can state that this is absolutely true. So universal is the belief that this is so, among those who have actually tried the exclusively raw-food diet (and so are entitled to speak upon the subject) that Professor Jaffa wrote,[4] "She believed, as do fruitarians generally, that people need far less raw than cooked food."[5]

(7) *All stimulants*—liquid and solid—*should also be discontinued immediately*, as these have a tendency to increase the appetite. See "Papers on Alcohol," p. 1., etc.

(8) *Think about the present mouthful, not the one just ahead.* We always have a tendency to forget the mouthful actually in the mouth, and being masticated, in preparing the next mouthful —at least, I have noticed this weakness in myself, and do not doubt that others are affected in a like manner. This bad habit— of always living in the future—instead of in the present—mouthful, is one great cause of over-eating, I am convinced, for the reason that it causes us to forget to give proper attention to the mouthful being masticated, at the time. I shall only say— experiment at the next meal, and I think you will find this to be the case. An elaboration of this idea I cannot attempt here.

(9) *Practice thorough—very thorough—mastication.* If food is masticated properly and thoroughly, hunger will be fully satisfied with far less bulk of food, and with greater gustatory pleasure and

[1] "Food and Diet," p. 24.
[2] "Food and Diet," p. 155.
[3] "Uncooked Foods," p. 46.
[4] "Nutrition Investigations Among Fruitarians and Chinese," p. 12, (Bulletin. U. S. Dept. of Agr.)
[5] See also Macfadden: "Natural Cure for Rupture," p. 39. Salt: "Logic of Vegetarianism," p. 63, etc.

benefit than when such mastication is neglected. Says Doctor Holbrook:[1] "Count Rumford calculated that one-fourth less food is required if it be perfectly masticated." This subject has, however, been so well and so exhaustively handled by Mr. Horace Fletcher, in his two books, that I need but mention the subject here, and refer the reader to the books in question

(10) Last but not least: *Use your will!*

"Eating for Strength," p. 58.

APPENDIX G

It is beginning to be realized that consumption is due (for its predisposing cause, at least,) to an excess of nutriment over the quantity of oxygen inhaled; to the quantity of food ingested over and above that properly aërated. Doctor Trall traces the causes of consumption so clearly, it seems to me, that I cannot do better than to quote his terse language in this place. In part, he says:

"First in the list of predisposing causes is constipation of the bowels. This is usually more or less connected with a torpid condition of the liver, because the same dietetic or other errors which occasion obstructions in the bowels, occasion, also, the same condition in the large depurating organ called the liver. When constipation of the bowels and liver exists, the kidneys and skin are compelled to perform extra duty in the work of eliminating morbid and effete materials from the system, in consequence of which they become, finally, exhausted and torpid. Then it is that the lungs have to sustain the chief burden of depuration, and the result of this is a disorganization or destruction of their tissue—consumption."

Accordingly, Doctor Trall came to this momentous conclusion —that the most prominent cause of consumption is:

"*Excessive alimentation;* or rather, *the disproportion between the aliment and respiration. It is the excess of food taken into the stomach, over and above the quantity of air taken into the lungs.*"[1]

Dr. C. H. Davis[2] stated that:

"Most people who have tuberculosis have some serious disturbance of their digestion and nutrition before the tubercular trouble shows itself. . . . There is not the slightest question but that tuberculosis is a disease of malnutrition."

All this is beginning to be recognized, as I have said, but the medical profession have attacked the problem from one side only. They have, *e.g.*, supplied the patient with an abundance of fresh air, which, when more or less continuously and forcibly breathed, will oxidize a larger proportion of the food material ingested than formerly; and this, by allowing none to accumulate in the system in a mal-assimilated form, greatly assists in the cure. This is all

[1] "Diseases of the Throat and Lungs," p. 13. See also "Prevention and Cure of Consumption," by David Wark, M.D., p. 30.

[2] "Self Cure of Consumption," pp. 75–76.

very well, so far as it goes; but, as I formerly said, it attacks one side of the problem only. Consumption being due to a disproportion of the food and oxygen taken into the system, doctors have sought to remedy this defect by increasing the one deficient —the oxygen; and so far, that is quite right and logical. But why not attack the disease from the other side also, and attempt to equalize the disproportionate factors by *decreasing the one in excess,* (the food-supply)? If all this is so, we can readily see that over-nutrition is the chief factor in the causation of this disease, and that fasting would be, *à priori,* the speediest and most certain method of curing such a diseased condition. Taken in conjunction with deep-breathing, and other hygienic, purifying measures, it would most assuredly effect a cure in the shortest possible time, and with almost infallible precision. And there are other authors who advise this plan also; Doctor Trall wrote,[1] "With regard to diet, no disease, not even dyspepsia, requires a more rigidly plain and abstemious course." Dr. Felix Oswald,[2] while considering consumption "the most curable of all chronic diseases" (when treated properly!) said that "a tendency to emaciation, the most characteristic symptom of tuberculosis, generally continues to counteract the normal effects of a liberal diet, even combined with continence and a tranquil mode of life . . . " Doctor Page gives a case of a patient "pronounced incurable, who was made convalescent by a voluntary and absolute fast of forty-three days—taking water freely, however, during that time—and following this by the bread-and-fruit-diet . . . "[3] Inasmuch as one lung has to do the work of both, when one is diseased—and so do the purifying work of both—we can clearly see how important it is not to over-work the lungs, at such a time, with a surfeit of food material calling for aëration.

I may add one or two words on the "milk diet," now so much in vogue. That many cases recover under this treatment there can be no doubt—though milk is unquestionably a highly unnatural food. The explanation is simple. The milk diet is practically a fasting cure! When we consider that from 84 to 90 per cent. of milk is water,[4] we can calculate easily enough that it is the fasting more than the special diet which effects the cure.

[1] "Hydropathic Encyclopædia," Vol. II., p. 163.
[2] "Household Remedies," p. 50.
[3] "Natural Cure," pp. 62-63.
[4] "Milk as Food," p. 5, (U. S. Dept. of Agr. Bulletin.)

APPENDIX H

AGAIN, I cannot too strongly protest against the current theories and treatment of *anæmia.* The view that tends to find, in all anæmic patients, under-nourished patients, is very far from being the truth—so far, indeed, as to be almost an inversion of the truth. The fact is that anæmic patients are almost invariably over-fed; but this we shall see more clearly as we proceed. I quote the following very excellent remarks upon this subject from Doctor Rabagliati's "Aphorisms, Definitions, Reflections, and Paradoxes," pp. 200–1. There he says:

"The anæmic girl is in a state of indirect, not of direct, anæmia. Her circulation is really blocked. It is in a state which may be called 'constipation of the circulation.' The muscular elements of the vessels, and particularly their transverse fibers, are hypertrophied, and being, besides, over-stimulated, they go into a state of excessive contraction. The effect of this is to narrow the lumen of the vessels, and to prevent the blood from flowing freely along them, and by this means, of course, a proper supply of blood is prevented from reaching the tissues. The consequence is that the girl appears pale and anæmic, and no doubt is so. But the cause is really an excess of food-supply, which in the first instance caused the muscular elements to hypertrophy, and, as the over-circulation of too much food . still continued, the hypertrophied transverse muscular fibers contracted and narrowed the lumen of the vessels. The process is really a beautifully adapted provision of Nature to limit the blood-supply to parts which have already been over-nourished, and which would tend to become still further hypertrophied if the nutritive process were carried still further. The process is plainly one of starvation, due to over-repletion, caused by contraction of hypertrophied or over-fed muscular fibers. And, obviously, the means of treatment proper to such a state is to restrict the diet until, some of the hypertrophy of the muscular fibers of the vessels having been removed, some of the spasm passes off, and blood flows more freely, and the anæmia is reduced. To recommend more food, as is so often done, is to do the precise opposite of what good treatment demands. The meals ought to be reduced in number and quantity, not increased."[1]

It will now be seen that even anæmia is, in reality, a curing process—an attempt to right a wrong. And this wrong is too much food, and food of the wrong kind. The one aspect of the problem we have just put before us; the other I now place before

[1] See also this author's "Air, Food and Exercises," pp. 238, 255–56, etc.

my readers in the form of a quotation from Dr. H. Lahmann's "Natural Hygiene," pp. 70–1, where he says:

"Lean dysæmia is generally artificially produced by a so-called 'generous' diet. This 'generous' diet consists in foods rich in albumen and poor in soda—meat, fowl, eggs, etc. The excess of insufficiently oxidized albumen gives rise to the formation of a considerable quantity of sulphuric acid which, unless it combines with alkalies, will attack the tissues: (comp gout and diabetes). Now, as there is a want of alkalies (bases) especially of soda, in the blood, the free sulphuric acid will attack the body material istelf, to draw the necessary bases from it, and will thus destroy it. This is the process which takes place in the so-called Banting cure, in which the tissues are destroyed by the sulphuric acid, formed from the excess of the albuminous food; a Banting cure is, therefore, constitutionally debilitating and cannot be called rational."

Doctor Densmore concluded that anæmia is the result of a "large quantity of carbonic acid in the blood."[1] This may be verv true, but it is coincidental, not casual—the ultimate cause being under-breathing, and food in excess, and of an improper quality.

Besides this general misapprehension—that anæmia is the result of under- and not over-feeding, there is the mistaken notion that it is largely due to lack of "iron" in the system. Now, even were this the case, (which is very doubtful, since the deficiency is probably due to the inability to utilize the iron already in the system rather than to a lack of this salt in the food eaten) we should supply this element in an *organic* (appropriable) and not in an inorganic (inappropriable) form. See the chapter on "Drug Medication." It is needless to say that the "iron tonics," etc., prescribed are worse than useless—they are positively injurious. Says Doctor Trall:[2]

"Iron in all its forms and preparations occasions a feverish condition of the system, and an inflammatory state of the blood. It is an irritant, a stimulant, a blood destroyer, a nerve-exhauster, a poison, as is alcohol."

The *apparently* beneficial effects which result from its administration, in certain cases, are doubtless those pointed out by Doctor Bellows, in his "Philosophy of Eating," p. 164, where he says:

" Scores of cases can be brought, where, under a different treatment, the results were the same, and even more striking, without using a particle of iron; and my explanation is, that the effect of iron was that of a mere stimulant, promoting sanguification, from food taken in the meantime containing iron."

[1] "Consumption and Chronic Diseases," p. 132.
[2] "True Temperance Platform," p. 61.

APPENDIX I

THE question of the health of babies is a very misunderstood one. Most persons have an idea that all babies must of necessity be sick more or less all of the time; and that, especially at the time of teething, sickness, bowel complaints, etc., are quite customary for babies, and are natural and to be expected! Doctor Page clearly pointed out the fallacy of this idea, and said:[1]

"It is the popular idea that when an infant begins to teeth he is peculiarly liable to intestinal and other troubles, and when the disorders occur at this period of infant life, the cause is at once said to lie in the fact that the baby is teething, and that, consequently, it is an unavoidable misfortune that the baby is sick. The only misfortune therewith is the ignorance of the physician and attendants. In no sense is sickness an incident of teething. It is simply coincident, and rises from the fact that it is at *about this age* that the system begins to break down under the excessive labor so long imposed upon the organs of digestion, assimilation, and excretion."

This is rendered all the more probable when we remember that the simple process of teething is (or should be) practically painless. Says Dr. George Black:[2]

"It (teething) is not, therefore, as the common expression of 'cutting the teeth' would indicate, a process of laceration, tearing, or cutting, but of removal of impeding tissue by absorption, which allows the passage of the teeth through the gums."

And just here might be the best place to make one or two remarks with regard to a very common but harmful fallacy. It is all but universally admitted that the pregnant or nursing woman should "eat for two" and the poor mother is constantly urged repeatedly to ingest great quantities of food during these periods in order to supply this additional loss. But, as Doctor Rabagliati pointed out:[3]

"As a newly born babe weighs from five to seven or nine pounds, and the placenta two or three pounds, there are, say, about nine pounds of tissue to be made up in, say, nine months. This comes to about one-half ounce daily;

[1] "How to Feed the Baby," p. 22.
[2] "The Mouth and the Teeth," p. 47.
[3] "Aphorisms," etc., p. 115.

and even if the baby and placenta were of giant size and weighed even eighteen pounds, which they do very rarely, there would only require to be made up about two pounds a month, or, say, one ounce a day during the period of pregnancy. To make up this amount the expectant mother takes perhaps one-half pound or more of extra food three times a day. What wonder if she has a bad labor, fevers, and takes pneumonia, or becomes septic, or has frightful laceration of the perineum at her confinement, the tissues being so loaded with effete material as to become easily lacerable?"

Dr. C. E. Page also insisted upon this aspect of the problem; see his "How to Feed the Baby," p. 86.

Dr. Joel Shew, indeed, insisted that *less* food was required at this time than at any other period—or rather, less should be eaten. He says;[1]

"Too much food, and that which is too exciting, will cause more harm in pregnancy than at other times, from the greater tendency to fever. The common belief among women is that more food is needed during pregnancy than at other times, because the food goes to furnish nourishment for two instead of one, that is, for the mother and the child within her. 'It is therefore,' says Doctor Dewees, 'constantly recommended to eat and drink heartily; and this she too often does, until the system is goaded to fever; and sometimes to more sudden and greater evils, as convulsions or apoplexy.'

"If, instead of full diet, women in pregnancy will but try the plan of eating less food, even of becoming very abstemious, they will most assuredly find that they get along better, suffer less from plethora and fullness, and enjoy greater comfort of body in every respect.

"There is a mechanical reason—one which females themselves can best understand—why less food should be taken during pregnancy than at other times; the abdomen is more full at this period; much more so toward the end of pregnancy. Hence it is that at this time a full meal will cause a greater sense of fullness, and in every respect a greater degree of discomfort, than when pregnancy does not exist."

Dr. M. L. Holbrook took a similar position, and wrote:[2]

"We habitually take more food than is strictly required for the demands of the body; we therefore daily make more blood than is really wanted for its support. A superfluity amply sufficient for the nourishment of the child is thus furnished—for a very small quantity is requisite—without the mother, on the one hand, feeling the demand to be oppressive, and, on the other, without a freer indulgence of food being necessary to provide it. Nature her self corroborates this opinion; indeed, she solicits a reduction in the quantity of support rather than asks an increase of it; for almost the very first evidence of pregnancy is the morning sickness, which would seem to declare that the system requires reduction rather than increase, or why should this subduing process be instituted?"

[1] "Water Cure in Pregnancy and Childbirth," pp. 55–56.
[2] "Parturition Without Pain," pp. 62–63.

This question of vomiting is a very interesting one. I should be glad to see a case of this kind that could withstand prolonged fasting; water drinking, and bathing, if such a case could be found. In cases of vomiting, both patients and physicians seem to be afraid of nothing so much as starvation. Hence the stomach is made the receptacle of all manner of things, clean and unclean—saying nothing of the inordinate dosing that is usually practiced on such occasions. It is no wonder that the vomiting continues under such treatment.

These remarks apply also to the practice of giving growing children large quantities of food, on the supposition that they require great bulk in order to replace the wastes of the system and to allow for the extra growth of the tissues. Doctor Rabagliati pointed out the absurdity of this practice, and said:

"The growing boy or girl may grow twelve pounds in a year, but six pounds is much more common. To make up the former weight, he requires one-half ounce of extra food a day; to make up the latter, he requires one-quarter ounce. To this end he is often supplied with one pound extra of food, or even one and one-half pounds daily. What wonder if, under these circumstances, he should have tonsilitis, tracheitis, broncho-pneumonia, pleurodynia, pleurisy, growing pains, or rheumatic fever, or even that he should be attacked by one of the continued fevers—his tissues being so loaded with effete material that they form a suitable nidus or resting place for the growth of the micro-organism which is associated with the cause of the disease?"

As Dr. T. L. Nichols said:[1]

"An ounce a day is nearly twenty-three pounds a year. No one expects to grow at that rate."

Dr. Dio Lewis also said:[2]

"The common notion, that when a child is growing, he needs unlimited quantities of food, is an error. It is true that, during this period he is adding, perhaps two ounces a day, to his weight, but the quantity he eats, in view of this increase of weight, is fearful to behold!"

[1] "Diet Cure," p. 21. [2] "Weak Lungs," p. 109.

APPENDIX J

In this place I desire to touch upon one or two aspects only of that momentous question—the causation of *cancer;* bearing in mind particularly the relation of cancer to food habits—since, to me, the connection is both close and distinct. It is frequently said that old wounds, blows, knocks, bruises, etc., cause cancer—but this is a mistake. They may *occasion* cancer, sometimes, perhaps, (though not so often as is generally supposed) but they do not *cause* it. And the distinction should be apparent to my readers. Why such blows, etc., occasion cancer is intelligible enough; it is for this reason: The bruise occasions a temporary obstruction in the minute blood vessels at that point, causing a congestion and temporary blockage or obstruction. If the system is surcharged with effete, mal-assimilated material, this will commence to "dam" and collect in that part, being caught and retained by the blockage in the blood vessels. This obstruction, since it is not removed, becomes chronic, and chronic congestion follows; inflammatory symptoms appear; the part is at once overfed and under-nourished, while oxidation and elimination are practically impossible within that area; continued accretion continues, while the old material is not removed; a growth is formed —perhaps a tumor, perhaps a cancer! As Doctor Trall put it:[1]

> " A blow, a bruise, a clot of blood, a floating impurity, a morbid humor, have disorganized a portion of the living organism, or formed a nucleus to which the organic atoms may be accreted or transformed by a new series of affinities . . . "

It is merely a question of time; of the condition of the organism; (of the quality and quantity of the effete material it contains) which determines what the growth will be; and it should be obvious from this, that, unless such conditions exist, and such impurities are present, any growth of the kind—simple or malignant[2]—would be impossible, for the reason that the true causal

[1] "Uterine Diseases and Displacements," p. 85.

[2] That simple and malignant growths are, in the ultimate analysis, one and the same thing, or rather that the causes of the one are invariably the causes of the other, is clearly shown in Dr. A. Rabagliati's "After-Medical Treatment in Cases of Ovariotomy and Other Surgical Operations."

agencies would be lacking[1] If the system were pure and free from such obstructing material; and, *e.g.*, a blow were struck, the resultant congestion would be merely transitory and quite harmless —passing off in a short time—and for the very obvious reason that there would be no impurities in the system to collect at any such point or nucleus—even provided such were formed. And so a growth of the kind would become an utter impossibility; and tumors, cancers, etc., are thus traced back to the one primary cause which is equally the cause of all diseases whatsoever. *It is the overplus of mal-assimilated material within the system; and it is this and not the blow, which is the real cause of the disease.* And the remedy also becomes apparent—the oxidation and elimination of the morbid material which caused the obstruction in the first place. Unfortunately, the tendency to regard cancer as a purely "local" disease makes the acceptance of this view of its causation all the more difficult of acceptance. As Dr. Samuel Dickson wrote:[2]

> "It is a very common error on the part of medical men, to state in their reports of cases, that a 'healthy' person presented himself with a particular tumor in this or that situation. Now, such practitioners, by the very expression, show how much they have busied themselves with artificial distinctions —distinctions which have no foundation in nature or reason—to the neglect of the circle of actions which constitute the state of the body termed Health. Never did a tumor spring up in a perfectly healthy subject. In the course of my medical career, I have witnessed tumors of every description, but I never met one that could not be traced, either to previous constitutional disturbance, or to the effect of local injury on a previously unhealthy subject . . . "

It should now be apparent that fasting, in the initial stages of this disease (cancer), should be capable of curing this terrible disease—for the reason that it would absorb, oxidize and eliminate the blocking and encumbering material—thus preventing its permanent presence, and final disorganization of the material lodged in the blood vessels. All the predisposing causes of the disease would thus be removed, and the disease itself rendered impossible. This idea I shall now attempt to elaborate and defend in some detail.

I need hardly say that, among the exponents and defenders of this view, Doctor Rabagliati—himself a cancer specialist—is one of the most prominent and persistent. His view is that "overfeeding is the predisposing cause of cancer."[3] He defends this

[1] See Page: "Natural Cure," p. 38.
[2] "Chrono-Thermal System of Medicine," etc., p. 129.
[3] "Air, Food and Exercises," p. 398.

view at length in his books, giving abundant evidence to show that such is in all probability the case, and asserts that fasting is the only hope for a permanent cure. Revolutionary as this may appear, he is not alone in this view. Dr. C. P. Newcombe[1] has stated his conviction of this fact, and recommends fasting as a cure. (p. 33.) Doctor Haig[2] stated that it is almost always in the highly fed that cancer appears, and that restriction of the diet is the only rational course to pursue. Dr. Robert Bell clearly traced the connection between cancer and over-feeding,[3] while this author hints that the causation of leprosy is also, probably, wrong diet.[4]

Doctor Rabagliati shows in great detail how this excess of food material must be the chief predisposing cause. Taking the accepted view that a cancer is the result of hypertrophy, or overgrowth,[5] he goes on to say:[6]

"The essence of the disease . . . is the hypertrophy; the occurrence of parasites the accident. Now, the question is, what is the chief predisposing cause of the overgrowth? Well, what *can* be the cause except an excess of materials in the blood? And if so, whence came the excess of material which is poured out of the blood in the form of the cancerous exudation? What source can there be but the environment of the organism? And of all the facts of environment, what so likely to be the chief cause of change in the body as the food?"

Says Doctor Newcombe:[7]

"Always bear in mind that your object and intention is to starve out your enemy by taking only what food you want for yourself with none to spare to feed the cancer, so that it may wither away."

This is, it will be observed, but another way of putting Doctor Dewey's dictum, "starve a sick man, and you have begun to starve, not the sick man but the disease." Doctor Keith quotes a case of a woman who recovered from cancer by living for two years on a small quantity of milk daily.[8] He noted a marked relief in all cases when an extremely light diet was allowed. (pp. 82–3.)

[1] "Diet Cure of Cancer," pp. 15–16.
[2] "Cancer and Uric Acid," pp. 3, 4, 7.
[3] "Constipation Prevented by Diet," by Albert Broadbent, pp. 5–6.
[4] "Fruits, Nuts and Vegetables," p. 7.
[5] I think I am right in saying this is now the all-but universally held theory; the older view that they are due to "wandering corpuscles becoming fixed and developing into epithelial cells," ("On the Structure of Cancerous Tumors and the Mode in which Adjacent Parts are Invaded," by J. J. Woodward, M.D., p. 20), being quite given up.
[6] "Air, Food and Exercises," pp. 397–98.
[7] "Diet Cure of Cancer," p. 37.
[8] "Fads of an Old Physician," p. 84.

Sir W. Banks, Doctor Kellogg, Dr. J. E. Gemmell, all take the stand that there is a close connection between cancer and wrong food habits.[1] Doctor Dewey defended this view; Sir Benj. Ward Richardson stated his conviction that cancer was closely connected with the excess of rich foods consumed.[2] Doctor Shew was convinced that fasting was the only hope for cancerous patients,[3] and many other writers are inclined to take a similar view, of late.

Doctor Robert Dawbarn, of New York, arrived at the conclusion that cancer and similar growths were due to excessive nutrition of the parts involved, owing to the fact that "malignant growths seem endowed with a relatively large number of blood vessels as one of their striking characteristics,"[4] so that, "when this mass of billions of cells is suddenly reduced to feeding upon no more blood than the adjacent healthy tissues get, then, because of their aggregate bulk, each individual malignant cell may be supposed to get less nourishment than does each cell of the adjacent healthy flesh. Consequently we might naturally expect them to be more nearly killed than are the latter." But since he had previously shown that "the more food, the greater activity" (of the growth), Doctor Dawbarn concluded that the only rational method of treatment was to decrease the blood-supply to the diseased part—to induce a local, peripheral anæmia, and for this reason he performed a number of operations—excising one external carotid artery. It was soon found, however, that even this failed to cut off the blood-supply sufficiently, and that the growth, although checked, was not eradicated. Accordingly, he finally resorted to excision of both external carotids! As might be expected, every one of the patients died! But I am not criticising Doctor Dawbarn or his work. He has got so far as to recognize that cancers and other malignant growths are the result of over-nutrition, and that is one step in the right direction, at least. But the treatment is open to at least two fatal objections, to which I would now call attention.

Doctors have not yet realized that operations, *per se*, do not and can not cure; they merely remove the *effect of a cause—a product*, so to speak.[5] Operations only remove the effects of causes—the cause being the real disease. No operation can, therefore, ever

[1] "Food and Strength," by the Hon. R. Russell, pp. 481–83.
[2] "Diseases of Modern Life," pp. 373.
[3] "Family Physician," pp. 584–85.
[4] "Starvation Treatment of Certain Malignant Growths," p. 118.
[5] See Doctor Hilton's "Lectures on Rest and Pain," p. 63.

cure any patient, unless the habits of life are at the same time changed, for the reason that the cause which rendered the first growth possible would, if allowed to operate in the system, produce the same growth in the same or some other place, or some other disease at a later time. The operation only removes the effects of this cause—which must be removed, if a real cure is ever to be effected. The *real* cure is the removal of the cause which rendered the operation necessary.

Second. As before stated, Doctor Dawbarn's idea was to check the excessive supply of nutrition to the affected parts—to "starve" them—and in this he was quite right. But, I ask, would it not be far more rational to withhold the food-supply at its source—the stomach—and so starve the parts in a natural and gradual manner, by general denutrition, and without the exhausting, dangerous and ultimately useless operations? Such would certainly seem to be the more rational theory. I cannot elaborate this idea here, for lack of space; but I think the theory should be sufficiently apparent, without such elaboration.

APPENDIX K

It would be impossible for me to oppose too strongly the system of giving food in diseased conditions of any character whatever; and I say this with full knowledge of the many cases that have been cured by giving a "full diet"—cases treated by the Weir-Mitchell treatment, etc. I am persuaded that most of these cures are more apparent than real, and that the patient either suffers from the same or some other disease before so many years or even months have passed—owing to the same cause being continually operative within the system—*viz.*, over-nutrition. Doctor Keith asserted his belief that, "The excess of food given to those on the Weir-Mitchell system does much more harm than good; but this shows what massage can do even when so strongly handicapped."[1] To the majority of medical men too little food means but one thing—increase the intake! They seem to be blind to the facts that go to point that it is rather the inability of the system to utilize the food already ingested that causes the trouble; and that this inability is caused, in nine cases out of ten, by over-eating in the first place. Thus, we are told that at the Hospital for Consumptives on Blackwell's Island, "there are nine hours of sleep, and the patients eat nine times a day. . . "[2] And Doctor Densmore tells us that:

> " . . Here are three features of the cure: nourishment, rest, and fresh air. Of the three, the over-feeding is by far the most important, for it is conceivable that a cure might be effected by this means alone, which could never be accomplished by rest and fresh air only."[3]

Is it not marvelous that any patients at all get well under such barbarous treatment? And what wonder that consumption is such a deadly disease—instead of having Trall's record of "hundreds of cases treated, and none lost."

And this extends to other diseases also. Doctor Partsch contended that the best way to prevent sea-sickness was to "keep

[1] "Fads of an Old Physician," p. 64.
[2] C. H. Davis, M.D., "Self-Cure of Consumption," p. 89.
[3] "Consumption and Chronic Diseases," p. 53.

the blood saturated with nutrient material," and said that food should be eaten every ten minutes! What wonder that people get sea-sick? Doctor Osborne, again,[1] gives instructions for feeding insensible persons!

As another example I quote the following from "The Lightning Doctor," by Benj. F. Weaver, M.D., p. 141, where, in speaking of typhoid fever, he says:

"Robertson marshals a strong array of facts in favor of more liberal feeding in typhoid fever. It is strange, in view of the fact that the exhaustive wasting is so pronounced in this disease, and since no specific remedy exists, that no determined effort is made to increase the resistance of the patient by systematic and judicious feeding. Fitz has shown by statistical study of the cases occurring in the Massachusetts General Hospital from 1821 to 1899—a period of seventy-eight years—that the mortality has varied little from the days when calomel, tartar emetic, and bleeding were practised, to the present time."

Indeed, one can quite see why this thould be the case!—and it is quite probable that no very great change *will* be noted until the fasting method be tried and adopted. In view of the fact that most persons assert that no physicians would think of giving solid food in typhoid, now-a-days, I think this quotation is interesting. Even so "orthodox" a writer as Dr. Burney Yeo realized that no food should be allowed in typhoid, and pointed out that the conditions present indicated clearly that we must "keep the intestines absolutely at rest, and allow no débris of food to pass through to excite peristaltic action."[2] The idea that the patient's strength is to be kept up by passing food-rubbish over tender, bleeding surfaces is palpably ridiculous. Even did we receive strength from our food, it should be clear that we could not do so under any *such* circumstances. But, as we have seen that we do not derive any strength whatever from food, at any time, or under any circumstances, this notion of feeding the typhoid patient becomes little less than barbarous.

[1] "First Aid," p. 128.
[2] "Food in Health and Disease," p. 323.

APPENDIX L

The narrative I am about to give was sent me by my friend, Miss Louise W. Kops, in whose word I have the completest confidence. Miss Kops is a good observer, and knows what is needed in observations of this kind. In many ways I consider this report of interest, both because of the suggestive remark as to the relative time for feeding chicks and babies; and because of the fact that a chick was apparently brought back to life when to all appearances dead—though probably not really so—thus illustrating, in a most interesting manner, Sir Benj. Ward Richardson's statement. The significance of the facts I leave to my readers: I merely give the report *verbatim*, as sent to me. In part, it is as follows:

"On Thursday, May 30th, 1907, I watched a batch of fifty eggs hatch out in an incubator. The first chick came out about 5 P.M., and the others started about 9 P.M., and continued all through the night. A chick would first peck a hole in the shell, and then stop for a second or two, and then continue to do some pecking, until it had a good sized hole in the shell; then it would rest for quite a few moments before commencing to struggle out of it. After one came out of the shell, it would rest some time before it would be strong enough to stand up. Of course, some seemed stronger than others, and got their balance quicker than they; yet even the weak chicks, who had to be taken out of the shells, sometimes proved as strong as the others; and one chick especially so. He was practically lifeless when taken from the shell, and we did not think he could live, but after the third day, (which is the length of time they are left in the incubator, after they come out of the shell, and the length of time a hen sits on her chicks, before she gets off to feed them), I took this little chick that had been so lifeless, and cared for him —giving him water from a spoon every ten minutes for the first day, and then feeding him on the yolk of an egg (warmed only) in a liquid form. I kept this up for about three days, giving him the egg about four times a day, but the water more often. He got stronger each day, and at the end of the week it was impossible to tell him from the others. I could distinguish him from the others at first because of the egg spilt down the front of him, from the spoon, while feeding him. There were others who were weak also, and these I would take up in my hand, and teach them to drink; sometimes they would appear to be very weak, but as soon as they had taken several drinks of water they would brighten up and become quite lively and attempt to pick for themselves. And so we cared for them all—and there were about fifty of them—for a week, and they grew to be fine little chicks and were very tame. The days when they had to stay in the brooder, they were not quite so lively, but as soon as they were put out of doors they would brighten up in less than ten minutes. .

"I wish to note here the method of setting of the hen—and of the incubator—when the eggs are first put under her for setting. She does not get off the eggs for three days; neither do you open the incubator. That is done to warm the eggs first, and then, after that, the hen gets off but once a day to feed and eat. After she has eaten, she turns her eggs over, and sits on them again until the next morning. When the eggs hatch out the chicks are left for another three days, with neither food nor water. After the third day they are put in a brooder, and those that are strongest begin to pick for food; and when they drink they will stand up and drink from the cup, several mouthfuls at a time. I quote this to show how much better animals are cared for (with regards to their eating) than babies, who are usually fed the first day.

"On Thursday, June 6th, one of the little chicks was hurt by being squeezed between the board of the brooder and the side, and was hurt quite badly. Mrs. H. took him out and held him for about an hour on her chest, and he seemed to revive. We then put him in a box, in the brooder, and a few hours later I found him practically lifeless. The other chicks had hopped in the box, and stood on the top of him, and he, being weak, was unable to help himself, or get out. When I took him in my hands he was *cold*, and lay over, apparently with no life. I held him in my hands, and took him over to the stove, and held my hands in the oven for a second or two. Then I gave him drops of water to drink every few minutes, and he revived so far that he could sit up. I then placed him in a small basket, and hung it by the door of the stove—taking him out every ten minutes and giving him water to drink. At the end of an hour and a half he stood up on the table and chirped! He was as bright as could be. I put him back in the basket, not giving him water quite so often. He lived for about six hours after he was hurt; then died. I think I made a mistake in leaving him too near the stove at the last part of his treatment; if I had wrapped him up and taken him out of doors, it seemed to me he would have lived. (This is only a supposition.) But he was quite bright for a whole hour after he came to, and only seemed to sink again after placing him near the oven at the last. Mrs. H. could prove the details, as she was there, and saw just what I did to the chick, and how I brought him back to life. I write this after copying the details from my diary, which I kept at West Willington, Conn.

"LOUISE W. KOPS."

APPENDIX M

The following paper I reprint *verbatim*, at the request of several persons, who heard it read. Under the auspices of the Health-Culture Club, of New York, of which I was then Treasurer, a debate was held on February 13th, 1906, the following being topic debated:

Resolved—*That the food-factor is the most important single factor in the maintenance of health.*

The affirmative was maintained by Mr. Eugene Christian and myself; the negative being taken by Doctors Patchen and Taylor. I am glad to say that the affirmative side won easily. The fol lowing is my paper as then read:

Ladies and Gentlemen:

It is, of course, most hard to pick out any one factor that is the *most* important in the maintenance of health—since *all* the laws of hygiene must be obeyed, in order that the greatest degree of physical and mental health may be preserved. The position I occupy to-night is, therefore, *not* that these other hygienic agencies are in themselves unimportant, or anything but of the greatest importance, but it is that if we are to choose any one factor, the food-factor is the *most* important, for the reason that the abuse of the laws relating to diet and food will, in the end, lead to more disastrous consequences to the organism, than the greater or lesser use of any other single physiological auxiliary in the maintenance of health. In occupying this ground, I shall, therefore, come at once to the point, and give my reasons for believing this to be so:

‡ 1. First, I would point out that, in lower organisms, biologists have always asserted that reproduction and nutrition are the two most important and most essential factors in the perpetuation of the race of any species; reproduction continuing the race, or perpetuating it; nutrition maintaining the physiological integrity of the individual living at any one time; and, though it will be seen that reproduction is all important to the race, nutrition is even more important, for the reason that, if the individual fails to receive its proper share, the race would die out promptly, since there would be no organisms left to reproduce their like. For the individual, therefore, nutrition is the most important factor entering into the case; reproduction merely subsidiary, and depending altogether upon it, in so far as it depends upon the organism that nutrition has maintained. And, in these lower organisms, and especially in those thriving in the *water*, air and breathing must certainly

be of altogether insignificant importance when compared with this question of nutrition—while, with them, all the exercise which they are called upon in their actual life to take is just as much exercise as is necessitated in their search for, and devouring of, food. Nutrition is, therefore, with them, the one primal all-important factor; and this aspect of the problem has, I think, been overlooked by those physiologists who would maintain that the food-factor is second to *any* in the order of importance.

‡ 2. I should now like to answer the most forcible objection that can be raised against this position—that food is the most important factor—and it would be in favor of breathing as against food; the position being, we shall be told, that, whereas one may live for many days without food, and for many hours without water, it is possible to live only for a few minutes without air; and this is a fact which I shall not, of course, attempt, for one minute, to dispute. At first sight, that proves conclusively that breathing is the most important factor, but I think it shows only that the complete arrest of the breathing function induces death somewhat *more rapidly* than the complete arrest of any other physiological function—since any one of these arrested completely would ultimately result in death. One might answer, indeed, that a blow on the head would terminate our life even more speedily than the cessation of the breathing process, and consequently that a sound brain is the most important factor in the maintenance of health; but I do not think that this reasoning can be carried to its logical conclusion on these lines. We must take the ultimate, all-day effects of any one process, and, in summing up the effects of the greater or lesser abuse of that process or functioning, and of its effects upon the organism, we will find, I think, that this process or function of breathing can be infringed upon and abused to a greater extent than the function of nutrition can be abused; and that its ultimate effects upon the organism will be less harmful. That is, I contend that breathing impure air, or too little air, though doubtless of great harm to the vital economy, is not *so* harmful as an equal proportion of abuse of the bodily nutrition; and in support of this view, I would call to your attention the following from Doctor Rabagliati's work: "Air, Food and Exercises," pp. 4–5.

"As a preliminary to the consideration of the question whether it is more likely that bad, vitiated air or wrong feeding is the more potent cause [of certain diseases], let us consider which of these two great sets of physiological processes most alters a man. A man emits as much carbonic acid gas through his respiration as would suffice to supply about half a pound of carbon daily, were it to be chemically separated from the carbonic acid gas. This is a large amount, and bears quite a considerable proportion to his body weight of say 140 pounds, or about 7 per cent. But if he takes what is generally considered the quite moderate allowance of two pounds of food daily, it is evident that he consumes his own weight of food in seventy days, or a little over two months; while if he takes three pounds of food daily, the quantity recommended by Dr. King Chambers, for the nursing mother, he consumes his own weight of food in forty-six days. Some physiologists contemplate with equanimity the consumption of five pounds of weight of food daily, and at this rate a man would eat his own weight in twenty-eight days. I hope to say something later regarding the very extensive quantities of fluid which in various forms pass into and out of the blood daily; but, referring now to food alone, as distinguished from water, I think I am justified in saying that, *à priori*, so to say, and on the general merits of the question, it is more likely that a man's body should be modified by food than by air. Of course, there are many other changes effected by the respiration than the mere emission of half a pound of carbon daily. Other organic materials, not to mention a quite considerable amount of watery vapour, are given forth by the lungs, but the total amount of change in the body effected by the respiration is very much less than the amount effected by the digestion and assimilation of food and water in the body. Whoever, therefore, should argue that food is probably a greater agent in producing health or disease in the body than air, founds his opinion on substantial facts of this kind; and, at any rate, no inherent improbability attaches to his contention."

‡ 3. The next point I would call to your attention is this: Food, and only food, *makes blood,* and blood, as we know, makes body; so that our bodily structure is dependent upon, and *only* upon, the food we eat. Breathing simply purifies that blood, or oxidizes it; exercise merely circulates it; but the food we eat is that which *makes* the blood, and in this respect food is certainly the most important factor that can possibly enter into the case from any point of view whatsoever. It may be claimed that proper breathing will oxidize all food material ingested, turning it into healthy blood, even if that material be at the start not of the best, and that insufficient breathing and exercise may render the best food unsuited to the organism, for the reason that it is not properly utilized, and remains, as it were, always mal-assimilated. To a certain extent this may be very true, but it only emphasizes the point that breathing and exercise are, in a sense, necessary, not that they are *more* essential than the food which they oxidize and circulate! Pure air cannot turn bad food into good blood. If the material used in the construction of a house be not of the best, no amount of careful plastering and no amount of ingenuity displayed by the contractors and builders can make that house as strong and as normal, so to speak, as if the material were, in the first place, the best. Moreover, I would insist upon the fact that breathing and exercise can never supply certain materials to the body, which, if lacking in the food, must be always lacking, and the body starve ultimately for lack of these materials. Thus, in those cases where the food lacks certain salts, in organic compound, the body dies, as we know, of saline starvation, and this would assuredly happen no matter how careful we were in breathing, or in exercise, or in mental attitude, or in any other manner whatever.

‡ 4. The position, then, which I assume is, that we may, with more or less impunity, neglect all other hygienic laws, as to exercise, breathing, etc., if we do take proper care of this great question of nutrition, or food supply—merely supplying to the body the proper quality and the proper quantity of food; and that this is no mere theory, but an actual demonstrable fact, is, I think, proved by some cases—notably, that of Mr. Horace Fletcher. In this case, as you will doubtless remember, Mr. Fletcher pays no particular attention to exercise, to breathing, to any of the great hygienic laws, except this one of the simplicity and reduction of the food supply. His daily exercise consists only in walks about town, yet, because he supplies the organism with only as much food as it actually requires, and does not overload and burden it with an unnatural excess, he is always in perfect physical condition, enabled to undertake the most strenuous physical exercises, such as those pursued by the athletes of our universities when in training for particular events, and *that* without any exhaustion at the time, or consequent stiffness and fatigue on the following day. And why? Simply because stiffness results from bringing to the surface, and lodging in the muscular tissues, mal-assimilated

food-material; and in *his* body there is no such material to bring to the surface; consequently, he is always in perfect physical training; and, further than that, he conserves, and is enable to expend in other ways, the immense amount of energy, which, in most cases, is utilized as "energy of digestion." And this practical case, supported as it is by others, less famous, perhaps, conclusively proves, it seems to me, the position I occupy—that if we were to give proper attention to our diet, all other agencies are of more or less inconsequence.

‡ 5. And this brings me to a simple practical point, which may, perhaps, have escaped your observation as yet, but the importance of which can hardly be over-estimated. It is this: that all these other hygienic auxiliaries are more or less dependent upon, and necessitated by, this question of the regulation of the food supply. Were the food simplified in quality and reduced in quantity, these other agencies would become unnecessary—for the reason that they are merely called upon to elimintae from the system a certain amount of mal-assimilated food material, which should never have been introduced. Thus; were we to have recommended to us a series of deep breathing exercises, this would merely prove, to my mind, that we must forcibly eliminate, through the lungs, a certain amount of nutritive material, over and above the amount that should normally have been carried there. Were we to have a series of exercises recommended, it would prove merely that it is necessary for us to forcibly oxidize or burn up, in this manner, an amount of material which is introduced into the body over and above its physiological requirements. Were there prescribed for us a greater quantity of water to be drunk daily, it would prove merely that the system needed cleansing, to a large extent, of material which should not have been present; and this applies throughout the list, as can readily be seen when we consider the reason for stimulating baths, enemas, etc. Now, the point I make is this: That were we not to introduce into the system, in the first place, the excessive food material, these other agencies would not be necessitated in order to oxidize, and get rid of, this super-abundance of material, that should never have)een introduced. And thus I contend that, of all the physiological, hygienic agencies that go to make perfect health, this one of the regulation, the simplifying and restriction of food supply, is by far the most important.

APPENDIX N

It is not my purpose to discuss here the momentous question of *insanity;* but I cannot refrain from offering one or two remarks upon one particular aspect of the question—that which connects insanity with the present food-habits of the people. Doctor Dewey contended most strongly, that such was the case, in his "No Breakfast Plan," pp. 157–70. He points out that, in many cases of insanity, no lesion of any kind is to be found that will explain the state of the mind existent. Now, it is known that excesses of all kinds are one of the great predisposing causes of insanity—anything that tends to deplete the vitality assisting in the work of destruction. Since, then, the digestive energies are the most severely taxed of all those in the body, as a rule, it will be seen that over-eating may be and probably is one of the chief causes of insanity to-day. This view has the support of Doctor Keith—a most cautious observer—for he says:[1]

"Believing as I do that rest is Nature's great cure for a damaged organ, I cannot help thinking that this rest of the brain might be a large element in the cure of the insane, and certainly the experiment of giving it would be a very safe one."

Doctor Rabagliati offers strong reasons for thinking that insanity is the direct outcome of the perverted food habits, and writes in part.[2]

" . One of the chief causes why such persons (the neurotic) not infrequently pass the border line between sanity and insanity, is, I believe, through the mismanagement of their food. I feel certain that many persons, especially women, are in asylums mainly through this cause. . . . If this be so, we can see how insanity is often brought on just as other diseases are, just in the same way, often, as an ordinary cold or sore throat is induced. . Sometimes love is said to make them go wrong, sometimes religion. The fact is, they are so disturbed that anything would or might have upset the balance. Love or religion may be the *occasion,* no doubt, but the condition of the nutrition is the main *cause.* The connective tissue inside the head

[1] "Fads of an Old Physician," p. 139.
[2] "Air, Food and Exercises," pp. 247–48; 319–20.

has become congested from improper nutrition, and has irritated the brain-cells, preventing their healthy action."

Doctor Page gives one very interesting case in which a patient recovered normal mental health by fasting forty-one days, after other treatment had miserably failed.[1] Even so orthodox a practitioner as Doctor Pereira,[2] insists that many insane patients are in no real condition to eat or properly digest food, and that:

"To force food into the enfeebled and dying stomach would not be sanctioned by any well-regulated hospital . and their distinction (between the refusal to eat food because of a morbid fancy of some kind and a truly diseased state) ought not to be overlooked because they occur in a hospital for the insane."

Let us take an example of this mal-treatment, as I conceive it to be, so far as the food habits of the insane patients go. Kraepelin, in his "Clinical Psychiatry," after admitting (p. 2), that "only a comparatively small percentage of mental cases are permanently and completely cured in the strictest sense of the term," and that *poisons* are frequently the direct cause of insanity—especially the poisons resultant from certain diseases (pp. 341–2), cites a number of cases in which patients had to be fed against their will, in all sorts of barbarous and villainous ways, and advises this method of treatment strongly! Yet it is obvious to any one reading the cases that the excessive food forced upon the system is one of the chief causes of the condition that is present, both from the description of the case, and from what the patient said. Thus: "He complained bitterly of the whole treatment, and especially of the artificial feeding, so long necessary, which he said had made him ill," runs one passage. Others could be mentioned *ad. lib.*, if necessary. On p. 343 it is acknowledged that "waste products" are one great factor in the causation of insanity. C. R. Krehbiel distinctly stated that "through intemperate eating I contracted a disease which brought me twice into the asylum."[3] Dr. Charles Mercier, in his "Text-Book of Insanity" (p. 46), admits that "by far the most important of the direct stresses, perhaps the most important of all the stresses which contribute to the production of insanity, is alteration in the composition of the blood by which the highest nerve regions are nourished." "Poisonous food" is spoken of as one of the causes of poisoned blood, and

[1] "Natural Cure," pp. 140–43.
[2] "Food and Diet," p. 256.
[3] "Memories and Experiences," by One Demented, p. 23.

hence insanity. It does not seem to have occurred to our authors that the best food, in excess, will produce the same poisoning effects upon the organism—a fact of unparalleled importance, yet one that is never or hardly ever recognized as a *vera causa* by the medical profession. Until this truth is thoroughly established and recognized, but little hope can be entertained that any great advancement will be made in the treatment of the insane.

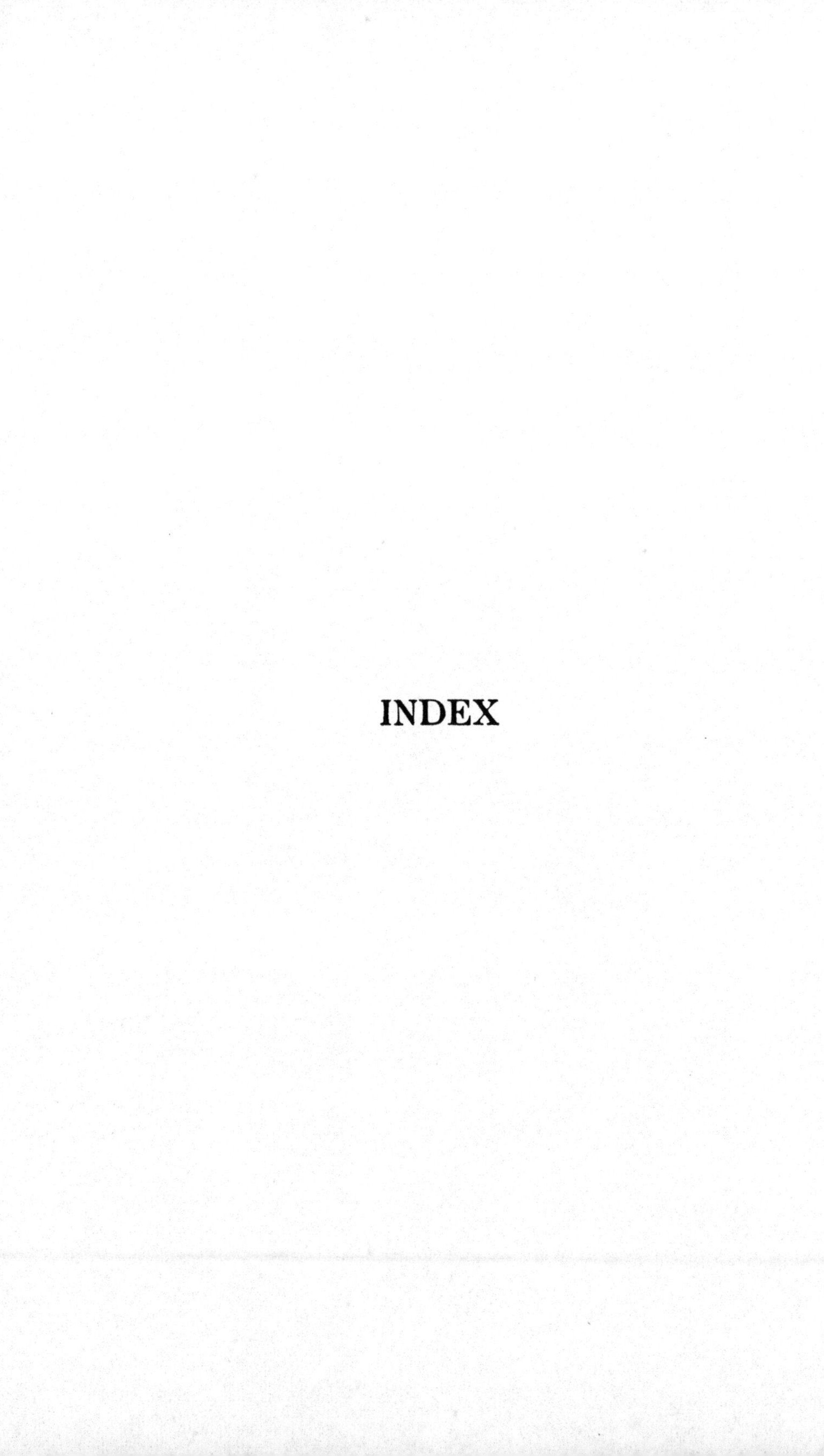

INDEX

INDEX

A., Mrs. T., Case of, 195–7
Abel, Mary H., on sugar injections and fatigue, 281
Abhedananda, Swami, on Yogi practices, 108
 on the connection of vital energy with the body, 322
Abnormal appetite, 551–3
Abnormally slow pulse, causes of, 528–9
 treatment of, 529
Abnormally rapid pulse, causes of, 530
 treatment of, 530–2
Acclimatization, 177–8
Acid, uric, *see* Uric acid
Action of drugs, 31–33
 of bowels, while fasting, 420–22
Active exercise, *see* Exercise
Acute and chronic disease, 60
Aëration, imperfect, as a cause of emaciation, 277
After-cures, 392
After effects of disease, 450
Aged, overfeeding of, 135
Air, impure, and bad diet, 89
 city and country, 89
 and food, proportion of, 120
 night, 315
 fresh, importance of, 351
 and food, 352
 impure, effects of, 353
 amount required by each person, 353
 changes of, in body, 353
 fresh, and pneumonia, 354–5
Alcohol, question of its efficacy, 34–41
 and energy production, 37–8
 stimulates appetite, 38
 differing action of, 40
Alcoholic thirst, 39
Alcoholism, rational cure of, 110–11
Alkali, same as a fasting, for uric acid, 157
Altered bodily conditions, and diet, 88
Amount of sleep required, while fasting, 319–22
Anæmia, cerebral, as a cause of sleep, 305
Anæmia of skin, cause of sense of chilliness, 375
Anæmia of skin, treatment of, 604–5
Anæsthetics, questionable use of, 26–
Anæsthetic, rapid breathing as an, 35
Anger, effects of, upon secretions, 42(
Animals, instinct of, to fast, 77–8
 lower, feeding habits of, 106–7
 number of meals for, 147
Antiseptics, 150
Appendicitis, 498
Appetite, stimulated by alcohol, 38
 influence of habit upon, 116, 11
 stimulation of, 170
 return of normal, 173
 loss of, case of cure of, 222
 after fasting, 492–4
 abnormal, 551–3
 creation of, 556
Arachnoid plexus, excessive functioning of, as a cause of sleep, 30
Arguments, summing up of, 572–4
Asiatic cholera, temperature during 448
Asthma, case of cure of, 222
Atmosphere, temperature of, 357
Atmospheric dampness, 357
Atomic grouping, difference in, as a cause of death, 331
Atwater, Prof. W. O., on source and equivalence of energy, 230–1
 on amount required in mental operations, 231
 on impossibility of measuring potential energy, 233
 on fuel value of foods, 344–5
 on heat and energy production in the body, 348
Atwater, Helen W., on certainty of energy supply, 243
Austin, Dr. Harriet N., on irrational clothing, 371
Auto-infection, as a cause of disease, 167
Auxiliaries, hygienic, importance of, while fasting, 539
Average loss of weight, while fasting, 468
Average length of life, 593–4
Aversion to food, by the sick, 171, 17?
 by the insane, 623
Awakening at a fixed hour, 305

B., Dr., case of, 208
B., J., case of, 188–9
B., Mrs., case of, 189
B., Robert, case of, 197–8
Babies, overfeeding of, 133–5
fasting for, 133
normal growth of, 134
treatment of, 606–8
Bacilli, *see* Germs
Bacteria, *see* Germs
Bad taste in the mouth, while fasting, 526
Bain, Prof. Alexander, on functions of food in the body, 236
on methods for increasing bodily energy, 237
Bailey, George M., on regularity at meals, 542
Baker, Dr. A. R., on atmospheric dampness, 357
Balbirnie, Dr. John, on normal hunger, 147
Balancing of circulation, *see* Circulation
Bandages, how administered, 365
Banks, Sir W., on diet and cancer, 612
Barker, Prof. Anthony, on fasting, 487
Barker, Prof., on drug medication, 584
Barling, Dr., on appendicitis, 498
Bathing, amount of, 360
and food habits, 362–3
Baths, cold, 361
medicated, 361
warm, 361
Beale, Prof. Lionel S., on distinctions of vital and chemical action, 249
on the nucleus as a source of energy, 294
Beaumont, Dr., case recorded by, 62
on length of time for digestion, 486
Bell, Dr. Robert, on diet and cancer, 611
Bellows, Dr. A. J., on heart failure, 167
on iron for anæmia, 605
Bernard, Claud, on vitality, 293
Berrier, M., on inflow of energy, 253
Besant, Annie, on the influence of bodily conditions upon mental life, 517
Best time for fasting, 108
Bichat, Prof., on drug medication, 583
Bible, on vegetarianism, 81
on fasting, 91
on the no-breakfast plan, 136
Bigelow, John, theory of sleep, 304
Black, Dr. George, on theory of sleep, 309
on physiological cleanliness, 366
on specific reaction of nerves, 599
on food for babies, 606
Blockage, as a cause of death, 331
Blood, impoverishing of, 109
black, in suffocation, 354

Burke, Dr. J. Butler, on dissimilarity of natural and created life, 287
on incertitude of experiments in spontaneous generation, 288
on crystals, 292
on the nucleus as a source of energy, 294
on organic rhythm, 323
on definition of life, 334

., Mrs. J. F., case of, 194–5
Cabanis, Dr., theory of sleep, 305
Cajal, Ramon y, theory of sleep, 305
alderon, Council of, on fasting, 91
Call, Annie P., on imperfect relaxation, 252
alories of heat, question of, 344–5
ancer, causes of, 609–13
blows and, 609
and diet, 611
nature of, 611
structure of, 611
how cured, 613
Cannon, Dr. W. B., on intestinal movements during injections, 417
on movements of the intestines during sleep, 486
Cappie, Dr., theory of sleep, 305
arotid artery, excision of, for cancer, 612
Carpenter, Dr. W. B., on remarkable gains in weight, 480
on sleep, 305
Cases, miscellaneous, 222–3
Catarrh, cases of cure of, 186, 188–9, 197–8, 223
Causes of death, *see* Death
Causes of disease, 6, 9–10, 13
Cerebral congestion, as a cause of sleep, 305
hyperæmia, as a cause of sleep, 305
Certainty, conditions of, 8
Chapman, Dr. N., on intestinal obstruction, 420
Chemical *vs.* vital action of drugs, 32
and vital forces, 293
theories of sleep, 305
Chest, carriage of, 359
protection of, 372
protectors, 372
Children, growing, amount of food required by, 608
Chilliness, sensation of, due to anæmic skin, 375
Chittenden, Prof. Russell H., on minimum food supply, 115, 116
on influence of habit upon appetite, 116
on the source of bodily energy, 234
on the relations of diet and the amount of water craved, 388

Consciousness, sleep a resting time of, 306
Conservation of energy, law of, 227–8
life wrongly included under, 228
new construction of, 297–8
Constipation, cases of cure of, 220–1
caused by insufficient water drinking, 390
universality of, 406
possible, with daily movements, 418–19
Constitutional treatment, 19
Consumption, cases of cures of, 194–5, 222
and carriage of chest, 359
causes of, 495–6
curability of, 603
milk diet for, 603
causes of, 602–3
overfeeding for, 614
Cooking, effects of, upon food, 87, 265
Cooley, Dr. J. S., on remarkable gains of weight, 479
Cornaro, Luigi, on cures by fasting, 92
case of, 113
on impossibility of disease, when in health, 127
Corning, Dr., theory of sleep, 305
Corns, cause of, 374
Corpuscles, blood, effects of fasting upon, 511
Correspondence of eating and breathing, 602–3
Corsets, question of, 373
Cosmic energy, 250
capacity to draw upon, 277–8
germs, 285
Cosmozoans, 285
Cough, *rationale* of, 12
Council of Calderon, on fasting, 91
Craig, Dr. J. M., on orange *vs.* lemon juice, while fasting, 405
Cramps, while fasting, 524
Crandall, Dr. Floyd M., on plurality of disease, 17
on germ diseases, 50
on diabetes, 187
Cravings and dislikes of the sick, 171
Cravings, abnormal, 552
Creation of appetite, 556
Creation of life, 286
criticism of experiments in, 288–9
Crises, *rationale* of, 518–19
comparative rarity of, during a fast, 536–7
Crosby, Ernest, on compression of the feet, 373
Crying, therapeutic value of, 352
Crystals, similarity of, to living organism, 291
distinctions between, 292
Crystals and vitality, 292
Cures, miraculous, 162, 299, 426
by lightning, 162
Curious phenomena, observed while fasting, 535–6
Cut throat, treatment of, 357–8

ewey, Dr. E. H., on waste of vitality in digestion, 103
on elimination of fat, by fasting, 132
on abnormality of morning appetite, 140
on the effects upon the stomach of unnecessary food, 144
on frequent eating, 146
on the origin of all disease, 149
on the evolution of disease, 153–4
on the philosophy of fasting, 155
on the discovery of the fasting cure, 160–1
on death from starvation, 161
on the non-waste of the nervous system, during a fast, 163–4
on the impossibility of feeding the body, while diseased, 165
on disease as a cause of bodily weakness, 270
on activity denoting an expenditure of energy, 274
on disease, a summing up, 326
on bathing, 361, 362
on exercise while fasting, 378
on water drinking during a fast, 402
on effects of mental states upon digestion, 437
on the character of the breath while fasting, 446
on fasting as a cure for over and under weight, 475
on thin and thick blood, while fasting, 510
on vomiting, during a fast, 534, 535
on death while fasting, 539
on natural and artificial hunger, 551
on breaking the fast, 559, 560, 562
on diet and cancer, 612
on the causes of insanity, 622
Dexter, Prof. Edwin G., on weather influences, 152
Diabetes, case of cure of, 187–8
Diagnosis, value of, 2
by means of blood, 508–9
facial, 589–91
Diarrhœa, while fasting, treatment of, 525
Diet, question of, 81–89
and altered bodily conditions, 88
bad, and impure air, 89
bad, and drunkenness, 110
influence of, upon mental life, 111–12
reduced, improvement under, 115
Japanese, 116
and exercise, 384–5
and work, 386

Dodds, Dr. Susanna, on thin and thick blood, 511
  on natural and artificial hunger, 550
Downie, George, ease of, 463
Draughts, question of, 355
Drinking at meals, 397, 599
Dropsy, case of cure of, 205–8, 223
Drug medication, fallacy of, 20–22
  opinions upon, 583–6
Drugs, poisonous, 22
  action of, 31–33
Drunkenness, and overfeeding, 110–11
  rational cure of, 110–11
  and fasting, 111
Dualism and monism, 432–3
Dubois, M. R., on physiological light, 293
Du Bois-Reymond, on origin of life, 285
Dunlop, Dr. Durham, on unity of disease, 17–18
  on small percentage of deaths under hygienic treatment, 73
Durant, Dr. Ghislani, on stimulation of appetite, 170
Durham, Dr., on theory of sleep, 305
Dutton, Dr. Thomas, on fasting for seasickness, 172
Duval, Dr., on theory of sleep, 305
Dynamometer, an indicator of increased strength, after sleep, 309
Dyspepsia, nervous and mental, 121
  case of cure of, 222

E., Mrs., case of, 208
Eales, Dr. I. J., case of, 216–20
Easily digested foods, 103–4, 275
Eating and breathing, must correspond, 602–3
Eating, frequent, 146
  before sleeping, danger of, 147
Ebbard, Dr. Richard J., on suggestion, 430
Eczema, cases of cure of, 220–1, 222
Edinger, Dr., on the limits of voluntary control of the food supply, 114
Edison, Thomas A., on drug medication, 585
Effects of cooking upon food, 87
Electric motor, body compared to, 249–50
Electricity, closely allied to life, 249
Emaciation, cause of, 121–2, 124, 474
  how cured, 474–5
  fasting, in cases of, 475–6
  checked by water, 480
  results from imperfect aëration, 277
Enema, how taken, 411
  positions for taking, 412
  author's method of taking, 412–15
  temperature of water, 412–13

Energy, connection of, with body, 322–3
and life, 330
percentage of, wasted, 387
increased, after breaking fast, cause of, 566–8, *see* Vitality
Energizing force of universe, 580
ngine, and body compared, 244–5
steam, compared with body, 117
steam, dissimilar to body, 249–50
nnui, cause of, 380
pidemics, 56–9
rrera, Dr. Leo, theory of sleep, 305
origin of life, 285
squimaux, food of, 341–2
strapper, Jr., J., case of, 469–70
vans, Dr. DeLacy, theory of vitality, 226
on causes of death, 331
on abnormal heat, 455
on drug medication, 586
volution of disease, 153–4, 326
xcess of food eaten, 101–35, 471–2
xercise, and energy, 273
and bodily heat, 335–6
on empty stomach, *rationale* of, 144–5
breaks down tissue, 248
water craved during, 273
limitations of meaning of, 378
question of, while fasting, 378, 382–4
definition of, 378
rationale of, 379
benefits of, 380
active and passive, 381
loss of weight from, 383
why necessary, 384
and diet, 384–5
Exhaustion, sexual, nature of, 282
rationale of, 282–3
from pain, 283
Experience, its worthlessness, 73
Experimental fasts, cases of, 216–20, 222
Experimenting upon health, 170
Exposure, supposed dangers of, 48
External energy, *see* Energy
External *vs.* internal causes of disease, 149–53
Eyesight, improvement of, while fasting, 205–8
Eyesight, bad, case of cure of, 220–21

Facial diagnosis, 589–91
Fæces, composition of, 421
Fainting, uses of, 437
during a fast, causes of, 523
treatment of, 523–4
Famine fever, 520–1
Fast, Christ's, 93
possibility of determining length of, 472–3

Fasting and consumption, 495–6
for strong sexual passions, 501
proper and improper, 519
effects of, upon mind of patient, 518–19
first days of, 519
increase of symptoms during, 519–23
vomiting during, 532–5
curious phenomena observed during, 535–6
causes of death, during, 537–9
unnecessary, if rules of health were followed, 541–3
varied duration of, 546
vs. starving, 563–4
for mental troubles, 575–6
as a panacea, 577
as a cure for cancer, 610–11
Fat, *vs.* thin persons, 121
a disease, 126–33
—— may starve in spite of presenee of, 128
not an indication of health, 131
how to dispose of, 132
digestive qualities of, 341
Fatty tissue, causes of increased, in married persons, 131
a product of overfeeding, 130
is retained excreta, 131
Fatigue, definition of, 278
theory disproved, 278–80
author's theory of, 279–80
and tissue poisoning, 279–80
nervous and muscular, 280
mental, not physical, 280–1
and multiple personality, 281–2
sugar injections and, 281
and sleep, 305
is disgusting, 315
upon awakening, 311–12, 315–17
Fayrer, Sir John, on comparative importance of temperature and food habits in hot climates, 152–3
Feet, cold, cause of, 123
cures by fasting, 123
Feet, compression of, 373–4
Fever, *rationale* of, 337
Filters, 390
Fireflies, 292–3
First days of fasting, 519
Fisher, Dr., theory of sleep, 305
Fisher, Dr. I. C., on open air treatment of pneumonia, 355
Fiske, Prof. John, on relations of mental life and bodily energy, 301–2
Flame, life compared to, 303
Flammarion, Camille, cases of paralysis cured by lightning, recorded by, 162

Food supply, all-importance of, 580
amount of, required by babies, 606–7
by nursing mothers, 607
by growing children, 608
most important factor, 618–21
aversion to, by insane, 623
Forbes, Sir John, on drug medication, 584
Forest, Dr. W. E., on purgatives, 409
on high temperature, 449
on stomachic conditions, 483
on colds, 587
Fox, Francis, on effects of impure air, 353
Franklin, Benjamin, on colds, 588
Frequent eating, 146
Fresh air, importance of, 351
Fruit and cold water, 396
Fruitarian diet, amount of food required in, 595
list of books on, 595–7
Fruitarianism, 86–9
Fuel value of foods, 344–5
Fumigation, 358–9

Gain of weight, *see* Weight—and loss from omitting a meal, 568–9
Gastric juice, secretion of, 488
influence of mind upon, 488
Gates, Prof. Elmer, on effects of mental states upon the organism, 426
Gaze, Harry, on immortality in the body, 327
Gemmell, Dr. J. E., on diet and cancer, 612
Generation, spontaneous, 284–5
George, Marion M., on sleep, 316
Germ theory, questioned, 46
Germ diseases, definition of, 49, 54
Germicides, 50–1
Germs, suitable soil for, 46–51
as scavengers, 50
and fasting, 51
benefactors, 51–2
poisons created by, 54–5
unimportance of, 55–6
real action of, 58–9
God, as energizing force of universe, 580
Good, Dr. John Mason, on drug medication, 584
Goodfellow, Dr. J., on altered bodily conditions and diet, 88
Graham, Dr. Sylvester, on unity of the organism, 17
on minimum food supply, 103
on fasting for the lean and the fat, 127
on the philosophy of fasting, 158
on experimenting upon health, 170
on stimulating foods, 268

Habit, influence of, upon appetite, 116–17
question of, 314
and water drinking, 403
hunger, 553–6
Haeckel, Prof. Ernst, on the nature of disease, 67
on the cause of death, 331
Haig, Dr. Alexander, on uric acid, 157
on stimulation *vs.* strength, 312–13
on the influence of bodily conditions upon mental life, 517
on the reaction of the skin, 545
on diet and cancer, 611
Hair, question of washing, 367
Hall, Dr. Marshall, theory of sleep, 305
Hammond, Dr. William A., theory of sleep, 305
on immortality in the body, 328
Hampson, Dr. William A., on the output of energy by radium, 254
Hancock, H. Irving, on the Japanese diet, 116
Hands, cold, cause of, 123
cured by fasting, 123
Hanish, Dr. O., on breaking the fast, 563
Hanney, P. M., on the dissimilarities of the body and steam engine, 244
Harm, from fasting, supposed, 487
Hartmann, Dr. Franz, on the cause of death, 331

Harvey, Dr. William, on the condition of the tongue, 442
Haskell, Charles C., on the impossibility of normal hunger more than twice daily, 145
on mental influences, during a fast, 439
on natural hunger, 549
Headaches, cause of, 28, 138, 139
cure of, 139
chronic, case of cure of, 189, 210–11
while fasting, treatment of, 525–6
Health, ideal, non-existent, 63
and bodily temperature, 350
Heart, failure, causes of, 167
strengthened, and increased energy, 278
weak, 500
effects of fasting upon, 500
pain in, 528
Heat, bodily, and alcohol, 35–6
and energy, souree of, 230–1
current theories of, 232–3
not dependent upon food supply, 333
correspondence of, to rate of vibration, 334–5
author's theory of, 335
and exercise, 335–6
and energy expended, 337
and foods, 337–8, 343–5
and sexual excitement, 348
Heath, Dr. F. M., on waste of life in digesting food, 105
Height, in proportion to weight (standard), 218
Hemiplegia, *see* Paralysis
Hemmeter, Dr., on the excess of food eaten, 101
Hemorrhoids, case of cure of, 220–1
Henderson, Mrs. Mary F., on the universality of disease, 593
Heredity, 150–1
Hibernation, 108
Higgins, Dr. H., on decrease of weight, with benefit, 130
Hindus, food habits of, 145
Hinton, Dr. James, on pain, 28
Hip baths, how administered, 365
Hippocrates, on the philosophy of fasting, 155
Histological theories of sleep, 305–6
Historic fasts, 90–5
Holbrook, Dr. M. L., on the effects of cooking upon food, 87
on fasting, 94
on the amount of food required, during pregnancy, 607
Holland, Dr., theory of sleep, 305
Holmes, Dr. Oliver Wendell, on drugs, 25, 30

nsane, feeding of, 623
nsanity, case of cure of, 223
causes of, 622–4
nsensible persons, feeding of, 615
nsomnia, case of cure of, 186
while fasting, treatment of, 526–8
nstantaneous energizing, during sleep, 246–7
nstinct, in animals, to fast, 77–8
for no-breakfast plan, 143–4
nternal muscular work, energy required by, 232
nternal *vs.* external causes of disease, 149–53
ntestine, disorders of, 209
movements of, during injection, 417
obstruction of, 418–20
amount of fecal matter contained by, 420
movements of, during sleep, 486
large, removal of, 499
ntoxication, physiological, as a cause of sleep, 305
ron, for anæmia, 605

., Mrs. T., case of, 209
ackson, Dr. James C., on stimulants, 35
on diphtheria, 53
on the real curative power, 66
on "agreement" of foods, 85
on no-breakfast plan, 143
on the causes of deafness, 198
on mineral waters, 391
on natural death, 593
affa, Prof., on cooked and uncooked foods, 600
ames, Prof. William, on effects of muscular tension upon the mental life, 252
on priority of nervous activity to circulation, 305
on phosphorus and nerve activity, 514
amison, Dr. A. B., on intestinal impurities, 406–7
on purgatives, 409
on the position for enema taking, 412
on the temperature of water for enema taking, 413
on journeys for health, 418
on the possibility of constipation with daily movements, 418
on the composition of the fæces, 421
on the quantity of the secretions, 504
apanese, diet, 116
rarity of heart failure among, 168
Johnson, Dr. James, on drug medication, 585
Joule, Prof., on the similarity of the body to electric motor, 250
Journeying for health, 418

Lactic acid, a cause of sleep, 305
Lahmann, Dr. H., on uric acid, 157
on anæmia, 605
Langemeyer, Dr., on sugar injections and fatigue, 281
Langlet, Dr., theory of sleep, 305
Langworthy, Dr., on phosphorus and fish, 514
Lateau, Louise, case of stigmata in, 427
Latson, Dr. W. R. C., on auto-infection, 167
on starvation from overfeeding, 418

Latson, Dr. W. R. C., on effects of diet upon the heart, 461
Lawrence, Dr., on the action of drugs, 31
Laws of nature, impossibility of deviating from, 592–4
Laxative foods, before fasting, 422
Laying on of hands, possible benefits from, 255
Laziness, a sign of disease, 315
LeConte, Prof. Joseph, on organic and inorganic elements, 22–3
  on the definition of vital force, 229
  on vital force as a product of decomposition, 287
LeFevre, Carrica, on the percentage of wasted energy, 387
Lemon *vs.* orange juice, during a fast, 404–5
Length of time we may continue without food and without sleep, 245
  of time for digestion, 482
  of life, normal, 593–4
Lepine, Dr., theory of sleep, 305
Leprosy, possible cause of, 611
Lewes, Dr. G. H., theory of sleep, 305
  on immortality in the body, 328
Lewis, Dr. Dio, on the impossibility of local diseases, 18
  on a short and a merry life, 64
  on the tables of the poor, 102
  on the influence of habit upon appetite, 117
  on the prevention of overfeeding, 598
  on the amount of food required by growing children, 608
Liebig, Prof., theory of bodily heat, 339
Life, presence of, temperature dependent upon, 334
  definition of, 334–5
  is innate, 337
  prolongation of, by will power, 434
  average length of, 593–4
  wrongly included in the law of conservation, 228, 297–8
  origin of, 284–5
  persistence of, 285
  creation of, 286
  dissimilarity of, in created and natural bodies, 287
  criticism of experiments in creation of, 288–9
  supposed dependence of, upon food supply, 300
  compared to a flame, 303
  and energy, 330
Light, physiological, 292–3
Lightning, cures by, 162
Live and dead foods, 265
Liver, congested, case of cure of, 195–7, 222
  diseased, 222
  effects of fasting upon, 497
Lloyd, Prof. John Uri, theory of vitality, 264
Local diseases, impossibility of, 17–19, 610
Locomotive, *see* Engine
Lodge, Sir Oliver J., on the creation of life, 289–90
  on monism and dualism, 432–3
Löhre, Rev. N. J., case of, 186
Long and short fasts, 568–71
Loss and gain, from omitting a meal, 568–9
Loss of flesh, in starvation, 160–1
  in fasting, 476–7
Loss of weight, from exercise, 383, *see* Weight
Low morning temperature, 319, 457–9
Low, Prof. Gilman, his endurance lifting test, 382–3
Lowell, Prof. Percival, theory of sleep, 309
Lower animals, feeding habits of, 106–7
Lung capacity (standard), 218
Lungs, effects of fasting upon, 495–7
Lymph vessels, indicators of limited food supply, 105–6
Lys, Dr., on death from mental causes, 162

Malcolm, Dr. J. D., on sudden death, 168
on the production of bodily heat, 347
on the correspondence of the temperature and the pulse, 462
Malignant growths, 609
Manaceine, Dr. Marie de, theory of sleep, 306
on increased strength after sleep, 309
Martin, Mrs., case of, 470
Martin, Prof. H. N., on the priority of nervous activity to circulation, 305
Mastication, importance of, 114
thorough, effects of, 114
importance of, 600–1
Material remedies *vs.* mental cures, 578–80
Matthews, Mrs. I., case of, 186
Mayer, Prof. L., theory of sleep, 305
Mayer, Prof. Robert, on the source of vital energy, 229–30
Meals, time interval between, 140
standing up at, 598
Medicated baths, 361
Melville, Rear Admiral George W., case reported by, 481
Mental cures, *vs.* material remedies, 578–80
Mental life, influenced by diet, 111–12
dyspepsia, *see* Dyspepsia
causes of death, 162–3
operations, require bodily energy, 231
operations, amount of energy required by, 235
states, influence of, upon the inflow of energy, 252–3
nature of fatigue, 280–1
life and bodily energy, 300–3
work, 386
cures, 430
and physical phenomena, 430–33
grasp of organism, 434
states, effects of, upon digestion, 437–8
effects of fast upon, 516–17
life, determined by condition of organism, 516
effects of bodily conditions upon, 517
factor, in disease, 578–80
cure of disease, 578–80
limitations of, 579–80
Mentality, and food habits, 107
and stamina, 434
Mercier, Dr. Charles, on the causes of insanity, 623
Metchnikoff, Prof. Elie, on the nature of disease, 67
on natural death, 325

Nails, toe, rate of growth of, 374
finger, as indicators of health, 544
Nasal discharge, case of cure of, 213–15
Natural hunger, *see* Hunger
death, 324–6
Nature, only curative agency, 64
laws of, impossibility of deviating from, 592–4
Nerves, and blood supply, 513–14
and phosphorus, 513–14
specific reaction of, 599
Nervous, dyspepsia, *see* Dyspepsia
system, does not waste during fast, 163–4
disorders, case of cure of, 222
prostration, case of cure of, 222
system, compared with wireless telegraph, 251
and muscular power, 433–4
system, effects of fasting upon, 511–16
system is physical, 512–13
diseases, full diet for, 512
treatment for, by fasting, 514–16
Newcombe, Dr. C. P., on diet and cancer, 611
on fasting for cancer, 611
New stomach, creation of, 490
Nichols, Dr. Mary, on improper clothing, 373
Nichols, Dr. T. L., on minimum food supply, 102–3
on strength and food supply, 284
on work in relation to diet, 386
on extraordinary gains in weight, 479, 480
on stomachic abuses, 484–5
on the amount of food required by growing children, 608
Night air, question of, 315, 356–8
Nightingale, Florence, on the nature of disease, 7
on drug medication, 30
on fumigation, 358–9
on the physiognomy of disease, 589
No-breakfast plan, objections to, 137
replies to the objections, 137–8
arguments for, 141–7
for the aged, 143
Nordau, Max, on pessimism, 517
Normal appetite, *see* Appetite
hunger, *see* Hunger
Nourishment, amount of, depends on assimilated, not ingested food, 118–19
Noyes, I. P., on weather influences, 153
Nozzle, size of, for enema taking, 413
Nucleus, as a source of energy, 294
Nursing mother, amount of food required by, 606–7

Oxygen, impoverishment of, as a cause of sleep, 305
inability of living tissues to absorb, directly, 353

Page, Dr. Charles E., on the unity of disease, 16
on germs, 51–2
on acute disease, 60
on similarity of human organisms, 84
on historic fasters, 94
on the secretions, 119
on fat as a disease, 128
on the number of meals daily for a baby, 133
on instinct for the no-breakfast plan, 144
on weather influences, 152
on fasting *vs.* stimulation, 168–9
on diet *vs.* exercise, 385
on the action of the bowels, while fasting, 420
on the composition of the fæces, 421
on scratching, 437
on the condition of the stomach, after fasting, 493–4
on abnormal appetite, 551
on habit-hunger, 554
on colds, 587–8
on proper diet, 594
on consumption, 603
on the treatment of babies, 606
on insanity, 623
Pain, nature and causes of, 25–9
theory of, 27
other theories of, 27–8
causes and cure of, 139
exhaustion from, 283
faint breathing during, 352
in the heart, causes of, 528
Panacea, possibility of, 574–8
Panspermia, 285
Paralysis, cured by lightning, 162
cured by fasting, 182
cases of cures of, 183–6, 189–94, 202–5, 208, 211–13, 220–1, 222
Parlow, Prof. J. P., on the effects of the mind upon the digestion, 488
on the artificial creation of appetite, 556
Partsch, Dr. H., on the necessity of eating in disease, 172
on overfeeding for seasickness, 614–15
Passive exercise, *see* Exercise
Patchen, Dr. G. H., on the unity of disease, 16
Patten, Dr., theory of pain, 28
Patterson, C. G., case of, 213–15

Proper diet, importance of, 594
Proportions of food, and air, 120
and exercise, 165
Psychical phenomena, objections to removed, by the theory of vitality defended, 303
Puller, Rev. F. W., on fasting before communion, 93
Pulse, rate of, controlled by suggestion, 425
how felt, 460
rate of, at various ages, 460
causes of variations in, 461
cause of abnormally slow, 461–2
and temperature, correspondence of, 462
variations in, while fasting, 462–5
rhythm of, 465
rate of, in brain, 515
abnormally slow, cause of, 528–9
treatment of, 529
rapid, cause of, 530
treatment of, 530–2
Purgatives, effects of, in fasting, 215
objections to use of, 409–10
true action of, 410
effects of, negated by suggestion, 425
Purinton, Edward Earle, on the best time for fasting, 108
on fatigue, 279
on diet and exercise, 385
on the quantity of water during a fast, 403
on laxative foods, before fasting, 422
on mental conditions during a fast, 439
on effects of fasting upon the mind, 501
on phosphorus and nerve activity, 514
on proper and improper fasting, 518
on the improper breaking of the fast, 560–1
Purity of water, during the fast, 404–5
Pyle, Dr. Howard, on the nature of fatigue, 280

Quain, Dr., on drug medication, 585
Quantity of water system requires, 397
of food required *per diem*, 470–1

R., Mrs. A. E., case of, 209–10
Rabagliati, Dr. A., on the unity of disease, 16
on local diseases, 18–19
on overeating by the poor, 109
on uric acid, 157
on the causation of paralysis, 182

Reinhold, Dr. A. F., on significance of increased weight, 129
theory of vitality, 225–6
on clothes, 375
Relapse, cause of, 176
Relation of life to organism, 297–8
Relaxation, imperfect, 252
Removal of colon, 499
Repose *vs.* movement, 314
Resistance to cold, 226
Rest and fasting, 43, 170
Restrictive clothing, 373–4
Retention of urine, while fasting, 525
Reversal of motor, theory of, 317
Rich foods, 345
Richards, Miss Ellen H., on stimulating foods, 600
Richardson, Dr. Benjamin Ward, on stimulants, 34–5
on vitality, 290–1
on reanimation, 291
on the causes of death, 331
on the wholesomeness of work, 386
on diet and cancer, 612
Richet, Prof. Charles, on the conditions of certainty, 8
Ritter, Henry, fasting cases conducted by, 222–3
Rheumatism, and fasting, 27
cured by lightning, 162
cases of cure of, 220–1, 222
Rhythm, organic, 323
Right thinking, 578–9
Rosenbach, Dr. O., on the germ theory, 48
on predisposition, 49
on the harmlessness of germs, 53
on epidemics, 59
on the causes of death, 331
Ruckhardt, Prof. Rabl, theory of sleep, 305
Russell, Henrietta, on fatigue, 315
on yawning, 352
Ryan, Dr. John, on medicines and poisons, 30
Rybilkin, Dr., experiments of, in suggestion, 428–9

S., Mr. G. W., case of, 211–12
St. Francis of Assisi, case of, 427
Sailors, shipwrecked, 270–2
Saline waters, 393–5
Salt, H., on material remedies *vs.* mental cures, 579
on the amount of food required on fruitarian diet, 595
Salt rub bath, 365
Salt, injurious effects of, 393–4
Samuels, Maurice V., experience of, with cold baths, while fasting, 296
Sargent, Dr. Dudley A., on the danger of eating before sleeping, 147

Shew, Dr. Joel, on fasting as a cure for toothache, 27
  on fasting as a cure for syphilis, 100
  on the philosophy of fasting, 154–5
  on the advantages of fasting for seasickness, 172
  on fasting *vs.* water cure, 363
  on the condition of the tongue, while fasting, 443–4
  on the cure of piles, by fasting, 498
  on the first days of fasting, 519
  on morbid appetites, 552–3
  on the amount of food required by pregnant woman, 607
  on fasting for caneer, 612
Short and long fasts, 568–71
Sieveking, Dr., theory of sleep, 305
Significance of hunger, 120
Simple and malignant growths, 609
Sitz bath, how administered, 365
Size of nozzle for enema taking, 413
Skeleton condition, 161–2
Skin, degree of activity of, 363–4
  reaction of, 545
Sleep, danger of eating before, 147
  organic changes during, 244
  ignored, in discussion of energy supply, 244
  more necessary than food, 245–6
  length of time possible to be without, 245
  instantaneous energizing during, 246–7
  as a period of greatest weakness, 263
  postponing, 304
  as an active and a passive process, 306
  author's definition of, 309
  depth of, 309
  why tired after, 311–12, 315–17
  length of time required for, 315
  hygiene of, 316
  amount required, in fasting, 319–22, 526–7
  more required in winter, 321
  intestinal movements during, 486
Sleeping on the ground, 252
Smidovich, Dr. V., on the universality of disease, 63
Smith, Dr. John, on stimulating foods and fasting, 268
Snyder, Carl, on immunity, 24
  on the recent knowledge of "true" medicine, 76
  theory of death, 325
Soap, question of, 360
Soil, for germs, 46–51
Sommer, Dr., theory of sleep, 305
Specific reaction of nerves, 599
Spencer, Herbert, definition of life, 334

S
S
S

Strength, "supported" in disease, 175–6
cases of increase of, during fast, 257
comparative, and food supply, 283–4
actual, *vs.* stimulation, 262, 312–13, 314, 458
after breaking fast, cause of, 564–6
Strong, Prof. C. A., on matter, 430–1
on idealism, 432
Structure of cancerous growths, 611
Stuffing a cold, 588
Sudden death, 11, 168, 324–5
Suffocation, death from, 354
Sugar injections, and fatigue, 281
Suggestion, present interest in, 424
pulse altered by, 425
temperature altered by, 425
relative value of, 430
and vital influx, 435
and stimulation, 435
Summary of Book I., 79–80
of arguments, 572–4
Sunshine, real food of body, 264
Suppression of symptoms, 10, 11, 12, 25
Susceptibility, question of, 60
Sweetser, Dr., on death from mental causes, 162
Symptoms, suppression of, 10, 11, 12, 25
increase of, during fast, 519–23
Syphilis, cured by fasting, 99–100

T., Mrs. R., case of, 210–11
loss of weight by, 475
Tait, Prof., on the similarity of the body to an electric motor, 250
Tanner, Dr., his fasts, 92–3
on water drinking, during a fast, 400–1
on capacity of the stomach, after a fast, 489
Tarchanoff, Dr., theory of sleep, 305
Teale, Dr., case recorded by, 448
Teeth, universal decay of, 63–4
Teething, 606
Teichmann, Dr. E., theory of death, 325
on natural death, 593
Temperature, bodily, and alcohol, 36
low, in morning, 319
uniformity of, 333
high and low, 336
regulation of, 342–3, 346
and health, 350
and atmosphere, 357
and water drinking, 399
of water, for enema, 412–13
altered by suggestion, 425
how taken, 448
normal, 448
in Asiatic cholera, 448
variations from normal, 449

Training, effects of, upon energy production, 276
Trall, Dr. R. T., on the nature of disease, 5–6, 7, 9, 29, 68–9
on foods *vs.* poisons, 22
on pain, 26
on drugs, 31
on the action of drugs, 32
on stimulants, 36–7, 39
on premature decay of teeth, 64
on the "seat" of diseases, 67–8
on the percentage of cases lost under hygienic treatment, 72–3
on experience, 73
on easily digested foods, 104
on the proportions of air and foods, 120
on starvation, despite presence of fat, 128
on weather influences, 153
on the wasting of disease, 179
on the unreliability of sensations, 262
on stimulating foods and fasting, 268–9
on increased energy and strength of heart-beat, 278
on laziness as a sign of disease, 315
on the definition of death, 331
on respiration during pain, 352
on too heroic water treatment, 361
on bathing, 362–3
on the bathing processes, 365
on the possible dangers of the Turkish bath, 368
on overwork, 386
on mineral waters, 391
on temperature of water for enema, 413
on the cause of consumption, 602, 603
on iron for anæmia, 605
on the causation of cancer, 609
Trance, hypnotic, 253
physiological aspects of, 107–8
Transmission of energy, theory of, 250
from one organism to another, 254–5
Treves, Sir Frederick, on the nature of disease, 13
on catarrh of the appendix, 498
Tropics, comparative influence of food habits and temperature in, 152–3
True, Prof. A. C., on Atwater's experiments, 344
Tuke, Dr. Hack, on the effect of anger upon the secretions, 426
Tumors, as local diseases, 610
Turkish bath, cleansing properties of, 366
instructions for taking, 367–9

Uni
Un

Varicose veins, case of cure of, 209–10
Varigny, Henri de, on life manifestations in variable temperatures, 334
on the inability of living tissues to absorb O. directly, 353
Vegetable life, cannot be forced, 253
Vegetarianism, 86–9
list of books on, 595–7
Venous stasis, as a cause of sleep, 305
Verworn, Dr., on cosmic germs, 285
Vibration, as the physical manifestation of life, 334
and bodily heat, correspondence of, 334–5
Vicars, Marie D., on fasting *vs.* starvation, 163
Virchow, Prof., on the movements of the stomach during sleep, 147
Vital *vs.* chemical action, of drugs, 32
force, is innate, 255–6
and chemical force, 293
functions, non-suspension of, 322
influx, and suggestion, 435
Vitality, always noted in its expenditure, 41
definitions of, 225
question of essence of, 225

Vitality, source of, 226
how lost, 226
how increased, 226–30
present theory of causation of, 242–5
cannot be manufactured, 250–3
hunger an indication of the presence of, 273
as a product of decomposition, 287
nature of, 290–1
and crystals, 292
not involved in the law of conservation, 297
and water drinking, 399, 401–2
analogy of, to army, 548–9
see Energy
Voit, Prof., theory of sleep, 305
Vomiting, during a fast, 532–5
treatment of, 533–4
during pregnancy, 608

W., Prof. F., case of, 187–8
Wait, Dr. C. E., on the similarity of individuals, 85
Wallace, Dr. A. R., on the improper administration of chloroform, 98–9
Wallace, Dr. Joseph, on the unity of disease, 16
Walsh, Dr. David, on the non-suspension of vital functions, 322
Walter, Dr. Robert, on stimulation, 42
on germs and fasting, 51
on acute and chronic disease, 61
on energy influx, 254
on strength and food supply, 283
on bodily heat, 350
War, mortality during, 592
Warm baths, 361
Waste matters, as a cause of death, 331
Waste of energy, in digestion, 103–5
per cent. of, 387
Wasting of disease, 124, 178–9
Water, craved during exercise, 273
hot, and bodily heat, 343
cure *vs.* fasting, 363
proportion of, in body, 388
percentage of, in foods, 388
amount craved, and diet, 388–9
amount of loss of, in excreta, 389
necessity of, in diseased conditions, 389
drinking, insufficient, cause of constipation, 390
quality of, 390–5
quantity of, 395–7
periodicity, 397–405
filtered, 390
boiled, 390
distilled, 390
mineral, 391–2
saline, 393–5

Wood, Dr. George B., on definition of disease, 3
Woodhead, Dr. G. S., on germs, 50
Woodward, Dr. J., on the structure of cancerous growths, 611
Work, in relation to diet, 386
Wounds, comparative rapidity of healing of, 150
Wright, Dr. A. E., on drug medication, 585
Wright, Dr. Laura M., on positions for enema taking, 412
on the temperature of water for enema, 412–13
Wright, Dr. Laura M., on the size o nozzle for enema taking, 413
on the difficulty of expellin enema water, 416
Wundt, Prof., theory of sleep, 306

Y., Mrs. G., case of, 202–5
Yawning, causes of, 352–3
Yeo, Dr. Burney, on organic and in organic elements, 23
aversion to food by the sick, 172
on condiments, 600
on feeding in typhoid, 615
Yogis, food habits of, 108

Made in United States
Orlando, FL
31 May 2024

47390819R00391